ADVANCES IN BRUCELLOSIS RESEARCH

Funds for publication of this book were provided

by

The Texas Agricultural Experiment Station

and

The United States Department of Agriculture -
Animal & Plant Health Inspection Service

ADVANCES IN BRUCELLOSIS RESEARCH

Edited by

L. Garry Adams

Texas A&M University Press
College Station

Library of Congress Cataloging - in - Publication Data

Advances in Brucellosis Research.
Includes Index.
1. Brucellosis in cattle--Congresses. 2. Brucellosis--Congresses.
3. Brucella--Congresses. I. Adams, L. Garry. II. Texas Agricultural
Experiment Station. III. International Symposium on Advances
in Brucellosis (1989 : Texas A&M University)
[DNLM: 1. Brucellosis--congresses. WC 310 A244 1989]
SF967.B7A38 1990 636.2'0896957--dc20 90-11118
ISBN 0-89096-447-5
9 78089 0964477

To world-wide fellow scientists committed to the quest of eradicating brucellosis,
to my colleagues in the Brucellosis Research Group at Texas A&M University,
to my parents, Hershel and Iris Adams,
to my wife, Gerry, and my children, Paige and Thad,
without whose confidence and support,
this book would not have been accomplished.

CONTENTS

LIST OF FIGURES

LIST OF TABLES

Foreword

The International Symposium on Advances in Brucellosis provides an historical bench mark for the Texas A&M group that organized and hosted this event. Our current research effort began in the College of Veterinary Medicine under sponsorship of The Texas Agricultural Experiment Station in the the summer of 1975. In February 1977, our first International Symposium, Bovine Brucellosis, was held. The intervening years have brought striking changes in 1) what we know about the interaction of the organisms, its hosts and the environment, 2) the prevalence of the disease in the United States, especially in Texas, and 3) attitudes of the beef cattle and dairy industries about the disease.

In 1977, as in 1989, the Texas A&M team used an international symposium to define the state of knowledge at that point, to define researchable issues for further study, and to stimulate creative thinking about the disease and its management. At the first symposium, much emphasis was placed on sorting out what was known about a series of diagnostic tools that were developed in previous decades, to separate epidemiologic facts from myths and to lay out an agenda for new research which would contribute to a reasoned regulatory program that was scientifically sound and economically affordable.

The second symposium offered the opportunity to assess the progress made in the intervening twelve years of international research toward understanding the fundamental nature of the disease and the development of new tools for diagnosis, immunization and management of infected animals and herds. In this interval, the applications of molecular biology to animal disease blossomed and were used as exciting new tools in brucellosis research. General principles learned from research on other diseases found application in bovine brucellosis. The specific application of these new methods has given us substantial insight into the genetic basis of the interactions between *Brucella abortus* and its host. It has provided an understanding of the basis of natural resistance to disease, which not only has major relevance to brucellosis, but spin-off implications for other animal diseases.

Reasoned use of the knowledge that existed at the beginning of this decade, coupled with almost immediate transfer and use of new technology that emerged from research over the intervening years has allowed major progress to be made on the eradication of bovine brucellosis in this country. As the new science based regulatory program has had demonstrable success, the confidence of people in the beef and dairy industries has increased, as has their understanding of the disease, its economic impact and its human health implications. For example, at the beginning of the 1980s, ranchers in Texas were very close to abandoning the existing regulatory program and taking the consequence of a threatened federal embargo on movement of cattle out of the state. Now, we find this same industry petitioning the federal regulatory authorities to engage in an accelerated program of eradication. This change in attitude and perspective could not have been forecasted ten years ago; it also seems fair to say that it would not have occurred without the introduction of new knowledge and tools that have come from research in this same period.

At the beginning of this decade, it was estimated that about 35% of all known infected herds were in Texas. Bovine brucellosis was clearly one of the most important diseases in terms of both economic and regulatory burden in the state. On a world-wide basis, research on this disease had diminished substantially in the '70s. Texas A&M University received new state funding to develop and maintain an expanded program of research in the early '80s. A team of interdisciplinary researchers in the Colleges of Veterinary Medicine and Agriculture, including more than a dozen scientists and a total of almost 30 people, have gradually built an expertise and developed contributions to knowledge about bovine brucellosis that have led them to a position of international recognition for their excellence.

This team has become competitive for research funds from both federal and private resources; team members have published, patented and placed into practice the results of a very fine set of interrelated studies that address a range of science from very fundamental knowledge of host-parasite relationships to applications of computer technology and new biology for management of the disease on a herd, regional, and national basis. Coincidentally, at the time of the 1989 symposium, the Texas A&M team was presented the USDA's award for excellence in team research by Secretary of Agriculture Clayton Yeutter in Washington D.C.

Excellent contributions to knowledge and progress on bovine brucellosis have also come from a number of comparable laboratories both in the U.S. and abroad. Our group has benefited immeasurably from the contributions of others and from collaborations with many colleagues located elsewhere. We are particularly appreciative for the active participation of these colleagues in our latest symposium. We hope and believe that this proceedings represents the same kind of current assessment that our first symposium provided in setting the agenda for application of recent knowledge and in charting the course for future studies.

While progress has been impressive in this decade the job is far from finished with respect to what we must learn about this disease. Unparalleled opportunities for progress lie ahead with further use and refinement of the tools of modern biology and computer science and with continued commitment to sustaining the effort needed to apply these tools to the studies of brucellosis and other animal diseases.

Finally, I wish to say from a personal perspective that it has been exciting, as an administrator, to watch the Texas A&M University team gain and expand their scientific skills and momentum and to successfully place the fruits of their labors into useful practice. I express appreciation to each of them for their efforts and congratulate them on a successful and very useful symposium.

Neville P. Clarke
Director, Texas Agricultural Experiment Station

Preface

In May, 1989 an international symposium for Advances in Brucellosis Research was hosted at Texas A&M University. The purpose of the symposium was to review the progress made in fundamental and applied research on brucellosis as a worldwide problem during the last decade. The scope of the symposium was designed to encompass the most recent findings of the tools of modern genetics, biochemistry, cell biology, immunology and molecular biology as they are being applied to infectious diseases as well as updating the level of understanding of the epidemiology and economics of brucellosis. In this book, the attention of the scientific community is focused on the most fundamental nature of Brucellae, their hosts and their environments bridging disciplines from the molecular genetics of *Brucella* spp. to applied epidemiology at the level of the producer. Consequently, the thirty chapters in this volume evolve from basic to applied sciences. It is recognized that research involving brucellosis is advancing rapidly, nonetheless, a courageous attempt is made to clearly describe the present aspects of the state of knowledge of research on brucellosis and integrate the latest phenomena at molecular, cellular and host levels as they have emerged since the last international symposium on bovine brucellosis was sponsored here in 1976.

The subject matter of brucellosis research is organized into seven parts, often with the first chapter of each part illustrating a current scientific approach to one aspect of an infectious disease with obvious implications in brucellosis research. Part I. Taxonomy and Molecular Biology of Brucellae considers the genetic analysis of *Salmonella* spp. and its utilization for studying *B. abortus*, in addition to the use of phylogenetic markers to describe Brucellae and their evolutionary development and taxonomy. Part I illustrates how modern molecular genetics can be used with conventional taxonomic methodology to develop a clearer understanding of not only the evolutionary development of the *Brucella* spp. but also host preference. Part II. Biological and Structural Properties of Brucellae demonstrates the structural relationship of membrane carbohydrate, lipid and protein moieties in the function of the outer and cytoplasmic membranes of *Brucella* spp. as compared to other Gram-negative bacteria. Part III. Pathogenesis and Host Parasite Interactions of Brucellosis is focused on the use of *in vitro* model systems as a strategy to unravel host-parasite interactions of mutated intracellular pathogens like *Brucella* spp.

with cultured mammalian cells leading to a clearer understanding of the pathogenetic mechanisms. Part IV. Natural and Acquired Immunity Against Brucellae compares the protective immune response against a number of intracellular bacteria to that known about *Brucella* spp. in cattle and the mouse model. This part carefully analyzes the status of knowledge with regard to humoral and cellular protective immune mechanisms as well as encompassing the function of phagocytes in resistance to brucellosis. The genetic basis of natural resistance to *Brucella* spp. is reviewed as are mechanisms of self-cure.

In the quest for new approaches to protecting against brucellosis Part V. Vaccination against Brucellosis reviews the rather meager progress that has been made in the development of improved vaccines against *Brucella* spp. Part V readily illustrates that recent approaches using well defined killed or replicating sub-unit vaccines can be applied to reducing the problem of persistent antibody titers and lack of immunity with existing vaccines and this part also outlines the protocols necessary for evaluation of traditional and new recombinant biological products. Part VI. Diagnosis, Epidemiology, and Economics of Brucellosis demonstrates the power of modern biotechnology in the application of DNA probes for diagnostic and epidemiologic analysis, particularly when applied with the new serologic methods disclosed in this section. This part also documents the new challenges of infectious diseases that society and its animals will face in the next decade. Part VI further contributes valuable information on evaluating economic losses, the role of wildlife in brucellosis, eradication of brucellosis at the herd level, and regulatory program decision making through epidemiologic and econometric simulation modeling. Part VII. National Program Policies reviews features of regulatory programs and the approaches presently being applied in national programs of brucellosis free countries as compared to other approaches in countries where brucellosis remains a significant disease problem. Part VII further documents the necessity for rapid and accurate detection of brucellosis in infected areas and how the information generated from regulatory programs can be used to construct national epidemiological electronic data bases for implementing and measuring the progress of control and eradication programs. Finally, the abstracts disclose the most recent international scientific results of research on brucellosis.

More than anything else, it is intended that this volume will stimulate those in pursuit of understanding the interaction of *Brucella* spp. with their hosts and environments in order to conceptualize future experimental approaches in broader terms encompassing the latest knowledge and most modern methodologies providing new insight and hence better solutions for the world-wide control and eradication of brucellosis.

L. Garry Adams

Acknowledgements

Many people have contributed to the publication of this volume. Foremost are the contributing authors who took time from their busy schedules to thoughtfully review the most recent accomplishments of research from their own and others laboratories as it applies to brucellosis. The publication of this volume and the hosting of the symposium was provided under the auspices of and with the funding of the Texas Agricultural Experiment Station with valued input in the organization of the scientific program by Director Dr. Neville P. Clarke and Deputy Director Dr. Robert G. Merrifield. I am indebted to numerous professional staff of the United States Department of Agriculture, Animal and Plant Health Inspection Service, namely Dr. John D. Kopec, Dr. Jan D. Huber, Dr. Andrea M. Morgan, Dr. Granville H. Frye, Dr. Billy Johnson, Dr. Saul T. Wilson, Jr. and Dr. James Glosser for their assistance in the organization of this symposium as well as the generous financial support for the publication of this volume. Support for the symposium was also provided by Dean John A. Shadduck of the College of Veterinary Medicine and as well as by Mr. Frank B. Wilkins and the staff of the Biomedical Learning Resources Center for the book cover design and technical assistance for artistic and graphic subjects . The careful typing by Miss Mary Cay Boatright and fastidious proofreading by Miss Julie Goecke are gratefully acknowledged. Invaluable information on the organization of materials and subject matter for the publication of this volume was provided by Editor-in-Chief, Mr. Noel R. Parsons of the Texas A&M University Press.

I am in the debt of the Granada Land and Cattle Company of Marquez, Texas and the Clayton Williams Alumni Center at Texas A&M University for hosting a special Texas barbecue and formal banquet for the participants of the symposium. I am also very grateful to the staff of the Rudder Tower and Theater Complex for providing excellent audio-visual programming and meeting conditions for the lectures and the poster sessions. I am particularly thankful for the technical assistance provided by Ms. Katherine Kelly and Mrs. Jan Patterson for organizing and arranging the poster session, to Mrs. Doris Hunter, Mr. Bruce Crooker and Dr. Randy Simpson for assistance in the detailed operation of the program and especially to Mrs. Katherine Smith for managing the financial matters pertaining to the symposium and the publication of this volume.

To my fellow colleagues of the Brucellosis Research Group of the Texas Agricultural Experiment Station and the College of Veterinary Medicine, Drs. Richard P. Crawford, Donald S. Davis, Thomas A. Ficht, Roger Smith III, Blair A. Sowa, Joe W. Templeton, and John D. Williams, I am forever in their debt for their assistance in organizing the symposium, reviewing and editing manuscripts, providing for the needs of speakers, and their commitment to many details to making the symposium a success and the publication of this volume worthwhile. Lastly, and most importantly, I simply must say that neither the symposium nor the publication of this book would have been possible without the commitment to the organization and management of the symposium and the preparation of quality manuscripts of the able, dedicated, and enthusiastic efforts of Mrs. Kay E. Sanders, Senior Secretary of the Brucellosis Research Group.

L. Garry Adams

The Contributors

L.G. Adams

Department of Veterinary Pathology
College of Veterinary Medicine
Texas Agricultural Experiment Station
Texas A&M University
College Station, TX 77843-4463

A.T. Adawi

General Organization for Veterinary Services
Dokki
Giza, Egypt

H. Adler

Veterinary Services and Animal Health
POB 12
Beit Dagan, Israel

S.H. Amosson

Texas Agricultural Extension Service
Farm Management
3971 Eaton Dr.
Amarillo, Texas 79109

J.B. Armstrong

King Ranch Corporation
P. O. Box 193
Kingsville, TX 78363

M. Banai

Veterinary Microbiology
Kimron Veterinary Institute
POB 12
Beit Dagan, Israel

V.C. Beal, Jr.

United States Department of Agriculture
Animal & Plant Health Inspection Service
Policy and Program Development
Hyattsville, MD 20782

S.W. Bearden

Department of Veterinary Microbiology
College of Veterinary Medicine
Texas Agricultural Experiment Station
Texas A&M University
College Station, TX 77843-4463

N. Buchmeier

Department of Molecular Biology
Scripps Clinic & Research Foundation
10666 North Torrey Pines Rd.
LaJolla, CA 92037

D.R. Bundle

Immunochemistry Section
Division of Biological Sciences
National Research Council of Canada
Ottawa, Ontario
Canada K1A OR6

P.C. Canning

Animal Health Research Department
Pfizer, Inc.
P. O. Box 88
Terre Haute, IN 47808

J.D. Clements

Department of Microbiology & Immunology
Tulane University School of Medicine
1430 Tulane Ave.
New Orleans, LA 70112

A. Cohen

Kimron Veterinary Institute
POB
Beit Dagan, Israel

R.P. Crawford

Department of Veterinary Public Health
College of Veterinary Medicine
Texas Agricultural Experiment Station
Texas A&M University
College Station, TX 77843-4463

M. Davidson

Ministry of AgricultureVeterinary Services
and Animal Health
POB 12
Beit Dagan, Israel

D.S. Davis

Department of Veterinary Pathology
College of Veterinary Medicine
Texas Agricultural Experiment Station
Texas A&M University
College Station, TX 77843-4463

R.A. Dietrich

Institute of Arctic Biology
University of Alaska
Fairbanks, AK99701

S. El-Gibaly

Animal Health Research Institute
Dokki
Giza, Egypt

F.M. Enright

Louisiana State University
Department of Veterinary Science
Rm 121
Baton Rouge, LA 70803

D.A. Espeseth

United States Department of Agriculture
Animal and Plant Health Inspection Service
Biotechnology, Biologics and Environmental
Protection
Veterinary Biologics
Hyattsville, MD 20782

A.S. Evans

Dept. of Epidemiology & Public Health
Yale University School of Medicine
60 College St.
box 3333
New Haven, CT 06510

S. Falkow

Department of Medical Microbiology
Sherman Fairchild Science Building
School of Medicine
Stanford University
Stanford, CA 94305

T.A. Ficht

Department of Veterinary Microbiology
College of Veterinary Medicine
Texas A&M University
College Station, TX 77843-4463

B.B. Finlay

Biotechnology Laboratory and Departments of
Microbiology & Biochemistry
University of British Columbia
Vancouver, B.C.,
Canada V6T 1W5

I.E.A. Flesch

Department of Medical Microbiology and
Immunology
University of Ulm
Albert-Einstein-Allee 11, D-7900
Ulm, FRG

P.C. Genho

General Manager
Deseret Ranches of Florida
13754 Deseret Lane
Melbourne, FL 32904

R.E.W. Hancock

Department of Microbiology
University of British Columbia
Vancouver, B.C., Canada V6T1W5

F. Heffron

Department of Molecular Biology
Scripps Clinic & Research Foundation
10666 North Torrey Pines Rd.
LaJolla, CA 92037

J.D. Huber

United States Department of Agriculture
Animal and Plant Health Inspection Service
Veterinary Services
Hyattsville, MD 20782

S.H.E. Kaufmann

Department of Medical Microbiology and
Immunology
University of Ulm
Albert-Einstein-Allee 11, D-7900
Ulm, FRG

S. Libby

Department of Molecular Biology
Scripps Clinic & Research Foundation
10666 North Torrey Pines Rd.
LaJolla, CA 92037

H. Marquis

Department of Veterinary Microbiology
College of Veterinary Medicine
Texas Agricultural Experiment Station
Texas A&M University
College Station, TX 77843-4463

N.L. Martin

Department of Microbiology
University of British Columbia
Vancouver, B.C., Canada V6T1W5

H.E. Metcalf

United States Department of Agriculture
Animal and Plant Health Inspection Services
Policy and Program Development
Hyattsville, MD 20782

M.E. Meyer

Department of Epidemiology and Preventive
Medicine
School of Veterinary Medicine
University of California at Davis
Davis, California

K.H. Nielsen

Agriculture Canada
Animal Disease Research Institute
P. O. Box 11300
Station H
Nepean, Ontario
Canada K2H 8P9

M.B. Perry

Immunochemistry Section
Division of Biological Sciences
National Research Council of Canada
Ottawa, Ontario

M. Plommet

Directeur de Recherche
Station de Pathologie de la Reproduction
Institut National de la Recherche
Agronomique
37380 Nouzilly, France

M.K. Refai

Department of Microbiology
Faculty of Veterinary Medicine
Cairo University
Giza, Eqypt

G.P. Shibley

United States Department of Agriculture
Animal and Plant Health Inspection Service
Biotechnology, Biologics and Environmental
Protection
Veterinary Biologics
Hyattsville, MD 20782

A. Shimshony

Veterinary Services and Animal Health
POB 12
Beit Dagan, Israel

R. Smith III

Department of Veterinary Pathology
College of Veterinary Medicine
Texas Agricultural Experiment Station
Texas A&M University
College Station, TX 77843-4463

B.A. Sowa

Department of Veterinary Pathology
College of Veterinary Medicine
Texas Agricultural Experiment Station
Texas A&M University
College Station, TX 77843-4463

J.W. Templeton

Department of Veterinary Pathology
College of Veterinary Medicine
Texas Agricultural Experiment Station
Texas A&M University
College Station, TX

S. Weber

Chief, Program Services
National Center for Animal Health
Information Systems
United States Department of Agriculture
Animal & Plant Health Inspection Services
555 S. Howes, Suite 300
Fort Collins, CO 80521

A.J. Winter

Department of Veterinary Microbiology,
Immunology and Parasitology
New York State College of Veterinary
Medicine
Cornell University
Ithaca, NY 14853

D.F. Wirth

Department of Tropical Public Health
Harvard School of Public Health
Harvard Medicine School
666 Huntington Ave.
Boston, MA 02115

P.F. Wright

Agriculture Canada
Animal Disease Research Institute
P. O. Box 11300
Station H
Nepean, Ontario
Canada K2H 8P9

ADVANCES IN BRUCELLOSIS RESEARCH

PART ONE

TAXONOMY AND MOLECULAR BIOLOGY OF BRUCELLAE

Chapter One

A Genetic Analysis of
Salmonella typhimurium:
Implications for Studying
Brucella abortus

Nancy Buchmeier

Steven Libby,

and Fred Heffron

This report compares the two facultative intracellular pathogens, *Brucella abortus* and *Salmonella typhimurium,* and suggests how experiments being carried out in our laboratory on *Salmonella* intracellular pathogenesis can be applied to the study of *Brucella*. *Brucella abortus, melitensis,* and *suis* are closely related members of the same genus.[1,2] They are extremely infectious pathogens capable of passing through unbroken skin,[3] have a very broad host range, and can cause a lingering disease in man that is difficult to diagnose and treat. *Salmonella typhimurium* is the principal cause of gasteroenterides in man in the United States but is rarely fatal. In mice, it causes a lethal systemic infection which is similar to typhoid fever in man caused by the *Salmonella paratyphi* and *typhi* serotypes. *Brucella* has been difficult to study because of its extremely infectious nature. Researchers trained in bacterial genetics and using modern containment facilities have recently begun work on this fascinating pathogen. The fact that *Brucella* has adapted so well to its role as a pathogen is precisely its allure to scientists interested in studying intracellular parasitism.

Much of what we have learned about *Salmonella* pathogenesis may serve as a guide to the examination of the molecular basis of *Brucella* infections. *Salmonella typhimurium* like *Brucella* is a facultative intracellular pathogen but is less infectious and therefore, much less hazardous to the investigator. *Salmonella* is one of the most extensively studied procaryotic organisms. *Salmonella, E. coli* and *Brucella* are all Gram-negative organisms that should permit the extensive genetic manipulations performed in *E. coli* to be carried out with *Brucella* genes.[4] The genome complexity of *Brucella* is low and a physical map is being worked out which will greatly aid genetic studies.[1] *Brucella* persistence in the mouse provides a simple animal model of infection.[5] *Brucella* also causes a severe disease in guinea pigs that is fatal at a sufficient infectious dose. Like *Salmonella, Brucella* will invade tissue culture cells[6] and survives in vitro in macrophages.[7-11]

Several genetic approaches have proved fruitful in studying *Salmonella* pathogenesis. The basic approach is to make mutations in the virulent parent bacteria, particularly transposon mutations, and screen these for virulence using *in vitro* assays and infections in mice. The *in vitro* virulence assays are based on invasion of tissue culture cells,[12,13] passage through polarized epithelial cells,[14] survival in phagocytic cells,[15] and direct observations on the interaction between *Salmonella* and the eukaryotic cell. Transposon generated mutants are well suited for these studies because they contain single hit mutations and allow recovery of the mutated gene. Methods of generating transposon Tn5 insertions in *Brucella abortus* have been developed.[16] Improved methods for generation of larger numbers of mutants are currently being developed in several laboratories. These methods utilize plasmids that cannot replicate in *Brucella* as delivery systems for the transposon.

The primary technique used in our laboratory to study *Salmonella* pathogenesis was to make random transposon mutations in the genome and screen these individually for those that affect survival in the macrophage.[15] In practice, *Salmonella* is first added to a monolayer of macrophages in a microtiter dish, the bacteria are phagocytized, and remaining extracellular bacteria are killed with low doses of gentamicin. Macrophages containing bacteria are then incubated for varying times (15 minutes to 2 days) and surviving bacteria quantitated by lysing the macrophages and counting colony forming units on bacterial plates.[15,17] Bacteria can also be visualized within the macrophage by using either immunofluorescence techniques[18] or electron microscopy.[19] Approximately 10,000 independent Tn10 insertion mutants were screened and about 80 identified that repeatedly survived less well than the parent within thioglycollate-elicited peritoneal murine macrophages (BALB/c). These macrophage-sensitive (MS) mutants survived poorly in four other sources of macrophages and were avirulent when tested in the mouse animal model.[20] The mutants were screened for secondary phenotypes to provide potential information about the function of the mutated gene. From this preliminary screening, we have identified groups of mutants that are sensitive to oxidizing and DNA damaging agents, complement, and auxotrophs. Most mutants had no secondary phenotypes other than increased sensitivity to macrophages.

The first group of six mutations studied in detail had a very high LD_{50} and a common phenotype (sensitivity to complement), V and mapped close to each other at 25 minutes on the *Salmonella* map. The clustering of insertions at this spot probably reflects a hot spot for Tn10 insertion similar to that observed within the *his* operon of *Salmonella*. By comparison of phenotypes, by careful transductional mapping against other genes within this region, and by direct DNA sequencing, we have shown that all six of these transposon mutations are found within the same gene, *phoP*.[21-23] This gene had earlier been shown to regulate expression of other genes, including the gene that encodes acid phosphatase. DNA sequence analysis revealed that *phoP* is related to a class of two component regulators.[22,24] A closely linked gene, *phoQ*, senses the low phosphate concentration within the cell. By analogy with other two component regulators, the *phoP* product is phosphorylated by *phoQ* and, in its phorphorylated state, acts as a transcriptional activator for a specific group of genes. Presumably, one or more of these regulated genes confer resistance to microbiocidal products made by the macrophage.

The *phoP* mutants are sensitive to complement. This suggests that a mutant of *phoP* might contain a membrane or lipopolysaccharide (LPS) defect that enables lysogenic molecules to penetrate the LPS layer or to disrupt the cell membrane. To test this, we compared the sensitivity of the *phoP* mutant to other microbicidal factors. We found that the *phoP* mutants were sensitive to whole granule extracts prepared from neutrophils and macrophages. In collaboration with Dr. Robert Lehrer, we have found that the *phoP* mutants are specifically sensitive to small cationic proteins, including defensins. Cationic microbiocidal proteins are present within the lysosomes of macrophages. Possible explanations for the macrophage sensitivity of these mutants is that *phoP* regulates the expression of genes which change the bacterial membrane so that cationic proteins either cannot insert or cannot disrupt the bacterial membrane or by preventing passage of cationic proteins through the LPS layer.

Identification of the *phoP* regulator suggested that regulated gene expression might be a common theme for bacterial intracellular survival. *Salmonella* proteins synthesized in culture medium were compared to bacterial proteins synthesized during macrophage infections. Macrophages were infected with *Salmonella* and treated with cyclohexamide to inhibit eukaryotic protein synthesis, then bacterial proteins were labelled with ^{35}S methionine. After labelling for one hour, the macrophages were lysed, bacteria pelleted, and bacterial proteins analyzed by two dimensional gel electrophoresis. Out of 500 proteins analyzed by computer techniques, over 25 bacterial proteins were induced at least four-fold within the macrophage and over 50 proteins were repressed within the macrophage (Figures 1-1 A and 1-1C). We have also analyzed the proteins synthesized by several MS mutants during macrophage infection. At least seven *Salmonella* proteins normally induced within the macrophage are missing in the *phoP* mutant (Figure 1-1D). Another mutant, MS4347, failed to synthesize six of the induced proteins. MS4347 may be part of a separate regulatory network because the proteins controlled by MS4347 differ from those controlled by *phoP*. These observations demonstrate that *Salmonella* protein synthesis is regulated by the macrophage environment, that the enhanced synthesis of *Salmonella* proteins is controlled by multiple regulators, and that it contributes to intracellular survival.

Maybe the most exciting result of this work was the discovery that the heat-shock proteins *GroEL* and *DnaK* are induced within the macrophage and are in fact the most abundant bacterial proteins synthesized within

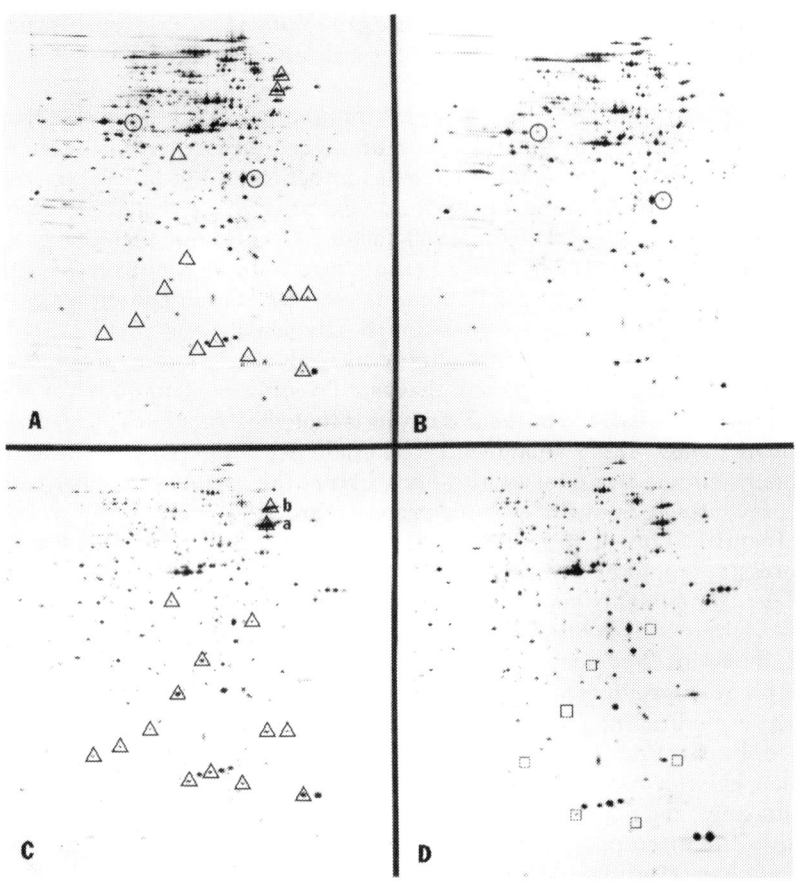

Figure 1-1. Autoradiographs of Two Dimensional Gels of ³⁵S Labeled Proteins from (A) *S. typhimurium* 14028 Grown in Methionine Free DMEM, (B) MS7953(*phoP*) Grown in Methionine Free DMEM, (C) *S. typhimurium* 14028 Infected Macrophages, (D) MS7953(*phoP*) Infected Macrophages. (O) Proteins with reduced synthesis in MS7953(*phoP*). (Δ) *Salmonella* proteins induced in macrophages. (□) *Salmonella* macrophage induced proteins which are reduced in MS7953 (*phoP*).

this environment. Heat-shock proteins are immunodominant antigens for many pathogenic microorganisms including *Salmonella*.[25] We propose that the high level of expression of stress response proteins within the macrophage, a major antigen processing and presenting cell, may contribute to the heightened immune response against them. This may also explain the superiority of immunizing with living attenuated vaccines, as compared to killed bacteria. To survive within phagocytic cells, living bacteria express new proteins which could be considered virulence determinants. Although many *Salmonella* survive within the macrophage, some bacteria are killed and presumably their antigens, including the newly induced ones, are processed and presented to T cells. The immune response generated by living bacteria would be directed against these abundant proteins (virulence determinants) instead of against non-protective antigens contained on bacteria grown in culture medium present on killed vaccines.

To understand how *Salmonella* survives inside macrophages, we have carried out cytological studies comparing the infection of MS mutant bacteria, *E. coli*, and virulent *Salmonella* strains within the macrophage.[20] Examination of thin sections has shown that *Salmonella* is not taken up by coiling phagocytosis as happens for *Legionnella pneumophila* (Figure 1-2A). Phagosome fusion with lysosomes was detected by incubating macrophages with thorotrast (thorium dioxide), an electron-dense compound that is specifically transported to lysosomes, before infection with *Salmonella*. Phagosomes that have fused with lysosomes can be easily distinguished from unfused phagosomes because they contain dark particles of thorotrast.

We found that *Salmonella* remains inside a membrane-bound phagosome in the macrophage. We observed *Salmonella* in both fused and unfused phagosomes (Figure 1-2B). The level of fusion at 14 hours was much less than for *E. coli*, suggesting that *Salmonella* partially inhibited phagolysosomal fusion. At 14 hours, undegraded *Salmonella* was still present in unfused vacuoles whereas *E. coli* was almost completely degraded in phagolysosomes (Figure 1-2C). At later times, we observed an increase in the percentage of *Salmonella* in unfused phagosomes which corresponded to an increase in viable bacteria within the cell. This suggests that *Salmonella* intracellular replication may preferentially take place in nonfused phagosomes. Multiple bacteria within the same unfused phagosome were never observed in the macrophage-like cell line J774 although *Salmonella* are clearly replicating inside these same macrophages. This suggests that division of the bacteria and the phagosome may occur in syncrony. This result is in contrast to *Salmonella* replication in epithelial cells where the endosome eventually becomes a bag of bacteria before the cell bursts. These observations suggest that the basic bacterial replication mechanism may be different in phagocytic and nonphagocytic cells.

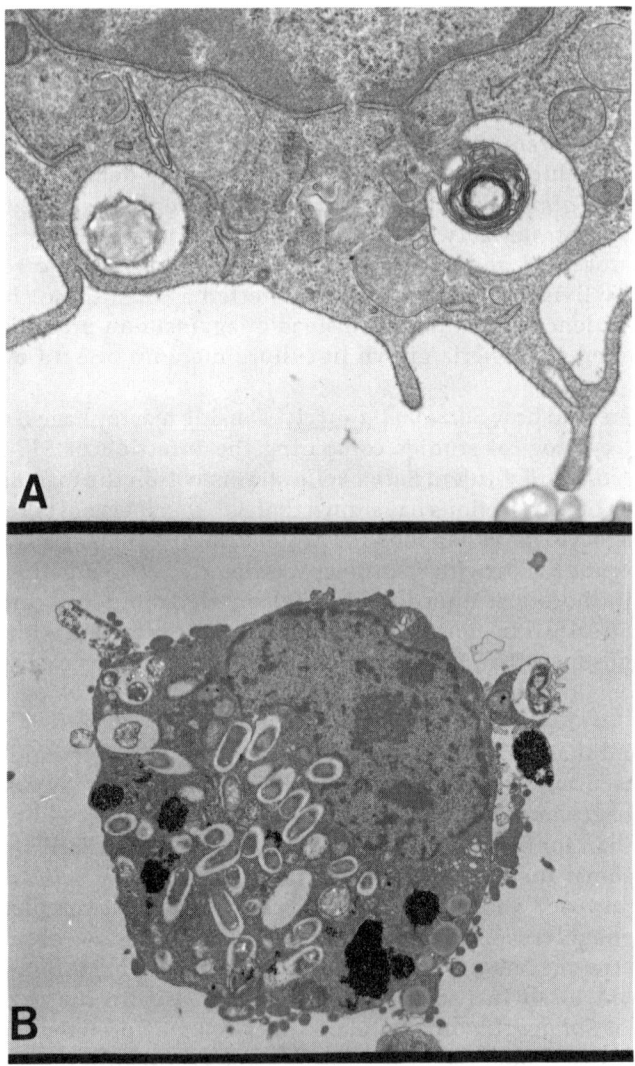

Figure 1-2. Electron Micrographs of Bacterial Infected Macrophages. (A) Bone marrow derived macrophage in the process of phagocytosis of *Salmonella*, 6.5 minutes after infection. (B) J774 macrophage infected for 14 hours with *Salmonella*, dark granules are thorium dioxide in secondary lysosomes.

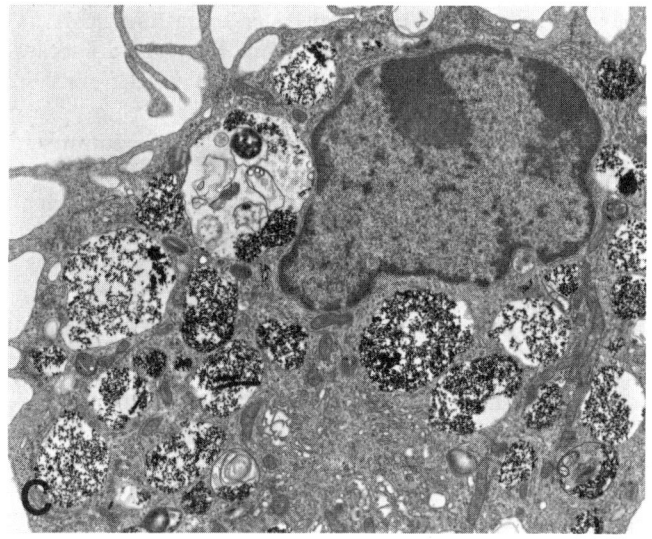

Figure 1-2. (C) Bone Marrow Derived Macrophage Infected 14 Hours with
E. coli.

We have observed differences between the survival of *Salmonella* within phagocytic and nonphagocytic cells. The MS mutants were identified because they could not survive within macrophages. We felt it probable that genes necessary for survival and replication in epithelial cells were a subset of those needed for survival in phagocytic cells. To test this, we compared the MS mutants with the parent and other strains of *Salmonella* for their ability to invade and replicate in epithelial cells.[26] All except one of the MS mutants contained defects specific to their survival in phagocytic cells and exhibited no defect in their replication in epithelial cells. One MS mutant appeared to be blocked in epithelial cell attachment and invasion.

The above approaches, which we have used in the study of *Salmonella*, should be useful to those working on *Brucella* pathogenesis. The basic genetic approach is surely not new and has been used successfully by hundreds of bacterial geneticists working on many different problems. The success of this approach is related to screening large numbers of mutants using simple *in vitro* assays for virulence. Mutants identified using *in vitro* assays can then be tested for virulence in the animal to verify that the gene is needed for virulence. Obviously, this approach also relies on the ability to make transposon insertion mutations and to return mutated genes to the organism for complementation studies. With the application of these techniques to *Brucella*, we can expect to identify new virulence determinants within this organism in the next few years.

References

1. Allardet-Servent A, Bourg G, Ramuz M, Pages M, Bellis M Roizes, G. DNA polymorphism in strains of the genus *Brucella*. *J Bact* 1988;170:4603-4607.
2. Hoyer BH, McCullough NB. Polynucleotide homologies of *Brucella* deoxyribonucleic acids. *J Bact*. 1968;95: 444-448.
3. CottonWE, Buck JM. Further researches on Bang's disease. *Journ Am. Vet. Med. Assoc.* 1932;33:342-355.
4. Davis RW, Botstein D, JR Roth. Advanced bacterial genetics, Cold Spring Harbor Laboratory, 1980.
5. Winter AJ, Howe GE, Duncan JR, Eis MJ, Widom J, Ganem B Morein B. Effectiveness of natural and synthetic complexes of porin and O polysaccharide as vaccines against *Brucella abortus* in mice. *Infect Immun* 1988;56:3251-3261.
6. Holland JJ, Pickett MJ. Intracellular behavior of *Brucella* variants in chick embryo cells in tissue culture. *Proc Soc Exp Bio Med* 1956;93:476-479
7. Braun W, Pomales-Lebron A, Stinebring WR. Interactions between mononuclear phagocytes and *Brucella abortus* strains of different virulence. *Proc Soc Exp Biol Med* 1958;97:393-397.
8. Freeman BA, Vana LR. Host-parasite relationships in brucellosis. I. Infection of normal guinea pig macrophages in tissue culture. *J Infect Dis* 1958;102:258-267.
9. Stinebring WR, Kessel R. Continuous growth of *Brucella abortus* in mononuclear phagocytes of rats and guinea pigs. *Proc Soc Exp Biol Med* 1959;101:412-415.
10. Freeman BA, Kross DJ, Circo, R. Host-parasite relationships in brucellosis: II. Destruction of macrophage cultures by *Brucella* of different virulence. *J Infect Dis*

1961;108:333-338

11. Freeman BA, Pearson GR, Hines WD. Host-parasite relationships in brucellosis. III. Behavior of avirulent *Brucella* in tissue culture monocytes. *J Infect Dis* 1964;114:441-449.

12. Finlay BB, Falkow S. Comparison of the invasion strategies used by *Salmonella cholerae-suis, Shigella flexneri* and *Yersinia enterocolitica* to enter cultured animal cells: endosome acidification is not required for bacterial invasion or intracellular replication. *Biochimie* 1988;70:1089-1099.

13. Isberg RR, Falkow S. A single genetic locus encoded by *Yersinia pseudotuberculosis* permits invasion of cultured animal cells by *E. coli* K12. *Nature* 1985;317:262-264.

14. Finlay BB, Starnbach MN, Francis CL, Stocker B, Chatfield S, Dougan G, Falkow S. Identification and characterization of Tn*pho*A mutants of *Salmonella* that are unable to pass through a polarized MDCK epithelial cell monolayer. *Molecular Microbiol* 1988;2:757.

15. Fields PI, Swanson RV, Haidaris CG, Heffron, F. Mutants of *Salmonella typhimurium* that cannot survive within the macrophage are avirulent. *Proc Natl Acad Sci USA* 1986;83:5189-5193.

16. Smith LD, Heffron F. Transposon Tn5 mutagenesis of *Brucella abortus. Infect Immun* 1987;55:2774-2776.

17. Lissner R, Swanson RN, O'Brien AD. Genetic control of the innate resistance of mice to *Salmonella typhimurium*: Expression of *ity* genes in peritoneal and splenic macrophages isolated in vitro. *J Immunol* 1983;131:3006-3013.

18. Buchmeier NA, Heffron F. Intracellular survival of wild-type *Salmonella typhimurium* and macrophage-sensitive mutants in diverse populations of macrophages. *Infect Immun* 1989;57:1-7.

Chapter Two

Evolutionary Development and Taxonomy of the Genus *Brucella*

Margaret E. Meyer

Development and Structure of the Genus

The isolation of the causal agent of Malta fever by Bruce[1] a century ago had a decisive and permanent impact on clinical medicine as well as on systematic bacteriology. Malta fever had been difficult to differentiate symptomatically and clinically from other fevers, i.e. the so-called typhoid-malarial complex, then endemic in countries of the Mediterranean littoral. Thus, to clinicians, the isolation of these organisms separated and defined Malta (undulant) fever as a distinct clinical entity. Since we have the advantage of historical hindsight, we now know that when Bruce[2] later named the causal organisms *Micrococcus melitensis*, he created the first species of *Brucella*.

Interestingly, the realization that undulant fever of man and brucellosis of animals were different manifestations of the same infection led to the creation of the genus *Brucella*. Evans[3] established that *M. melitensis* was, in fact, a small rod (coccobacilli) rather than a coccus and that it was morphologically, culturally, and biochemically essentially indistinguishable from *B. abortus*. Because these two organisms shared the distinctive in vivo capabilities of producing abortion in animals and undulant fever in man, Meyer and Shaw[4] found unacceptable Evan's suggestion that they be classified in the genus *Bacterium*, which included the typhoid-dysentery group of intestinal organisms. To accommodate the distinctive features of *M. melitensis* and *B. abortus* and to commemorate the work of David Bruce, they gave them separate rank as the genus *Brucella*.

From its formation in 1920 until 1963, one additional species, *B. suis* was incorporated into the genus,[5,6] as were several biotypes.[6-11] During these 43 years, there were various critical assessments as to the naming and numbering of biotypes and as to whether these were aberrant, atypical, and/or transitional strains of brucellae.[7,12-17] Nonetheless, the genus membership remained stabilized with the three species of *Brucella abortus*, *Brucella suis* and *Brucella melitensis*, now frequently referred to as the three classical species.

Since 1966, three additional species have been added to the genus, *Brucella neotomae*, *Brucella ovis*, and *Brucella canis*, now appropriately referred to as the three new species. *Brucella neotomae* was accepted without controversy[18] as it has an essentially smooth colonial morphology, fits other criteria by which *Brucella* organisms can be identified,[19] and also has a distinctive metabolic pattern.[20]

The flow of thought that prevailed concerning both the structure of the genus and the pedigree required for admission into it was abruptly interrupted with the descriptions of *B. ovis*[21] and the accompanying suggestion that it was a *Brucella* organism, and that it should be considered a new species.[22] In fact, 18 years of doubt and controversy[23] reigned regarding the true identity of *B. ovis* before it was ultimately admitted into the genus *Brucella*. *Brucella ovis* had not previously been assigned to a taxonomic niche because it differed markedly from the existing criteria for generic recognition of brucellae and because the manifestations of infection it caused in individual animals, as well as in flocks of sheep, did not fit the classical disease pattern associated with brucellosis. Further, it contradicted the conventional wisdom that only smooth brucellae were virulent and could long maintain themselves in populations of host/reservoir animals. The same circumstances initially clouded the identity of *B. canis*.[24-27]

Hoyer and McCullough[28] ushered in the "high-tech" era in this genus in 1968 by being the first to explore species relatedness at the genome level. The results of their DNA-DNA hybridization experiments established that the four brucellae species then accepted (*B. abortus*, *B. suis*, *B. melitensis*, and *B. neotomae*) had 100% homology in their polynucleotide sequences, that *B. ovis* had 94% homology with the other species, and that the base composition of G+C of 56 to 58 mole percent was the same in all five species. In a subsequent paper,[29] they established that *B. canis* had DNA homology with the three classical species and, by reciprocal DNA-DNA hybridization, established that the difference in *B. ovis* was not due to a rearrangement of 6% of the sequences, but that they were actually missing from the genome. On the basis of these results, they concluded that *B. ovis* was a deletion mutant of one of the classical species and that all the species are closely related.

Recently, Verger et al.[30] examined the DNA homologies of the polynucleotide sequences in 51 strains of *Brucella*, which included representatives of the six species and several strains of biotypes within each of the classical species. There are no reported biotypes within the three new species. In DNA-DNA reassociation experiments using labeled DNA strands from *B. melitensis* 16M to determine its homology with the other 50 strains, they reported relative binding ratios (percent homology) of 84 to 100% percent. In their results on reciprocal DNA-DNA relatedness, they reported percentages ranging from 87 to 104 percent. Even though their 23% range in percentages of binding ratios and 17% range in reciprocal ratios considerably exceeded the reported standard error of 3% in DNA relatedness results,[31,32] they nonetheless denied the validity of Hoyer and McCullough's finding concerning the 6% difference between *B. ovis* and the other species.

However, by using a different molecular genetic technique, De Ley et al.[33] established with certainty the genetic similarity of the six species. These investigators previously had found that genome sizes (i.e. molecular complexes) are similar among different strains within a single, well-defined species (standard deviation of a group of averages is less than 14.5%). When the same techniques were applied to the six species of *Brucella*,[34] they found genome molecular complexities of 2.37 x 10[9], with standard deviation of 8%, indicating an intimate genetic relationship. Their data on DNA ribosomal RNA hybridization also shows, via a similarity map, few measurable differences among the species. Thus, by all available molecular genetic techniques for ascertaining relatedness at the genome level, it is clear that the relationship among all brucellae is exquisitely close.

Current Taxonomic Status of the Genus

What, then, is the current taxonomic status of this genus? Taxonomy seems to mean different things to different people. However, in its purest sense, it means having a scheme of hierarchical classification that reflects and reveals the evolutionary relatedness of the organisms, ideally at all taxon levels; i.e., biotypes, species, genus and family. As distinct from the evolutionary relatedness imbued in a taxonomy, the taxonomic process obviously includes a workable identification key and a system of nomenclature.

For many years, the genus *Brucella* was sequestered in the family *Brucellaceae*,[35] which also included many other genera (i.e. *Bordetella*, *Pasteurella*, etc.). Through DNA-DNA hybridization studies and G+C base ratio determinations, the genus *Brucella* was found to be unrelated to the other family members and, in fact, most of the genera in the family were found to be unrelated to each other. In the most recent edition of Bergey's Manual,[36] the genus is not subsumed to any family but is free-floating in a group of Gram-negative rods and cocci.

However, based on recent results calculated from DNA-ribosomal RNA reciprocal hybridizations, De Ley et al.[34] reported that the genus *Brucella* and plant pathogens in the agrobacterium-rhizobium complex of organisms have a "rather close phylogenetic origin and they sprang from the same ancestor." These investigators also commented that this unique finding would have to be examined further with other sophisticated genetic techniques. Nonetheless, the genus may now have a family affiliation and a very unexpected one at that.

Because of the exquisite closeness of the genetic relationship among all brucellae, there is no question but that the boundaries of this genus are elegantly defined. Based on all these genetic lines of evidence, the suggestion has been made that all *Brucella* strains are biotype (biovars) of a single species and should be renamed to reflect this fact.[30,37] This may well be true, but all these sophisticated molecular techniques have revealed only genome similarities and no attempt has been made to account for the discrete and substantial differences known to exist among these organisms. Additionally, these techniques have revealed only two evolutionary clues: *B. ovis* is probably a deletion mutant of one of the classical species and the genus may be descended from some plant pathogens.

Differences Among the Species

The differences between and among the species described below could be useful in ascertaining evolutionary pathways.

1. Differences in the number of biotypes within a species: Even though the current classification scheme recognizes but eight biotypes (biovars) within the species *B. abortus*, at least 22 have been reported.[38-41] In the species *B. suis* there are four recognized biotypes, and a fifth has been reported.[42] In the species *B. melitensis,* there are no reported biotypes, but there are three serotypes. There are no reported biotypes or serotypes within the species *B. neotomae, B. ovis,* or *B. canis.* Thus, the species *B. abortus* is genetically labile, while the others are relatively stable in respect to the numbers of biotypes.

2. Differences in colonial morphology at time of initial isolation: Each of the three classical species and *B. neotomae* are smooth on initial isolation. *Brucella ovis* and *B. canis* are non-smooth (i.e. mucoid), but not fully rough.

3. Differences in metabolic patterns: Each of the six species has a characteristic and definitive pattern of oxidation on an array of 14 amino acid and carbohydrate substrates. In addition, in the species *B. suis,* the oxidative pattern also is discrete for the biotypes.[14-17,20,27,43,44]

4. Patterns of growth on appropriate concentrations of the dye, basic fuchsin and thionin: Even though these dyes are man-made products derived from coal tar and are substances the organisms are unlikely to encounter in nature, nonetheless, there is a consistent pattern of growth that recurs throughout the species and their biotypes. Possibly the ring structures of these dyes are mimetic of substrates naturally occurring in mammalian tissues.

5. Need for CO_2 and serum for growth, especially on initial isolation: Serum and/or CO_2 is required only by some of the biotypes of *B. abortus* and *B. ovis,* however, it is an inherent environmental pabulum unneeded by other genus members and is important in considering lines of decen-

dancy both of the species and of the biotypes.

6. Susceptibility to B. abortus bacteriophage, strain 3, also known as the Tbilisi phage: Several strains of phage have been found that lyse various of the species of Brucella[45] but strain 3 has provided the most consistent and precise results and also is highly correlated to the metabolic patterns.[46] As such, it may also offer clues to evolutionary dependency.

7. Biological behavior in nature: Each of the three classical species has a preferential reservoir of infection and each differ in their host ranges.[47,48] Certainly, each occasionally infects other animals but they do not perpetuate themselves indefinitely in non-reservoir, non-preferential hosts. In contrast to the host ranges exhibited by the three classical species, each of the three new species B. neotomae, B. ovis, and B. canis, has a very limited host range. As far as is known, each is restricted respectively to wood rats, sheep (especially rams) and dogs. Also, of probable significance all the biotypes of B. abortus have the same host range while in B. suis, hosts of the biotypes differ. On the other hand, the host ranges of B. suis biotypes may reflect the geographic range of the hosts. Additionally, no disease in man has been attributed to B. suis, type 2, B. neotomae, or B. ovis. Also, brucellosis in man is but rarely caused by either B. canis or B. abortus, type 5.

It is thus abundantly clear that there are marked and substantial differences in nature in the biological behavior of the organisms in this genus. Even though classification purists and numerical taxonomists insist that host not be considered when ordering a classification hierarchy, there is experimental evidence to indicate, at least in the genus Brucella, that such behavior can provide clues to the mechanism of evolutionary decendancy.

As it has been established by several lines of evidence that all organisms in this genus share an exquisitely close genetic relationship, it is biologically reasonable to assume, as a working hypothesis, that they arose from a common "stem" or progenitor organism. Also, since "new species" are of apparent recent origin, it is reasonable to assume that the progenitor is an extant organism. The genus member that is biologically most capable of serving in this role is B. abortus, type 2. It is sensitive to both basic fuchsin and thionin and requires both CO_2 and serum for growth. Thus, in vitro its environmental demands are the strictest among the three classical species and, except for B. ovis, all derivative organisms are less environmentally demanding. In addition, all other Brucella organisms either share the pattern of dye sensitivity of B. abortus, type 2 or are less sensitive.

There is strong evidence considering B. ovis a derivative organism of B. abortus, type 2. An organism essentially indistinguishable from B. ovis in its colonial morphology, environmental requirements, and metabolic pattern was derived in vitro from a culture of B. abortus, type 2. The mechanism of derivation was the induction of L-forms by steroid hormones

Model for Evolutionary Derivation of *Brucella* Organisms with Supporting Evidence

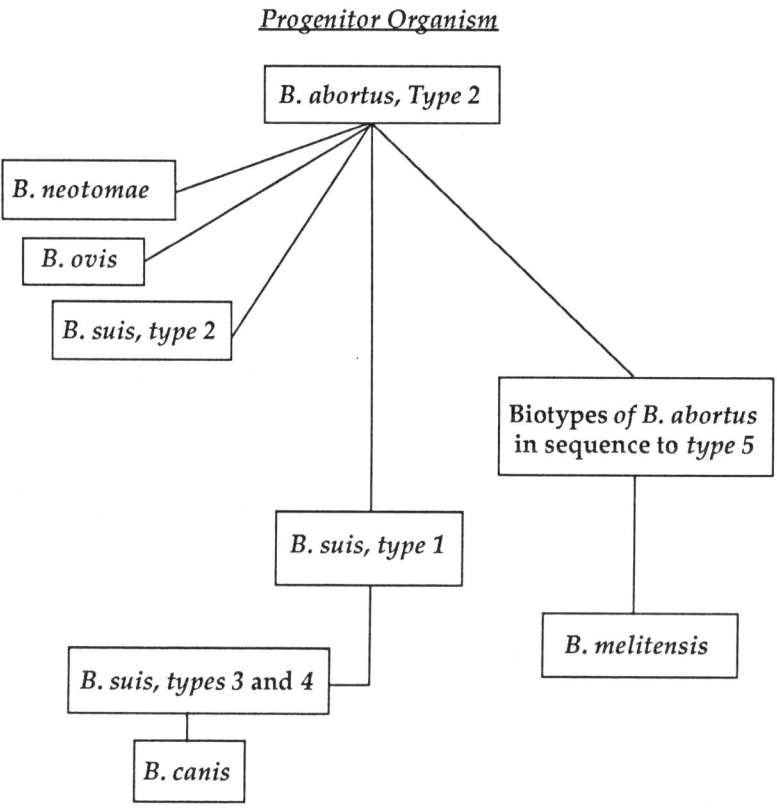

and the subsequent incomplete reversion of these L-forms to their parental forms. There are substantial reasons to believe that the laboratory lineage of B. ovis parallels its natural lineage. B. abortus, type 2 is the only extant Brucella organism that requires both CO_2 and serum for growth and, thus, is the only species and/or biotype that could transmit these characteristics to a derivative. Hoyer and McCullough[29] hypothesized that the 6% deletion in polynucleotide sequences occurred as a result of multiple, small stepwise losses. Under laboratory conditions, the derivation occurred following a single exposure to the inducing agent and the resultant derivative was at the most, two generations removed from its parent-one generation on progesterone and one generation for reversion.[49-50] The same brevity of time and events must have occurred in nature. If the loss of polynucleotide sequences happened over a period of time with many small losses, then strain variants of B. ovis should be found. Such variants have not been found. In fact, the characteristics of all reported isolates of B. ovis are of such uniformity as to have prompted investigative comment,[51] and also a separate report on the matter.[52] Further, this uniformity has been confirmed at the genome level by O'Hara et al.[53] who, after analyzing 33 strains of B. ovis DNA with 11 different restriction endonucleases, concluded that B. ovis is a very homogenous species, and that B. abortus, B. melitensis, and B. canis are more closely related to each other than each is to B. ovis. One lesson learned from this derivation of B. ovis is that the order of decendancy from a progenitor is not necessarily linear.

Derivation of the Biotypes of Brucella abortus

Table 2-1 shows the taxonomic ordering of the biotypes of B. abortus according to the sequential flow of their characteristics by the conventionally measured characteristics. Table 2-2 shows those biotypes arranged in six groups according to loss of a characteristic. B. abortus, type 2 has the greatest environmental demands (need for serum and CO_2) and is the most sensitive to basic fuchsin and thionin, other dyes[41] and a variety of antibiotics.[54]

The greatest change in biotype characteristics occurs between biotypes 1 and 2, where there is a loss of the environmental demands and a concurrent loss in sensitivity to numerous dyes and antibiotics. Since these changes cannot be attributed to a massive occurrence of simultaneous and multiple mutations, this change in sensitivities may well indicate an alteration in permeability and/or structure of the cell surface, wall, or membranes. In any event, the change is dramatic and shared by all subsequent biotypes of B. abortus. Even though the metabolic pattern of all biotypes is identical, including type 2, there are changes that are substantial and can be measured by alterations in the sensitivity to basic fuchsin and thionin. When arranged in sequential order, it can be seen

Table 2-1. Biotypes of *Brucella abortus* Taxonomically Ordered According to the Sequential Flow of Their Characteristics

Brucella abortus Current Biotype Designation	Line Number	Number of Strains Examined (Total 613)	Serum Required for Growth (■=Yes □=No)	Basic Fuchsin (■=growth □=No growth) 10	20	Thionin 10	20	50	H₂S Produced (■=Yes □=No)	CO₂ Required for Growth (■=Yes □=No)	Lysis by Bacteriophage (■=Yes □=No) RTD	10⁴xRTD	Agglutination A(abortus)	M(melitensis)
2	1	38	■	□	□	□	□	□	■	■	■	■	■	□
—*	2	35	■	□	□	□	□	□	■	■	■	■	□	■
2	3	18	■	□	□	□	□	□	■	□	■	■	■	□
2	4	11	□	□	□	□	□	□	■	■	■	■	■	□
2	5	9	□	□	□	□	□	□	■	□	■	■	■	□
2	6	8	□	□	□	□	□	□	■	■	■	■	□	■
1	7	163	□	■	■	□	□	□	■	■	■	■	■	□
1	8	108	□	■	■	□	□	□	■	■	■	■	■	□
—*	9	3	□	■	■	□	□	□	■	□	■	■	□	■
4	10	43	□	■	■	□	□	□	■	■	■	■	□	■
3	11	20	□	■	■	■	□	□	■	■	■	■	■	□
3	12	21	□	■	■	■	■	□	■	■	■	■	■	□
9	13	13	□	■	■	■	■	□	■	■	■	■	□	■
9	14	5	□	■	■	■	■	□	■	□	■	■	□	■
—*	15	2	□	■	■	■	■	□	■	■	■	■	□	■
6	16	2	□	■	■	■	■	□	■	□	■	■	■	□
6	17	17	□	■	■	■	■	□	□	□	■	■	■	□
7	18	2	□	■	■	■	■	□	□	□	■	■	■	□
5	19	95	□	■	■	■	■	□	□	□	■	■	□	■

*Strains with combinations of characteristics not previously described

(Table 2-1) that *B. abortus,* type 2 is the only possible progenitor of the biotypes in *B. abortus,* and that *B. abortus,* type 5 is, so to speak, the end of the line.

Possible Derivation of *Brucella melitensis*

By all the conventional determinative methods, *B. melitensis* is indistinguishable from *B. abortus,* biotype 5. However, in its metabolic pattern, it differs on three carbohydrate substrates (arabinose, galactose, and ribose). There is evidence though that utilization of arabinose and galactose are interdependent, i.e., all species and biotypes either oxidize both or neither of these substrates. Additionally, it is known that one of the by-

TABLE 2-2

Biotypes of Brucella abortus Divided Into 6 Groups

Line Numbers on Table I	Characteristics By Conventional Determinative Methods ■=Yes □=No					
	Needs Serum for Growth	Sensitive to Basic Fuchsin	Sensitive to Thionin	Produces Hydrogen Sulfide	Needs Carbon Dioxide for Growth	Susceptible to Phage
Group 1 Lines 1,2	■	■	■	■	■	■
Group 2 Lines 3,4,5,6	1st Loss	■	■	■	■/□*	■
Group 3 Lines 7,8,9,10		2nd Loss	■	■	■/□	■
Group 4 Lines 11,12	3rd Loss		■	■	■/□	■
Group 5 Lines 13,14,15,16			4th Loss	■	■/□	■
Group 6 Lines 17,18,19				5th Loss	□**	■

*Need Variable; **Loss becomes permanent.

products of arabinose oxidation is galactose.[55] Thus, alteration in oxidation of one of these two substrates may reflect only one change. The second difference being oxidation of ribose.

Another difference that separates *B. melitensis* from *B. abortus,* biotype 5 is susceptibility to *B. abortus,* phage strain 3. In view of the fact that there is now extant a strain of *B. abortus* that is known to be resistant to this phage, and many strains of *B. melitensis* show lysis from without on exposure to this phage, differences in phage susceptibility may not mark as decisive a difference as previously believed. Nonetheless, there is essentially a permanent change in the phage susceptibility of *B. melitensis,* perhaps reflecting only a change in the phage receptor sites on the cell surface. Differences in cell surface may also be involved in the differing host responses (i.e., the preferential reservoir situation) to *Brucella* organisms, and may be related to both host susceptibility and lack of maintenance in nature among the non-preferential hosts. In any event, according to all available measures of similarity, *B. melitensis* is a close relative of *B. abortus,* type 5. This biotype is rarely pathogenic for man, a characteristic which may be a good indicator of the impending differences between the preferential hosts of *B. abortus* and *B. melitensis.*[13]

Derivation of *Brucella suis*

The first steps in the derivation of *B. suis* type 2, i.e. loss of need for CO_2 and serum, are identical to the first steps in derivation of *B. neotomae* and the biotypes of *B. abortus.* Thereafter, all of the biotypes of *B. suis* are derived in the same pattern of sequential flow of characteristics as are the biotypes of *B. abortus.* The loss of sensitivity to basic fuchsin by the biotypes of *B. suis* is the mirror image of the loss of sensitivity to thionin by the biotypes of *B. abortus.* In the species *B. suis,* type 3 and 4 (type 4 quantitatively has some M antigen) are apparently the "end of the line." The essential difference in the metabolic pattern between *B. abortus* and *B. suis* is the oxidation of amino acids in the urea cycle by *B. suis.*

It appears that whatever happens in nature to spark the initiation of altering the characteristics in *B. abortus,* type 2, the critical change can be measured by whether the first loss occurs as a loss of sensitivity to thionin, in which event the organism becomes characteristic of what we recognize as the species of *B. suis* and its descendant biotypes. On the other hand, if this first loss is measured as a loss of sensitivity to basic fuchsin, the organisms become characteristic of what we recognize as the species *B. abortus* and its descendant biotypes. After this first critical alteration, the biotypes then occur in a sequential and essentially linear decendancy for each successive biotype.

The change that is measured by the dyes is only mimetic and not duplicative of the changes that occur in nature. By using the techniques of providing selective environments, it is not difficult to obtain mutants with altered dye sensitivities. However, other changes, such as altered sensitivities to other dyes, antibiotics, or alterations in metabolic pattern, do not accompany changes in growth on these two dyes. Obviously, elucidation of the nature of this first critical alteration in *B. abortus*, type 2 is crucial for the recapitulation of the evolution of members in this genus.

Origin of *Brucella canis*

There is strong circumstantial evidence to indicate that *B. suis*, type 3 is the progenitor organism of *B. canis*, and that it arose by the same natural phenomenon as did *B. ovis*. By all the conventional determinative methods, it is indistinguishable from *B. suis*, type 3, and it also has the metabolic pattern that characterized the species *B. suis*. Further, it has the identical colony morphology (i.e., mucoid) as does *B. ovis* and, similarly, has a very restricted host range.

Derivation of *Brucella neotomae*

The characteristics of *B. neotomae* indicate that this species also could have been derived from *B. abortus*, type 2, in a fashion similar to *B. suis*, type 2, i.e. loss of the need for CO_2 and serum and loss of sensitivity to thionin. It also is similar to *B. suis* in that it is susceptible only to high concentrations of *B. abortus* bacteriophage, strain 3, and oxidizes one of the major substrates in the urea cycle. As with other "new species," it is not pathogenic for man and has a limited host range.

Thus, the model accounts for the known and possible lineages of all organisms in the genus *Brucella* and provides a structural working hypothesis for future investigations.

Mechanisms that Could Account for Alterations in Characteristics of Members of the Genus *Brucella*

Incomplete Reversion of L-forms, Producing Strains with Altered Characteristics

This phenomenon has already been confirmed experimentally in the case of *B. ovis* and may well occur with other organisms within this genus, especially in consideration of the fact that L-forms can be induced by steroid hormones. Since the preferred habitat of brucellae is the reproductive tract, especially the gravid uterus, there is no doubt about the organisms encountering these hormones in vivo.

In fact, a naturally occurring cell wall defective variant of *B. abortus* has been isolated from bovine tissue.[58] Significantly, this organism required serum for growth, the colonies were non-smooth, and the animal had a history of having been treated with stilbestrol.[58,59]

The phenomenon of incomplete reversion in the genus *Brucella* was first encountered in a culture of *B. melitensis*[49] so the mechanism certainly is not confined to the species *B. abortus*. Nor is it confined to this genus. It has been reported to occur in *Streptococcus faecalis*,[60] and is responsible for changes in features of *Escherichia coli*,[61] *Salmonella typhimurim*,[62] and β-hemolytic streptococci.[63]

There is no evidence to indicate that all incomplete and/or altered revertants undergo a full 6% loss in polynucleotide sequences and the possibility certainly exists that nucleotide changes could be more subtle, i.e. less than 3%, and only detectable by the most sensitive DNA techniques.

Activity of Plasmids

In the brucellosis laboratory at the University of California, Davis, we have examined 600 strains of *Brucella*, which included strains of all species and biotypes, using the Kado,[64] Guerry,[65] and Clewer[66] methods on essentially equal numbers of strains and found no evidence of plasmids. Simon[67] also reported negative results in his search for plasmids. However, it recently has been shown that via conjugation, *B. abortus* can accept and maintain certain broad host range plasmids from *E. coli*, i.e., pTHIO (Incp), pSa (Inc W) and R751 (Inc P). These plasmids have no effect on characteristics used for biotyping.[68]

Conventional Mutational Events Involving Discrete Characteristics

In view of the repeatedly expressed speculations on the mutability of the *Brucella* species, (see review by Meyer),[57] surprisingly little has been reported on the mutation of discrete characteristics. It is known that under laboratory conditions, mutations are responsible for the change from smooth to rough colonial morphology,[69] loss of CO_2 requirement in *B. abortus* type 6,[70] and alterations in sensitivities to various dyes,[71,72] erythritol,[73] and penicillin[74] and in hydrogen sulfide production.[75]

No mutants of mucoid colonial morphology comparable to the morphology of colonies of B. *ovis* and B. *canis* have been found to occur under laboratory conditions and we now know that laboratory-selected mutants with altered sensitivities to basic fuchsin and/or thionin are not comparable to the wild type mutants. However, the essentially minute changes among the species biotypes could easily be accounted for by one-step sequential mutations.

Activity of Bacteriophages

The potential impact that bacteriophages may have on causing alterations in strain characteristics is under active investigation. There are several approaches that can be used. One is to "cure" strains of any indigenous phage and check the before and after results. Another is to infect non-infected strains using a variety of phages and ascertain the before and after characteristics. Both of these, and other avenues for exploring the molecular biology of Brucellae have been reported by Rigby et al.[76,77]

Another avenue of approach in the investigation of the relationship of phages to alterations in strain characteristics is to further explore the possible role of sticky white *Brucella* phage carrier colonies. These types of colonies and their associated lytic activity have been reported by Renoux and Suire,[78] McDuff et al.,[79] and Meyer,[69] who also commented that carrier phage may be involved in the incomplete reversion process since sticky white colonies and lytic activity invariably accompanies this phenomenon.

Further Use of Restriction Endonucleases

Restriction endonuclease analysis has shown that there is a very close relatedness among all the *Brucella* species and also that B. *canis*, B. *suis*, and B. *melitensis* are more closely related to each other than to B. *ovis*.[53,80] However, we should now be looking for a technique that will help account for the observed differences.

Activity of Porins

The existence of porin channels in the outer membrane of brucellae was first suggested by Verstreate et al.[81] and further elucidated by Douglas et al.,[82] Verstreate and Winter[83] and Santos et al.[84] The relative sizes of the porin channels differ among the species, being wide in B. *canis*, medium in B. *abortus*, and narrow in B. *melitensis*. These findings may partially account for the differing permeability of the dyes basic fuchsin and thionin and may be reflected in the differing patterns of organism sensitivity to these dyes. However, before any conclusions can be drawn about porins, the critical strains remain to be examined, i.e., *B. abortus,* type 2 and 5, *B. neotomae,* and *B. suis,* type 2.

Use of Gas Chromatography to Ascertain Differences in Constituent Fatty Acids

Tanaka et al.[85] examined the 16 *Brucella* reference strains and 66 field isolates by gas chromatography for quantitative comparisons of 15 cellular fatty acids. Using the resulting data, they did a numerical taxonomic analysis to determine interspecies similarity matrices and also intraspecies matrices on the species *B. abortus, B. melitensis, B. suis,* and *B. canis.* Since only one strain each of *B. ovis* and *B. neotomae* were included in the study, the same type of analysis could not be done on the two later species. These investigators found that *B. abortus* and *B. melitensis* are quite similar to each other, *B. ovis* and *B. neotomae* are more similar to *B. abortus* than to the other species, *B. suis* had overall similarity but was a distinctive group, and *B. ovis* had greater similarity to *B. suis* than to the other species. Within the species, there was great similarity among biotypes within *B. abortus* and *B. melitensis* and complete homogeneity among strains of *B. canis.* In the *B. suis,* species, *B. suis* biotype 3 was distinctly different.

In a later study on the fatty acid content of *B. canis* and *B. suis* by Dees et al.[86] the presence of large amounts of 19-carbon cyclopropane acid was present in all strains of *B. suis* and absent in all strains of *B. canis.* The significance of these findings on the fatty acids lies in the following. If *B. canis* is a derivative of *B. suis* via the route of incomplete reversion of L-forms, then one of the losses must be 19-carbon cyclopropane acid. The marked difference observed in *B. suis* type 2 goes hand in hand with the fact that its behavior in nature is different, i.e., it has a restricted host range and is non-infectious for man. Additionally, *B. suis* type 2 colonies differ subtly but perhaps significantly from the classical fully smooth forms. They are neither fully smooth nor fully mucoid. Other investigators have also commented on the colonial morphology of *B. suis,* type 2.[87] This organism may well be from an L-form that has not completely reverted, but has reverted more fully than *B. canis* and *B. ovis.*

Since *B. suis,* type 2 is so remarkably different from *B. suis* biotypes 1, 3, and 4, the model shows these biotypes arising independently rather than sequentially.

Exploration of the Ribosomes

One of the newer and significant additions to the elucidation of the process of evolution in prokaryotic cells is the concept that RNA, i.e., ribosides and the ribosome, preceded nucleotides and DNA in the evolutionary development of prokaryotes. Thus there is not just a duality consisting of genotype and phenotype but a trinity of genotype, ribotype, and phenotype.[88] Or, as stated by Stanier[89] "at the level of gene products, information is accumulating which shows that the gene composition of phenotypically similar strains is closely related to ribosomal protein composition." Also, see Stanier,[90] Darnell,[91] and Woese.[92]

One of the common techniques for ascertaining differences in ribosomal structure/function is to examine ribosomes extracted from disrupted cells, or to ascertain the responses of intact cells and mutants thereof with antibiotics known to affect the ribosome, i.e., erythromycin and/or chloramphenicol. This approach has been fruitful in determining discrete ribosomal differences in such organisms as *E. coli*[93,94] and *B. subtilis*.[95-97]

In the brucellosis laboratory at the University of California, Davis, we have examined all the species and biotypes for their sensitivity to erythromycin and chloramphenicol using both a low and high concentration via antibiotic discs and measuring zones of inhibition in mm with calipers. All strains of *B. abortus*, type 2 were sensitive to erythromycin, all other *B. abortus* biotypes were resistant; all biotypes of *B. suis* were susceptible, as was *B. ovis*, *B. melitensis*, *B. canis*, and *B. neotomae* were sensitive only to the higher concentrations. All species and biotypes were equally sensitive to chloramphenicol.

These results indicate that there certainly may be marked ribosomal differences between *B. abortus*, type 2 and all its derivative biotypes. Additionally, there must be subtle but discrete and measurable differences in ribosomal structure/function that ebb and flow through this genus (possibly switched on and off?). Be that as it may, it is known that the differences between sensitivity and resistance to erythromycin are due to changes in the ribosomal structure resulting in a lower binding affinity to this antibiotic.[97] It would appear, therefore, that one of the critical points of inquiry to help account for and to recapitulate the lineage of the species and biotypes of *Brucella* is to further ascertain the importance and occurrence of these ribosomal differences. The isolation and functional determinations of individual and/or groups of genes is very much in its early infancy. Still, there are a few reports concerning gene isolation and expression of function.[98-100]

Current Taxonomic Status of the Genus *Brucella*

There should be an orderly sequence of processes in establishing the systematics of genus, i.e., strain descriptions, identification key, and hierarchal ordering of the organisms into a classification scheme based on known and observed evolutionary relationships. Clearly, taxonomy is a dynamic and ongoing rather than a static process.

The present classification scheme that sequesters this genus is actually a determinative identification key and, as such, it obscures rather than reveals the evolutionary relationships that must exist among the member organisms. Additionally, the species and biotypes have been intercalated into the scheme in the chronological order in which they have been isolated and described. Further disorder has been introduced in the scheme by virtue of the fact that there is no consensus on what constitutes a biotype. There is also now the recommendation that the nomenclature be changed to reflect the closeness or DNA-DNA homology,[30] and the genus be considered as one species.

What Course of Action?

The bottom line is that no one is certain about what constitutes a bacterial species. It is generally and somewhat loosely defined as a group of organisms sharing a mutuality of characteristics as measured phenotypically and that phenotypic discontinuities separates them into species.

In an hierarchal ordering of members of this genus, the great genetic plasticity of the species *B. abortus*, lesser plasticity of *B. suis*, and almost lack of plasticity in *B. melitensis* should be accounted for, as should be the phenotypic discontinuities between each species. The working model and submodel account for those differences, and also account for the origin of *B. ovis* and possibly of *B. canis*. Should the genus be considered as a single species based on DNA-DNA homology?

DNA-DNA homology of polynucleotide sequences may give the illusion of being more genetically precise than it actually is. For example, human beings and chimpanzees have 98% homology among their nucleotide sequences[88] and 99% of the amino acids in the proteins are the same.[101] At the bacterial level, among the serovars of *Listeria monocytogenes*, DNA relatedness has been found to be heterogeneous[102] and the serotypes have been divided into "genomic groups." Intragroup relatedness varies from 90 to 100% homology while intergroup relatedness falls to 25%.

In view of these disconcerting and somewhat confounding facts, before the species concept in this genus is altered, we should perhaps do what other phylogeneticists and molecular biologists are doing:

1) Even though overall polynucleotide homology does not separate humans from other primates, a fastidious examination of the DNA base sequences per se revealed altered positions of the protein (amino acid sequences) and these alterations, though very minimal, do separate man from African apes, orangutans and gibbons.[103]

2) Use of recombinant DNA techniques; as stated by Slatkin: "Even if we were presented with a complete DNA sequence of every individual of

every species, we would still not be able to discern what makes species differences. We need to be able to modify genes to see if we can produce new traits and even new species, and to see whether the species act as if they possess some inertia, resisting modification. The tools for this exist in using recombinant DNA."[101]

Use of DNA Fingerprinting

A benchmark paper on DNA polymorphism, as determined electrophoretically, recently was published on the genus *Brucella*. Significantly, each of the five species so examined (*B. abortus, B. suis, B. melitensis, B. ovis,* and *B. canis*) had a specie-specific DNA fingerprint. Further, the electrophoretic profile clearly placed *B. canis* evolutionarily near *B. suis* and also indicated *B. ovis* was a discrete species. The authors further state that these electrophoretic DNA fingerprints of polymorphism unexpectedly confirm the natural host as a phenotypic characteristic for classifying *Brucella*. They conclude additionally that, from a phylogenetic point of view, four of the five species (*B. abortus, B. suis, B. melitensis,* and *B. ovis*) arose from a common ancestor and that *B. canis* can be considered an authentic strain of *B. suis* or a strain recently evolved from this species.[100]

Bringing Order into the Taxonomy of the Genus *Brucella*

To do this will require consensus and consistency among members of the International Committee on Systematic Bacteriology, Subcommittee on Taxonomy of *Brucella*. Thus far, there has been little consistency and no consensus. In its 1970 meeting, even though it defined *B. suis* by both the conventional determinative methods and metabolic patterns, it assigned *B. canis* as an additional species, and simultaneously accepted an organism as a biotype of *B. suis* (type 5) that had not been adequately shown even to be a Brucella organism.[104] This organism later was decisively excluded from the genus.[105,106] There is no uniformity on the definition of a species and Pinigin, et al.[107] are still making a plea to have *Brucella suis* type 4 considered a separate species.[107,108]

Further, indecision has been caused by Corbel[109] who suggested that *B. abortus*, biotypes 3 and 6 be considered a single biotype because the only significant difference between them was a sensitivity to thionin. However, in 1984 he suggested strains of *B. suis* with slightly altered resistance to basic fuchsin be considered an additional biotype of this species.[42]

There has also been a suggestion that the species *B. melitensis* can be subdivided into five biovars on minute differences in the oxidative rates of five amino acids.[110] Since it has already been established[111] and observed many times over, that age, i.e., number of previous subculturings, and lyophilization tend to cause an increase in utilization rates (but do not alter the basic metabolic pattern) it is really not possible to distinguish metabolic biovars of *B. melitensis* by their oxidative metabolism.

Change in Nomenclature

Verger has proposed that, since he considers the genus *Brucella* to be a single species, *B. melitensis*, the names of the constituent organisms reflect this monospecies concept.[30] Thus, *B. abortus* would become *B. melitensis* biovar *abortus*. In view of what we do know about the evolutionary paths in this genus, this nomenclature is terribly misleading.

Until more is elucidated about the species and biotype derivations and lineages, it seems to be a good idea to adhere to the advice given in *Bergey's Manual*[36] i.e., "the advantage of adopting a restrictive species definition must be weighed against its potential impact on well-established and accepted bacteria groups." Thus, it seems the time to consider changing the structure of the genus is when we have more finite and discrete genetic and evolutionary information, especially as to what accounts for the substantial differences among these organisms.

In summary, the development of the infrastructure of the genus *Brucella* is traced briefly from its beginnings with Bruce to its present composition. A taxonomic ordering of the member organisms according to known and probable evolutionary relationships and lines of descent is presented with experimental and documentary evidence. The present nomenclature and taxonomy of the genes is discussed in relationship to proposed changes.

References

1. Bruce D. Note on the discovery of a microorganism in Malta Fever. *Practitioner* 1887;39:161.
2. Bruce D. Sur une nouvelle forme de fievre. *Ann Inst Pasteur* (Paris) 1893;7:289.
3. Evans AC. Further studies on *Bacterium abortus* and related bacteria. II. A comparison of *Bacterium abortus* and *Bacterium bronchesepticus* and with the organism which causes Malta Fever. *J Infect Dis* 1918;22:580.
4. Meyer KE, Shaw EB. A comparison of the morphological, cultural, and biochemical characteristics of *B. abortus* and *B. melitensis*. *J Infect Dis* 1920;27:173.
5. Traum J. Report of the Chief of the Bureau of Animal Industry, U.S. Department of Agriculture, U.S. Department of Agriculture, Washington, D.C. 1914:14.
6. Huddleson IF. The differentiation of the species in the genus *Brucella*. Michigan State College of Agriculture Experiment Station Technical Bulletin No. 100, East Lansing, Michigan, 1929.
7. Wilson GS. The classification of the *Brucella* group: a systematic study. *J Hyg* 1933;33:516.

8. Van der Schaff Roza M. Brucellosis en onchocerciasis in verband met un chronish gewrichtelijden bij runderen. *Ned Ind Bl* Diergenseek 1940;52:1.

9. Stableforth AW, Jones LM. Report of the subcommittee on taxonomy of the genus *Brucella*. *Int Bull Bacteriol Nomencl Taxon* 1962;13:145.

10. Meyer ME, Cameron HS. Identification of the causative agents and epidemiology of porcine brucellosis. *Bulletin, World Health Organization* 1963;28:499.

11. Meyer ME. Species identity and epidemiology of *Brucella* strains isolated from Alaskan Eskimos. *J Infec Dis* 1964;114:169.

12. Renoux G. La notion d'espece dans le genere *Brucella*. *Ann Inst Pasteur* (Paris) 1958;94:179.

13. Stableforth AW. Brucellosis in Infectious Diseases of Animals. I. Diseases Due to Bacteria. Stableforth A W, Galloway IA, eds. London: Butterworth Scientific Publications, 1959.

14. Meyer ME, Cameron HS. Metabolic characterization of the genus *Brucella*. I. Statistical evaluation of the oxidative rates by which type 1 of each species can be identified. *J Bacteriol* 1961;82:387.

15. Meyer ME, Cameron HS. Metabolic characterization of the genus *Brucella*. II. Oxidative metabolic patterns of the described biotypes. *J Bacteriol* 1961;82:396.

16. Meyer ME. Metabolic characterization of the genus *Brucella*. III. Oxidative metabolism of strains that show anamolous characteristics by conventional determinative methods. *J Bacteriol* 1961;82:401.

17. Meyer ME, Morgan WJB. Metabolic characterization of *Brucella* strains that show conflicting identity by biochemical and serological methods. *Bulletin World Health Organization* 1962;26:823.

18. International Committee on Nomenclature of Bacteria, Subcommittee on the Taxonomy of *Brucella*. Minutes of the Meeting of August 1970, *Int J Syst Bacteriol* 1971;21:126.

19. Stoenner HG, Lackman DB. A new species of *Brucella* isolated from the desert wood rat, *Neotoma lepida* Thomas. *Am J Vet Res* 1957;69:947.

20. Cameron HS Meyer ME. Metabolic studies on *Brucella neotomae* (Stoenner and Lackman). *J Bacteriol* 1958;76:546.

21. Buddle MB, Boyes BW. A *Brucella* mutant causing genital disease in sheep in New Zealand. *Aust Vet J* 1953;29:145.

22. Buddle MB. Studies on *Brucella ovis* (n.Sp.) a cause of genital disease of sheep in New Zealand and Australia. *J Hyg* 1956;54:351.

23. Meyer ME, Cameron HS. Studies on the etiological agent of epididymitis in rams. *Amer J Vet Res* 1968;64:495.

24. Carmichael LE, Bruner DW. Characteristics of newly recognized species of *Brucella* responsible for canine abortions. *Cornell Vet* 1968;48:579.

25. Diaz R, Jones LM, Wilson JB. Antigenic relationship of the Gram-negative organism causing canine abortion to smooth and rough brucellae. *J Bacteriol* 1968;95:618.

26. Jones LM, Zanardi M, Leong D, Wilson JB. Taxonomic position in the genus *Brucella* of the causative agent of canine abortion. *J Bacteriol* 1968;95;625.

27. Meyer ME. *Brucella* organisms isolated from dogs: comparison of characteristics of members of the genus *Brucella*. *Am J Vet Res* 1969;30:175.

28. Hoyer BH, McCullough NB. Polynucleotide homologies of *Brucella* deoxyri-

bonucleic acids. *J Bacteriol* 1968;95:444.

29. Hoyer BH, McCullough NB. Homologies of deoxyribonucleic acids from *Brucella ovis*, canine abortion organisms, and other *Brucella* species. *J Bacteriol* 1968;96:1783.

30. Verger JM, Gremont F, Gremont PAD, Grayon M. *Brucella*, a monospecific genus as shown by deoxyribonucleic acid hybridization. *Int J Syst Bact* 1985;35:292.

31. Grimont PAD, Popoff MY, Grimont F, Coynault C, Lemelin M. *Current Microbiol* 1980;4:325.

32. Grimont PAD, Popoff MY. Use of principal component analysis in interpretation of deoxyribonucleic acid relatedness. *Current Microbiol* 1980;4:337.

33. De Ley J, Gillis M, de Voss P. Range of the molecular complexities of bacterial genomes within some well established bacterial species. *Zentralbe Bacteriol Hyg* I Abt Orig Reihe 1981;2:263.

34. De Ley J, Mannheim W, Segers P, Lievens A, Denijin M, Vanhouke M, Gillis M. Ribosomal ribonucleic acid cistron similarities and taxonomic neighborhood of *Brucella* and CDC group Vd. *Int J Syst Bact* 1987;37:35.

35. Breed RS, Murray EGD, Smith NR, eds. *Bergey's Manual of Determinative Bacteriology*. 7th ed. Baltimore: The Williams and Wilkins, Co., 1957.

36. Buchanan RE, Gibbons NE, eds. *Bergey's manual of determinative bacteriology*. 8th ed. Baltimore: The Williams and Wilkins Co., 1974.

37. Verger JM, Grimont F, Grimont PAD, Grayson M. Taxonomy of the genus *Brucella*. *Ann Inst Pasteur Microbiol* 1987;138:235.

38. Meyer ME. Evolution and taxonomy in the genus *Brucella*: Contemporary evolutionary status of the species *B. abortus*. *Am J Vet Res* 1976;37:203.

39. Harrington R, Bond DR, Brown G M. Smooth phage resistant strain of *Brucella abortus* from bovine tissue. *J Clin Microbiol* 1977;5:63.

40. Ewalt DR, Forbes LB. Atypical isolates of *Brucella abortus* from bovine tissue. *J Clin Microbiol* 1977;5:633.

41. Farrell ID, Robertson L. The sensitivity of the biotypes of *Brucella abortus* to three antibiotics used in selective media, and the description of a new biotype. *J Hyg* 1967;65:165.

42. Corbel, MJ. Taxonomic studies on some atypical strains of *Brucella suis*. *Brit Vet J* 1984;140:34.

43. Meyer ME. Phenotypic comparison of *Brucella ovis* to the DNA-homologous *Brucella* species. *Am J Vet Res* 1969; 30:1757.

44. Philippon, A. Identification de *Brucella abortus*: metabolisme oxidatif et lysotypie. *Ann Inst Pasteur* 1968;115:367.

45. Corbel MJ. Brucella phages: Advances in the development of a reliable phage typing system for smooth and non-smooth *Brucella* isolates, in *Brucella* and brucellosis, an update. *Ann Inst Pasteur Microbiol* 1987;138:70.

46. Meyer ME. Metabolic characterization of the genus *Brucella*: IV. Correlation of oxidative metabolic patterns and susceptibility to *Brucella* bacteriophage, type abortus, strain 3. J Bacteriol 1961;82:950,

47. Meyer ME. The epizootiology of brucellosis and its relationship to the identification of *Brucella* organisms. *Am J Vet Res* 25:553 date.

48. Meyer ME. Host-parasite relationships in brucellosis. 1. Reservoirs of infection and interhost transmissibility of the parasite. Proc. U. S. Livestock Sanitary Assoc

1966:129.

49. Meyer ME. Evolution and taxonomy in the genus *Brucella*: Steroid hormone induction of filterable forms with altered characteristics after reversion. *Am J Vet Res* 1976;37:207.

50. Meyer ME. Evolution and taxonomy in the genus *Brucella*; Progesterone induction of filterable forms of *Brucella abortus*, type 2 with revertant characteristics essentially indistinguisable in vitro from those of *Brucella* ovis. *Am J Vet Res* 1976;37:221.

51. Todoriu C. D. Position of *Brucella ovis* (Buddle 1956) in bacterial taxonomy. (In Bulgarian) Lucr. Inst. Cerc. Vet. Biorep. Pasteur 1966;3:199.

52. Kaitmazova EI, Kurdina DS, Dranovskaya EA, Grekova NA, Sachnovski UG. Characteristics of cultures of *B. ovis*. (In Russian) *Veterinaria* (Moscow) 1971;48:44.

53. O'hara MJ, Collins DM, DeLisle, GW. Restriction endonuclease analysis of *Brucella ovis* and other *Brucella* species. *Vet Microbiol* 1985;10:425.

54. Robertson L, Farrell ID, Hinchliffe PM. The sensitivity of *Brucella abortus* to chemotherapeutic agents. *J Med Microbiol* 1973;6:549.

55. Kaitmazova IE, N N Ostrovskaya. Concerning the characteristics of *Brucella* isolated in USSR territory (In Russian) *Zh Mikrobiol* 1967;44:12.

56. Corbel MJ. Thomas EL, Garcia-Carillo C. Taxonomic studies on some atypical strains of *Brucella suis*. *Br Vet J* 1984;14:34.

57. Meyer ME. Evolution and taxonomy in the genus *Brucella*: Concepts on the origins of the contemporary species. *Am J Vet Res* 1976;37:199.

58. Corbel MJ, Scott AC. Properties of a cell-wall defective variant of *Brucella abortus* of bovine origin. *J Hyg Camb* 1980;85.

59. Ross HM. Isolation of a cell-wall defective strain of *Brucella abortus* from bovine tissue. *Vet Record* 1980;106;247.

60. Hoyer BH, King JR. Desoxyribonuclic acid sequence losses in a stable Streptococcal L-form. *J Bacteriol* 1969;9:1516.

61. Rhadakova ED. Properties of *E. coli* cultures reversed from L-forms. (In Russian) *Zh Mikrobiol* 1971;48:14.

62. Levina GL. Reversion peculiarities of penicillin induced L-forms of causative agent of mouse typhoid fever. (In Russian) *Antibiotiki* 1972;17:714.

63. Kagan G, Gryzlova ON, Mikhailova VS, Levashev VS. Some peculiarities of the cultures reversed from the L-forms of β Hemolyic streptocci. (In Russian) *Zh Mikrobiol* 1961;33:86.

64. Kado CI, Liu ST. Rapid procedure for detection and isolation of large and small plasmids. *J Bacteriol* 1981;145:1365.

65. Guerry P, Le Bank DJ, Falkow F. General method for the isolation of plasmids and deoxyribonucleic acid. *J Bacteriol* 1973;116:1064.

66. Clewel DB, Helenski DR. Supercoiled circular DNA protein complex in *Escherichia coli*: purification and induced conversion to an open circular form. Proc. Natl. Acad. Sci. USA 1969;62:1159.

67. Simon F. Contribution a' l'etude des bacteriophages du genera *Brucella*. Aspect morphilogiques, serologiques et physiologiques. (In French) Thesis, University of Paris.

68. Rigby CE Fraser ADE. Plasmid transfer and plasmid mediated genetic exchange on *Brucella abortus*. *Can J Vet Res* 1989;53:326-330.

69. Braun W. Dissociation in *Brucella abortus*: A demonstration of the role of inherent and environmental factors in bacterial variation. *J Bacteriol* 1946;51:327.

70. Marr AG, Wilson JB. Genetic aspects of the added carbon dioxide requirements of *Brucella abortus*. Proc So Ex Biol Med 1950;75:438.

71. Braun W, G Ogelsby. On the problem of naturally occurring aberrant strains of *Brucella*. Proc Soc Exp Biol Med 1954;86:757.

72. Shibata S, Isayama Y, Shimuzu T. A possibility in variation in *Brucella abortus* from type II to type I. Natl Inst An Hlth Organ. (Tokyo) 1962;2:20.

73. Jones LM, Montgomery V, Wilson JB. Characteristics of carbon dioxide-independent cultures of *Brucella abortus* isolated from cattle vaccinated with strain 19. *J Infect Dis* 1965;115:312.

74. Kraft ME. The identification of *B. abortus* strain 19 by penicillin tolerance. *Am J Vet Res* 1955;16:295.

75. Huddleson IF. Emergence during growth of *Brucella* strains on dye-agar media of cells that show changes in sulfur metabolism. Bull World Health Organization 1961;24:91.

76. Rigby EC, Fraser ADF, Garcia MM, Brooks BW. Studies on the molecular biology of *Brucella*. Brucellosis Symposium, Animal Disease Research Institute, Nepean, Ontario, Canada.

77. Rigby CE, Cerqueira-Campos ML, Kelly, HA, Surujballi OmP. Properties and partial genetic characterization of Nepean (NP) phage and other lytic phages of *Brucella* spp. *Can J Vet Res* (In press).

78. Renoux G, A Suire. Spontaneous lysis and phage-carrier state in *Brucella* cultures. *J Bacteriol* 1963;186:642.

79. McDuff CR, Jones L M, Wilson JB. Characteristics of *Brucella* phage. *J Bacteriol* 1967;91:324.

80 McGilvery, et al. Restriction endonuclease analysis of *Brucella abortus*. *Res Vet Sci* 1988;45:251.

81. Verstreate DR, Creasy MT, Caveney NT, Baldwin CL, Blab MW, Winter A J. Outer membrane proteins of *Brucella abortus*: Isolation and characterization. *Infect Immun* 1982;35:979.

82. Douglas JT, Rosenberg EY, Nikaido H, Verstreate DR, Winter AJ. Porins of *Brucella* species. *Infect Immun* 1984;44:16.

83. Verstreate DR, Winter AJ. Comparison of sodium dodecyl sulfate-polyacrylamide gel electrophoresis profiles and antigenic relatedness among outer membrane proteins of 49 *Brucella abortus* strains. *Infect Immun* 1984;146: 182.83.

84. Santos JM, Verstreate DR, Perera VY, Winter AJ. Outer membrane proteins from rough strains of four *Brucella* species. *Infect Immun* 1984;46:188.

85. Tanaka S, Suto T, Isayama Y, Azuma R, Hatakeyama H. Chemo-taxonomical studies on fatty acids of *Brucella* species. *Ann Sclavo* 1977;19:67.

86. Dees SB, Hollis DG, Weaver RE, Moss CW. Cellular fatty acids of *Brucella suis* and *Brucella canis*. *J Clin Microbiol* 1981;14:111.

87. Moreira-Jacobs, M. New group of virulent bacteriophages showing differential affinity for *Brucella* species. *Nature* 1968;219:752.

88. Barbieri, M. The Semantic Theory of Evolution. New York: Harwood Academic Publishers, 1985.

89. Stanier RY. Phototropic green and purple bacteria: a comparative systematic survey. Pfenning R, ed. *Am Rev Microbiol* 1977;31:296.
90. Stanier RY. Some aspects of the biology of cells and evolutionary significance, in Organization and Control. In: Charles HP, Knight BC, eds. *Prokaryotic and EuKaryotic Cells*. Cambridge: Cambridge University Press, 1970.
91. Darnell JED. RNA. *Scientific American* 1985;253:68.
92. Woese CR. Bacterial evolution. *Microbiol Rev* 1987;51:221.
93. Saltzman L, Aperion D. Bending of erythromycin to the 50S ribosomal subunit is affected by alterations in the 30S ribosomal subunit. *Molec Gen Genet* 1976;143:301.
94. Mao JCH, Robishaw EE. Erythromycin, a peptidyltransferase effector. *Biochem* 1972;11:4864.
95. Taubman SB, Jones NR, Young FY, Corcoran JW. Sensitivity and resistance to erythromycin in *Bacillus subtilis* 168; the ribosomal binding of erythromycin and chloramphenicol. *Biochem Biophys Acta* 1966;123:438.
96. Oleinick N, Wilhelm JM, JW Corcoran. Nonidentity of the site of action of erythromycin A and chloramphenicol on *Bacillus subtilis* ribosomes. *Biochem Biophysica Acta* 1968;155:290.
97. Oleinick NL, Corcoran JW. Two types of binding of erythromycin to ribosomes from antibiotic-sensitive and -resistant *Bacillus subtilis* 168. *J Biol Chem* 1969;244:727,
98. Mayfield IE, et al. The cloning, expression, and nucleotide sequence of a gene coding for an immunogenic Brucella protein. *Gene* 1988;63:1.
99. Ficht TA, Bearden SW, Sowa BA, Adams LG. A 36 kilodalton *Brucella abortus* cell envelope protein is encoded by repeated sequences closely linked in the genome of DNA. *Infect Immun* 1988;56:2036.
100. Bellis M, Roizes G. DNA polymorphism in strains of the genus *Brucella*. *J Bact* 1988;170:4603.
101. Slatkin M. The descent of genes. In Science 85, American Association for the Advancement of Science 1985;6:80.
102. Racourt J, Grimont F, Grimont PAD, Seeliger HPR. DNA relatedness among serovars of *Listeria monocytogenes sensu lato*. *Current Microbiol* 1982;7:383.
103. Wilson AC. The molecular basis of evolution. *Scientific American* 1985;253:164.
104. Renoux G, Philippon A. Position taxonomique dans le genre *Brucella* de bacteries isolees de brebis et de vaches. *Ann Inst Pasteur* 1969;117:524.
105. Morris IA. The use of polyacrylamide gel electrophoresis in taxonomy of *Brucella*. *J Gen Microbiol* 761;231:1973.
106. Corbel MJ. Examination of two bacterial strains designated "*Brucella suis* biotype 5." *Hyg Cam* 71; 271:100.
107. Pinigin AF, Petukhova OS, Therinov SP. Taxonomic status of *Brucella* strains isolated from reindeer. *Zh Mikrobiol* 1983;11;103.
108. Pinigin AF, Petukhora, OS, Merinov SP, Verishilova PA, Dranovskaya EA. A new species, *Brucella rangiferi*. *Zh Mikrobiol* 1986;6:98.
109. Tolari F, Thomas EL, Corbel MJ. On the differentiation of *Brucella abortus* biotypes 3 and 6. *Annali Sclavo* 1981;23:320.
110. Arnaud-Bosq, Brousson-Ialaguir J, Veron M, Roux J. Determination des biovars de *Brucella melitensis* par les caracteres manometriques: interet epidemiologique et relation avec les serovars. *Ann Inst Pasteur/Microbiol* 1987;138:189.

111. Meyer ME. Characterization of *Brucella abortus* strain 19 isolated from human and bovine tissues and fluids. *Am J Vet Res* 1985;46:902.

Chapter Three

Phylogenetic Markers to
Describe *Brucella abortus*

Thomas A. Ficht,

Scott W. Bearden,

and Hélène Marquis

The organisms of the genus *Brucella* maintain a close taxonomic relationship but can be distinguished through rigorous metabolic, antigenic, and biochemical analysis. Due to the diversity of this group of organisms, extensive phenotypic analysis has been used to establish their taxonomic relationships. Most researchers have concluded that, although divided into distinct forms, the *Brucella* represent an almost infinite number of variants. With the advent of molecular techniques, the resemblance among *Brucella* species was found to extend to the genetic level at which all species share greater than 90% DNA homology, and a genome size of 2.6 x 10^6 base pairs (bp).[14] As a result, some molecular biologists maintain that by definition the *Brucella* must be considered as a monospecific genus.[3] This proposal has been met with considerable opposition since the phenotypic differences used to define the *Brucella* species are useful epidemiologically, and have been thought to represent stable phylogenetic differences. It must also be pointed out that there are numerous examples demonstrating that DNA sequence and function do not necessarily evolve at the same rate.

Biotype Analysis

The phenotypic properties used to characterize *Brucella* include colony morphology, antigenicity, virulence, growth rate, viability, bacteriophage and salt sensitivity, and resistance to antibiotics and dyes.[5] These characteristics, and the adaptation to various hosts have been used to separate the *Brucella* into six species, three of which have been further subdivided into biovars (Table 3-1). Each of these phenotypic properties has been found to vary individually, but there are reports suggesting a high degree of association of changes in certain characteristics.[6,7] This is not an unusual observation; Atwood, et al. showed that serial transfer of *E. coli* resulted in the appearance of new types presumably with selective advantage.[8] Evidence has been presented to suggest that intra- and inter-species switching

Table 3-1. *Brucella* Biotype Analysis

Species	Biovar	CO₂	Erythritol 1	Erythritol 2	H₂S	Urease	Thionine Blue d	Thionin a	Thionin b	Thionin c	Fuchsin a	Fuchsin b	Fuchsin c	Aggl. A	Aggl. M	Aggl. R	Lysis by phage Tb 10,000x RTD
B. abortus	1	+/-	+	+	+	+	+	-	-	-	+	+	+	+	-	-	+
	2	+	+	+	+	+	-	-	-	-	+	-	-	+	-	-	+
	3	+/-	+	+	+	+	+	-	-	+	+	+	+	+	-	-	+
	4	+/-	+	+	+	+	+	-	-	-	+	+	+	-	+	-	+
	5	-	+	+	-	+	+	-	+	+	+	+	+	+	+	-	+
	6	-	+	+	+/-	+	+	-	+	+	+	+	+	+	+	-	+
	7ᵉ	-	+	+	+/-	+	+	-	-	-	+	+	+	+	+	-	+
	9	+/-	+	+	+	+	+	-	-	-	+	+	+	+	+	-	+
S19	1	-	+	-	+	+	-	-	-	-	+	+	+	+	-	-	+
thioʳ S19		-	-	-	+	+	-	+	+	+	+	+	+	+	-	-	+/-
thioʳ biovar	1	+/-	+	+	+	+	+	+	+	+	+	+	+	+	-	-	+/-
thioʳ biovar	2	+	+	+	+	+	-	+	+	+	-	-	-	+	-	-	+/-
B. suis	1	-	+	+	+	+	+/-	+	+	+	-	-	-	+	-	-	-
	2	-	+	+	+/-	+	-	+	+	+	-	-	-	+	-	-	-
	3	-	+	+	-	+	+	+	+	+	+	+	+	+	-	-	-
	4	-	+	+	-	+	-	+	+	+	-	+	+	+	+	-	-
	5	-	+	+	-	+	-	+	-	-	-	-	-	-	+	-	-
B. melitensis	1	-	+	+	-	+	+	+	+	+	+	+	+	+	-	-	-
	2	-	+	+	-	+	+	+	+	+	+	+	+	-	+	-	-
	3	-	+	+	-	+	+	+	+	+	+	+	+	+	+	-	-
B. neotomae		-	+	+	+	+	+	-	-	+	-	-	+	+	-	-	-
B. canis		-	+	+	-	+	+/-	+	+	+	-	-	+/-	-	-	+	+
B. ovis		+	-	-	-	-	-	+	+	+	+	+	+	-	-	+	-

occurs.[a] Moriera-Jacob found both species and biovar switching in 64 isolates out of a collection of 300.[9] In on group of 35 isolates of *B. melitensis* stored for one year on slants, 12 were reported to switch to *B. abortus*, 9 to *B. intermedia*, 11 to *B. suis* and 3 to B. 'strain AM'[b] (*B abortus* of M-serotype). Similar changes were recorded for the other species. However, these switches remained unsubstantiated in the absence of any stable, defined phylogenetic markers.

Frequent identification of atypical isolates both in the United States and Canada, such as the *B. abortus* biotype 2 (M-antigen) isolated by Ewalt et al., suggests that switching may occur *in vivo* as well.[10] Numerous reports of the isolation of species different from the infecting organism are also consistent with phenotypic instability. However, most *Brucella* bacteriologists maintain that the current *Brucella* species and biovars represent stable forms with sufficient phenotypic variability so that a genotype can be represented by more than one phenotype, and that careful maintenance of bacterial stocks will prevent the observed variation.

Phylogenetic Characterization

Taxonomic classification based on phenotypic properties requires the identification of those properties that remain stable and reflect a single genotype. For the *Brucella*, species and biotype classification have depended on numerical analysis of unstable phenotypic features. Until recently the best evidence to suggest a distinct phylogeny for each of the *Brucella* species has been the differences in virulence observed when infecting a common host. In the guinea pig and in human infections, the apparent order of virulence is *melitensis≈ suis>>abortus*.[11,12] This is thought to reflect differences in the genetic content of these organisms with regard to structural genes encoding virulence factors, or regulatory elements that govern expression. The self-limiting infections of *B. suis* and *B. melitensis* in cattle are consistent with the concept of species adaptation. Adaptation to a particular host is supported by the frequency of isolation of individual species, however a broad host range has been demonstrated for each of the *Brucella* species.[13]

The establishment of stable phylogenetic markers via genetic methods would help to better describe the Brucellae. This can be performed through characterization of multilocus enzyme electropherotypes or DNA

---

a.   Switching used instead of original terminology, "reversion" which implies knowledge of original form.
b.   Used to describe organisms of intermediate character, later separated into distinct biotypes.

profiles that do not change, despite the apparent switch in species or biovar as judged by evaluation of phenotypic parameters. The benchmark in *Brucella* taxonomy is the work of Allardet-Servent et al., who demonstrated that differences in electrophoretic profiles of total genomic DNA confirm the use of the preferred (or natural) host as a phenotypic characteristic for classifying *Brucella* strains.[4] According to the scheme proposed, five electropherotypes were identified in five reference strains from different species using a combination of low-cleavage-frequency enzymes such as Xba I, and pulse field gradient electrophoresis. From their work, Allaradet-Servent et al. made the following conclusions:

    1. *B. abortus, B. melitensis,* and *B. suis* each have species-specific DNA fingerprints.

    2. Electrophoretic profiles clearly place *B. canis* near *B. suis.*

    3. DNA fingerprints of *B. ovis* separated this species from all others.

    4. Differences between biovars within given species or strains are not constant and consequently are not sufficient to serve as markers for accurate epidemiological studies.

Similar results have been obtained via examination of restriction fragment length polymorphisms (RFLPs) at the *omp* 2 porin locus. Using this method we have been able to separate the *Brucella* into groups which coincide with classical species designations determined by biotype analysis.[14] In addition, the *omp* 2 porin protein profiles, can be used to classify the *Brucella* species.[14,15]

    The work described here reveals the presence of RFLPs in *Brucella* chromosomal DNA at the *omp* 2 porin gene locus; the RFLPs can be used to distinguish two classes of *B. abortus.* The potential significance of this observation lies in the fact that these two groups are also distinguished by their thionine sensitivity, and geographic distribution. Attempts to correlate all three parameters are described.

Results and Discussion

Characterization of the *omp* 2 Porin Gene Locus of *Brucella abortus*

    The cloning of the *omp* 2 locus of *B. abortus* has been described previously.[16,17] Briefly, two homologous genes, identified as *omp* 2a and *omp* 2b, reside on a 6.5-kbp (Kilobase pair) Bam HI fragment (Figure 3-1). Sequence alignment reveals that the two regions share more than 90% overall DNA homology, and the presence of several insertions/deletions (i.e., 3, 6, 9, 18, and 108 kbp) distributed in both genes.[17] The largest dif-

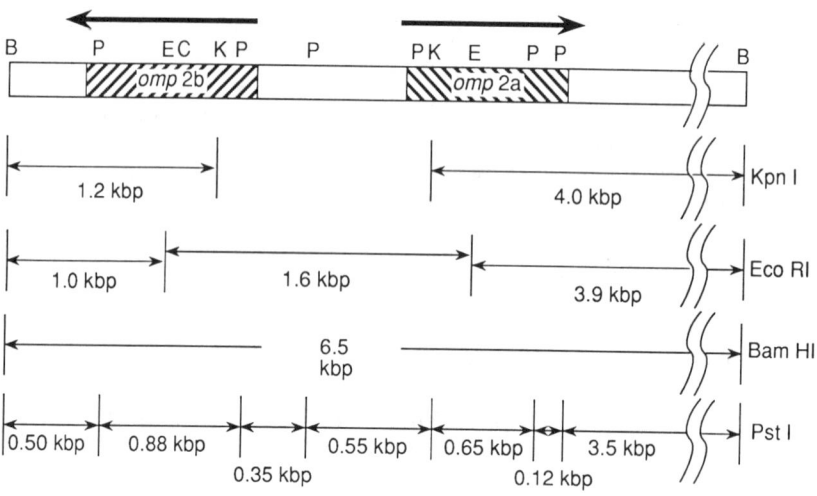

Figure 3-1. Restriction Map of *B. abortus omp* 2 Locus. Pst I, Eco RI, Cla I, and Bam HI restriction maps of the *omp* 2 locus which spans a 3.5 kbp stretch of *B. abortus* genomic DNA on a 6.5 kbp Bam HI fragment.

ference between the two genes is due to the absence of a 108 kbp segment from the middle of *omp* 2a. The two genes have identical Shine-Delgarno sequences, ATG start codons, and signal peptides; and the homology between the two structural genes extends 50 nucleotides upstream of the translation start codon. Identification of the canonical promoter sequences upstream from either gene is not possible.[18] This is not an unexpected result since porin genes, such as *omp* F and *omp* C in *E. coli*, are positively regulated, and generally have poor consensus promoter sequences.[19,20] As a result, characterization of promoter activity was performed via a functional assay.[17] Neither osmoboxes, related to those in the *E. coli* porin genes, nor invertible regions, such as in the *Salmonella* pilin genes were detected by homology search with any of the available nucleotide libraries.[20,21]

Expression and Description of the
B. abortus omp 2 Gene Products

Recombinant plasmids pAGF101 and pAGF201 containing the *omp* 2 locus of *B. abortus* biovar 1 (strains 19 and 2308) encode a 36-kDa protein in *E. coli* which comigrates with the native *Brucella* porin, BaomIIb1, on SDS-PAGE.[17] Inversion of the unique Kpn I fragment presumably containing the *omp* 2b promoter and alignment with the *omp* 2a structural gene results in the production of a 33-kDa protein in *E. coli*. There is no evidence of a lower molecular weight protein produced in laboratory-grown *Brucella*. Expression of the *omp* 2a gene product in a porin deficient *E. coli* strain ECB611(*lam* B⁻ *omp* F::Tn5 *omp* C::Tn10) permits the growth of this organism on high molecular weight maltodextrins (Figure 3-2). In contrast the *omp* 2b gene product does not stimulate such growth. These data suggest that expression of *omp* 2a results in a change in outer membrane pore size. Changes of this kind may represent adaptation to environmental changes, such as occur following macrophage engulfment. *E. coli* expressing the *omp* 2a gene product exhibited increased sensitivity to erythromycin and rifampin, suggesting some change in the hydrophobic character of the outer membrane.[22] However, excluding the two notable exceptions described above, the antibiotic and detergent sensitivities of these cells were not found to be significantly altered. Similar results were observed by Benson and DeCloux with *E. coli* porin mutants which had significantly larger porin channel diameters.[23]

The only block to expression from the *omp* 2a gene in *E. coli* appears to be the absence of a functional promoter. Whether this is also the case in *B. abortus* remains to be demonstrated. This situation may not maintained among all species; *B. melitensis* contains a 36-kDa *omp* 2 gene product similar to *B. abortus*; however, *B. ovis* contains a 40-kDa *omp* 2 gene product and *B. suis, B. canis,* and *B. neotomae* contain both 36- and

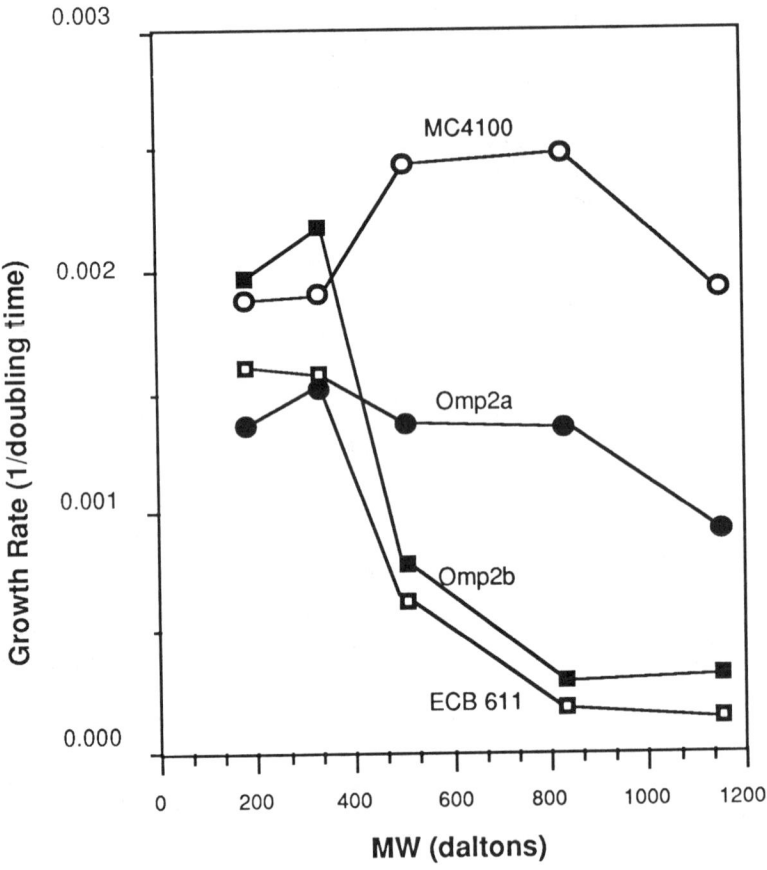

Figure 3-2. Complementation of a Porin Deficient *E. coli* by the Cloned *Brucella* Porin Genes. *E. coli* ECB611 was transformed with plasmids containing *B. abortus omp* 2 locus with the promoter containing fragment in the native or inverted configuration, Omp 2b or Omp 2a, respectively. Cells containing the plasmid with the promoter containing fragment deleted give the same results as cells lacking plasmid (*E. coli* ECB611).

38-kDa *omp* 2 gene products under laboratory conditions of growth.[14] Expression from these genes in *E. coli* has not been examined, and the physiological significance of this variation is not known.

Conservation of the *omp* 2 Operon

Although silent in *B. abortus*, the conservation of the open reading frame in *omp* 2a suggests that the gene could be expressed at some time during infection, perhaps under specific environmental conditions. If silenced for an extended period of time it is suspected that additional mutations would occur, some effectively blocking expression. The absence of such blocks is consistent with either a recent silencing of the *omp* 2a gene or the expression of this gene under certain conditions. In the absence of any data to support expression in laboratory grown *B. abortus*, an alternative approach was sought to predict the importance of both genes to the viability of the *Brucella*. Specifically, the conservation of the *omp* 2 gene arrangement in all species and isolates of *Brucella*, and the amount of genetic diversity permitted at this locus.

Figure 3-1 illustrates a restriction map of the *omp* 2 locus cloned from *B. abortus* biovar 1 (Strains 19 and 2308). This map indicates that digestion with Pst I produces restriction fragments which can be used to distinguish *omp* 2a from *omp* 2b, 650, and 880 bp fragments, respectively. Similar digests were used to examine the arrangement of these genes in the DNA of all other *Brucella* species[14] and *B. abortus* biovars (Table 3-2). The results of the Pst I digestion are shown in Figures 3-3a and 3-3b and are summarized in Figure 3-4. Comparison of *Brucella* species will be presented elsewhere and will not be discussed here.[14]

The *B. abortus* biovars can be divided into two RFLP sub-groups: the first group contains biovars 1, 2, and 4; the second group contains biovars 3, 5, 6, and 9. Biovars 7 and 8 do not exist.[5] The difference can be correlated with two phenotypic properties, geographic distribution and growth in the presence of thionine. Biovars 1, 2, and 4 are the predominant biovars isolated from cattle infected with *B. abortus* in the continental United States and are closely associated in other geographic locals.[24] Similarly, biovars 3, 5, 6, 7, and 9 are geographically associated (G.G. Alton, personal communication). The basis for this distribution is not known.

Thionine sensitivity is one of several tests currently used to classify *Brucella* according to species and biovar. Thionine is a relatively hydrophilic dye with a minimum diameter of 0.7 nm. It has been proposed that the porin channels are the major pathway for penetration by this dye.[25] The inability to grow in the presence of thionine correlates with the loss of a 108 bp segment from the silent structural gene for *omp* 2a. This sequence contains an additional Pst I site; as a result, DNA containing this sequence

Table 3-2. *Brucella* Type Strains and Isolates

Species	Biovar	Strain	Host	Geographic Origin
B. abortus	biovar 1	19	cattle	United States
	biovar 1	2308	rough derivative 2308[a]	United States
	biovar 1	RB51	rough derivative45/0	United States
	biovar 1	45/20	cattle, bison	England
	biovar 2	86/8/59T (ATCC# 23449)	"	England
	biovar 3	TulyaT (ATCC# 23450)	"	Uganda
	biovar 4	292T (ATCC# 23451)	"	England
	biovar 5	B3196T (ATCC# 23452)	"	England
	biovar 6	870T (ATCC# 23453)	"	Africa
	biovar 7	63/75T (ATCC# 23454)		
	biovar 9	C68T (ATCC# 23455)		England
B. melitensis	biovar 1	16MT (ATCC# 23456)	goat	United States
B. neotomae		(ATCC# 23459)	desert wood rat	United States
B. canis		RM6/66T (ATCC# 23365)	dog	United States
B. ovis		63/290T (ATCC# 25840)	sheep	Africa
B. suis	biovar 1	1330T (ATCC# 23444)	pig	United States

[a] Isolated by G.G. Schurig

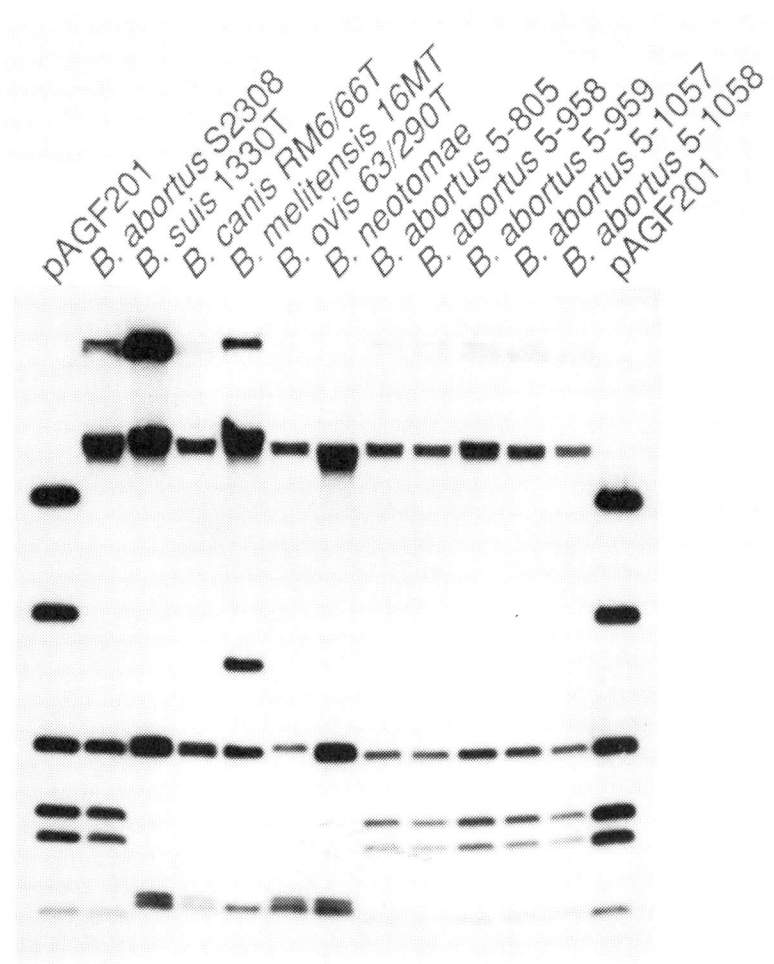

Figure 3-3a & 3b. Restriction Polymorphism at the *omp* 2 Locus of the *Brucella* Species. Southern blot analysis of genomic DNAs extracted from the type strains of all *Brucella* species (panel a) and *B. abortus* biovars (panel b) and digested with Pst I. Hybridization was performed with the complete *omp* 2 locus derived from *B. abortus biovar* 1 cloned into pBR322 and referred to as pAGF201. Hybridization to the cloned genes is shown in the outside/marker lanes.

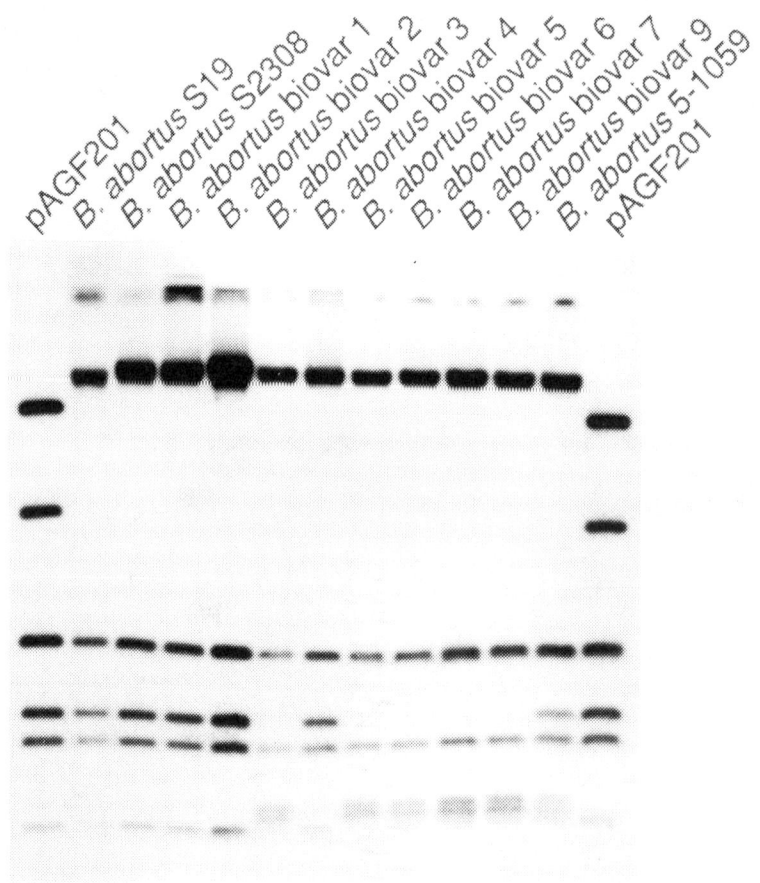

Figure 3-3a & 3b. Restriction Polymorphism at the *omp* 2 Locus of the *Brucella* Species. Southern blot analysis of genomic DNAs extracted from the type strains of all *Brucella* species (panel a) and *B. abortus* biovars (panel b) and digested with Pst I. Hybridization was performed with the complete *omp* 2 locus derived from *B. abortus biovar* 1 cloned into pBR322 and referred to as pAGF201. Hybridization to the cloned genes is shown in the outside/marker lanes.

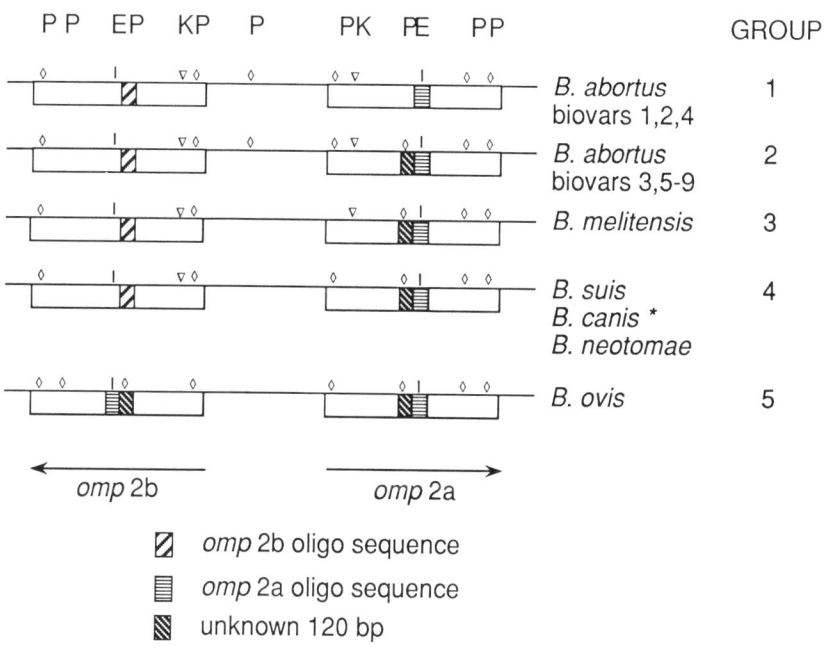

Figure 3-4. Restriction Maps of the *omp* 2 Locus of the *Brucellae*. Derivation of these Maps is Described Elsewhere (Ficht, et al, 1989). Strains used were type strains obtained from ATCC (Table 3-2). Conservation of these produces 390-and 370-bp fragments, while DNA lacking this sequence patterns in field strain isolates was performed for *B. abortus* biovar 1. Pst I(◊), Kpn I (Δ) and Eco RI (I).

produces a 650-bp fragment (Figures 3-3 and 3-4). All *Brucella* containing the 108-bp segment from the silent structural gene for *omp* 2a. This sequence contains an additional Pst I site; as a result, DNA containing this sequence produces 390-and 370-bp fragments, while DNA lacking this sequence produces a 650-bp fragment (Figures 3-3 and 3-4). All *Brucella* containing the 108-bp segment in *omp* 2a grow in the presence of thionine, whereas organisms lacking this insert in *omp* 2a are inhibited by thionine. To test the effect of the 108-bp insertion/deletion on thionine sensitivity, the *omp* 2a DNA from thio^r *B. abortus* biovar 1 (S19) isolates was analyzed. This organism is normally sensitive to thionine and, if there is a direct correlation between the absence of the 108-bp sequence and thionine sensitivity, perhaps due to large pore diameter, any significant ($\geq$50-100 nucleotide) DNA rearrangement will be revealed by Southern blot analysis.

B. *abortus* biovar 1 (strain 19 and other strains) revertants to thionine resistance (thio^r) arise at a frequency of 10^{-9} to 10^{-10}. The revertants are stable during several passages on TSA plates in the absence of thionine. Biotype analysis of these organisms indicates that the thio^r biovar 1 isolates are now best defined as *B. abortus* biovar 6 (Table 3-1). Slight to substantial changes in Tb phage sensitivity have been noted in subsequent biotype analysis. It is apparent that, by this criteria, thio^r *B. abortus* biovar 2 revertants might be considered as *B. suis* isolates, except for the notoriously unstable CO_2 requirement (Table 3-1). The identification of atypical isolates rather than low-level contaminants can be substantiated using additional markers; however, this is only possible with strain 19 thio^r mutants which remain sensitive to erythritol, thionine blue, and penicillin, or biovar 2 (thio^r) mutants which remain sensitive to Tb phage. In most cases, these phenotypes are also unstable; for example, erythritol-resistant variants arise at an unusually high frequency of 10^{-4} to 10^{-5}.

The result shown in Figure 3-5 indicates that there are no DNA rearrangements which accompany the shift from thio^r to thio^r. Although other changes may have occurred, they are not detectable using the assay described. These results point out the usefulness of the DNA profiles in classifying the Brucellae. In light of significant changes in phenotypic properties which would confuse biotype analysis, identification of this organism from the DNA profile is unambiguous. Future work will be designed to distinguish the individual biovars present in each group shown in Figure 3-4.

Phylogeny of the Brucellae

The two most significant observations in the work presented are 1) *B. abortus* biovars can be separated into two groups based on their RFLP pattern at the *omp* 2 locus, and 2) the RFLP pattern is stable despite phenotypic alterations that would confuse biotype analysis. These results ex-

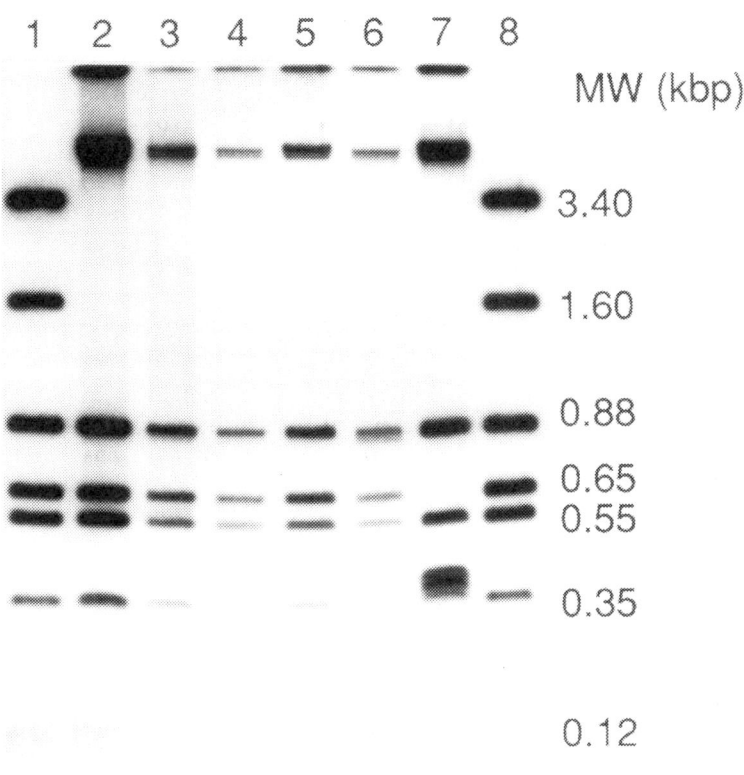

Figure 3-5. Analysis of *omp* 2 Locus of Thionine Resistant Biovar 1. The Southern blot was prepared as described in the legend to Figure 3-3. Pst 1 digested pAGFL01 (cloned omp 2 locus), lanes 1 and 8; *B. abortus* S19 (genomic DNA), lanes 2 and 6; *B. abortus* biovar 6 (genomic DNA), lane 7; *B. abortus* S19 thio^r (genomic DNA) selected on thionine plates at 10 µg/ml, 20 µg/ml and 40 µg/ml, lanes 3, 4, and 5, respectively.

tend the work of Allardet-Servent, and further demonstrate that the DNA sequences in the form of RFLPs can be used to describe *Brucella* species and even biovars. The significance of the subdivision of *B. abortus* into two classes is not known; however, its correlation with geographic distribution may suggest recent emergence of group 1 (biovars 1, 2, and 4).

A molecule whose sequence changes randomly with time can be considered a chronometer. To be a useful chronometer, a molecule must meet certain specifications.[26] A molecular chronometer should be representative of the overall rate of evolutionary change in a line of descent. The best chronometer is not necessarily a genetic segment upon which there are no selective constraints since they would be so rapid as to cover only a restricted phylogenetic distance. The more useful molecules for phylogenetic measurement represent highly constrained functions. Unfortunately, strict clock-like behavior is difficult to find. Unless functional constraints remain strictly constant, selected sequence changes accumulate, over and above randomly introduced ones, artificially increasing phylogenetic distances. A second difficulty with highly constrained chronometers is the extremely different rates at which various positions in a sequence tend to change.

The use of porin genes as chronometers has not been investigated primarily because of their high conservation in most organisms.[19] We propose to use these genes as molecular chronometers based on the observed duplication and conservation in all *Brucella* species examined. Correlation of genetic diversity at a single locus with evolutionary selective pressures has been disputed by Milkman and others;[27] however, Woese and co-workers have used the ribosomal RNA sequences to perform just such analysis.[26] Although rRNAs are considered the ultimate chronometer, the changes within the genus *Brucella* are presumably too few to provide a valid assessment of the derivation of species. In this case, the porin genes show diversity which correlates with classical biotype analysis. Adaptation to specific hosts (selective pressures) may result in abrupt changes in DNA sequence while highly conserved function will minimize any changes. Comparison of these results with multilocus enzyme electrophoresis and RFLP profiles from various regions of the genome will help to establish its usefulness as a chronometer. The apparent absence of genetic transfer between species or with other bacteria makes this group an excellent candidate for examination of bacterial evolution. The chances of there being genetic chimeras are insignificant. Furthermore no homology has been detected with a number of different bacteria.

If *omp* 2a is truly silent, changes in this gene should occur at a higher frequency than those in *omp* 2b and can be used to gauge any unusual or discontinuous events. If both genes are expressed, which would mean a high level of conservation for each, then both can be used to verify the clock-like activity and to serve as independent domains. In either case, the study of *omp* 2 locus should contribute appreciably to the understanding of the phylogeny of the Brucellae.

References

1. Hoyer BH, McCullough NB. Polynucleotide homologies of *Brucella* deoxyribonucleic acids. *J Bacteriol* 1968;95:444-448.
2. Hoyer B H, McCullough NB. Homologies of deoxyribonucleic acids from *Brucella ovis*, canine abortion organisms, and other *Brucella* species. *J Bacteriol* 1968;96:1783-1790.
3. Verger JM, Grimont F, Grimont PAD, Crayon M. *Brucella*, a monospecific genus as shown by deoxyribonucleic acid hybridization. *Int J Syst Bacteriol* 1985;35:292-295.
4. Allardet-Servent A, Bourg G, Ramuz M, Pages M, Bellis M, Roizes G. DNA polymorphism in strains of the genus *Brucella*. *J Bacteriol* 1988;170:4603-4607.
5. Alton GG, Jones LM, Angus RD, Verger JM. Techniques for the Brucellosis Laboratory. Paris: Institut National de la Recherche Agronomique,1988.
6. Wilson G.S. The classification of the *Brucella* group: a systematic study. *J Hyg (Camb)* 1933; 33:516-541.
7. Braun W. Variation in the genus *Brucella*. In: *Symposium on Brucellosis*. Washington: AAAS, 1955:26-36.
8. Atwood KC, Schneider LK, Ryan FJ. Periodic selection in *Escherichia coli*. *Genetics* 1951; 37:146-155.
9. Moriera-Jacob M. In vitro species (or type) transformation among strains of *Brucella*. *Nature* 1963;197:406.
10. Ewalt DR, Forbes LB. Atypical isolates of *Brucella abortus* from Canada and the United States characterized as dye sensitive with M antigen dominant. *J Clin Microbiol* 1987;25:698-701
11. Braude AI. Studies in the pathology and pathogenesis of experimental brucellosis. I. A comparison of the pathogenicity of *Brucella abortus, Brucella melitensis* and *Brucella suis* for guinea pigs. *J Infect Dis* 1951; 89:76-86.
12. Meyer KF, Fleischner EC. The pathogenicity of *Brucella melitensis* and *Brucella abortus* for guinea pigs. *J Infect Dis* 1922;31:159-197.
13. Spink WW. In *The Nature of Brucellosis*. Minneapolis: The University of Minnesota Press, 1956:65-79.
14. Ficht TA, Bearden SW, Sowa BA, Marquis H. Genetic variation at the *omp* 2 porin locus of the *Brucellae* species specific markers. *Mol Microbiol* Submitted for publication.
15. Santos JM. Verstreate DR, Perera VY, Winter AJ. Outer membrane proteins from rough strains of four *Brucella* species. *Infect Immun* 1984;46:188-194.
16. Ficht TA, Bearden SW, Sowa BA, Adams LG. A 36-kilodalton *Brucella abortus* cell-envelope protein is encoded by repeated sequences closely linked in the genomic DNA. *Infect Immun* 1988;56:2036-2046.
17. Ficht TA, Bearden SW, Sowa BA, Adams LG. DNA sequence and expression from the 36 kDa outer membrane protein gene locus of *Brucella abortus*. *Infect Immun* 1989;57:In press.
18. McClure W. Mechanism and control of transcription initiation in prokaryotes. *Ann Rev Biochem* 1988;54:171-204.
19. Mizuno T, Chou M-Y, Inouye M. A comparative study on the genes for three porins of the *E. coli* outer membrane: DNA sequence of the osmoregulated *omp* C gene. *J Biol Chem* 1983;258:6932-6940.
20. Ramakrishnan G, Comeau DE, Ikenaka K, Inouye M. Transcriptional control of

gene expression: osmoregulation of porin protein synthesis. In *Bacterial Outer Membranes as Model Systems*. New York: John Wiley and Sons, 1987:3-16.

21. Plasterk RHA, Brinkman A, van de Putte P. DNA inversions in the chromosome of *Escherichia coli* and in bacteriophage Mu: relationship to other site-specific recombination systems. *Proc Natl Acad Sci USA* 1984;81:5355-5359.

22. Nikaido H, Vaara M. Bacterial membrane permeability. *Microbiol Rev* 1985;49:1-32.

23. Benson SA, DeCloux A. Isolation and characterization of outer membrane permeability mutants in *E. coli* K-12. *J Bacteriol* 1985;161:361-367.

24. Thimm BM. Brucellosis: Distribution in man, domestic and wild animals. Springer-Verlag, Berlin 1982.

25. Douglas JT, Rosenberg EY, Nikaido H, Verstreate DR, Winter AJ. Porins of *Brucella* species. *Infect Immun* 1984;44:16-21.

26. Woese CR. Bacterial evolution. *Microbiol Rev* 1987;51:221-271.

27. Milkman R. Two elements of a unified theory of population genetics and molecular evolution. In: *Population Genetics and Molecular Evolution*. Ohta T, Aoki K, eds. 1985:65-83.

PART TWO

BIOLOGICAL AND STRUCTURAL PROPERTIES OF BRUCELLAE

Chapter Four

Function and Structure of the Major Components of the Outer Membrane of Gram-Negative Bacteria

N.L. Martin

and R.E.W. Hancock

In this review we have briefly outlined the major functional and structural aspects of the components of the outer membrane of Gram-negative bacteria. The functions of the major classes of proteins in the outer membrane are discussed, as are more general features such as antibiotic permeation pathways, receptors, protein excretion, and cell surface interactions. Structural information of a basic nature has been presented on the major proteins and other constituents of the cell wall. Included wherever possible are comparisons of the information available on *Brucella* with that of other Gram-negative species. We have chosen to present functional aspects of the Gram-negative cell wall first, leaving the more recent information concerning the structure of various outer membrane components to the second half of this review.

The Typical Gram-Negative Outer Membrane

The Gram-negative outer membrane profile (Figure 4-1), derived largely from studies of *Escherichia coli* and *Salmonella typhimurium*, serves as a standard for comparison of other enteric and non-enteric Gram-negative bacteria. The apolar (hydrophobic) region of the membrane, with a thickness of 4.5 nm,[1] provides an anchor for proteins and forms a structural and functional barrier between the periplasm and the exterior of the cell. The outer membrane is supported by an underlying layer of peptidoglycan. Current research suggests the peptidoglycan is a hydrated mesh approximately three molecular layers thick.[2] Approximately one-third of the Braun's outer membrane lipoprotein in *E. coli* is covalently attached to the peptidoglycan and thereby anchors and stabilizes the outer membrane.[3] However, it is not exposed to the external surface.[4] The remaining two-thirds of the Braun's lipoprotein in the cell is embedded in the outer membrane, but not covalently attached to the peptidoglycan. Other outer membrane proteins are noncovalently associated with the peptidoglycan. One of these proteins, OmpA, also plays a role in stabiliz-

ated. General porins function as channels to the interior of the cell for the diffusion of compounds below a limiting molecular weight (the exclusion limit) and thus determine the molecular seiving function of the outer membrane. Other porins demonstrate selectivity for specific solutes. Other proteinaceous components of the outer membrane include proteases,[6] phospholipase A,[7] pili,[8] flagella, and proteins induced under specific conditions such as the divalent cation-regulated protein, H1, in *Pseudomonas aeruginosa*,[9] and the iron-regulated receptors for iron-siderophore complexes.[10]

Two major classes of molecules present in the outer membrane, lipopolysaccharide (LPS) and phospholipids, are asymmetrically arranged. The LPS is present only in the external monolayer of the outer membrane and the majority of lipids are located on the periplasmic side of the outer membrane bilayer. For enteric bacteria, this arrangement of lipids seems wise as the bacteria exist in an environment full of bile salts and lipases in the intestine.[5] The phospholipids have only two fatty acid chains connected to polar head groups while LPS has six or seven fatty acid chains linked to a diglucosamine phosphate backbone.[11] Also, LPS molecules have many negatively charged groups in the rough core oligosaccharide and on membrane-proximal sugars such as 3-deoxy-D-manno-octulosonic acid (KDO) as well as chains of repeating sugar units extending various lengths into the environment surrounding the cell.[11]

Function of Outer Membrane Components

Structural Proteins

Two classes of outer membrane proteins have been demonstrated to be involved in both outer membrane and cell structure and growth in low-osmolarity media. These are represented in *E. coli* by Omp A and Braun's lipoprotein.[12] Loss of both of these proteins confers upon the cell a rounded shape and a growth defect in certain media (without any observable changes in penicillin-binding protein 2). Either protein will reverse both properties such that single mutants are rod-shaped and grow well in most media.[13] Interestingly, it is the covalently peptidoglycan-associated form of lipoprotein that appears to be most important for maintaining structural stability in *E. coli*. In *P. aeruginosa* PAO1, the Braun lipoprotein-equivalent is not apparently covalently peptidoglycan-associated and it seems that cell shape is maintained, at least in part, by OprF. *Pseudomonas aeruginosa* PAO1 *oprF::W* mutants demonstrate rounded morphology and a growth defect in low-osmolarity media.[14] This structural role of OprF and the fact that OprF and OmpA have substantial homology throughout their C-terminal halves, cross-react immunologically, and have many common physical properties,[14,15] lends additional support to OprF having an important role in maintaining cell shape and stability. In addition, OprF

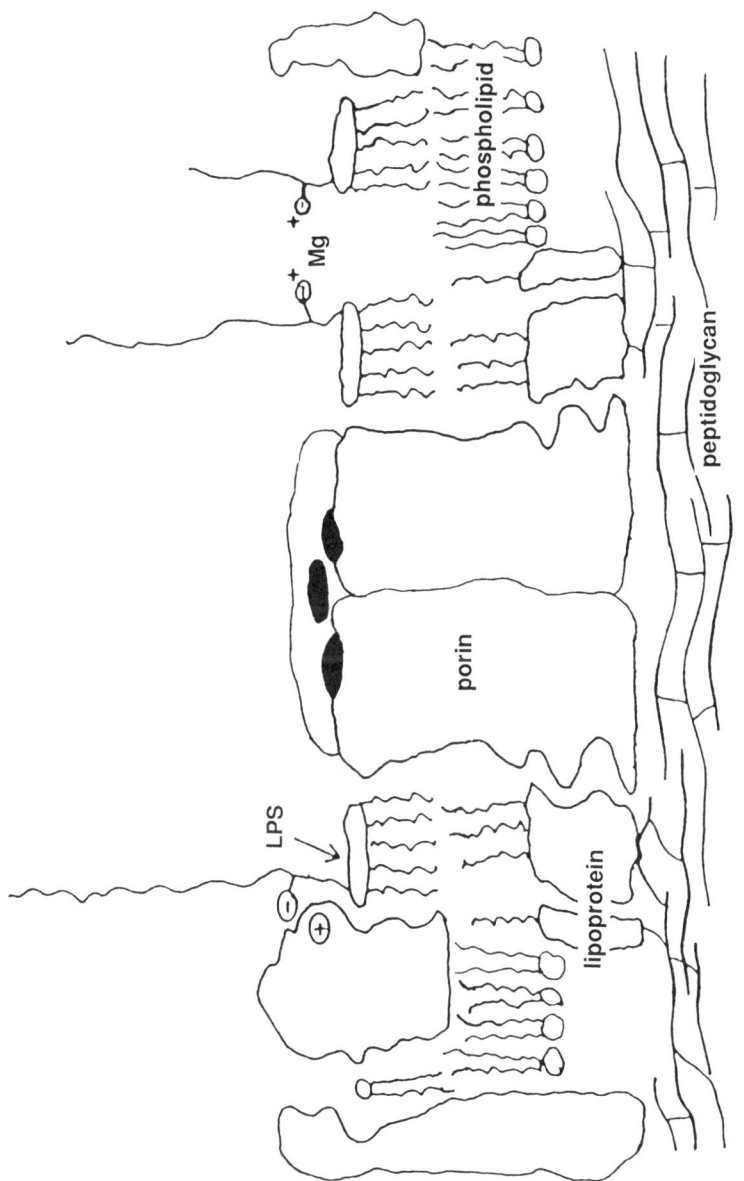

Figure 4-1. Schematic Diagram of the Gram-Negative Outer Membrane.

expressed from the cloned *oprF* gene will restore elongated morphology to an *E. coli* strain devoid of OmpA and Braun lipoprotein.[14]

In the *Brucella* spp. a peptidoglycan-associated lipoprotein that cross-reacts im-munologically with Braun lipoprotein has been demonstrated.[16] While there have been no specific studies of proteins related to OmpA in *Brucella*, it is possible that the group 3 proteins are the OmpA-equivalent in these species. In addition to *P. aeruginosa*, both *Haemophilus influenza* and *Neisseria gonorrhoeae* contain proteins that cross-react immunologically with the *E. coli* OmpA protein.[14,17]

One other outer membrane protein found in a variety of species is the peptidoglycan-associated lipoprotein,[18] equivalent to protein H2 of *P. aeruginosa*. The function of this species is unknown.

General Porins

To date, porins have been found in every Gram-negative species in which they have been sought. The porins are usually identified by their ability to reconstitute channels in lipid bilayers by one of four reconstitution methods discussed in previous reviews.[6,19] Their substantial structural stability and resistance to detergent denaturation have been extremely helpful in this regard. However, it must be stressed that these reconstitution methods are technically difficult. Based on such techniques, there is currently a dispute as to the channel size and nature of the major porin (OprF) of *P. aeruginosa*.[6,20] The problem may stem in part from the relatively low outer membrane permeability of *P. aeruginosa* compared to *E. coli*. Techniques for the examination of *E. coli* must be suitably adjusted to allow them to be applicable to *P. aeruginosa*. We feel that such disputes can only be solved by genetic experiments which confirm the nature of an outer membrane protein as a porin for antibiotics, for example. Thus, if a defined protein alteration (preferably a point mutation, or small deletion or addition to the gene) can be definitively associated with antibiotic resistance and/or a loss of *in vitro* porin activity, and these properties can be genetically cotransferred to another strain, this would represent proof of porin function. With the application of sophisticated molecular genetics to studies of porins, such mutations can be created *in vitro* and then recombined into the chromosome.[15] However, in the case of the OprF protein from *P. aeruginosa*, transposon or interposon insertion into the oprF gene, while causing modest increases in antibiotic resistance, was not entirely satisfactory due to the substantial effects of the deletion of OprF on the structure[14,20] and non-specific permeability[15] of *P. aeruginosa*.

With the above limitations, model membrane studies have allowed one to build up a very detailed picture of how general porins function.[21,22] They contain channels which are weakly selective for cations over anions, or vice versa, due to the presence of charged amino acid residues.[23] There are some suggestions that certain porins are voltage regulated,[24] but these have been disputed.[19,25] With respect to *Brucella* porins (group 2 proteins), the available evidence suggests that they fit into the Gram-negative "norm" in that they are apparently oligomeric, SDS-resistant, peptidoglycan-associated porins with pore sizes similar to *E. coli* porins.[26,27] Their strong peptidoglycan association and heterogeneous banding on SDS-PAGE represent variations on the general porin theme.

Specialized Porins

There are a limited number of known "specialized" porins. These are proteins which have channels containing specific binding sites for given molecules (Figure 4-2). The two best-studied cases are the phosphate-selective protein P (OprP) of *P. aeruginosa*[19,23,28,29] and the maltose/maltodextrin-selective LamB protein of *E. coli*.[23,30] In each case, these channels have some permeability towards other solutes, but the possession of specific binding sites allows substantially enhanced uptake at a low substrate concentration of molecules which bind, compared to molecules that do not bind (Figure 4-3). Indeed, at these low, physiologically relevant concentrations the specialized porins are orders of magnitude more effective in the uptake of their particular substrate than the general porins which possess substantially larger channels. Important features of the above two channels are that their production is regulated by their specific substrates and they are coregulated with a complex transport system.[23,31]

Other specialized porins have been less well studied. They include the glucose-selective protein D1[32] and the imipenem-selective protein D2[33] of *P. aeruginosa*, as well as the nucleoside-selective tsx protein of *E. coli*.[23,34] In addition, the iron-regulated outer membrane proteins of *E. coli* contain binding sites for specific iron-siderophore complexes, but there is no definitive data demonstrating that they are porins.[23,35] The NosA protein of *P. stutzeri* apparently contains a copper-binding site and is a porin, but the porin channel is not copper selective.[36]

Antibiotic Permeation Pathways

In most Gram-negative bacteria, porins constitute a major permeation pathway across the outer membrane for hydrophilic antibiotics. The exclusion limit and activity of the porin channels determine the efficiency of the porin pathway (also called the hydrophilic pathway). For example, it has been suggested that *P. cepacia* is antibiotic resistant due to its low outer membrane permeability, which is caused by the small size of its major porin channels.[37] Similarly, the majority of *P. aeruginosa* protein F channels are small and presumably impermeable to antibiotics, though a small percentage (<1%) have been proposed to be large and antibiotic permeable (but see above and references 6,20,22, and 38 for discussion). In *E. coli* the OmpF channel represents the major conduit for β-lactam antibiotics.[11,39] However, even in this case considerations such as the frictional

A

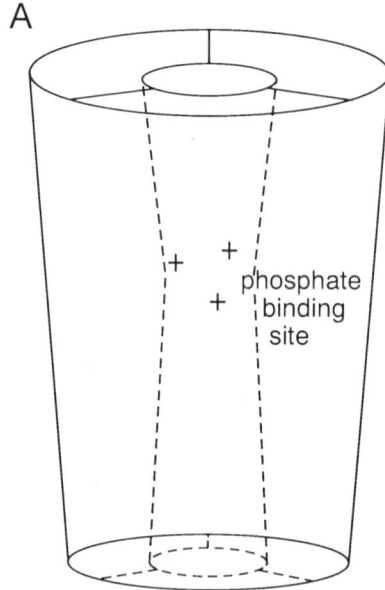

B

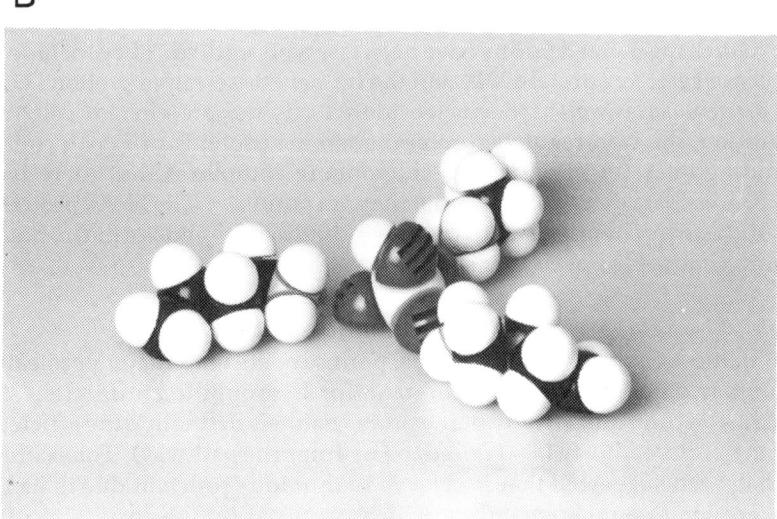

Figure 4-2a & 2b. Schematic Diagram of OprP. A. Showing the phosphate binding site. The binding site B, as diagramed here, is proposed to consist of three lysine side chains, one amino acid residue being from each monomer, which extend into the channel forming a positively charged cloud shell that would effectively bind HPO_4^2. There is a 3-fold symmetry of the HPO_{42}^- centered around the phosphate atom.[29]

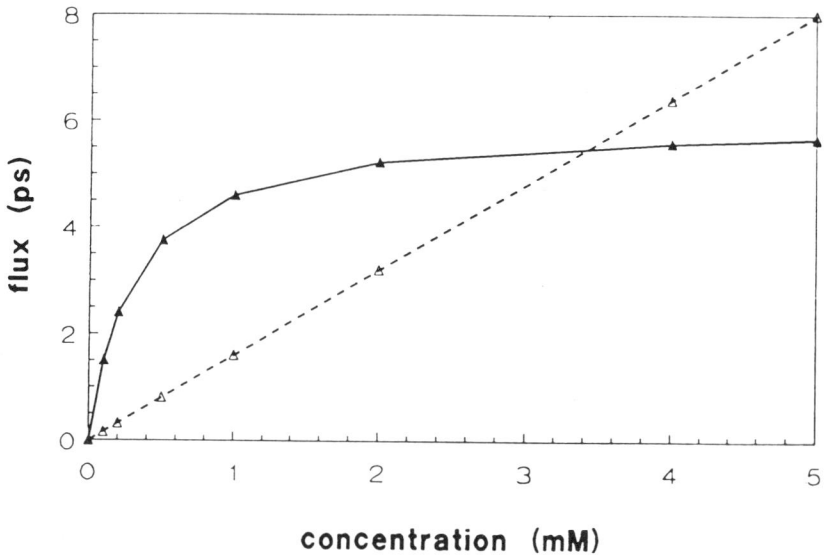

Figure 4-3. Phosphate Flux as a Function of the Concentration of Phosphate for OprP ▲ and PhoE △. The half-saturation constant Ks is 0.30 mM for OprP.

interactions between the sides of the OmpF channel and the permeating β-lactams, as well as the relatively small proportion of total outer membrane surface area that represents porin channels, means that the outer membrane reduces the rate of passage of β-lactams into the periplasm.[11,19] Thus, together with secondary defences like periplasmic β-lactamases, the molecular sieve nature of the outer membrane contributes substantially to the intrinsic resistance of Gram-negative bacteria to antibiotics.[39] The moderate susceptibility of *Brucella* spp. to hydrophilic antibiotics is consistent with model membrane studies showing similar porin sizes for *Brucella* and *E. coli.*[27]

There are two other well-defined antibiotic pathways across the outer membranes of Gram-negative bacteria, the hydrophobic pathway and the self-promoted uptake pathway.[9,11,40] The hydrophobic uptake pathway involves the uptake of hydrophobic or amphipathic molecules by direct passage through the outer membrane bilayer. Gram-negative bacteria like *S. typhimurium, E. coli,* and *P. aeruginosa* wild-type strains do not have a predominant hydrophobic permeation pathway.[6,41]

Studies with mutants of these bacteria (often LPS-altered) that are supersusceptible to hydrophobic agents, and with divalent cation chelators or polycations that increase the permeability of wild type strains to antibiotics, have indicated that the exclusion of hydrophobic antibiotics is mediated by the outer membrane in these strains.[9,41,40] It has been suggested that the outer membrane is stabilized by the strong interaction of LPS (the major, if not sole, lipidic component of the outer monolayer of the outer membrane) with itself, via divalent cation crossbridging, and with outer membrane proteins.[9,11,40] In contrast to these above bacteria, however, several pathogens, including *N. gonorrhoeae, N. meningitidis, H. influenzae,* and *B. pertussis,* have outer membranes which do take up hydrophobic compounds.[9] Symptomatic of a hydrophobic permeation pathway is high susceptibility to moderately hydrophobic agents including erythromycin and rifampicin. Based on the high susceptibility of *Brucella* spp. to these antibiotics we can assume that *Brucella* also possesses a relatively efficient hydrophobic permeation pathway.[42]

The other well-defined outer membrane permeation pathway is the self-promoted uptake pathway.[9,43] In this pathway, polycationic agents or chelators competitively displace or remove divalent cations from sites on the outer membrane where these divalent cations cross-bridge adjacent LPS molecules. The consequent destabilization of the outer membrane has been proposed to permit the enhanced uptake of the destabilizing compound, hence the name self-promoted uptake. The pathway is utilized by polycationic antibiotics such as polymyxins and, in some bacteria, amioglycosides.[9,43] Polycationic peptides called defensins (which are part of the non-oxidative killing arsenal of phagocytic cells),[44] and the fluoroquinolone antibiotic fleroxacin also use the pathway.[45] Self-promoted uptake, and consequent killing by these agents, can be inhibited by excess divalent cations in the medium, by LPS alterations possibly in negatively charged phosphate residues, or by induction of an LPS-associated protein which has been proposed to replace divalent cations in stabilizing outer membranes.[46] Also, *P. fluorescens* cells grown under phosphate-limiting conditions are resistant to polymyxins and produce large amounts of an ornithine amine lipid in contrast to *P. fluorescens* grown in a phosphate-rich medium.[47]

Brucella outer membranes are resistant to the destabilizing effects of the divalent cation chelator EDTA[48] and *Brucella* spp. are also resistant to the polycation polymyxin B.[32] Thus, we can assume that *Brucella* does not have a self-promoted uptake system. *Brucella* spp. have been shown to contain a high content of an ornithine lipid (17 to 32% of total lipid)[49] and we propose that this molecule replaces divalent cations as the chief outer membrane stabilizing agent, thus explaining the resistance of *Brucella* to polycations and EDTA. Since *Brucella* is a facultative intracellular parasite that can survive in phagocytic cells, we assume that this property is required for *Brucella's* resistance to the polycationic peptides and proteins of neutrophil granules.[50]

In addition to the above, we have recently argued, based on data in mutants, that there are other potential non-porin pathways.[9] The above-mentioned imipenem-selective protein, D2 of *P. aeruginosa*, also creates a precedent for the existence of a selective porin for a given group of antibiotics. Another group of β-lactams contain catechol groups and are thought to be taken up and across the outer membrane by iron-siderophore uptake systems.[51]

Receptor and Enzymatic Functions

Outer membrane macromolecules, both various proteins and LPS, also serve as cell surface receptors for adsorption of phages and bacteriocins.[5] Since this results in killing of cells, we can assume these are not the normal physiological functions of these molecules. In addition, outer membrane molecules are involved in binding of conjugative pili in genetic transfer.[5] A class of high molecular weight, iron-regulated, outer membrane proteins that have been identified in most bacteria examined function as receptors for iron-siderophore complexes and in subsequent permeation of these complexes across the outer membrane.[52] Such proteins are considered important in pathogenesis since it is generally held that bacteria grow *in vivo* under iron-deprived conditions.[53] Similarly, other outer membrane proteins in *Neisseria* sp. and *H. influenzae* function in binding and subsequent removal of iron from iron-loaded transferrin or lactoferrin.[54] The btuB protein serves as a receptor for vitamin B-12 as part of the vitamin B-12 uptake pathway of *E. coli*.[5] All of these receptors have been reasonably well characterized with regards to their binding function and in many cases mutants lacking these proteins have a clearly defined loss of uptake of the substate that binds to this receptor. However, little is known about the actual mechanism of translocation of the substrates across the outer membrane. Outer membranes have also been shown to contain proteins with a variety of enzymatic functions including phospholipase A1, esterase, and proteases.[1,5]

Role in Protein Excretion

A feature of many Gram-negative bacteria is their ability to excrete a variety of different proteins, including certain exotoxins, proteases, lipases, phospholipases, nucleases, haemolysins, etc, into the external medium. It was once assumed that such excretion might involve outer membrane breakdown and release of the enzyme from a periplasmic pool, but this is now known not to be generally true.[55,56] At least four pathways have been proposed for the mechanism of transit of excreted proteins across the outer membrane. These include secretion into the periplasm as a proprotein, followed by proteolytic removal of the "pro" sequence during passage across the outer membrane, secretion into the periplasm in a native form followed by release across the outer membrane, excretion of specific proteins associated with blebs of outer membrane material, and excretion through Bayer adhesion zones.[56]

Interaction with Environmental Surfaces

Various cell surface molecules have been described as being involved in adhesion to environmental surfaces (including adhesion to eukaryotic cells). Such adhesins include cell surface polysaccharides, fimbriae or pili, and fibrillar adhesins. However, only recently has there been good evidence to suggest a presumptive role for outer membrane proteins in adhesion. This evidence arose from genetic studies of E. coli P fimbriae, which like other fimbriae or pili, are anchored in the outer membrane. P fimbriae mediate binding of E. coli to the globoside receptor on epithelial cells.[57] It has been demonstrated that the receptor binding ligand for these fimbriae is not contained on the papA pilin protein that makes up the shaft of the P fimbriae, but rather is contained on a pair of proteins, papF and papG, which are usually located at the tip of the fimbriae. Mutants lacking the fimA protein, which presumably express the papF and papG proteins on the surface of the outer membrane, are still able to bind to globoside receptors. Although direct evidence is lacking, this creates a precedent suggesting that outer membrane proteins may be specifically involved in binding to environmental surfaces.

Structure of the Components of the Outer Membrane

Structural Proteins

It is interesting to note that predictive models of the E. coli OmpA protein based upon its primary structure[58] and mapping of surface exposed regions[59] suggest that only the N-terminal portion of this protein is embedded in the membrane.[60] Searches for similarities between the *P. aeruginosa* major outer membrane protein, OprF, and other proteins have found that the C-terminal half of OprF is very similar to the C-terminal half of OmpA from *E. coli* and *Enterobacter aerogenes*, and the pIII protein from *N. gonorrhoeae*.[14,61] It is this C-terminal region of OmpA which is thought not to be exposed on the surface of, or embedded in the outer membrane.[59] This is not true in the case of OprF since molecular genetic manipulation of the gene has permitted localization of the surface-exposed epitope of monoclonal antibody MA5-8 to the carboxy terminal half of the molecule (Woodruff, W.A. and R.E.W. Hancock, unpublished data). Interestingly, comparison of the antigenic index, which is calculated by summing several weighted measures of secondary structure (hydrophilicity, surface probability, flexibility, and the Chou-Fasman and Robson-Garnier predictive methods), shows a better correlation between OmpA and OprF in the N-terminal half of these proteins than in the C-terminal half which is more closely related at the primary sequence level (Figure 4-4). Group 3 proteins from *Brucella*, the proposed OmpA equivalent,[16] do not have any porin activity,[27] but no further studies on this particular group of proteins have been carried out in order to conclusively determine their structure or functional properties.

Another protein offering structural stability to the outer membrane, the Braun's lipoprotein, is not essential for growth, but mutants lacking lipoprotein produce increased amounts of outer membrane vesicles and release periplasmic enzymes.[65] A third of the lipoprotein present in the cell wall is covalently attached to the peptidoglycan through the ε-NH_2 group of the C-terminal lysine.[3] The protein portion of the molecule is mostly α-helical[4,63] and the N-terminal cysteine residue is substituted with a diglyceride on the sulfhydryl group and its α-NH_2 group is substituted with an amide linked fatty acid residue.[4] In *Brucella* the covalently peptidoglycan linked lipoprotein has an amino acid composition which is similar to that of *E. coli*[64] and seems to share antigenic epitopes with *E. coli* lipoprotein.[16]

Porins

General diffusion pores appear to be constitutively expressed, but the amount of expression seems to vary with the cell's needs. OmpF has long been regarded as the major porin of *E. coli*, however, expression of the *ompF* gene is regulated in response to the osmolarity of the medium and is predominant only under conditions of low osmolarity. At high osmolarity OmpC is predominantly expressed. Recent studies have shown that at intermediate salt concentrations there are actually OmpF/OmpC heterotrimers formed which cannot be distinguished from homotrimers by SDS-PAGE, but can be separated by anion exchange chromatography.[65] Considering the large degree of homology of the amino acids between OmpF and

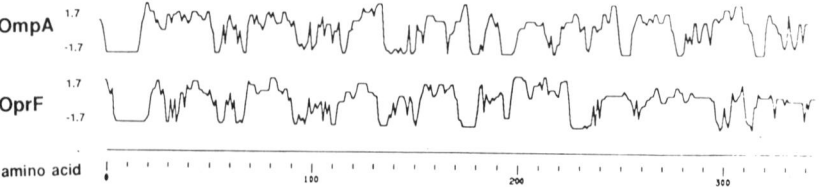

Figure 4-4. Plot of the Antigenic Index for Proteins OmpA and OprF. Note the similar peaks and valleys in the first 150 amino acids with much less similarity in the remaining C-terminal portions of the two proteins.

OmpC,[66] it seems feasible that the monomers would be interchangeable to form heterotrimers. This work, along with data which suggests that porin trimers are assembled via a dimeric intermediate,[67] suggests that bacterial cells are capable of "fine tuning" the outer membrane permeability characteristics by structurally altering porin types within the membrane.

A large amount of research has been directed towards establishing a molecular model for bacterial porins in the past few years. The crystallization of a porin and the concommitant resolution of that crystal structure will provide eagerly anticipated answers concerning the nature of the pore within these proteins, but technical problems such as protein purity (i.e. homogeneity), the need to crystallize in a detergent solution, and the difficulty of obtaining isomorphous heavy metal derivatives have proven to be significant obstacles. Nevertheless, a number of alternate techniques have been utilized to derive informative models of porin structure. Regions of cell surface exposed protein have been extensively mapped by molecular genetic studies of mutants selected using both antibody techniques and bacteriophages specific for PhoE[68,69] and LamB.[70,71,72] In addition, a series of hybrid genes generated by *in vivo* recombination between the *phoE* and *ompC* genes were characterized with respect to the binding of PhoE and OmpC specific bacteriophages and monoclonal antibodies raised against PhoE.[73,74] For PhoE, the data was consolidated and a model formulated in which eight hydrophilic regions are exposed on the external surface of the protein. Each of these regions is separated by approximately forty amino acids. These are stretches of amino acids long enough to cross the membrane twice, for a total per PhoE molecule of sixteen transmembrane segments.[66] The data for LamB suggest a folding model with eighteen membrane spanning segments.[66] These membrane spanning segments are thought to be arranged in β-pleated sheet conformation in porin proteins. There are none of the long segments of hydrophobic residues which have been shown to form membrane spanning α-helices in other membrane proteins.[75] The absence of hydrophobic segments could reflect a necessity for translocation to the outer membrane in Gram-negative bacteria. MacIntyre et al.[76] have shown that the addition of a segment of 16 to 18 hydrophobic residues inserted between amino acids 153 and 154 of OmpA blocked translocation, leaving this protein anchored in the cytoplasmic membrane.

Analyses of circular dichroism data on various bacterial porins,[77,78] infrared absorption and high angle x-ray diffraction,[79] Raman spectroscopy,[80] x-ray diffraction,[81] and Fourier transform infrared linear dichroism,[82] have all indicated a high content of β-sheet structure in OmpF, LamB, OprP, OprF, and the N-terminal 177 amino acids of OmpA. A model for the orientation of these anti-parallel β-pleated sheet structures[79] has been proposed by Nabedryk et al.[82] They suggest that the porin monomer consists of at least two β-sheet domains, both with planes perpendicular to the membrane. The strands of one sheet are lying nearly parallel to the membrane normal and the strands of the other are inclined at a small angle away from the membrane plane.

Extensive studies using electron microscopy have also provided a great deal of structural information about porins. Dorset et al.[83] examined the structure of OmpF trimers from *E. coli* by forming two-dimensional crystals of protein packed into lipid bilayers followed by reconstruction of optical diffraction patterns. Since the resolution of these experiments was limited to 2.2 nm, the shape of the transmembrane channels could not be determined, but they found lattice constants in one crystal form to be similar to those obtained from three-dimensional crystals.[81] They also found that the amount of phospholipid associating with the protein in a small hexagonal crystal form was comparable to the amount of LPS bound to membranous sheets generated by SDS extraction of undisassociated outer membrane from *E. coli*[84,85] indicating that porin packing in two-dimensional crystals is similar to the arrangement of porin in native outer membranes. To date, electron microscopy via both optical and electron diffraction techniques has been used to generate three-dimensional images from two-dimensional specimens of OmpF,[83,86,87,88] LamB,[89] and PhoE[90] to a maximum reconstructed resolution of approximately 0.6 nm. At this resolution it has been reported that there are three channels per trimer on the external surface of the protein which merge to form one channel at the periplasmic side for proteins OmpF and LamB, or merge, but do not converge, in the case of PhoE. It now seems likely that the OmpF channel arrangement is similar to PhoE (R.M. Garavito, personnel communication) in that the channels do not actually merge, but rather narrow and bend closer together at the periplasmic side of the membrane (Figure 4-5). A similar structural arrangement among the porins of *E. coli* would be consistent with their extensive homology at the primary level.

Other methods used to determine porin structure include chemical modification of specific amino acids and analysis of the resulting changes in solute permeability through the porin. For example, it has been demonstrated that OprP from *P. aeruginosa* has a fixed, anion binding site within the channel[28,29] and that the channel has an effective sieving diameter of approximately 0.5 - 0.6 nm[29] (Figure 4-2). Various methods were used to modify charged groups within the channel and the resulting conductance was analyzed via black lipid bilayer studies. Similar studies on PhoE from *E. coli* suggested that this protein does not have a specific binding site for phosphate.[91] These results have been confirmed recently by using PhoE mutants and black lipid bilayer techniques.[92] Chemical modification has also been used to demonstrate that porin channels have constrictions[28] and that charged amino acid residues are responsible for the weak ion selectivity of general diffusion pores.[29] Modification with bulky reagents such as trinitrobenezenesulphonate does not alter the exclusion limit of the OprP channel, which suggests that the charged residues responsible for selectivity are not located in the most constricted part of the channel.[93]

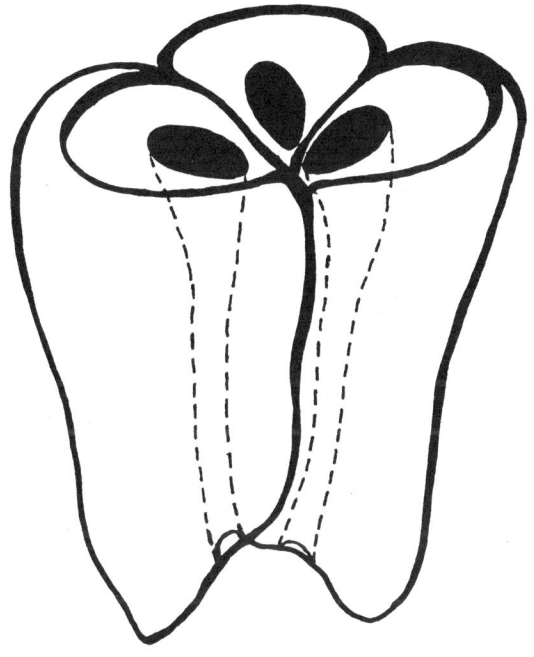

Figure 4-5. Schematic Diagram of a General Diffusion Porin with Three Separate Channels.

The properties of *Brucella* porins have been studied by Douglas et al[27] using liposome swelling assays. They found a range of pore sizes in different strains of *Brucella* with *B. canis* having the largest pores (larger than OmpF from *E. coli*), a middle range of pore sizes in several smooth and rough strains of *B. abortus*, and the smallest pore size in *B. melitensis* group 2 proteins. Except for the *B. canis* group 2 protein which had a lower mobility on SDS gels,[27] all of these proteins run as multiple bands at a molecular weight of 37,000-42,000.[27] All of these multiple bands give similar patterns in peptide mapping experiments. Explanations for the differing mobilities may be the heat modifiability of these proteins or the possibility of having different amounts of LPS remaining tightly associated with the proteins and causing them to run at slightly different positions on SDS gels.[94] The unusually strong association between protein and LPS is well documented for both smooth and rough *Brucella* strains[26,49,95,96] and seems not to be mediated by divalent cations[26] as it is in *E. coli* and other Gram-negative bacteria.[92,98,99,100]

Lipopolysaccharide

In addition to proteins, a major portion of the exterior surface area of the Gram-negative outer membrane consists of LPS. Most Gram-negative bacteria, including *Brucella*, produce both the rough and smooth types of LPS. Most enteric organisms have LPS structures consisting of similar lipid A, core oligosaccharides, and O-poly-saccharides, but *Brucella* LPS has a very different lipid A structure from that of enteric bacteria.[101] In *E. coli* all of the fatty acid chains attached directly to the disaccharide backbone of the LPS are 3-OH-tetradecanoic acids (primarily 3-hydroxymyristic acid). There are additional fatty acid residues linked to these 3-hydroxy groups forming a characteristic 3-acyloxyacyl structure.[11] *Brucella* lipid A contains amide linked, acyloxyacyl residues, 3-O(16:0)12:0, 3-O(16:0)13:0, 3-O(16:0)14:0, 3-O(18:0)14:0, 3-OH-16:0, and 3-OH-14:0, and an unusual 2,3-diamino-2,3-dideoxy-D-glucose as a backbone sugar which is similar to the lipid A of several photosynthetic bacteria.[102] There seems to be no phosphate associated with the core region although there is KDO. The lack of phosphate is interesting in light of the unusually strong association between LPS and proteins in *Brucella*. It is generally thought that LPS-protein interactions in many other bacteria may be mediated by charged residues on the LPS molecule.[11] In addition, the presumed low phosphate content of *Brucella* LPS is consistent with the lack of a self-promoted uptake pathway (see above).

In summary, the outer membrane of the Gram-negative cell wall must be traversed by every compound entering into or exiting from the bacterial cell as well as serving as a barrier against potentially harmful compounds. In this respect, the elements of the outer membrane are both functionally and structurally specialized. This review discusses the functions of the major proteins of the outer membrane in the context of permeability, structural stability, protein excretion, and cell surface interactions. In order to understand the function of a membrane at a molecular level it is necessary to know its structure. To this end, the structure of the major proteins, lipopolysaccharide, and lipoproteins are briefly discussed. As most of the information presented here is derived from studies of *Escherichia coli* and *Pseudomonas aeruginosa,* the available research on *Brucella* spp. is included for comparison wherever possible.

Acknowledgments

The authors' own research has been generously supported by the Natural Sciences and Engineering Research Council of Canada and the Canadian Cystic Fibrosis Foundation.

References

1. Lugtenberg B, Alpen LV. Molecular architecture and functioning of the outer membrane of *Escherichia coli* and other gram-negative bacteria. *Biochim Biophys Acta* 1983;737:51-115.

2. Glauner B, Höltje JV, Schwarz U. The composition of the murein of *Escherichia coli.* *J Biol Chem* 1988;263:10088-10095.

3. Inouye M, Show J, Shen C. The assembly of a structural lipoprotein in the envelope of *Escherichia coli.* *J Biol Chem* 1972;247:8154-8159.

4. Braun V. Covalent lipoprotein from the outer membrane of *Escherichia coli.* *Biochim Biophys Acta* 1975;415:335-377.

5. Nikaido H, Nakae T. The outer membrane of Gram-negative bacteria. *Adv. Microb Physiol* 1979;20:163-250.

6. Nikaido H, Hancock REW. Outer membrane permeability of *Pseudomonas aeruginosa* In *The Bacteria,* Vol. X Academic Press 1986;145-193.

7. Nishijima M, Nakaike S, Tamori Y, et al. Detergent-resistant phospholipase of *Escherichia coli* K-12. Purification and properties. *Eur J Biochem* 1977;73:115-124.

8. Paranchych W, Sastry PA, Vogel K, et al. Fimbriae (pili):molecular basis of *Pseudomonas aeruginosa* adherence. *Clin Invest Med* 1986;9:113-118.

9. Hancock REW, Bell A. Antibiotic uptake into Gram-negative bacteria. *Eur J Clinical Microbiol and Infect Dis* 1988;7:713-720.

10. Braun V. Iron supply as a virulence factor. In *The Pathogenesis of Bacterial Infections,* Bayer-Symposium VIII, Springer-Verlag 1985;68-176.

11. Nikaido H, Vaara M. Molecular basis of bacterial outer membrane permeability. *Microbiol Rev* 1985;49:1-32.

12. Henning U, Hindennach I, Haller I. The major proteins of the *Escherichia coli* outer cell envelope membrane: evidence for the structural gene of protein II*. *FEBS Lett* 1976;61:46-48.

13. Sonntag I, Schwarz H, Hirota Y, et al. Cell envelope and shape of *E.coli* multiple mutants missing the outer membrane lipoprotein. *J Bacteriol* 1978;136:280-285.

14. Woodruff WA, Hancock REW. *Pseudomonas aeruginosa* outer membrane protein F: structural role and relationship to the *Escherichia coli* OmpA protein. *J Bacteriol* 1989;171:in press.(June).

15. Woodruff WA, Hancock REW. Construction and characterization of *Pseudomonas aeruginosa* porin protein F-defficient mutants after *in vivo* and *in vitro* mutagenesis of the cloned protein F gene in *Escherichia coli.* *J Bacteriol* 1988;170:2592-2598.

16. Gómez-Miguel MJ, Moriyón I, López J. *Brucella* outer membrane lipoprotein shares antigenic determinants with *E.coli* Braun lipoprotein and is exposed on the cell surface. *Invest Immun* 1987;55:258-262.

17. Gotschlich E, Seiff M, Blake M. The DNA sequence of the structural gene of gono-coccal protein III and the flanking region containing a repetitive sequence: homology of protein III with enterobacterial OmpA proteins. *J Exp Med* 1987;165:471-482.

18. Mizuno T. A novel peptidoglycan-associated lipoprotein found in the cell envelope of *Pseudomonas aeruginosa* and *Escherichia coli*. *J Biochem* 1979;86:991-1000.

19. Hancock REW. Model membrane studies of porin function. In *Bacterial Outer Membranes as Model Systems*. John Wiley and Sons 1986;187-225.

20. Gotoh N, Wakebe H, Yoshihara E, et al. Role of protein F in maintaining structural integrity of the *P. aeruginosa* outer membrane. *J Bacteriol* 1989;171:983-990.

21. Yoshimura F, Zalman LS, Nikaido H. Purification and properties of *Pseudomonas aeruginosa* porin. *J Biol Chem* 1983;258:2308-2314.

22. Benz R and Hancock REW. Properties of large ion-permeable pores formed from protein F of *Pseudomonas aeruginosa* in lipid bilayer membranes. *Biochim Biophys Acta* 1981;646:298-308.

23. Benz R. Structure and function of porins from gram-negative bacteria. *Ann Rev Microbiol* 1988;42:359-393.

24. Dargent B, Hoffman W, Pattus F, et al. The selectivity filter of voltage-dependent channels formed by phosphorin (PhoE) from *E. coli. EMBO J* 1986;5:773-778.

25. Sen K, Hulman J, Nikaido H. Porin channels in intact cells of *E.coli* are not affected by Donnan potentials across the membranes. *J Biol Chem* 1988;263:1182-1187.

26. Moriyón I, Berman DT. Isolation, purification and characterization of *Brucella abortus* matrix protein. *Infect Immun* 1983;39:394-402.

27. Douglas JT, Rosenberg EY, Nikaido H, et al. Porins of *Brucella* species. *Infect Immun* 1984;44:16-21.

28. Hancock REW, Poole K, Gimple M, et al. Modification of the conductance, selectivity and concentration-dependent saturation of *Pseudomonas aeruginosa* protein P channels by chemical acetylation. *Biochim Biophys Acta* 1983;735:137-144.

29. Hancock REW, Benz R. 1986. Demonstration and chemical modification of a specific phosphate binding site in the phosphate-starvation-inducible outer membrane porin protein P of *Pseudomonas aeruginosa*. *Biochim Biophys Acta* 1986;860:699-707.

30. Benz R, Schmid A, Vos-Scheperkeuter GH. Mechanism of sugar transport through the sugar-specific LamB channel of *Escherichia coli* outer membrane. J *Membrane Biol* 1987;100:21-29.

31. Poole K, Hancock REW. Phosphate transport in *Pseudomonas aeruginosa*. Involvement of a periplasmic phosphate binding protein. *Eur J Biochem* 1984;144:607-612.

32. Hancock REW, Carey AM. Protein D1-a glucose inducible, pore-forming protein from the outer membrane of *P. aeruginosa*. *FEMS Microbiol Lett* 1980;8:105-109.

33. Quinn JP, Dudek EJ, DiVincenzo CA, et al. Emergence of resistance to imipenem during therapy for *Pseudomonas aeruginosa* infections. *Infect Dis* 1986;154:289-294.

34. Maier C, Bremer E, Schmid A, et al. Pore-forming activity of the Tsx protein from the outer membrane of *Escherichia coli*. Demonstration of a nucleoside specific binding site. *J Biol Chem* 1988;263:2493-2499.

35. Bauer K, Schmid A, Boos W, et al. Pore formation by *pho*-controlled outer membrane proteins of various *Enterobacteriaceae* in lipid bilayers. *Eur J Biochem* 1988;174:199-205.

36. Lee HS, Hancock REW, Ingraham JL. Properties of a *Pseudomonas stutzeri* outer membrane channel-forming protein (NosA) required for production of copper-containing N_2O reductase. *J Bacteriol* 1989;171:2096-2100.

37. Parr TR, Moore RA, Moore LV, et al. Role of porins in intrinsic antibiotic resistance of *Pseudomonas cepacia*. *Antimicrob Agents Chemother* 1987;31:121-123.

38. Woodruff WA, Parr TR, Hancock REW, et al. Expression in *Escherichia coli* and function of *Pseudomonas aeruginosa* outer membrane porin protein F. *J Bacteriol* 1986;167:473-479.

39. Hancock REW. Role of porins in outer membrane permeability. *J Bacteriol*

1987;169:929-933.
40. Hancock REW. Alterations in outer membrane permeability. *Annu Rev Microbiol* 1984;38:237-264.
41 Nikaido H. Outer membrane of *Salmonella typhimurium*:transmembrane diffusion of some hydrophobic substances. *Biochim Biophys Acta* 1976;433:118-132.
42. Hall WH, Manion RE. *In vitro* susceptibility of *Brucella* to various antibiotics. *Appl Microbiol* 1970;20:600-604.
43. Moore RA, Woodruff WA, Hancock REW. Antibiotic uptake pathways across the outer membrane of *P.aeruginosa*. *Antibiotics and Chemother* 1986;39:172-181.
44. Sawyer JL, Martin NL, Hancock REW. The interaction of macrophage cationic proteins with the outer membrane of *P. aeruginosa*. *Infect Immun* 1988;56:693-698.
45. Chapman JS, Georgopapadakou NH. Routes of quinolone permeation in *Escherichia coli*. *Antimicrob Agents Chemother* 1988;32:438-442.
46. Nicas TI, Hancock REW. Alteration of susceptibility to ethylenediaminetetraacetate, polymyxin B and gentamicin in *Pseudomonas aeruginosa* by divalent cation regulation of protein H2. *J Gen Microbiol* 1983;129:509-517.
47. Dorrer E, Teuber M. Induction of polymyxin resistance in *Pseudomonas fluorescens* by phosphate limitation. *Arch Microbiol* 1977;114:87-89.
48 Moriyón I, Berman DT. Effects of nonionic, ionic and dipolar ionic detergents and EDTA on the *Brucella* cell envelope. *J Bacteriol* 1982;152:822-828.
49. Kreutzer DL, Robertson DC. Surface macromolecules and virulence in intracellular parasitism comparison of cell envelope components of smooth and rough *Brucella abortus*. *Infect Immun* 1979;23:819-828.
50. Kreutzer DL, Dreyfuss LA, Robertson DC. Interaction of polymorphonuclear leukocytes with smooth and rough strains of *B. abortus*. *Infect Immun* 1984;23:737-742.
51 Watanabe NA, Nagasu T, Katsu K, et al. E-0702, a new cephalosporin, is incorportated into *Escherichia coli* cells via the *ton*B-dependent iron transport system. *Antimicrob Agents Chemother* 1987;32:497-504.
52. Neilands JB. Microbial envelope proteins related to iron. *Annu Rev Microbiol* 1982;36:285-309.
53. Griffiths E, Stevenson P, Joyce P. Pathogenic *Escherichia coli* express new outer membrane proteins when growing *in vivo*. *FEMS Microbiol Lett* 1983;16:95-99.
54. Schryvers AB. Characterization of the human transferrin and lactoferrin receptors in *Haemophilus influenzae*. *Molecular Microbiol* 1988;2:467-472.
55. Poole K, Hancock REW. Phosphate transport in *Pseudomonas aeruginosa*. Involvement of a periplasmic phosphate-binding protein. *Eur J Biochem* 1984;144:607-612.
56. Hirst TR, Welch RA. 1988. Mechanism for secretion of extracellular proteins by Gram-negative bacteria. *Trends Biochem Sci* 1988;13:265-269.
57. Lindberg FP, Lund B, Normark S. Genes of pyelonephritogenic *E. coli* required for digalactoside-specific agglutination of human cells. *EMBO J* 1984;3:1167-1173.
58. Beck E, Bremer E. Nucleotide sequence of the gene omp_A coding the outer membrane protein II* of *Escherichia coli* K-12. *Nucl Acids Res* 1980;8:3011-3024.
59. Morona R, Klose M, Henning U. *E coli* K-12 outer membrane protein (OmpA) as a bacteriophage receptor: analysis of mutant genes expressing altered proteins. *J Bacteriol* 1984;159:570-578.
60. Schweizer M, Hindennach T, Garten W, et al. Major proteins of the *E. coli* outer cell envelope membrane. Interaction of protein II with lipopolysaccharide. *Eur J Biochem* 1978;82:211-217.
61. Duchene M, Schweizer A, Lottspeich F, et al. Sequence transcriptional start site of the *P. aeruginosa* outer membrane porin protein F gene. *J Bacteriol* 1988;170:155-162.
62. Suzuki H, Nishimura Y, Yasuda S, et al. Murein-lipoprotein of *Escherichia coli:* a protein involved in the stabilization of bacterial cell envelope. *Mol Gen Genet* 1978;167:1-9.
63. Braun V, Rotering H, Ohms J-P, et al. Conformational studies on murein lipoprotein

from the outer membrane of *Escherichia coli*. *Eur J Biochem* 1976;70:601-610.

64. Gómez-Miguel MJ, Moriyón I. Demonstration of a peptidoglycan-linked lipoprotein and characterization of its trypsin fragment in the outer membrane of *Brucella* spp. *Infect Immun* 1986;53:678-684.

65. Gehring KB, Nikaido H. Existence and purification of porin heterotrimers of *E. coli* K12 OmpC, OmpF, ånd PhoE proteins. *J Biol Chem* 1989;264:2810-2815.

66. Tommassen J. Biogenesis and membrane topology of outer membrane proteins in *Escherichia coli*. In *Membrane Biogenesis*, Vol. H16. Springer-Verlag,1988.

67. Reid J, Fung H, Gehring K, et al. Targeting of porin to the outer membrane of *Escherichia coli*. Rate of trimer assembly and identification of a dimer intermediate. *J Biol Chem* 1988;263:7753-7759.

68. Van der Lay P, Struyvé M, Tommassen J. Topology of outer membrane pore protein PhoE of *Escherichia coli*. Identification of cell surface-exposed amino acids with the aid of monoclonal antibodies. *J Biol Chem* 1986;261:12222-12225.

69. Korteland J, Overbeeke N, De Graaff P, et al. Role of the Arg-158 residue of the outer membrane PhoE pore protein of *Escherichia coli* K-12 in bacteriophage TC45 recognition in channel characteristics. *Eur J Biochem* 1985;152:691-697.

70. Desaymard C, Déborbouillé M, Jolit M, et al. 1986. Mutations affecting antigenic determinants of an outer membrane protein of *E.coli*. *EMBO J* 1986;5:1383-1388.

71. Charbit A, Clément J-M, Hofnung M. Further sequence analysis of the phage lambda receptor site. Possible implications for the organization of the LamB protein in *Escherichia coli* K-12. *J Mol Biol* 1984;175:395-401.

72. Gehring K, Charbit A, Brissaud E, et al. Bacteriophage l receptor site on the *Escherichia coli* K-12 LamB protein. *J Bacteriol* 1987;169:2103-2106.

73. Tomassen J, Van der Ley P, Zeiyl Van M, et al. Localization of functional domains in *Escherichia coli* K-12 outer membrane porins. *Embo J* 1985;4:1583-1587.

74. Van der Ley P, Burm P, Agterberg M, et al. Analysis of structure-function relationships in *E coli* K-12 outer membrane porins with the aid of ompC-phoE and phoE-ompC hybrid genes. *Mol. Gen. Genet.* 1987;209:589-591.

75. Deisenhofer J, Epp O, Miki K, et al. Structure of the protein subunits in the photosynthetic reaction centre of *Rhodopseudomonas viridis* at 3Å resolution. *Nature* 1985;318:618-624.

76. MacIntyre S, Freudl R, Eschbach M-L, et al. An artificial hydrophobic sequence functions as either an anchor or a signal sequence at only one of two positions within the *E.coli* outer membrane protein OmpA. *J Biol Chem* 1988;263:19053-19059.

77. Worobec EA, Martin NL, McCubbin W, et al. Large scale purification and biochemical characterization of crystallization-grade porin protein P of *Pseudomonas aeruginosa*. *Biochim Biophys Acta* 1988;939:366-374.

78. Rosenbusch JP. Characterization of the major envelope protein from *Escherichia coli*. Regular arrangement of the peptidoglycan and unusual dodecyl sulphate binding. *J Biol Chem* 1974;249:8019-8029.

79. Kleffel B, Garavito RM, Baumiester W, et al. Secondary structure of a channel-forming protein: porin from *E.coli* outer membranes. *EMBO J* 1985;4:1589-1592.

80. Vogel H, Jähnig F. Models for the structure of outer membrane proteins of *Escherichia coli* derived from Raman spectroscopy and prediction methods. *J Mol Biol* 1986;190:191-199.

81. Garavito R, Jansonius J, Jenkins J, et al. X-ray diffraction of matrix porin, an integral membrane protein from *E. coli* outer membranes. *J Mol Biol* 1983;164:313-327.

82. Nabedryk E, Garavito RM, Breton J. The orientation of β-sheets in porin. A polarized Fourier transform infrared spectroscopic investigation. *Biophys J* 1988;53:671-676.

83. Dorset D, Engel A, Häner M, et al. Two-dimensional crystal packing of matrix porin a channel forming protein in *E.coli* outer membranes. *J Mol Biol* 1983;165:701-710.

84. Rosenbusch JP, Garavito RM, Dorset DL, et al. Structure and function of a pore-forming transmembrane protein: high resolution studies of a bacterial porin. In

Protides of Biological Fluids, pp 171-174 Pergamon Press, 1982.
85. Steven AC, Jeggeler ten B, Müller R, et al. Ultrastructure of a periodic protein layer in the outer membrane of *Escherichia coli. J Cell Biol* 1977;72:292-301.
86. Engel A, Massalski A, Shindler H, et al. Porin channel triplets merge into single outlets in *Escherichia coli* outer membrane. *Nature* 1985;317:643-645.
87. Engel A, Massalski A. 3-dimensional reconstruction from electron micrographs: its potential and practical limitations. *Ultramicroscopy* 1984;13:71-84.
88. Massalski A, Sass HJ, Zemlin F, et al. High-resolution low-dose electron cryomicroscopy of negatively stained matrix porin, a transmembrane protein from *Escherichia coli* outer membranes. In *Proceedings of the 45th Annual Meeting of the Electron Microscopy Society of America.* San Francisco Press, pp. 788-789, 1987.
89. Lepault J, Dargent B, Tichelaar W, et al. Three dimensional reconstruction of maltoporin from electron microscopy and image processing. *EMBO J* 1988;7:261-268.
90. Jap BK. High resolution electron diffraction of reconstituted PhoE porin. *J Mol Biol* 1988;199:229-231.
91. Darveau RP, Hancock REW, Benz R. Chemical modification of the anion selectivity of the PhoE porin from the *Escherichia coli* outer membrane. *Biochim Biophys Acta* 1984;774:67-74.
92. Bauer K, Van der Ley P, Benz R, et al. The *pho*-controlled outer membrane porin PhoE does not contain specific binding-sites for phosphate or polyphosphate. *J Biol Chem* 1988;263:13046-13053.
93. Hancock REW, Schmidt A, Bauer K, et al. Role of lysines in ion selectivity of bacteial outer membrane porins. *Biochim Biophys Acta* 1986;860:263-267.
94. Verstreate DR, Winter AJ. Comparison of sodium dodecyl sulfate-polyacrylamide gel electrophoresis profiles and antigenic relatedness among outer membrane proteins of 49 *Brucella abortus* strains. *Infect Immun* 1984;46:182-187.
95. Santos JM, Verstreate DR, Perera Y, et al. Outer membrane proteins from rough strains of four *Brucella* species. *Infect Immun* 1984;46:188-194.
96. Verstreate DR, Creasy MT, Caveney NT, et al. Outer membrane proteins of *Brucella abortus*: isolation and characterization. *Infect Immun* 1982;35:979-989.
97. Matsushita K, Adalhi O, Shinagawa E, et al. Isolation and characterization of outer and inner membranes from *Pseudomonas aeruginosa* and effect of EDTA on the membranes. *J Biochem* 1979;83:171-181.
98. Schnaitman CA. Effect of EDTA, Triton X-100, and lysozyme on the morphology and chemical composition of isolated cell walls of *Escherichia coli. J Bacteriol* 1971;108:553-563.
99. Garrard WT. Selective release of proteins from *Spirillum itersonii* by tris (hydroxymethyl)aminomethane and EDTA. *J Bacteriol* 1971;105:93-100.
100. Johnston KH, Gotschlich EC. Isolation and characterization of the outer membrane of *Neisseria gonorrhoeae. J Bacteriol* 1974;119:250-257.
101. Moreno E, Pitt MW, Jones LM, et al. Purification and characterization of smooth and rough lipopolysaccharides from *Brucella abortus. J Bacteriol* 1979;138:361-369.
102. Moreno E, Borowiak D, Mayer H. *Brucella* lipopolysaccharides and polysaccharides. *Annales de L'Institut Pasteur Microbiol* 1987;138:102-105.

Chapter Five

Lipopolysaccharide Antigens
and Carbohydrates of *Brucella*

Malcolm B. Perry
and David R. Bundle

Over the past 50 years an abundance of papers and reviews have been written on the antigenic components of *Brucella* strains and their importance in diagnosis, serological classifications, cross-reactions, and virulence, and their potential role in immunity.[1-8] It is not possible in this short review to give credit to all the researchers who have made their contribution to the present state of knowledge of *Brucella* cellular compositions. However, the work of Wilson, Miles, and Pirie[9-11] stands as a landmark. They postulated that the serologically characterized *Brucella* A and M antigens are associated with a single complex molecule analyzed as an "aminopolyhydroxy component containing formyl residues" present in the lipopolysaccharides (LPS) of *Brucella abortus* and *B. melitensis*. Following this incisive work, little more was added to the picture over the next 30 years. Subsequent research publications describing the results of chemical fractionations and characterizations of *Brucella* cellular components are difficult to summarize because of the variety of extraction and purification procedures employed and, in particular, the failure to provide chemical and elementary physical data which would have permitted comparative evaluations to be made.

Until a few years ago, the complex and confusing serological cross-reactions described between *Brucella* LPS and preparations termed native hapten (NH)[4] and polysaccharide B (poly B, PB)[12,13] were difficult to explain. Similarly, the reasons for the cross serological reactivities between *Brucella* species, and between *Brucella* and other bacteria such as *Vibrio cholerae*, *Escherichia coli* O157, *Salmonella* (Group N, O:30), *Yersinia enterocolitica* O:9, *Pseudomonas maltophilia* 555,[14] and *Escherichia hermannii*[15,16] could not be explained owing to the lack of structural information on their cross reacting antigens.

Many of the above problems were resolved when the structures of the *Brucella* carbohydrate antigens had been determined. Fortunately, the newer methods of carbohydrate analysis, in particular the use of high-resolution nuclear magnetic resonance spectroscopy, and the analytical use of specific monoclonal antibodies, proved to be ideally suited to the solution of the structural base of antigenic specificities. This review decribes some of the results obtained in our laboratory which have led to an explanation of the main aspects of the structural chemistry involved in the immunobiological properties of *Brucella* species. cribes some of the results obtained in our laboratory which have led to an explanation of the main aspects of the structural chemistry involved in the immunobiological properties of *Brucella* species.

Discussion

Designation of *Brucella* strains as serologically A or M has been interpreted as the predominant expression of either antigen at the cell surface of *B. abortus, B. melitensis,* and *B. suis.*[1] Since both antigens were considered to be present on all smooth (S-LPS) *Brucella* strains, their classification as A or M positive was regarded as a difference in the quantitative distribution of the A and M antigens as estimated by antisera rendered essentially monospecific by cross-absorption. Early work had indicated that the A and M specific antigenic activities of *Brucella* resided in their respective LPS and experiments involving inhibition of antibody-LPS[8,11] reactions by isolated *Brucella* O-polysaccharides using ELISA methods confirmed the fact that the antigenic determinants resided in the O-polysaccharide moieties of their LPS.[17]

In light of the above information, attention was first directed towards the determination of the structures of the LPS O-polysaccharide portions of *B. abortus* 1119-3[18] and *B. melitensis* 16M, respectively regarded as species type A and M strains, and of the LPS O-polysaccharide of *Y. enterocolitica* O:9[19,20] which showed unusually strong specific cross serological activity with the LPS of *Brucella* species. Extraction of *B. abortus* 1119-3 and *Y. enterocolitica* O:9 cells by the hot aqueous phenol methods followed by ultracentrifugation of the dialysed and concentrated separated phenol phases yielded smooth LPS. SDS-PAGE analysis of the LPS and detection by the periodate-silver nitrate staining method showed similar continuous staining in the S-LPS region typical of LPS having an O-polysaccharide moiety composed of a uniquely linked single repeating monosaccharide unit. Both LPS were cleaved by hot 5% (v/v) acetic acid to yield free O-polysaccharides which were recovered by Sephadex G-50 column gel-filtration. Attempts to determine the O-polysaccharide component glycoses by classical hydrolysis procedures resulted in extensive decomposition; this no doubt accounts for the earlier difficulties encountered in attempts to characterize the antigen. The detection of low yields (ca 2%) of 2-amino-2,6-dideoxyglucose, D-mannose, D-glucose and 3-deoxy-D-manno-octulosonate (3:1:1:1) in the *Brucella* O-chain hydrolysates arises from the core moiety of the LPS.

Application of ¹H and ¹³C NMR analysis showed the spectra of the B.

abortus 1119-3 and *Y. enterocolitica* O:9 polysaccharides to be essentially identical and characteristic resonances in the ^{13}C-NMR spectrum (Figures 5-1 and 5-2). The anomeric resonance with a distinctive coupling constant ($^1J_{C-H}$ = 173Hz) indicated that the polymers were composed of a single α-linked 4-amino-4,6-dideoxyhexopyranosyl repeating unit in which the amino group was N-formylated. The presence of the N-formyl group gives rise to spectra showing more resonance signals than would be expected from a uniformly linked homopolymer since this N-acyl substituent causes microheterogeneity as a consequence of rotational isomerism of the formate group. This isomeric effect is not present in the spectra of the corresponding N-acetylated O-polysaccharides made by selective N-ace-tylation of the free amino O-polysaccharides produced by N-deformyla-tion of the native O-chains by hot aqueous sodium hydroxide.

Identification of 4,6-dideoxy-4-formamido-D-mannose (D-Rhap4 NFo) as the monosaccharide component of the *B. abortus* 1119-3 and *Y. enterocolitica* O:9 LPS O-chains was established following its almost quantitative liberation by cleavage with cold anhydrous hydrofluoric acid from the N-acetylated polymeric antigen. The liberated glycose proved to be identical with an authentic sample with respect to its specific optical rotation, ^{13}C and ^{1}H-NMR spectra, and GLC-MS analysis of its 2,3-di-O-acetyl-4-acetamido-4,6-dideoxy-D-mannitol-l-d derivative. Methylation analysis of the N-acetylated O-polysaccharides gave 4,6-dideoxy-3-O-methyl-4-(N-methylamino)-D-mannose identified by GLC-MS as its 2-O-acetyl-4,6-dideoxy-3-O-methyl-4-(N-methylacetamido)-D-mannitol-l-d derivative.

From a consideration of the combined methylation, NMR, positive optical rotation, and serological[20] data, it was concluded that the O-polysac-charides were homopolymers of 1,2-linked 4,6-dideoxy-4-formamido-a-D-mannopyranosyl units with an approximate chain length of 100 glycose residues terminated at the reducing end groups by approximately 2% of core oligosaccharide. Subsequent more rigorous analysis revealed that, whereas the *Y. enterocolitica* O:9 O-polysaccharide was an entirely 1,2 linked polymer, the *B. abortus* 0119-3 O-polysaccharide contained a very low percentage of 1,3 linked residues. The *Yersinia* O-polysaccharide proved to be a valuable homogeneous reference material in later investi-gations involved in defining the structural nature of *Brucella* A and M antigens.

In an endeavor to define the structural features that determine the *Brucella* M antigen, the structure of the O-polysaccharide of the LPS produced by *B. melitensis* 16M was examined in detail.[21] Unlike the LPS of *B. abortus* 1119-3, the LPS of *B. melitensis* 16M was liberated, over six days at 4C, into a 2% (w/v) phenol saline solution of the suspended cells from which solution the LPS was recovered by ultracentrifugation. The O-polysaccharide was obtained after hydrolysis of the LPS with 5% (w/v) acetic acid in the same way as that described for the preparation of the *B. abortus* O-chain. By chemical analysis, the O-chain was also found to be

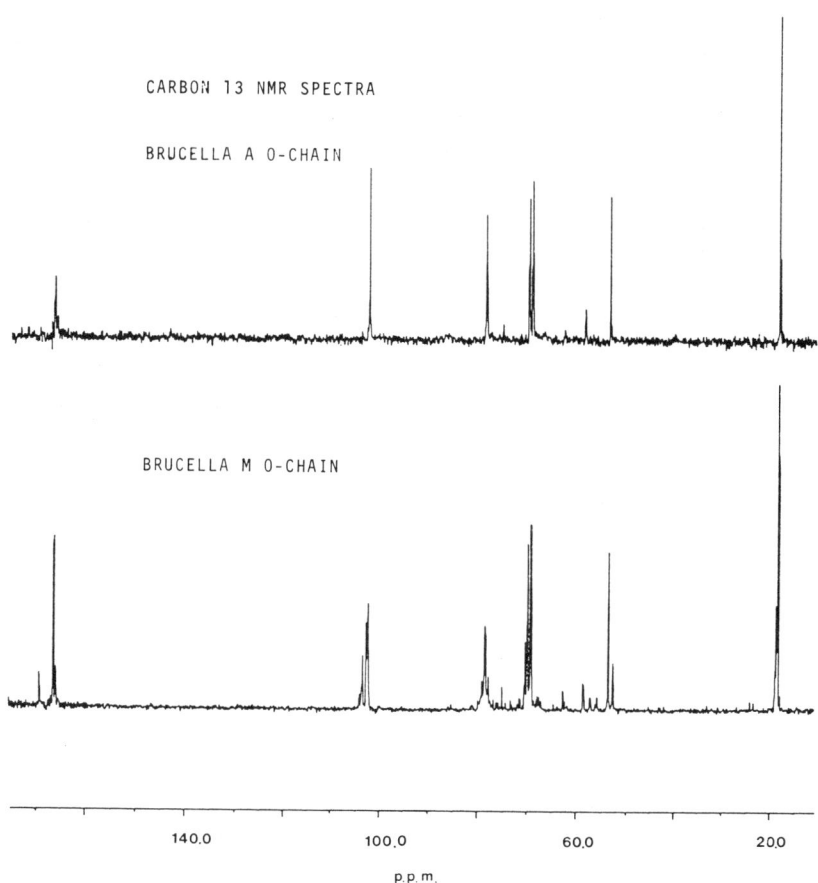

Figure 5-1.   Carbon-13 NMR Spectra of the LPS O-Polysaccharides of
B. abortus **1119-3 and** *B. melitensis* **M16.**

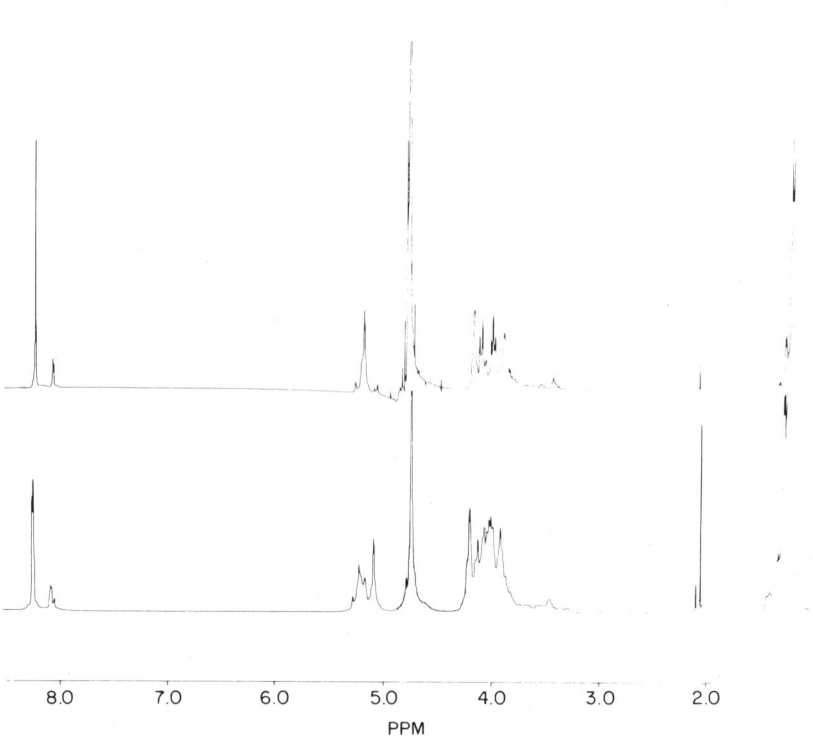

Figure 5-2. Proton NMR Spectra of the LPS O-Polysaccharides of *B. abortus* 1119-3 and *B. melitensis* M16.

composed of the D-Rha4NFo residues. The first indication that the LPS O-polysaccharides from *B. abortus* 1119-3 and *B. melitensis* 16M were not identical, despite their common glycose constituent, came from their specific optical rotations which were respectively [a]$_D$ +28° and [a]$_D$ +56°. Another difference was the patterns exhibited in the SDS-PAGE analysis of the native LPS where the *B. melitensis* 16M gave a ladder banding typical of a smooth LPS with an O-polysaccharide composed of a possible pentasaccharide unit. Supporting evidence for the postulated difference was the observation that the ¹³C and ¹H-NMR spectra of the *B. melitensis* O-polysaccharide showed complex multiple signals located around the resonance frequencies of the signals seen in the corresponding spectra of the *B. abortus* O-polysaccharide (Figures 5-1 and 5-2).

Structural analysis of the *B. melitensis* O-polysaccharide by NMR methods was difficult due to the apparent microheterogeneity of the repeating unit, which was in fact caused by the presence of rotational isomers of the N-formyl substituents and different glycosidic linkages. This problem was resolved by chemical modification of the polysaccharide to its free amino and N-acetyl derivatives. The 500-MHz ¹H and 125-MHz ¹³C spectra of these derivatives could be analyzed in terms of a unique structure through application of pH-dependent β-shifts and two-dimensional techniques that included COSY, relayed COSY, and NOESY experiments, together with heteronuclear C/H shift correlation spectroscopy. On the basis of the NMR experimental data and supportive methylation and periodate oxidation results, the structure of the *B. melitensis* 16M LPS O-polysaccharide was deduced as an unbranched linear polymer of repeating pentasaccharide units consisting of four 1,2 and one 1,3 linked D-Rhap4NFo residues.

The quantitative physical determination of the proportion of 1,3- and 1,2-linked a-D-Rhap4NFo residues in *Brucella* O-polysaccharides can be made from the integration of the C-4 and formamido carbonyl resonances in their high-resolution ¹³C-NMR spectra. In the C-4 resonance region (50 to 60 ppm), 2-O-substituted a-D-Rhap4NFo residues show signals at 57.7 and 52.7 ppm, whereas the 3-O-substituted residues show signals at 56.3 and 51.7 ppm. In the C=O region, signals at 168.8 and 165.9 ppm are characteristic of 2-O- substituted residues as opposed to signals at 165.3 from 3-O- substituted a-D-Rhap4NFo units.

Three-dimensional models deduced for the linear hexasaccharide fragments of the A and M antigens (Figure 5-3) that are consistent with NMR-NOE data and potential energy algorithm (HSEA and GESA) calculations demonstrate how the introduction of a 1,3 linkage into the otherwise 1,2 linked O-polysaccharide alters the direction of chain propagation and hence the topography presented by the O-polysaccharide to specific antibodies. The nearly identical antigen surface presented by the tetrasaccharide sequences exclusively involved in 1,2 linkages of the M antigen should be capable of reacting with a major population of antibodies generated in response to the *Brucella* A antigen. As a corollary, polyclonal antibodies generated by the M antigen would contain a significant proportion of antibodies cross-reacting with the A antigen in addition to antibodies specific for the unique structural features of the M antigenic epitopes. Monoclonal antibodies generated to *Brucella* A and M antigens do, in fact, show this pattern of reactivities.[22,23] While the elucidated structural features of the *Brucella* A and M antigens allow a structural explanation of the long-established serological cross-reactivities, the question of whether both antigenic determinants may be carried on a single molecule remained. It is interesting to note that recent chemical evidence has given proof that some strains of *Salmonella* produce several separate chemically similar but structurally distinct LPS that differ in their unique O-chains.[24,25]

By SDS-PAGE analysis, convincing evidence was obtained for the heterogeneity of LPS among 16 smooth *Brucella* strains.[26] Profiles present in biovars M≥A were a close succession of regularly spaced narrow bands; the second, present in biovars M≥A, showed regularly spaced doublets separated by barely visible bands. LPS from the type and reference strains of five of the six *Brucella* nomenspecies, *B. abortus*, *B. melitensis*, *B. suis*, *B. canis*, and *B. neotomae* were analyzed by SDS-PAGE, in conjunction with immunoblotting and immunostaining with specific A and M *Brucella* monoclonal antibodies and showed banding characteristics for A, M, or mixed A and M antigens.[21] A and M structural features were confirmed on analysis of the ^{1}H and ^{13}C-NMR spectra of the LPS O-polysaccharides. The A antigen was shown to possess a fine structure that involved, albeit a low frequency of, α-1,3 linked D-Rhap4NFo residues in an otherwise α-1,2 linked polymer, a feature previously attributed to the *Brucella* M antigen. *B. melitensis* biotype 3, and *B. suis* biotype 4 LPS showed mixed A and M antigenic characteristics on NMR and EIA analyses.

Immunoabsorption of O-polysaccharides from either of these strains using an affinity column prepared from A-specific monoclonal antibodies enriched antigen O-chains with A characteristics but did not completely remove M epitopes. Composite A and M characteristics observed for cells of these two biotypes were considered to result from a heterogeneous population of bacterial cell surface O-polysaccharides in which the frequency of α-1,3 linkages, and hence M characteristics, were variable.

Since all biotypes assigned as A⁺M⁻ expressed one or two α-1,3 linked D-Rhap4NFo residues per polysaccharide O-chain, the paradigm of Wilson and Miles that stipulated the presence of A and M epitopes on a single molecule is shown to be essentially correct. M-Antigens (M⁺A⁻) also possess epitopes in common with all A antigenic structures. *B. canis* and *B. abortus* 40/20, which are both rough strains, express A antigen on low molecular weight O-chains.

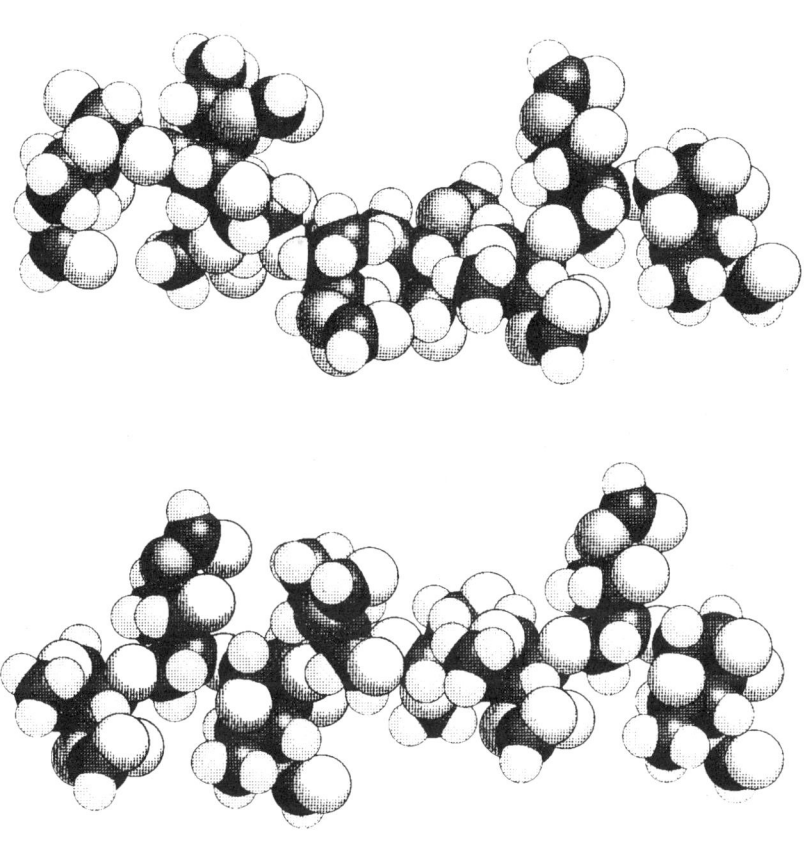

Figure 5-3. Space-Filling Models of the *Brucella* A and M Antigens Displayed as Hexasaccharide Units in the Preferred Conformations Predicted from Potential Energy Calculations.

The binding profiles of nine monoclonal antibodies generated in response to *B. melitensis* 16M were characterized using the defined reference O-polysaccharides of *B. abortus* 1119-3, *B. melitensis* 16M, *Y. enterocolitica* O:9,[21] and an extensive series of synthesized $\underline{D}$-Rhap4NFo oligosaccharide analogues of the A and M antigens.[27,28] In competitive binding studies, three distinct binding patterns were characterized for the M antibodies and previously reported A antibodies. Antibody that was specific for the A antigen required at least five contiguous α-1,2 linked $\underline{D}$-Rhap4NFo residues while antibodies that had equal affinity for A and M epitopes were effectively inhibited by α1,2-linked tri- and tetrasaccharides. Specificity for the M epitope correlated with binding that involved the crucial element α-$\underline{D}$-Rhap4NFo-(1-3)-α-$\underline{D}$-Rhap4NFo- bracketed by α-1,2 linked $\underline{D}$-Rhap4NFo residues. Three monoclonal antibodies demonstrating these described binding specificities can be used as standards for the detection and identification of *Brucella* A and M antigens. Their analytical use confirmed the linkage distributions in *Brucella* O-polysaccharides found from the results of chemical studies.

Polysaccharides referred to as native haptens (NH)[4] which show serological relationships to A and M antigen have been described as products of *B. abortus* and *B. melitensis*. Analysis of NH from *Brucella* strains revealed that they had chemically identical structures with the O-polysaccharides derived from the LPS of the respective homologous organisms. The observation that they were terminated at their reducing ends by core regions of typical *Brucella* glycose composition strongly suggested that NH are artifacts derived from originally intact LPS molecules.[29]

Products of *Brucella* species refered to as polysaccharide B (Poly B, PB)[12,13] and described as having serological activity with A or M antisera have been reported. An analysis of PB preparations revealed that these materials were nonreducing cyclic $\underline{D}$-glucans composed exclusively of 1,2 linked β-$\underline{D}$-glucopyranosyl residues having an average ring size of 20 glycose units.[30] The purified cyclic $\underline{D}$-glucans showed no serological activity with *Brucella* antisera. Crude preparations of PB contained polysaccharide having A or M activity which would account for reported serological activities. Experiments have shown that the *Brucella* cyclic $\underline{D}$-glucans form strong non-covalent complexes with *Brucella* O-polysaccharides to the extent that the $\underline{D}$-glucan, despite its relatively low molecular weight, is eluted with the O-polysaccharide at the void volume of a Sephadex G-50 gel filtration system.

With the acquired knowledge of the structures of the *Brucella* A and M antigens, it is of interest to discover the structural reasons for the observed serological cross-reactions recorded with other bacterial species.[14] An analysis of the cross-reacting bacteria revealed that, in every case, the LPS O-polysaccharides were the antigens responsible for cross-reactions seen in the use of polyclonal antisera. From the structures of the respective LPS O-chains shown below, it can be seen that the common feature is the presence of N-acyl derivatives of a-D-Rhap4N residues in their repeating units and these units almost certainly are involved in the epitopes responsible for serological cross-reactivities with *Brucella* antisera.

LPS O-polysaccharide structures:

Yersinia enterocolitica O:9[19]

-2) - α - D - RhapFo-(1-

Escherichia coli O157[31]

-4 - β - D - Glcp - (1-3) - α - D - GalpNAc -(1-2)- α- D -Rhap4NAc-(1-3) - α- L - Fucp - (1-

Salmonella Group N (O:30)[32,33]

-4 - β - D - Glcp - (1-3) - α - D - GalpNAc -(1-2)- α- D -Rhap4NAc-(1-3) - α- L - Fucp - (1-

and

-4 - β - D - Glcp - (1-3) - α- D - GalpNAc -(1-2)- α- D -Rhap4NAc-(1-3) -
α- L - Fucp - (1-   4
                                |
                                1
                          b-D -Glcp

Pseudomonas maltophilia 555[34]

-3) - α - D - Rhap4NAc -(1-3) α - D -Rhap4NAc-(1-2)- α -D - Rhap-(1-3) - α -D - Rhap4NAc - (1
                                2
                                |
                                1
                          α-D -Fucp3NAc

Vibrio cholerae[35]

-2) - α - D - Rhap4N(3-deoxy - L -tetronic acid) - (1-

Escherichia hermannii[15,16]

-2) - α - D - Rhap4NAc - (1- . . . . -3) - α - D - Rhap4NAc - (1-   (1:5 and 1:6)

The *E. hermannii* strains described were those that gave serological cross-reaction with polyclonal *E. coli* O157 antisera but not with specific monoclonal *E. coli* O157 antisera. It is interesting that these *E. hermannii* LPS O-chains show a close structural similarity to the *Brucella* M antigens although the amino groups of the common α-D-Rhap4N residues are N-acetylated in the *E. hermannii* O-chains and N-formylated in the case of the *Brucella* M antigens, and the ratio of 1,2 to 1,3 glycosidic linkages varied among different isolates.

Summary

Chemical and physical analyses of the O-polysaccharide moieties of *Brucella* lipopolysaccharides (LPS) has shown that they are polymers of 4,6-dideoxy-4-formamido-α-D-mannopyranosyl (α-D-RhapNFo) residues and that the A and M antigenic expressions are related to the proportion of 1,2 and 1,3 linkages present in the unbranched linear O-chains. The SDS-PAGE analysis of the LPS and the analytical use of monoclonal antibodies of determined A and M specificities and inhibition studies using synthetic *Brucella* oligosaccharides, supports the conclusion that the A specificity resides in an essentially 1,2 linked sequence of α-D-Rhap4NFo residues whereas the epitope characteristic of the M antigen resides in a sequence involving a 1,3 linked α-D-RhapNFo residue abutted by 1,2 linked a-D-RhapNFo units.

Analysis of *Brucella* carbohydrate antigens termed native haptens (NH) revealed that these polymers were identical in all respects with the O-polysaccharides derived by mild acid hydrolysis of the homologous *Brucella* LPS. Analysis of a *Brucella* glycan, termed polysaccharide B (poly B, PB), revealed that this product was a family of nonreducing cyclic polymers of β-D-glucopyranosyl residues of an average ring size of 20 glycose units which showed a strong non-covalent binding with free *Brucella* LPS O-polysaccharides.

The serological cross-reactions between the *Brucella* LPS O-polysaccharides and the LPS of *Y. enterocolitica* O:9, *E. coli* O157, *E. hermannii*, *V. cholerae*, *P. maltophilia* 555, and *Salmonella* Group N (O:30) can be related to the occurrence of N-acylated derivatives of α-D-RhapN residues present in the repeating units of their respective LPS O-chains.

References

1. Wilson G. *Brucella. In:* Wilson G, Parker M, eds. *Principles of Bacteriology, Virology and Immunity.* London: Edward Arnold, 7th Ed. 1984;2:406-421.
2. Raybould PJ. Antigens of diagnostic significance in *Brucella abortus. Can J Microbiol* 1982;28:557-566.

3. Holman PJ, Schurig G, Douglas JT. Development of monoclonal antibodies to *Brucella* cell surface antigens. In: Macario AJL, Macario EC, eds. *Monoclonal Antibodies Against Bacteria*. Vol. II New York: Academic Press, 1985;389-393.
4. Moreno E, Speth SL, Jones LM, et al. Immunochemical characterization of *Brucella* lipopolysaccharides and polysaccharides. *Infect Immun* 1981;31:214-222.
5. McCullough NB. Identification of the species and biotypes within the genus *Brucella*. In: Bergan E, Norris JR, eds. *Methods of Microbiology*. New York: Academic Press, 1978;10:201-225.
6. Brucella Forum. *Ann Inst Pasteur Microbiol* 1987;138:27-148.
7. 3rd International Symposium on Brucellosis. Karger S, ed. *Devl biol Stand* 1983;56:1-779.
8. Diaz R, Jones LM, Leong Wilson JB. Surface antigens of smooth brucella. *J Bact* 1968;96:893-901.
9. Wilson GS, Miles AA. The serological differentiation of smooth strains of the *Brucella* group. *Br J Exp Path* 1932;13:1-13.
10. Miles AA, Pirie NW. The properties of antigenic preparations from *Brucella melitensis*: IV. The hydrolysis of the formamido linkage. *Biochem J* 1939;33:1709-1715.
11. Miles AA, Pirie NW. The properties of antigenic preparations from *Brucella melitensis*. V. Hydrolysis and acetylation of the amino-polyhydroxy compound derived from the antigen. *Biochem J* 1939;33:1716-1724.
12. Diaz R, Toyos J, Salvo S, et al. Studies on the polysaccharide B and native haptene of *Brucella* and *Yersinia entercolitica* serotype 9. *Dev Biol Stand* 1983;56:213-320.
13. Fernandez-Lago, Moriyon I, Toyos J, et al. Immunological identity of of *Brucella* native hapten, polysaccharide B, and *Yersinia enterocolitica* serotype 9 hapten. *Infect Immun* 1982;38:778-780.
14. Corbel MJ, Stuart FA, Brewer RA. Observations on serological cross-reactions between smooth *Brucella* species and organisms of other genera. *Dev biol Stand* 1984;56:341-348.
15. Borczyk AA, Lior H, Ciebin B. False positive identification of *Escherichia coli* O157 in foods. *Int J Food Microbiol* 1987;4:247-249.
16. Perry MB, Bundle DR, Gidney MAJ, et al. Identification of *Escherichia coli* O157 strains by using a monoclonal antibody. *J Clin Microbiol* 1988;26:2391-2394.
17. Cherwonogrodzky JW, Perry MB, Bundle DR. Identification of the A and M antigens of *Brucella* as the O-polysaccharides of smooth lipopolysaccharides. *Can J Microbiol* 1987;33:979-981.
18. Caroff M, Bundle DR, Perry MB, et al. Antigenic S-type lipopolysaccharide of *Brucella abortus* 1119-3. *Infect Immun* 1984;46:384-388.
19. Caroff M, Bundle DR, Perry MB. Structure of the O-chain of the phenol phase soluble cellular lipopolysaccharide of *Yersinia enterocolitica* O:9. *Eur J Biochem* 1984;139:195-200.
20. Bundle DR, Gidney MAJ, Perry MB, et al. Serological confirmation of *Brucella abortus* and *Y. enterocolitica* O:9 antigens by monoclonal antibodies. *Infect Immun* 1984;46:389-393.
21. Bundle DR, Cherwonogrodzky JW, Perry MB. Structural elucidation of the *Brucella melitensis* M antigen by high-resolution NMR at 500 MHz. *Biochemistry* 1987;26:8717-8726.
22. Meikle PJ, Perry MB, Cherwonogrodzky JC, et al. The fine structure of A and M antigens from *Brucella* Biovars. *Infect Immun* 1989;57:2870-2828.
23. Bundle DR, Cherwonogrodzky JC, Gidney MAJ, et al. Definition of *Brucella* A and M epitopes by monoclonal typing reagents and synthetic oligosaccharides. *Infect Immun* 1989;57:2829-2836.
24. Brisson JR, Perry MB. The structures of the two lipopolysaccharide O-chains produced by *Salmonella boecker*. *Biochem Cell Biol* 1988;66:1066-1077.

25. Di Fabio JL, Brisson JR, Perry MB. Structural analysis of the three lipopolysac-charides produced by *Salmonella madelia*. *Biochem Cell Biol* 1989;67:78-85.

26. Dubray G, Limet J. Evidence of heterogeneity of lipopolysaccharides among *Brucella* biovars in relation to A and M specificities. *Ann Inst Pasteur/Microbiol* 1987;138:27-37.

27. Peters T, Bundle DR. Synthetic antigenic determinants of the *Brucella* A polysac-charide: A disaccharide thioglycoside for block synthesis of pentasaccharide and lower homologues of a-1, 2 linked 4,6-dideoxy-4-formamido-a-$\underline{D}$-mannose. *Can J Chem* 1989;67:491-496.

28. Peters T, Bundle DR. Block synthesis of two determinants of the *Brucella* M antigen using thioglycoside methodologies. *Can J Chem* 1989;67:497-502.

29. Zygmunt MS, Dubray G, Bundle DR, et al. Purified native haptens of *Brucella abortus* B19 and *B. melitensis* 16M reveal the lipopolysaccharide origins of the antigens. *Ann Inst Pasteur/Microbiol* 1988;139:421-434.

30. Bundle DR, Cherwonogrodzky JW, Perry MB. Characterization of *Brucella* poly-saccharide B. *Infect Immun* 1988; 56:1101-1106.

31. Perry MB, MacLean L, Griffith DW. Structure of the O-chain of the phenol-phase soluble lipopolysaccharide of *Escherichia coli* O:157:H7. *Biochem Cell Biol* 1985;64:21-28.

32. Bundle DR, Gerken M, Perry MB. Two-dimensional nuclear magnetic resonance at 500 MHz: the structural elucidation of a *Salmonella* serogroup N polysaccharide antigen. *Can J Chem* 1986;64:255-264.

33. Perry MB, Bundle DR, MacLean L, et al. The structures of the antigenic lipopoly-saccharide O-chains produced by *Salmonella urbana* and *Salmonella godesberg*. *Carbohydr Res* 1986;156:107-122.

34. Di Fabio JL, Perry MB, Bundle DR. Analysis of the lipopolysaccharide of *Pseudomonas maltophilia* 555. *Biochem Cell Biol* 1987;65:968-977.

35. Keene L, Lindberg B, Unger P, et al. Structural studies of the *Vibrio cholerae* antigen. *Carbohydr Res* 1982;100:341-349.

Chapter Six

Membrane Proteins of
Brucella spp.

Blair A. Sowa

Why study the membrane proteins of the genus *Brucella*? Recent advances in molecular biology and biotechnology have focused attention on the role of bacterial outer membrane proteins as safer vaccines and more effective diagnostic reagents.[1] When one considers that the cell envelope is the site where host and pathogen do battle, it becomes evident that the molecular basis for many of the properties that make the Brucellae unique must be located on or in the outer membrane.

Survival in the host is dependent on the integrity of the bacterial membrane; once it is breached by the host the bacterium no longer survives. Host defenses can only act on exposed components of the membrane. Thus virulent *Brucella* are constantly undergoing strong selective pressure to maintain a membrane structure capable of resisting host defense mechanisms. Selective pressure on genes coding for internal or cytoplasmic proteins is bound to be less severe, since the environment for these proteins is enclosed and protected from the host by the bacterial membrane.

The bacterial membrane contains proteins and protein products, and we would expect to find located in this structure virulence factors and antigens that are unique to *Brucella*. Further understanding of virulence mechanisms may ultimately lead to methods of neutralization to provide protection against infection. Study of surface proteins may be expected to identify antigens which might be manipulated to stimulate protective immunity or simplify diagnosis. In the last 10 years numerous researchers have studied the membrane proteins of *Brucella* spp. and their findings are reviewed below.

The membrane composition of *Brucella* is often compared to that of *Escherichia coli*, as considerably more is known about this Gram-negative bacterium. Many excellent reviews of the Gram-negative cell envelope have been published and we are brought up to date by Robert Hancock in chapter four of these proceedings, *Function and Structure of the Major Components of the Outer Membrane*. The *E. coli* model is useful as a reference to describe how the Brucellae differ.

Studies of bacterial membrane proteins have traditionally begun with separation of the cell envelope (CE) into its component membranes, the outer membrane (OM) and the inner or cytoplasmic membrane (CM). The OM consists of a mixed bilayer; on the distal surface it is largely the lipid A portion of lipopolysaccharide (LPS) and on the proximal side it is phospholipid. The CM consists of a phospholipid bilayer. Sandwiched between the CM and OM are the periplasmic space and the peptidoglycan layer (PG) which is closely associated with the OM. Proteins, which may contain lipid and/or glycosyl adducts, are inserted into the OM and CM bilayers. LPS or endotoxin is anchored to the OM by insertion of the lipid A moiety into the distal surface of the OM bilayer which positions the O-antigen distal to the OM surface. Transmembrane pores that extend thru the OM are formed by trimers of porin proteins. Strong hydrophobic regions on these proteins serve to link the monomer into trimers and position them to span the OM bilayer. Also typically located in the OM are the lipoprotein and matrix protein(s).

In E. coli approximately 30% of the lipoprotein has been reported to be covalently bound to PG by the C-terminus while lipid moieties bound to the N-terminus to anchor it in the OM. This arrangement serves to secure the OM to the PG. The term matrix proteins typically refers to proteins that are present in large quantities in the OM and are believed to contribute to the structural integrity of the membrane. These may include proteins for which no other function is known, as well as porins. Functionally, the rigid OM-PG serves to protect the more vulnerable CM from osmotic and other environmental challenges.

In a review of membrane fractionation methods, Sarvas[2] notes that typically separation of OM from CM has been accomplished by the methods of differential centrifugation or particle electrophoresis. Of the two, differential centrifugation which makes use of differences in the buoyant density of OM and CM either before or after digestion of PG with lysozyme is the most rational. Particle electrophoresis relies on differences in surface charges of OM and CM to effect differential migration of disrupted membrane components in the influence of an electric field. Because of the need for specialized equipment it is used infrequently.

In reviews, Sarvas[2] and others[1,3] further note that differential solubilization in detergents has been used for the purpose of isolating specific OM or CM membrane proteins such as porins. Detergent solubilization seeks to exploit differences between OM and CM proteins and is based on empirical observations that some OM proteins resist solubilization in various detergents. Extraction of CM and non-porin OM proteins with detergent is highly variable and affected by complex interactions including protein to detergent ratio, temperature, duration of extraction, and salt concentration which affect detergent efficacy and concentration by altering critical micelle concentration. Thus reports of differential solubility of CM versus OM are highly dependent on the identity and ratios of the buffer salts and components as well as bacterial fractions. The observed differences are not consistent between species and the resulting preparations contain only a small fraction of the proteins originally contained in the OM or CM lipid bilayers; the lipids and a majority of non-porin membrane proteins are dissolved by such treatment. That one cannot obtain intact *Brucella* OM after using detergents was noted by Moriyón et al.[4]

In the last 10 years approximately a dozen studies describing the major outer membrane proteins of *Brucella* have been published. Because of early reports that lysozyme was incapable of reaching and digesting PG in intact *B. abortus* cells, researchers resorted to the less desirable methods of differential solubilization in detergents to attempt to obtain relatively pure preparations of outer membranes and the proteins contained therein. As a result, almost all of the studies have focused mainly on the porins and other highly hydrophobic proteins tightly associated with the PG. In reviewing these studies it is important to note that SDS-PAGE (sodium dodecylsulfate-polyacrylamide gel electrophoresis) technology which has enabled visualization of the complexity of the protein content of *Brucella* cell envelope fractions was undergoing continuous development and refinement during this time.

A Ten-Year Review

Early on, French researchers reported that SDS-insoluble sacculi composed of proteins and polysaccharides strongly bound to cell wall peptidoglycan from *Brucella* were capable of inducing reasonable protective immunity in mice,[5] guinea-pigs,[6] and farm animals.[7] Most likely as a result of these early reports, almost all studies on *B. abortus* membrane proteins have employed detergent solubilization to isolate OM proteins which bound strongly to PG. As a result, this small group of important OM proteins was studied in detail while other SDS-soluble OM proteins were largely ignored until recently.

In 1980 Dubray and Bezard[8] reported the isolation of three *B. abortus* cell wall antigens (Table 6-1) exhibiting molecular weights of 37 kilodalton (kDa) (band I), 25 kDa (band II), and 15 kDa (band III) on SDS-PAGE from lysozyme-treated peptidoglycan sacculi remaining after extraction of cell walls of *B. abortus* Strain 99 with boiling 4% SDS. They identified another minor band having an apparent molecular weight of 31 kDa in this preparation and reported that bands I and II were composed of multiple "subbands." Band I was reported to contain 40 kDa, 38 kDa, 37 kDa, and 34 kDa sub-bands, while band II was reported to contain 27 kDa, 26 kDa, 25 kDa, and 23 kDa sub-bands. When stained with carbocyanine dye, band I exhibited a red color indicative of protein, band II exhibited a blue color indicative of acidic glycoprotein, and band III showed a yellow color indicative of lipoprotein or lipid plus protein. Each of the three proteins was isolated from SDS-PAGE and was statistically not different from killed whole cells, PG sacculi, and PG sacculi after lysozyme treatment in ability to lower the number of viable *Brucella* found in spleens of challenged mice.[8]

Verstreate et al.[9] in 1982, reported three major groups of proteins from *B. abortus* strains S19, 2308, 45/20, C-10, and Y having similarity to structural outer membrane proteins of *E. coli*. Using SDS-PAGE of lysozyme-treated cell envelopes previously extracted with N-laurylsarcosinate and dipolar ionic detergent, they demonstrated the presence of three outer membrane proteins having apparent molecular weights of 94 kDa (group 1), 41 and 43 kDa (group 2), and 30 kDa (group 3). Separated by column chromatography, the zwitergent-solubilized group 2 proteins displayed heat modifiability and amino acid composition comparable to *E. coli* OmpF. Group 3 proteins exhibited no altered migration on SDS-PAGE after heating but had amino acid composition similar to that of *E. coli* OmpA. Hydrophobicity of group 2 proteins was 892 ± 30 calories/mole and 980 ± 54 calories/mole for the group 3 proteins. Calculated polarity index of 42% for both groups of proteins agreed with published values of outer membrane proteins from other gram-negative bacteria.

In the same year Moriyón and Berman[10] demonstrated that, in contrast to *E. coli*, cell envelope proteins and/or LPS of *B. abortus* 1119.3, 45/20 and *B. melitensis* B115 were resistant to extraction with nonionic detergents after attempted destabilization by chelation of divalent cations with ethylene diamine tetracetic acid (EDTA). They further demonstrated that EDTA-lysozyme spheroplasts were not formed in *Brucella* and concluded that, in contrast to *E. coli*, *Brucella* LPS and membrane proteins are not stabilized by divalent cations. They postulated that the observed resistance to nonionic detergent extraction could be due to the unusually high concentration of long-chain fatty acids in the *Brucella* membrane. Through the use of the more efficient ionic detergents, sarcosinate and zwittergent 3-16, they were able to extract some but not all proteins from the envelopes of cells surface labeled with ^{125}I by the lactoperoxidase method. Autoradiography of an SDS-PAGE gel containing extrinsically labeled *Brucella* contained 23 to 25 sarcosinate resistant bands.

Working with peptidogylcan sacculi prepared by extracting cell envelopes (5 mg protein) in 1 ml 0.7% SDS (SDS:protein = 1.4:1) at 50°C, Moriyón and Berman in 1983[11] identified a 38-kDa matrix protein in *B. abortus* strains 45/20 and 1119.3 which was tightly associated with PG and yielded a V8 protease map containing some peptides of similar molecular weights to those obtained from *E. coli* K-12 matrix protein. Apparent molecular weight of matrix protein from 45/20 was reported to be somewhat less than that from 1119.3 on SDS-PAGE, but similar V8 protease patterns were obtained from each of these proteins. Using extrinsic ^{125}I lactoperoxidase labeling, they demonstrated that the matrix protein in both the rough and smooth strains was exposed to the *B. abortus* surface. They concluded that this 38-kDa matrix protein and the group 2 cluster identified by Verstreat et al.[9] were the same.

Dubray and Charriaut[12] in 1983 elaborated on earlier work and identified, by SDS-PAGE of lysozyme-treated PG sacculi of *B. abortus* Strain 99, two major groups of three proteins each, having molecular weights of 38, 37, and 36 kDa and 27, 26, and 25 kDa. In SDS-PAGE of cell walls previously extracted with 2% triton, they observed an additional major band exhibiting a molecular mass of 40 kDa and 39 additional outer membrane proteins present in lesser quantities. They concluded that the CE of *Brucella* contained at least these 40 SDS-soluble proteins as well as the two groups of PG bound proteins.

In the following year Douglas et al.[13] working with *B. abortus* Strains 19, 2308, 45/20 and 1119.3, *B. melitensis* Strain B115, and *B. canis* Strain RM666, demonstrated in vitro porin activity by the incorporation of group 2 proteins (approximately 37-42 kDa) in liposomes composed of egg phospholipids. Liposomes containing a mixture of group 2 proteins exhibited porin activity in both a swelling assay employing isotonic sugar solution and an assay based on the eflux of radiolabeled dextran and oligosaccharide. Similarly isolated group 3 proteins did not exhibit porin activity in these assays. Swelling rates obtained from group 2 proteins ranked from fastest to slowest as follows: *B. canis, B. abortus* S19, 1119.3, 2308, 45/20 and *B. melitensis*. The rates observed demonstrated a strong dependence on molecular size; the group 2 protein of *B. canis* being clearly larger than the rest. However the *B. abortus* and *B. melitensis* preparations contained mixtures of at least three group 2 proteins and the relative contribution of each of these was not assessed. Similar V8 protease maps obtained from group 2 proteins from *B. abortus* strains 45/20 and 2308 indicated that the multiple bands represented forms of a single protein.

The following year Santos, Verstreate, Perera, and Winter[14] compared the major PG bound outer membrane proteins of 15 rough and two smooth strains of *B. abortus, B. canis, B. ovis,* and *B. melitensis* using SDS-PAGE. Lysozyme digestion was used to solubilize proteins remaining attached to PG after extraction of crude membranes with either Triton X-100 or sodium deoxycholate. In *B. abortus, B. ovis,* and *B canis,* three protein groups were observed as follows: group 1, average molecular weight 94 to 88 kDa; group 2, average molecular weight 39-35 kDa; and group 3, average molecular weight 31-25 kDa; *B. melitensis* contained a protein band at 48 kDa in addition to proteins from groups 1, 2, and 3. Verstreate and Winter[15] in a comparison of outer membrane SDS-PAGE profiles from 49 *B. abortus* strains observed the following three groups of proteins to be present in all strains: group 1, 94-88 kDa; group 2, 40-35 kDa; and group 3, 30-25 kDa. Gómez-Miguel and Moriyón[16] identified an 8-kDa fragment obtained by treating SDS-extracted PG sacculi with trypsin. The fragment was reported to have a molecular weight and isoelectric point similar to the Braun lipoprotein of *E. coli*, to have similar amino acid composition, and to contain both ester- and amide-linked fatty acids.

Exploiting the observation that periplasmic and non-porin outer membrane proteins may be extracted from bacteria by saline extraction, Tabatabai and Deyoe[17] use HPLC to identify 12 *B. abortus* membrane-associated proteins which ranged in molecular mass from 10 to 51 kDa. These soluble proteins were demonstrated to be antigenic in guinea pigs, rabbits, and cattle and immunogenic in lemmings, guinea pigs, and cattle. All but the 14.5-kDa molecular weight protein were most likely periplasmic, as only the 14.5 kDa protein contained label when surface-labeled *B. abortus* cells were extracted with saline. Mayfield et al.[18] isolated and cloned the gene for the 31-kDa protein from this group, BCSP31, superoxide dismutase from *B. abortus* Strain 19, and expressed it in *E. coli*. From a partial N-terminal amino acid sequences and from amino acid sequence predicted by the DNA sequence, the protein is predicted to be slightly basic, to contain 24% alanine plus glycine, and to have no major hydrophobic segments.

Ficht et al.[19] through the use of an λgt11 expression library and oligonucleotide probe specific for the N-terminal end of an SDS-soluble 36 kDa major OM protein, identified and cloned from *B. abortus* two homologous genes tentatively named *omp2b* and *omp2a* which respectively encode 36 kDa and 33 kDa group 2 proteins. The predicted amino acid compositions are similar to that reported by Verstreate for the group 2 porins. The predicted gene products of *omp2b* and *omp2a* were identical over the first 100 amino acids including a 22-amino acid signal sequence and differed primarily by a 108-nucleotide deletion from the smaller. The authors postulated that these genes might represent an active and a silent or cryptic porin gene, or two active porin genes which are expressed under different environmental conditions.

Table 6-1 contains a summary of the *Brucella* outer membrane protein isolations described above. With the few exceptions noted, the majority of proteins identified were tightly associated with peptidoglycan and were released only after lysozyme treatment. In most cases, the cell envelope preparation was disrupted and partially solubilized prior to analysis through the use nonionic or ionic detergents in an attempt to differentially remove CM and its associated proteins.

An Alternative Approach

Seeking to avoid OM bilayer destabilization and protein losses associated with differential detergent solubilization of CM, we attempted to obtain intact CE from sonically disrupted *B. abortus* by a modification

Table 6-1. Synopsis of Outer Membrane Proteins Identified from
Brucella Species During the Last 10 Years.

Author	group 1	band I group 2	band II group 3	band III low MW
Dubray '80		37k*	25k*	15k*
Verstreate '82	94k	43,* 41k*	30k*	
Moriyon '82	88k	38k	30k	
Moriyon '83	88k	38k*		
Dubray '83	94k	43k, 38,* 37,* 36k*	31,* 27,* 26,* 25k*	
Douglass '84		37-42k*	26k*	
Santos '84	94-88k*	39-35k*	31-25k*	
Verstreate '84	94-88k*	40-38*	30-25*	
Gómez-Miguel '86				8k*§
Mayfield '88			31k‡	
Ficht '88		36k		

*released from protein-peptidoglycan sacculi by lysozyme
§tryptic fragment
‡salt extracted, most likely periplasmic

of the method of Lutkenhaus.[20]

However, we were unable to further fractionate the pellet obtained, and several methods of analysis lead to the conclusion that the modified Lutkenhaus procedure when applied to *B. abortus* yields only an OM-PG (outer membrane-peptidoglycan) complex. The most compelling data supporting this argument are that the Lutkenhaus preparation OM-PG complex pellet is identical to the OM-PG buoyant in 55% sucrose obtained by density gradient centrifugation of sonicated whole *B. abortus* cells (Figure 6-1). As expected, the whole lysate contained cytosolic proteins in

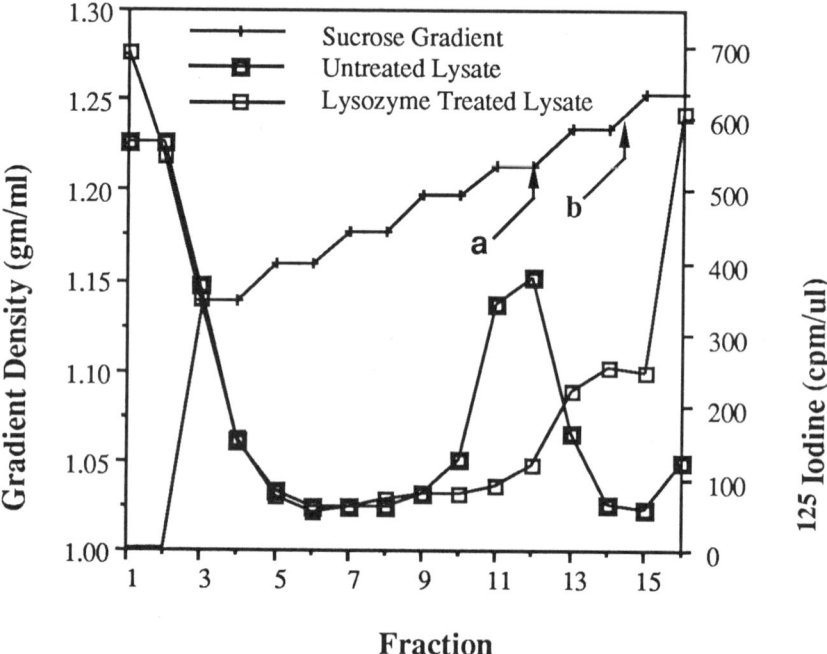

Figure 6-1. Distribution of ^{125} Iodine from Sonically Disrupted Surface-Labeled *B. abortus* RB51 Cells in a 35 to 65% Sucrose Density Gradient. Notes: a = buoyant density of pellet from Lutkenhaus preparation, b = buoyant density of pellet from Lutkenhaus prepation after lysozyme treatment.

the sample application buffer and a CM band exhibiting a density of 1.15 gm/ml, as well as a denser OM-PG band. The Lutkenhaus preparation contained only the dense band. When treated with lysozyme, both the Lutkenhaus pellet and the OM-PG band obtained by density gradient centrifugation increased to a buoyant density equal to 60-65% sucrose (1.25 gm/ml) and banded as a single layer having the same SDS-PAGE profile (Sowa et al., submitted for publication). The density values obtained for the CM and OM are in reasonable agreement with those obtained for *Salmonella typhimurium*[21] and no evidence of CM proteins was observed in the Lutkenhaus preparations. A reasonable explanation for this is presented in the review of membrane fractionation procedures by Sarvas[2] who states:

> Sonication extensive enough to disrupt most Gram-negative bacteria also breaks the CM into very small vesicles, which are not pelleted by high speed ultracentrifugation (>200,000 x g) even for several hours. The OM-peptidoglycan complex remains after sonication mainly as large, easily sedimentable fragments and vesicles.

Sonication followed by differential centrifugation has been used to obtain small quantities of OM which are essentially free of CM.[22,23] Considering the severity of sonication required to lyse *B. abortus*, it is not surprising that the CM fraction was absent from the Lutkenhaus preparation and that relatively pure OM-PG are obtained from *B. abortus* by this method.

When OM-PG obtained from unlabeled as well as surface biotinylated cells were analyzed by SDS-PAGE (Figure 6-2) or western blot (Figure 6-3), at least 67 SDS-soluble OM proteins were visible in the O-antigen deficient strain without the use of lysozyme. The identification of this number of SDS-soluble proteins in addition to eight PG-bound proteins (Figure 6-4) in the OM reflects the isolation procedure used and is in agreement with current knowledge of the protein population of the OM of *E. coli*.[24] Present in major amounts were single bands exhibiting apparent molecular weights of 88 kDa (I), 36 kDa (IIB), and 26 kDa (III) daltons corresponding to previously described proteins belonging to groups 1, 2, and 3, as well as a major protein (IIA) having a molecular weight of 40 kDa (Figure 6-2). When strains 2308 and 19 were compared, greater amounts of two low molecular weight proteins of 8.8 kDa and 7.5 kDa were observed in the virulent strain. Differences in molecular weights of several OM proteins observed in the rough versus the smooth strains were no longer apparent when SDS-PAGE was loaded with minimal amounts of protein and visualized with silver stain. It was concluded that the rough versus smooth differences observed in conventionally loaded Coomassie Brilliant Blue stained SDS-PAGE were artifacts induced by the presence of large amount of LPS (Sowa et al., submitted).

We also noted that no additional forms of group 2 or group 3 proteins could be extracted from the Lutkenhaus OM preparations by exhaustive

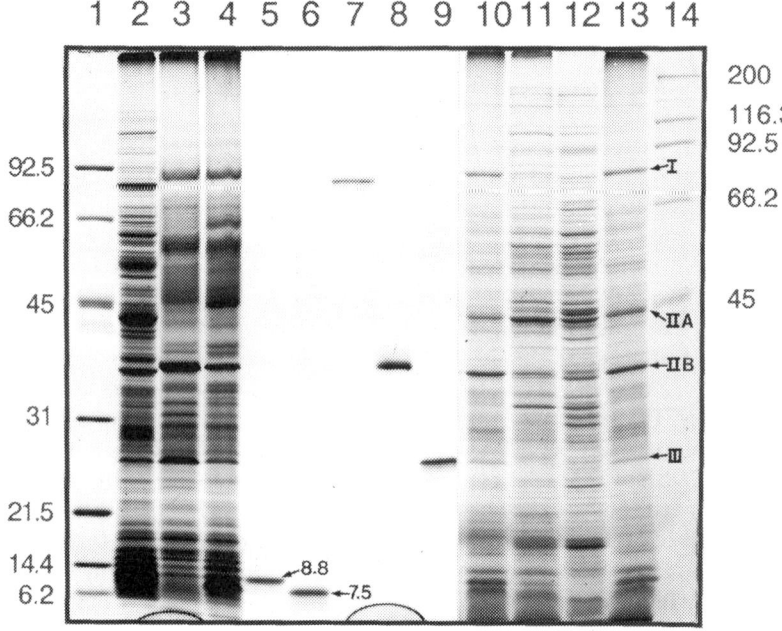

Figure 6-2. SDS-PAGE of OM-PG Obtained from *B. abortus* Strains RB51, 19, and 2308,Lanes 2, 3, and 4 Respectively (40 ug of Protein was Loaded in Each Lane). Also shown are purified Baom 8.8 kd (lane 5), Baom 7.5 (lane 6), BaomI (lane7), BaomIIB (lane 8), BaomIII (lane 9). Lanes 10 and 13 contain OM-PG pellet (18 ug protein) obtained from RB51 by the Lutken-haus method, while lanes 11 and 12 contain respectively the cytosolic and CM membrane fractions remaining after this isolation.

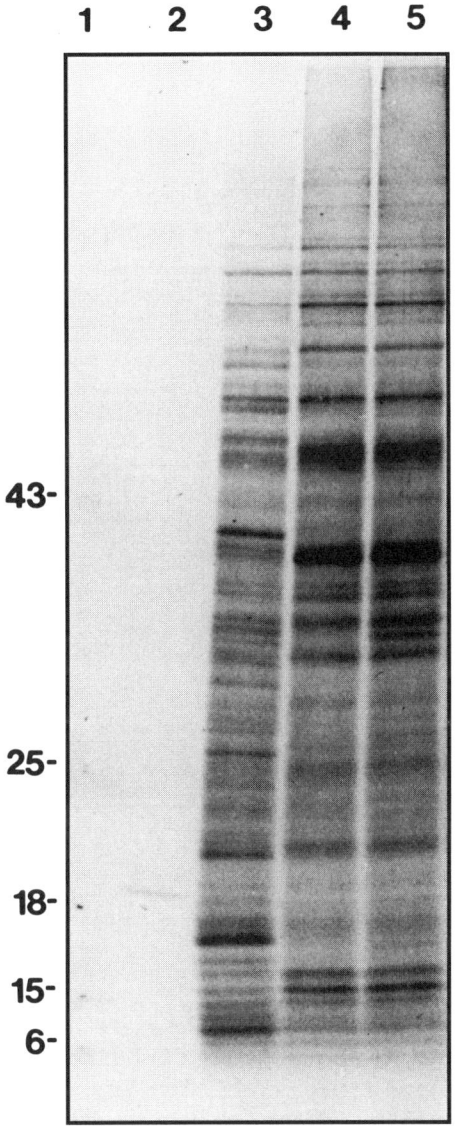

Figure 6-3. Alkaline Phosphatase Stained Western Blot of SDS-PAGE of Surface Biotinylated RB51 Cells. Lanes contain: 1) Prestained molecular mass standards, 2) unlabeled control, 3) surface biotinylated whole cells, 4) OM-PG prepared from surface biotinylated cells, 5) lysozyme treated OM-PG from surface biotinylated whole cells.

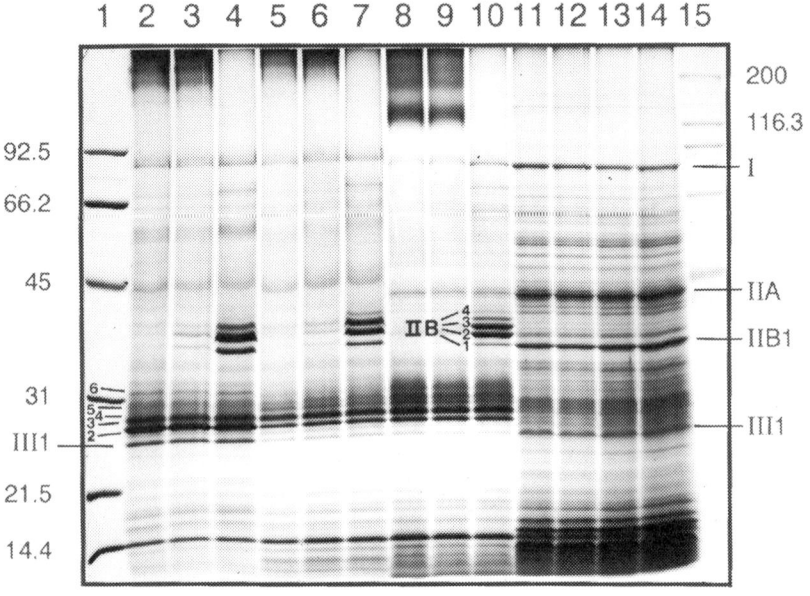

Figure 6-4. SDS-PAGE of SDS-Soluble Versus PG-Bound Proteins. Lanes 2, 3, and 4 contain lysozyme treated OM-PG from Strain 19. Lane 2 was heated to 50°C, lane 3 to 75°C, and lane 4 to 100°C in SDS-PAGE sample buffer. Lanes 5, 6 and 7 contain lysozyme treated OM-PG from strain 2308 heated at 50°, 75°, and 100°C respectively. Lanes 8, 9, and 10 contain lysozyme treated OM-PG from strain RB51 heated at 50°, 75° and 100°C respectively. Lanes 11 thru 14 contain OM-PG without lysozyme treatment from strain RB51 after boiling in SDS-PAGE sample buffer for 5, 10, 30, and 60 minutes respectively.

virulent strain. Differences in molecular weights of several OM proteins observed in the rough versus the smooth strains were no longer apparent when SDS-PAGE was loaded with minimal amounts of protein and visualized with silver stain. It was concluded that the rough versus smooth differences observed in conventionally loaded Coomassie Brilliant Blue stained SDS-PAGE were artifacts induced by the presence of large amount of LPS (Sowa et al., submitted).

We also noted that no additional forms of group 2 or group 3 proteins could be extracted from the Lutkenhaus OM preparations by exhaustive boiling in SDS-PAGE sample buffer containing 0.25M NaCl. However, when the PG sacculi remaining after exhaustive extraction with SDS-PAGE sample buffer were treated with lysozyme, three additional group 2 proteins and five additional group 3 proteins were released. Additional treatment with lysozyme did not alter the number or relative proportions of these proteins. When examined on SDS-PAGE, the group 3 proteins were solubilized equally well by SDS-PAGE sample buffer at 50°, 75°, and 100°C, but the group 2 proteins remained as higher molecular weight polymers unless they were heated to 100°C. They then exhibited molecular weights of 36.7 kDa, 37.7 kDa, and 39 kDa (Sowa et al., submitted).

Nomenclature

The conclusions presented in the following section regarding post-translational modifications of the *B. abortus* outer membrane proteins based on specific DNA and amino acid sequence data published[19] and submitted for publication, mandated assignment of unambiguous names to the outer membrane proteins. In the absence of any consistent precedent,[1] and until some proteins are more appropriately named to reflect function, we propose the use of the prefix name of Baom (*B. abortus* outer membrane [protein]) followed by either a molecular weight, or in the case of the previously named groups, a Roman numeral, as first used by Dubray,[8] to indicate the group number.

Where needed to positively identify different forms of the same protein, we have employed the standard convention for outlining. Thus, the 94-88kDa proteins (group 1) are named BaomI, the 36-40kDa proteins (group 2) are named BaomIIA, and BaomIIB1-4 and the 26-30kDa proteins (group 3) are named BaomIII1-6. This nomenclature permits sufficient sub-classification to encompass the observed post translational products Baoms IIB2-4 and Baoms III2-6 described below, as well as providing a system of nomenclature for homologous genes and gene products which may be expressed in response to environmental conditions as has been postulated by Ficht et al.[19] (Chapter 3) for the tentatively named *omp2b* and *omp2a* copies of the porin gene. Thus, the gene coding for the porin protein

BaomIIB is *baomIIBb* and the partially homologous "silent" or unexpressed gene is tentatively named *baomIIBa* until evidence for its expression is found.

Post-translational Processing

Amino acid sequences of the major SDS-soluble and PG-linked OM proteins obtained by automated Edman degradation of N-termini and CNBr fragments (Table 6-2) demonstrated that the BaomIIB1-4 group consisted of one SDS-soluble and three additional PG-bound proteins encoded by the tentatively named *omp2b* gene. No evidence for expression of the shorter *omp2a* gene was seen in the amino acid sequences obtained by us or others included in Table 6-2 for comparison. The three PG-linked forms exhibited blocked N-termini. No evidence of immature BaomIIB protein containing uncleaved signal peptide was found in the OM-PG preparation.

Similarly, by determining amino acid sequences of N-termini and of CNBr fragments, BaomIII1-6 were found to consist of six forms of a single protein; the smallest being SDS-soluble, not bound to PG, and possessing a free N-terminus. The additional five were PG-linked and contained blocked N-termini. We postulated that BaomIIB1 and BaomIII1 are N-terminally modified and covalently linked to PG in a series of post-translational modifications (Sowa et al., submitted for publication). We are currently working to determine if the bond to PG occurs at the N-terminal end of these proteins or at the C-terminus as in the case of the *E. coli* lipoprotein. Efforts are underway to determine the chemical identity of the N-terminal and possible C-terminal adducts responsible for the formation of BaomIIB2-4 and BaomIII2-6 and to determine if the enzymes responsible for these modifications respond to environmental conditions such as media composition and osmolarity.

In conclusion, having obtained a relatively quick and efficient method to purify *B. abortus* OM, we are currently engaged in examining this structure and its protein components for their ability to stimulate protective immunity in cattle. Preliminary vaccine challenge experiments have indicated that the intact OM-PG complex can stimulate significant protective immunity. We are currently evaluating individual OM-PG proteins for their ability to stimulate immunity and ultimately for incorporation into safer and more effective biosynthetic vaccines.

Table 6-2. Partial Amino Sequences and Homologies of *B. abortus* Membrane Proteins.

Protein, Source Strains	Sequence (N→C)

- Determined amino acid sequences (Sowa BA, et al, submitted for publication)

  SDS-Soluble

BaomI,	2308,RB51	AVVSRIEVRGNTRVDAQTI
BaomIIA,	2308,RB51	blocked
BaomIIB1,	2308	ADAIVAPEPEAVEYVRVCDAYGAGYFYIPGTET-LRV-GYVRYDVKGGDDVY
BaomIII1,	2308	ADAIQEQPPVPAPVEVAPQY
Baom8.8,	2308	?EASEKLGKLEEKI
Baom7.5,	2308	AEANINDIQQALEKQIAEMRTTLKGMI

  SDS-Soluble - CNBr Fragments

BaomIIA,	12.0 kDa, RB51	FGKLLVQ
BaomIIA,	18.0 kDa, RB51	blocked
BaomIIB1,	24.8 kDa, RB51	ADAIVAPEPEAVEY
BaomIIB1,	14.5 kDa, RB51	PDVVGGLKYAGG-GSI--V
BaomIII1,	6.0 kDa, 2308	PYLTAGIAGSQIKLN

  Peptidoglycan Linked

BaomIIB2,	RB51	blocked
BaomIIB3,	RB51	blocked
BaomIIB4,	RB51	blocked

  Peptidoglycan Linked - CNBr Fragments

BaomIIB2,	27.8 kDa, RB51	blocked
BaomIIB3,	27.0 kDa, RB51	blocked
BaomIIB4,	26.0 kDa, RB51	blocked
BaomIIB2,	14.5 kDa, RB51	PDVVGGLKYAGG-GSIAGVVAYDSV--E--AKVR-D--I
BaomIIB3,	14.5 kDa, RB51	PDVVGGL-YAGG--SI
BaomIIB4,	14.5 kDa, RB51	PDVVGGL-YAGG-GSIAGVVAYDSV
BaomIII6,	6.0 kDa, 2308	PYLTAGIAGSQIKLN

- Determined and <u>predicted</u> aa sequence (Mayfield JE, et al, 1988)[18]

  Periplasmic

BCSP31,	S19, N-term→	QAPTFF<u>RIGTFFTAGTVVPIGGLI...301</u>

- Determined and <u>predicted</u> aa sequences (Ficht TA, et al, 1989[19] and Sowa BA, et al, submitted)

omp2a,	S19,2308, N-term→	<u>ADAIVAPEPEAVEYVRVCDAYGAGYFYIPGTETCLRVHGYVRYDVKGGDDVY...</u>
omp2b,	S19,2308, N-term→	ADAIVAPEPEAVEYVRVCDAYGAGYFYIPGTET<u>CLRVHGYVRYDVKGGDDVY...</u>
omp2a,	...176(met)→	<u>PHVVGGLKYAGGWGSIAGVVAYDSVIEEWATKVRGDVNIT...299</u>
		|*||||||||||||||||||||||||*||||||||
omp2b,	...217(met)→	<u>PDVVGGLKYAGGWGSIAGVVAYDSVIEEWAAKVRGDVNIT...340</u>

  CNBr Frags from above

		||||||||||||-||||||||||||||--|--||||-|--|
BaomIIB1,	14.5 kDa	PDVVGGLKYAGG-GSI--V
BaomIIB2,	14.5 kDa	PDVVGGLKYAGG-GSIAGVVAYDSV--E--AKVR-D--I
BaomIIB3,	14.5 kDa	PDVVGGL-YAGG--SI
BaomIIB4,	14.5 kDa	PDVVGGL-YAGG-GSIAGVVAYDSV

Notes: Amino acids without underlining were determined by Edman degradation, underlined amino acids were predicted from DNA sequences, vertical lines (|) indicate homology, asterisks (*) indicate lack of homology, hyphens (-) indicate undetermined amino acids, question marks (?) indicate an unidentified adduct or uncommon amino acid.

Acknowledgments: I thank Katherine Kelly and Jan Patterson for their excellent technical assistance. I also thank Garry Adams and the other members and advocates of the bovine brucellosis research team at Texas A&M University for their cooperation and collaboration; for as is increasingly true of a great deal of biological research, the work described herein was greatly facilitated by the team approach. Support was provided in part by Texas Agricultural Experiment Station H-6194 funds and grants AG1001 from the Texas Advanced Technology Research Program and 58-6125-5-4 from the USDA/ARS/NADC.

References

1. Smyth CJ. Immunology of outer membrane proteins of gram-negative bacteria. In: *Immunology of the Bacterial Cell Envelope* eds. Stuart-Tull, DES and Davies, M. New York: John Wiley & Sons, 1985;177-201.

2. Sarvas M. Membrane fractionation methods. In: eds. Korhonen TK, EA Dawes, PH Mäkelä. *Enterobacterial Surface Antigens: Methods For Molecular Characterization.* Elsevier Science Publishers, Biomedical Div, 1985;111-122.

3. Hancock REW. Model membrane studies of porin function. In: ed. Inouye M. *Bacterial Outer Membranes as Model Systems,* New York: John Wiley & Sons, 1986;188-189.

4. Moriyón I, Gamazo C, Díaz R. Properties of the outer membrane of *Brucella*. *Ann Inst Pasteur* (Microbiol) 1987;138:89-91.

5. Dubray G, Bosseray N, Plommet M. Propriétés vaccinales de fractions de *Brucella*. C R Acad Sci (Paris) 1974;277:2281-1808.

6. Bosseray N. Immunity to Brucella in mice vaccinated with a fraction (F8) or a killed vaccine (H38) with or without adjuvant. Level and duration of immunity in relation to dose of vaccine, recall injection and age of mice. *Br J Exp Pathol* 1978;59:354-365.

7. Plommet M, Bosseray N. Le contrôle des vaccins antibrucelliques par dénombrement des *Brucella* dans la rate de souris, vaccinées ou non, innocullées par voi intrapéritonéale. *J Biol Stand* 1977;5:261-274.

8. Dubray G, Bezard G. Isolation of three *Brucella abortus* cell-wall antigens protective in murine experimental brucellosis. *Ann Rech Vet* 1980;11:367-373.

9. Verstreate DR, Creasy MT, Caveney NT, Baldwin CL, Blab MW, Winter AJ. Outer membrane proteins of *Brucella abortus*: Isolation and characterization. *Infect Immun* 1982;35:979-989.

10. Moriyón I, Berman, DT. Effects of nonionic, ionic and dipolar ionic detergents and EDTA on the *Brucella* cell envelope. *J Bacteriol* 1982;152:822-828.

11. Moriyón I, Berman, DT. Isolation, purification and partial characterization of *Brucella abortus* matrix protein. *Infect Immun* 1983;39:394-402.

12. Dubray G, Charriaut C. Evidence of three major polypeptide species and two major polysaccharide species in the *Brucella* outer membrane. *Ann Rech Vet* 1983;14:311-318.

13. Douglass J, Rosenberg E, Nikaido H, Verstreate D, Winter AJ. Porins of *Brucella* species. *Infect Immun* 1984;44:16-21.

14. Santos JM, Verstreate DR, Perera VY, Winter AJ. Outer membrane proteins from rough strains of four *Brucella* species. *Infect Immun* 1984;46:188-194

15. Verstreate DR, Winter AJ. Comparison of sodium dodecyl sulfate-polyacrylamide gel electrophoresis profiles and antigenic relatedness among outer membrane proteins of 49 *Brucella abortus* strains. *Infect Immun* 1984;46:182-187.

16. Gómez-Miguel MJ, Moriyón I. Demonstration of a peptidoglycan-linked lipoprotein and characterization of its trypsin fragment in the outer membrane of *Brucella* spp. *Infect Immun.* 1986;53:678-684.

17. Tabatabai LB, Deyoe BL. Biochemical and biological properties of soluble protein preparations from *Brucella abortus*. 3rd International Symposium on Brucellosis, Algiers, Algeria, *Develop biol Std* 1983;56:199-211.

18. Mayfield JE, Bricker BJ, Godfrey H, Crosby RM, Knight DJ, Halling SM, Balinsky D, Tabatabai LB. The cloning, expression, and nucleotide sequence of a gene coding for an immunogenic *Brucella abortus* protein. *Gene* 1988;63:1-9.

19. Ficht TA, Bearden SW, Sowa BA, Adams LG. DNA sequence and expression of the 36-kilodalton outer membrane protein gene of *Brucella abortus*. *Infect Immun* 1989;57:3281-3291.

20. Lutkenhaus JF. Role of a major outer membrane protein in *Escherichia coli*. *J Bacteriol* 1977;131:631-637.

21. Osborn MJ, Gander JE, Parisi E, Carson J. Mechanism of assembly of the outer membrane of *Salmonella typhimurium*. *J Biol Chem* 1972;247:3962-3972.

22. Crowlsmith I, Gamon K, Henning U. Precursor proteins are intermediates *in vivo* in the synthesis of two major outer membrane proteins, the OmpA and OmpF proteins, of *Escherichia coli* K12. *Eur J Biochem* 1981;113:375-380.

23. Palva ET. Major outer membrane protein in *Salmonella typhimurium* induced by maltose. *J Bacteriol* 1978;136:286-294.

24. Mizushima S. Assembly of membrane proteins. In: Inouye M. *Bacterial Outer Membranes as Model Systems* ed. New York: John Wiley & Sons, 1986;63-185.

25. Smyth CJ. Immunology of outer membrane proteins of gram-negative bacteria. In: Stuart-Tull, DES, Davies, M. *Immunology of the Bacterial Cell Envelope* eds. New York: Johh Wiley & Sons, 1985;177-201.

PART THREE

PATHOGENESIS AND HOST-PARASITE INTERACTIONS OF BRUCELLOSIS

Chapter Seven

Salmonella: A Model to Study Intracellular Parasitism

B. Brett Finlay
and Stanley Falkow

Diseases caused by *Salmonella* species (salmonellosis) pose major health problems throughout the world. In the United States, *Salmonella* infections account for 40,000 reported cases, 500 deaths and health care costs exceeding $50 billion annually.[1] It is thought that the number of un-reported cases is nearly ten-fold greater than those reported. Salmonel-losis is a serious disease in immunosuppressed patients and, with more im-munocompromised individuals (including AIDS and bone marrow trans-plant patients) appearing in hospitals setting, the number of non-typhoid *Salmonella* infections is rising.[2] Given the morbidity and mortality of salmonellosis, it is unfortunate that so little is known about the virulence factors of *Salmonella*. [3,4]

Salmonella bacteria are considered facultative intracellular parasites. Most *Salmonella* infections arise from oral ingestion of tainted food or water. After passing through the stomach, viable bacteria proceed to the distal small bowel and interact with the intestinal mucosa.[5] The bacteria subsequently enter the intestinal epithelial cells within a membrane-bound inclusion.[6] Once inside, the bacteria can replicate and pass through (transcytose)[7] the enterocytes to enter the underlying lamina propria. Within the lamina propria, the *Salmonella* first encounter cells of the reticuloendothelial system including macrophages and polymorphonuclear leucocytes. These cells can ingest the *Salmonella*, but, in the case of macrophages, do not necessarily kill the bacteria. In some cases, infected macrophages migrate to the regional lymph nodes, where the *Salmonella* replicate further before escaping these cells and entering the blood to disseminate throughout the body.

Very little is known about how *Salmonella* species enter into eukar-yotic cells, and once inside, how *Salmonella* responds to the new intracel-lular environment it encounters. It has been suggested that non-invasive *Salmonella* are avirulent,[8] indicating the importance of the ability to invade cells. The recent development of several *in vitro* model systems has provided new tools to dissect this host-parasite interaction at the molecular and cellular level.

Tissue Culture Model Systems

Several workers have used *in vitro* tissue culture monolayers to examine bacterial interactions with eukaryotic cells, including bacterial invasion (or entry).[9,10] These systems have the advantage of consistency and are easier to use than primary isolates of eukaryotic cells. We have used tissue culture models to study *Salmonella* interactions with eukaryotic cells, especially epithelial cells.[7,11-15] *Salmonella* species can invade MDCK (Madin Darby canine kidney epithelial cells), HEp-2 (human larynx epithelial cells), CACO-2 (human intestinal epithelial cells) and CHO (Chinese hamster ovary fibroblast cells) cells in a manner similar to that described for bacterial entry into the intestinal epithelium.[6] These bacteria initially adhere to the tips of the microvilli (Figure 7-1a), and enter into the cells in a membrane bound inclusion (Figure 7-1b). *Salmonella*-infected epithelial cells subsequently lose their microvilli[7] (Figure 7-1b).

Salmonella species replicate within cultured epithelial cells[12,13] (Figure 7-2). By using various inhibitors and mutant cell lines it has been demonstrated that endosome acidification is not required for bacterial entry or intracellular replication.[12] In contrast, a low pH of the endosome is essential for entry of enveloped viruses and many bacterial toxins. Microfilaments but not microtubules are required for bacterial entry.[12-14]

Although growth of tissue culture cells on plastic supports permits the study of bacterial entry, it does not conceivably permit the examination of later intracellular events such as penetration through the cell and exit to the opposite surface, processes essential to *Salmonella* penetration of the intestinal epithelium. To facilitate study of these processes, we have used polarized monolayers of MDCK and CACO-2 epithelial cells grown on filters[7] (Figure 7-1c). Such polarized monolayers of cells mimic an epithelial barrier;[16] they have defined apical (top) and basolateral (bottom) surfaces separated by tight junctions, and are impermeable to molecules as small as ions. Within four hours of addition, *S. choleraesuis* can pass through (transcytose) the apical surface of this epithelial barrier and enter the medium bathing the basolateral surface, reaching a maximal rate of 14 bacteria/MDCK cell/hour after nine hours.[7] However, when the intracellular trafficking of these bacteria is monitored, most of the intracellular organisms remain within the monolayer.[14] A small percentage (8.7%) exit to the apical surface, while only 1.3% transcytose and enter the basolateral medium eight hours after infection.

Although other *Salmonella* species, including *S. typhimurium* and *S. enteritidis* behaved similarly to *S. choleraesuis* in this system, non-invasive *E. coli*, which were added to the same epithelial cell samples, do not penetrate the tissue culture cells. *S. choleraesuis* bound as much as 100 times more efficiently to the apical surface than the basolateral surface of cells, perhaps indicating a concentration of specific bacterial receptors at

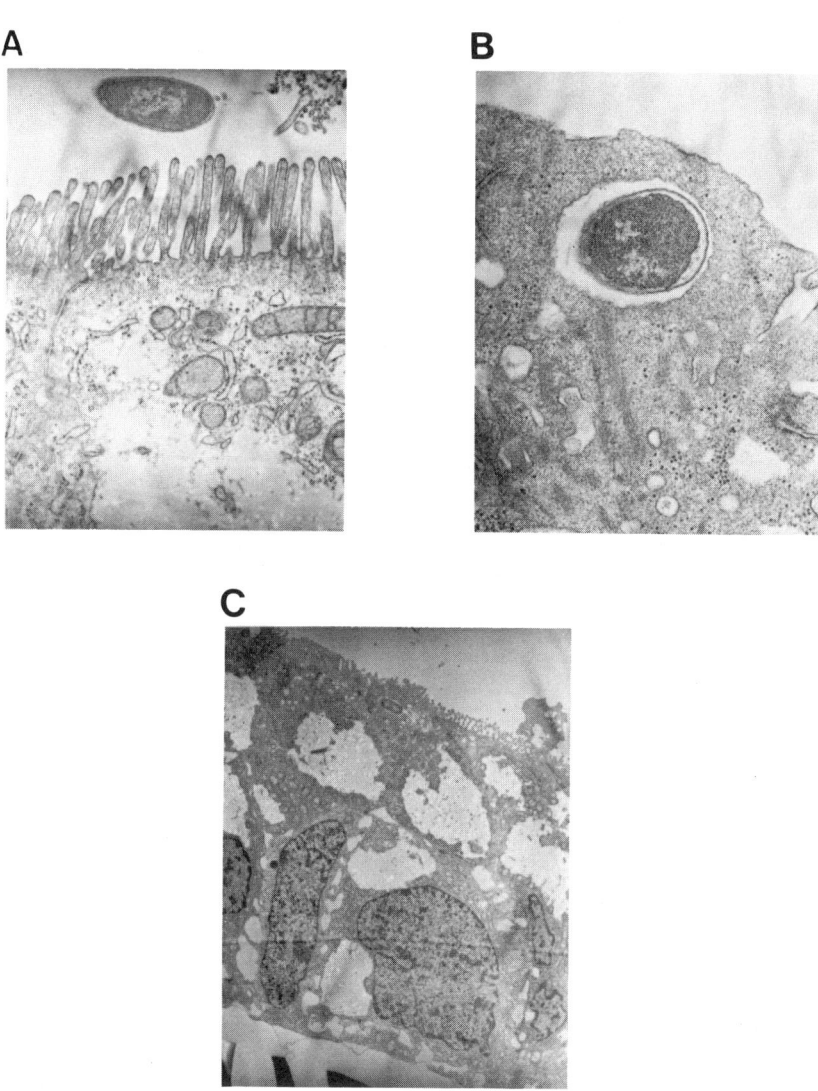

Figure 7-1. *Salmonella typhimurium* Interactions with Polarized Human Intestinal Carcinoma CACO-2 Cells. A) *S. typhimurium* adhering to the apical epithelial surface, which contains a well-defined brush border. B) *S. typhimurium* internalized into CACO-2 cells within a membrane-bound inclusion. C) Polarized CACO-2 cells grown on a filter with 3 μm pores.[7] An intracellular bacteria is visible near the apical surface, as is the disrupted brush border and microvilli in the infected cell.

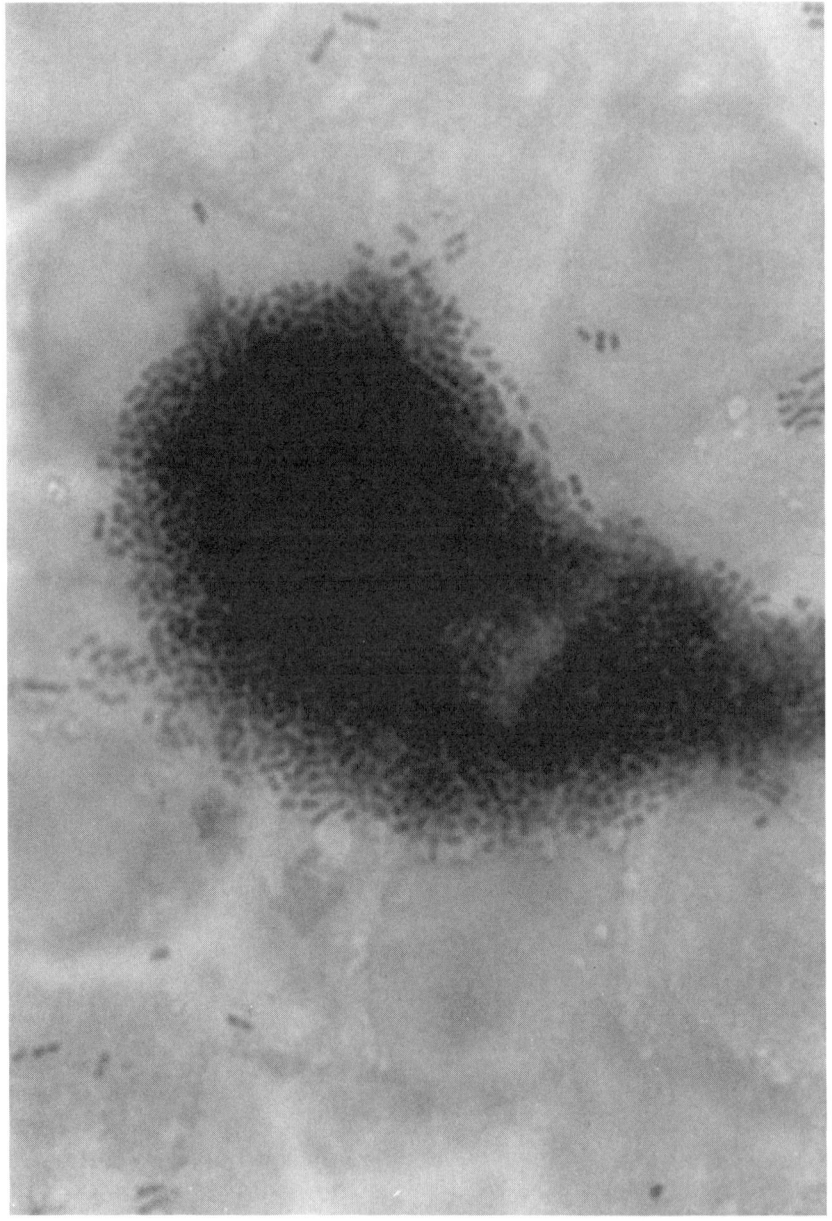

Figure 7-2. *S. typhimurium* Replicating within MDCK Cells. Monolayers were infected for 12 hours[12] and then visualized by light microscopy after Geimsa staining.

that surface. Measurement of the electrical resistance across these mono-layers showed that *Salmonella* disrupts the epithelial tight junctions in both MDCK and CACO-2 cells, causing a loss in resistance across the monolayer. Thus the examination of two polarized epithelial model systems has allowed us to begin to address several of the events involved in epithelial penetration by *Salmonella*.

Epithelial Cell Surfaces Induce *Salmonella* Adherence/Invasion Proteins

Several new bacterial proteins are induced when *S. typhimurium* or *S. choleraesuis* interacts with the eukaryotic cell surface.[11,14] Previous experiments suggested that bacterial RNA and protein synthesis are required for *Salmonella* adherence, invasion, and transcytosis.[7,17] By measuring the kinetics of bacterial-host cell interactions, we found that *Salmonella* adherence and invasion of MDCK cells requires about four hours before high levels of adherence or invasion were observed,[11] suggesting that the bacteria were required to synthesize proteins in order to adhere and invade. When bacteria that were interacting with glutaraldehyde-fixed or viable epithelial cells were labelled with ^{35}S methionine, several new proteins were synthesized, while numerous other bacterial proteins were "turned off."[11] This pattern of regulation is indicative of global regulatory networks, systems designed to sense environmental changes and adjust required protein levels accordingly.[18,19]

Originally these bacterial proteins were identified by using bacteria added to glutaraldehyde-fixed MDCK monolayers. These same proteins are regulated in the presence of other viable eukaryotic epithelial cells treated with cycloheximide or emitine, inhibitors of eukaryotic protein synthesis (These inhibitors have no effect on bacterial invasion).[11] Bacteria induced by interaction with eukaryotic cells could be transferred to another monolayer and adhere rapidly, without the normal four-hour lag period usually observed. We interpret this to mean that this incubation time induced the necessary proteins required for adherence and invasion so that the bacteria could adhere at once to animal cells. These data also indicate that the host cell receptor is normally exposed on the eukaryotic cell surface.

These polarized epithelial monolayers can be treated with modifying agents before fixation to attempt to determine the nature of the eukaryotic receptor. We found that treatment of these monolayers with periodic acid (which disrupts surface sugar molecules), trypsin (which cleaves surface proteins), or neuraminidase (which removes surface sialic acid residues) before fixation decreased bacterial adherence, and ultimately, bacterial entry (or invasion).[11,14] These data suggest that *Salmonella* probably interacts with glycoprotein-like structures on the epithelial cell surfaces.

Scanning electron micrographs of bacteria adherent to fixed epithelial cell surfaces indicate that the surface morphology of S. *choleraesuis* undergoes striking changes after adhering to these surfaces. When the bacteria initially interact with epithelial cell surfaces, flagellae are the only visible appendages and the bacterial surface is "smooth" (Figure 7-3a). However, after interacting with fixed epithelial surfaces for a few hours, several hair-like structures are visible spanning between bacteria, and between bacteria and the epithelial cell surface (Figure 7-3b). Additionally, several "knob-like" structures are apparent on the bacterial surfaces (Figure 7-3b). How these appendages contribute to adherence and invasion is under investigation.

Characterization of Genes Required for *Salmonella choleraesuis* Penetration

Other investigators have successfully introduced gene banks from the invasive bacteria *Yersinia pseudotuberculosis* and *Yersinia enterocolitica* into non-invasive E. *coli* and identified recombinants which were now able to enter into tissue culture cells.[10,20-22] However, we (and others) have been unsuccessful in using these methods to isolate *Salmonella* invasion factors, presumably in part because these genes are under regulatory control and are induced by epithelial cell surfaces.

To identify the genes needed for bacterial entry, we used transposon mutagenesis of S. *choleraesuis* with Tn*phoA*.[15] The transposon Tn*phoA* was used because it allows the identification of bacterial genes which encode proteins that are exported beyond the cytoplasm,[23] and we reasoned that gene products that interact with eukaryotic cells would be exposed on the bacterial surface. Tn*phoA* mutants in exported genes (PhoA+) were identified and screened for their ability to penetrate through a polarized epithelial monolayer of MDCK cells.[7] Although S. *choleraesuis* penetrates this barrier by four hours, mutations in genes required for adherence, invasion, intracellular survival and exit would all appear negative by this screening method.

We screened 626 PhoA+ mutants and found 42 that were unable to transcytose epithelial monolayers.[15] Through further characterization, these mutants were divided into six classes (Table 7-1). Classes 1 and 2 were mutants defective in lipopolysaccharide (LPS) O-side chain or LPS core synthesis, respectively, indicating that LPS is required for this process. However, mutants belonging to classes 3 through 6 had normal LPS profiles, suggesting that other surface gene products are also required. All classes of transcytosis mutants were also unable to adhere or invade, indicating that initial adherence is coupled with invasion and transcytosis.

A

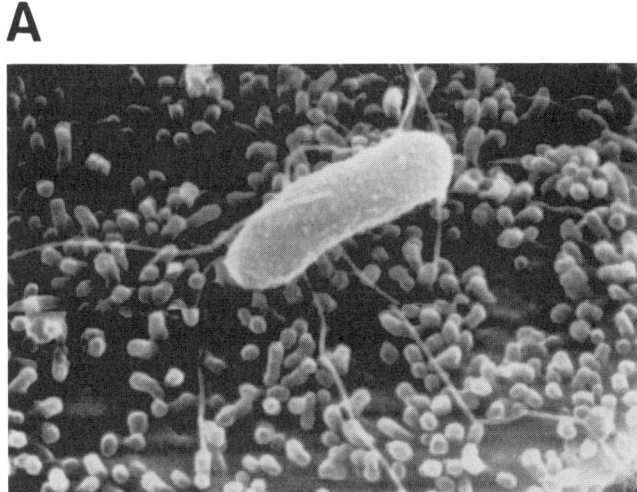

B

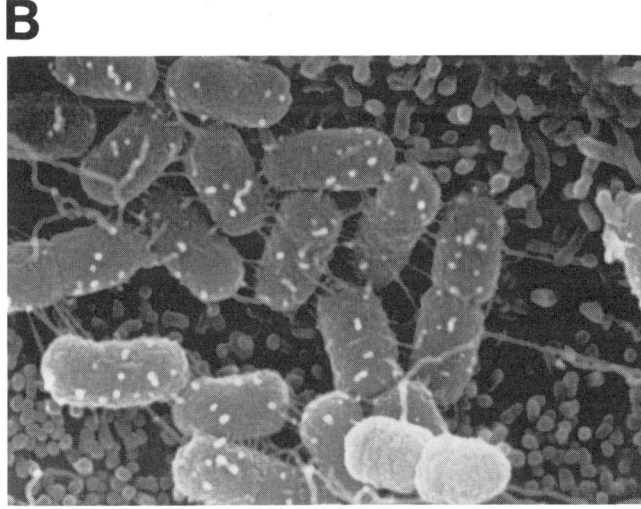

Figure 7-3. Scanning Electron Micrographs of *S. choleraesuis* Interacting with the Apical Surface of Polarized MDCK Cells which had been Previously Fixed in Glutaraldehyde to Prevent Bacterial Internalization. A) 2 hours post-infection. B) 6 hours post infection. Several morphological changes on the bacterial surface are now visible.

Mutants belonging to classes 1, 2, 4 and 5 were avirulent when fed orally to mice, indicating that epithelial penetration is indeed a virulence property of *Salmonella*. Interestingly, if the Class 4 mutant was injected intraperitoneally into mice, the mice died (unpublished data), suggesting that if epithelial penetration is bypassed, these *Salmonella* retain their virulence.

In the course of characterizing these Tn*phoA* mutants we identified a mutant that was unable to replicate intracellularly.[15] This mutant strain enters and transcytoses epithelial cells at the same rate as the parental strain. The mutant grows in minimal medium, suggesting that this strain is not an auxotroph. However, this *S. choleraesuis* mutant is avirulent in mice, suggesting that these organisms must be able to multiply intracellularly to be virulent.

In summary, *Salmonella* species are capable of entering eukaryotic cells and functioning as intracellular parasites, steps essential to their pathogenesis. These bacteria are ideally suited for examining host-parasite interactions since many aspects of *Salmonella* biology and biochemistry have already been characterized in detail. Several tissue culture models can be used to study *Salmonella* invasion (entry) and intracellular life. These include polarized epithelial cells and macrophages, two cell types encountered by these organisms within the host. Using these *in vitro* systems, the role of the host cell can be examined, including the involvement of host cytoskeletal structures, endosome acidification and intracellular trafficking. Transposon mutagenesis of these bacteria has been useful for identifying the bacterial components necessary for entry, intracellular survival, and replication within host cells. The use of appropriate animal models has enabled investigators to determine the contribution of these bacterial genes to *Salmonella* virulence.

Conclusions

To study intracellular parasites, the host-parasite interactions must be examined at several levels, and both the parasite and the host must be equally considered.[24] *In vitro* model systems make such studies considerably easier. In addition, these models allow investigators to examine a single step (or a series of steps), rather than being confined to studying virulence in an animal model. Animal death is a harsh experimental endpoint when one is attempting to dissect stages of host-parasite interactions. However, animal models are still essential because they enable the investigator to determine the contribution to pathogenesis of various factors, especially if mutations can be constructed in the gene of interest and the mutant strain compared to the isogenic parent strain. *Salmonella* species are facultative intracellular parasites, and make excellent systems for probing host-parasite interactions. We have used several *in vitro* tissue cell culture systems to examine the interactions of these organisms with

Table 7-1. Summary of *S. choleraesuis* Tn*phoA* Mutants Unable to Penetrate Polarized MDCK Epithelial Cells*

Mutant Class	LPS	Adherence	Invasion	Transcytosis	Transepithelial Resistance	Virulence
Wild Type	W.T.	+	+	+	-	+
1	O⁻	-	-	-	-	-
2	Core⁻	-	-	-	-	-
3	W.T.	-	-	-	-	+
4	W.T.	-	-	-	-	-
5	W.T.	-	-	-	+	-
6	W.T.	-	-	-	+	+

*This table is adapted from Finlay et al. 1988.

epithelial cells. Other workers have studied the interaction of these bacteria with macrophages *in vitro*.[25] Since *Salmonella* are easy to manipulate genetically, mutants can be constructed and screened for their inability to enter cells, and then tested in mice for virulence.

The strategies used to study *Salmonella* species should be applicable to studying other intracellular parasites including *Brucella*. Susceptible cell lines (either epithelial or macrophage-like) could be identified and host-parasite interactions examined. In addition, transposon Tn5 mutants can be generated in *Brucella*,[26] and various phenotypes of mutations could be isolated. These studies would provide useful information about the mechanisms used by *Brucella* to function as an intracellular parasite. It should be instructive to learn in which ways the pathogenic *Brucella* resemble *Salmonella* and, perhaps more importantly, how the *Brucella* uniquely interact with susceptible animal cells.

Acknowledgments

We would like to thank N. Ghori, D. Corwin, and S. F. Hayes for their excellent technical assistance with the electron microscopy studies. This work was supported by grant AI 26195 from the National Institute of Health to SF. BBF is a recipient of a post-doctorate Fellowship from the Alberta Heritage Foundation for Medical Research.

References

1. Cohen ML, Tauxe RV. Drug-resistant *Salmonella* in the United States: an epidemiologic perspective. *Science* 1986;234:964-9.
2. Sperber SJ, Schleupner CJ. Salmonellosis during infection with human immunodeficiency virus. *Rev Infect Dis* 1987;9:925-34.
3. Stocker BA, Makela PH. Genetic determination of bacterial virulence, with special reference to *Salmonella*. *Curr Top Microbiol Immunol* 1986;124:149-72.

4. Finlay BB, Falkow S. Virulence factors associated with *Salmonella* species. *Microbiol Sci* 1988;5:324-327.
5. Rubin RH, Weinstein L. *Salmonellosis: Microbiological, Pathogenic and Clinical Features.* New York, NY:Stratton Intercontinetal Medical Book Corp., 1977.
6. Takeuchi A. Electron microscope studies of experimental Salmonella infection.I. Penetration into the intestinal epithelium by *S. typhimurium. Am J Pathol* 1967;50:109-36.
7. Finlay BB, Gumbiner B, Falkow S. Penetration of *Salmonella* through a polarized Madin-Darby canine kidney epithelial cell monolayer. *J Cell Biol* 1988;107:221-30.
8. Giannella RA, Formal SB, Dammin GJ, Collins H. Pathogenesis of salmonellosis. Studies of fluid secretion, mucosal invasion, and morphologic reaction in the rabbit ileum. *J Clin Invest* 1973;52: 441-53.
9. Giannella R, Washington O, Gemski P, Formal S. Invasion of HeLa cells by *S. typhimurium*: a model for study of invasiveness of *Salmonella. J Infect Dis* 1973;128:69-75.
10. Miller VL, Finlay BB, Falkow S. Factors essential for the penetration of mammalian cells by *Yersinia. Curr. Top. Microbiol. Immunol.* 1988;138:15-39.
11. Finlay BB, Heffron F, Falkow S. Epithelial cell surfaces induce Salmonella proteins required for bacterial adherence and invasion. *Science* 1989;243:940-3:
12. Finlay BB, Falkow S. Comparison of the invasion strategies used by *Salmonella cholerae-suis, Shigella flexneri* and *Yersinia enterocolitica* to enter cultured animal cells: endosome acidification is not required for bacterial invasion or intracellular replication. *Biochimie* 1988;70:1089-1099.
13. Finlay BB, Falkow, SA. Comparison of microbial invasion strategies of *Salmonella, Shigella* and *Yersinia* species Horowitz, MA *Bacteria-host cell interaction.* New York, Alan R. Liss Inc., 1988.
14. Finlay BB, Fry J, Rock EP, Falkow S. Passage of *Salmonella* through polarized epithelial cells: role of the host and bacterium. *J Cell Sci* 1989;Suppl. 11:99-107.
15. Finlay BB, Starnbach MN, Francis CL, Stocker BAD, Chatfield S, Dougan G, Falkow S. Identification and characterization of TnphoA mutants of *Salmonella* that are unable to pass through a polarized MDCK epithelial cell monolayer. *Molecular Microbiol* 1988;2:757-766.
16. Simons K, Fuller S. Cell surface polarity in epithelia. *Ann Rev Cell Biol* 1985;1:243-88.
17. Lindquist BL, Lebenthal E, Lee PC, Stinson MW, Merrick JM. Adherence of *Salmonella typhimurium* to small-intestinal enterocytes of the rat. *Infect Immun* Dec 1987;55:3044-50.
18. Gottesman S. Bacterial regulation: global regulatory networks. *Annu Rev Genet* 1984;18:415-41.
19. Miller JF, Mekalanos JJ, Falkow S. Coordinate regulation and sensory transduction in the control of bacterial virulence. *Science* 1989;243:916-22.
20. Isberg RR, Falkow S. A single genetic locus encoded by *Yersinia pseudotuberculosis* permits invasion of cultured animal cells by *E. coli* K-12. *Nature* 1985;317:262-4.
21. Isberg RR, Voorhis DL, Falkow S. Identification of invasin: a protein that allows enteric bacteria to penetrate cultured mammalian cells. *Cell* 1987;50:769-78.
22. Miller VL, Falkow S. Evidence for two genetic loci in *Y. enterocolitica* that can promote invasion of epithelial cells. *Infect Immun* 1988;56:1242-8.
23. Manoil C, Beckwith J. TnphoA: a transposon probe for protein export signals. *Proc Natl Acad Sci USA* 1985;82:8129-33.
24. Moulder JW. Comparative biology of intracellular parasitism. *Microbiol Rev* 1985;49:298-337.
25. Fields P, Swanson R, Haidaris C, Heffron F. Mutants of *S. typhimurium* that cannot survive within the macrophage are avirulent. *Proc Natl Acad Sci* 1986;83:5189-93.
26. Smith LD, Heffron F. Transposon Tn5 mutagenesis of *Brucella abortus. Infect Immun* 1987;55:2774-6.

PART IV

NATURAL AND ACQUIRED IMMUNITY AGAINST BRUCELLAE

Chapter Eight

Cell-Mediated Immunity Against Intracellular Bacteria

Inge E.A. Flesch and Stefan H.E. Kaufmann

Intracellular bacteria are endowed with the capacity to replicate within mononuclear phagocytes, cells which are well equipped for engulfing, killing, and degradating invading microorganisms. For intracellular survival, these pathogens have developed potent evasion mechanisms. In principle, three evasion mechanisms can be distinguished (these need not be mutually exclusive): 1) resistance to lysosomal enzymes and/or reactive oxygen intermediates, 2) prevention of phagosome-lysosome fusion and 3) escape from the phagosome into the cytoplasm.[1] The pathogens that use each mechanism are listed in Table 8-1. Some of these pathogens also inhabit host cells other than mononuclear phagocytes; e.g., *Mycobacterium leprae* also lives in Schwann cells, and *Trypanosoma cruzi* also lives in heart muscle cells. After invasion of host cells bacteria are shielded from extracellular defense mechanisms, including opsonization by antibodies and complement.

During intracellular growth, some microbial antigens may be processed and presented by the infected macrophage in association with major histocompatibility complex (MHC) gene products. T lymphocytes can recognize bacterial products plus MHC molecules and are activated to proliferate and differentiate into effector T cells. Activated T cells recirculate in the host and, in response to an inflammatory signal, invade sites of bacterial implantation and interact with mononuclear phagocytes presenting bacterial antigens for a second time. As a corollary, interleukins (IL) are secreted that attract and activate blood monocytes. A granuloma is formed where microbes are confined to discrete foci and prevented from dissemination through the body. Figure 8-1 summarizes the major steps leading to granuloma formation and to protective immunity against intracellular bacteria.[2]

In this report, evidence will be presented showing that both helper T cells and cytolytic T cells can interact with infected mononuclear phagocytes and contribute to protection against intracellular bacteria. As models for facultative intracellular infections, pathogenic listeriae and mycobac-

Table 8-1. Some Intracellular Bacteria and the Evasion Mechanisms that Permit their Intracellular Growth

• Escape from phagosome:
  Trypanosoma cruzi
  Rickettsia spp.
  Mycobacterium leprae
  Listeria monocytogenes

• Resistance to lysosomal enzymes and/or O_2 metabolites:
  Listeria monocytogenes
  Mycobacterium tuberculosis
  Salmonella typhimurium
  Leishmania spp.
  Yersinia pestis
  Coxiella burnettii

• Prevention of phagosome-lysosome fusion:
  Mycobacterium tuberculosis
  Legionella pneumophila
  Toxoplasma gondii
  Chlamydia psittaci

teria were used. *Listeria monocytogenes* was first isolated by E.G.D. Murray et al. in 1926. It is a Gram-Positive, facultatively anaerobic rod which is widely distributed in nature and occasionally causes food-borne outbreaks of listeriosis.[3] Mycobacteria are acid-fast bacilli which include the etiologic agents of tuberculosis, *M. tuberculosis, M. bovis,* and *M. africanum* and the cause of leprosy, *M. leprae,* as obligate pathogens, as well as the opportunistic species *M. avium* and *M. intracellulare.*[4] Tuberculosis is still a major health problem in underdeveloped countries. In addition, due to increasing numbers of immunodeficient patients, the incidence of *M. tuberculosis* infections has increased again in developed countries.

Results

Role of T Lymphocytes in Antibacterial Immunity

T cells can be divided into two subclasses: helper T cells and cytolytic T lymphocytes. Helper T cells bearing the CD4 molecule (T4 in man; L3T4

EVENT

① Stimulation of
protective T cells
specific for epitopes
(in association with
self)

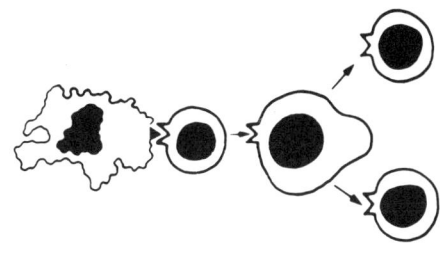

② immigration of
specific T cells into
sites of inflammation
and specific interaction
with macrophages

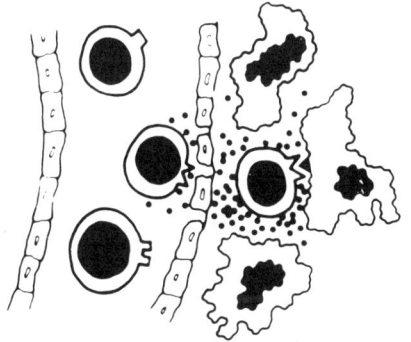

③ Attraction and
activation of
mononuclear cells
by lymphokines

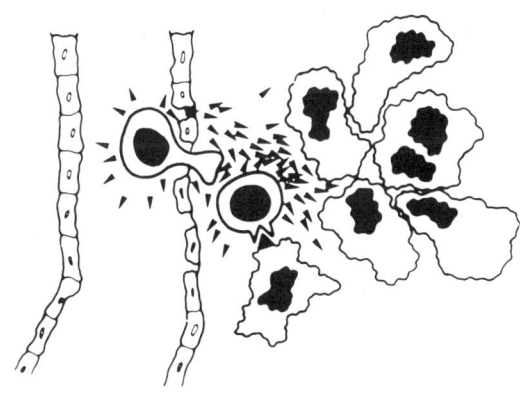

Figure 8-1. Simplified Scheme of the Major Steps Leading to Protective Immunity Against Intracellular Bacteria.[2]

in mice) recognize foreign antigen in association with class II MHC molecules. They produce a variety of soluble mediators called interleukins (or lymphokines) which can activate target cells, including mononuclear phagocytes, to perform their effector functions. It has been suggested that, on the basis of their interleukin secretion, murine CD4 T cells can be further divided into T_{H1} cells, which preferentially secrete interferon-γ (IFN-γ) and IL-2, and T_{H2} cells, which preferentially secrete IL-4 and IL-5.[5] Some T cell clones of the CD4 phenotype have been shown to express cytolytic functions. Cytolytic T lymphocytes bearing the CD8 molecule (T8 in man; Lyt2 in mice) recognize foreign antigens in association with class I MHC molecules. They lyse their target cells through direct cell contact and were assumed to recognize internally synthesized proteins only.

Originally it was thought that T cells contribute to protection by secreting interleukins which activate macrophage antibacterial mechanisms. Since lymphokine secretion is typical for CD4 T cells, it was generally accepted that helper T cells represent the relevant T cell population of antibacterial immunity. The first evidence that CD4 as well as CD8 T cells are involved in the protective mechanisms against listeriosis came from an *in vivo* experiment.[4] Peritoneal exudate T lymphocytes from *L. monocytogenes*-immune mice were treated with either anti-Lyt1 or anti-Lyt2 antibodies plus complement to select for helper or cytolytic T cells. T cell populations were transferred into recipient mice that were subsequently infected with viable *L. monocytogenes*. Protective activity against *L. monocytogenes* was only transferred by unselected T lymphocytes but not by T cells treated with either anti-Lyt1 or anti-Lyt2 antibodies plus complement.

To get more detailed information about the functional role of L3T4⁺ and Lyt2⁺ T cells in the immune response against listeriosis, T-cell clones were generated from infected mice and analyzed for their functional capacities.[7] In the presence of the listerial antigen and accessory cells, *L. monocytogenes*-specific L3T4⁺ T-cell clones were found to produce IL-2 and IFN-γ. At high cell numbers, these T cells were capable of inducing protection after adoptive transfer into recipient mice that had been infected with live *L. monocytogenes* organisms. Protective immunity against *L. monocytogenes* was also induced by systemic application of recombinant (r)-IFN-γ,[8] a finding which supports the notion that IFN-γ is involved in the induction of acquired resistance to *L. monocytogenes*. *L. monocytogenes*-specific Lyt2+ T cell clones secreted significant amounts of IFN-γ only after co-stimulation with r-IL-2 plus infected stimulator cells. These T cells were capable of lysing peritoneal macrophages from *L. monocytogenes*-infected mice as well as bone marrow-derived macrophages (BMM∅) primed with *L. monocytogenes* organisms *in vitro*.[9,10]

The involvement of both CD4 and CD8 T cells in the acquired resistance against intracellular bacteria was also found in the tuberculosis system.[11-13] Thymectomized mice were treated with monoclonal antibodies with specificity for the CD4 or CD8 molecule and afterwards were infected with viable organisms of *M. tuberculosis*. After 3 weeks, spleens were removed and mycobacterial numbers were determined. Treatment of mice with either anti-L3T4 or anti-Lyt2 monoclonal antibodies led to a marked increase of mycobacterial numbers in the spleen. Depletion of both T cell subsets did not worsen the disease. These results indicate that both T cell subsets participate in the acquisition of effective resistance against tuberculosis.[11]

Mycobacterium tuberculosis-specific L3T4+ T cell clones were established from *M. tuberculosis*-immunized mice and analyzed for their functional capacities.[12] After stimulation with antigen plus accessory cells, they produced the lymphokines IL-2 and IFN-γ. Culture supernatants from these T-cell clones activated normal BMMØ to inhibit the intracellular growth of *M. bovis*, which points to the relevant role of CD4 T cells in antituberculous immunity.

To examine the function of CD8 T cells in tuberculosis, Lyt2+ T-cell lines were established from *M. tuberculosis* and *M. bovis*-immune mice.[13] After appropriate stimulation, some of the Lyt2+ T cell lines were found to produce IFN-γ which is capable of activating anti-mycobacterial capacities in BMMØ. In addition, these Lyt2+ T cells were capable of lysing BMMØ primed with mycobacterial antigen. As shown in Table 8-2, lysis of mycobacteria-infected BMMØ by specific CD8 T cells leads to tuberculostasis. In this assay, r-IFN-γ was ineffective and anti-IFN-γ antibodies did not reverse mycobacterial growth inhibition. Obviously, cytotoxic T lymphocytes can induce tuberculostasis independent from IFN-γ and parallel to lysis of infected host cells.[14]

The Mononuclear Phagocyte as Effector Cell

The final effector cell in the elimination of intracellular bacterial pathogens is the mononuclear phagocyte. Mononuclear phagocytes exhibit a great diversity of functional potential. They are able to lyse tumor cells in an antibody-dependent and -independent fashion; they destroy extracellular bacteria by release of reactive oxygen metabolites and lysosomal enzymes; and they contribute to immune regulation by production of arachidonic acid metabolites. For the performance of these functions, mononuclear phagocytes have to be activated by interleukins produced by specific T cells.[15,16]

The crucial lymphokine for the activation of numerous macrophage capacities including tumor cell lysis has been shown to be IFN-γ, which is mainly produced by CD4 T cellc and also by CD8 T cells.[15] For analysis of anti-mycobacterial macrophage functions, we used murine BMMØ cultured in vitro for 9 days under serum-free conditions.[17] In contrast to peri-

Table 8-2. Growth Inhibition of M. *bovis* in Normal BMMØ Induced by Mycobacteria-Reactive Lyt2⁺ T Cells

T lymphocytes	Cell number x 10⁻⁴	³H-uracil (cpm)	% Inhibition
Control	-	18 580	-
M. *tuberculosis*-	45	2 230	87
reactive T cell	15	10 300	44
line	5	18 510	1
	1.5	20 300	-8

BMMØ were infected with viable M. *bovis* and 4 days later T cells were added. After 18 hours, cells were lysed and viability of mycobacteria was assessed by ³H-uracil uptake as described in reference 17. Percent inhibition = (1- ³H-uracil uptake after culture with T cells/ ³H-uracil uptake after culture without T cells) x 100. Data reproduced with permission from reference 13.

toneal macrophages, these cells represent a quiescent homogenousmacrophage population. As typical macrophage markers, Mac-1 antigen, Fc-receptors, and nonspecific esterase were analyzed. After appropriate activation these cells can be rendered tumoricidal. The BMMØ were stimulated with r-IFN-γ or with IFN-γ-containing supernatants from antigen- or mitogen-stimulated T cells for 24 hours and subsequently infected with viable organisms of M. *bovis* BCG, M. *tuberculosis* H37Rv, or M. *tuberculosis* Middelburg. Viability of intracellular bacteria was assessed after 4 or 5 days by two read-out systems, namely, determination of colony-forming units (CFU) or incorporation of ³H-uracil into the RNA of mycobacteria. Both read-out systems gave comparable results. As shown in Figure 8-2, growth of M. *bovis* BCG and M. *tuberculosis* H37Rv was inhibited significantly by IFN-γ-activated BMMØ; however, replication of M. *tuberculosis* Middelburg was not affected. From these results two conclusions can be drawn. First, r-IFN-γ can activate antimycobacterial macrophage functions and second, different M. *tuberculosis* strains vary in their susceptibility to IFN-γ-activated BMMØ.[17]

In the same assay system, namely, activation of BMMØ for 24 hours and subsequent infection with mycobacteria, other lymphokines were tested for their ability to activate macrophage antituberculous functions. As shown in Table 8-3, none of these lymphokines, except IFN-γ, was able to activate BMMØ for growth inhibition of M. *bovis*.[18]

By using another assay system, namely, infection of BMMØ with mycobacteria and subsequent stimulation with lymphokines, a different picture emerged. The IFN-γ induced lower but still significant tuberculostsis.

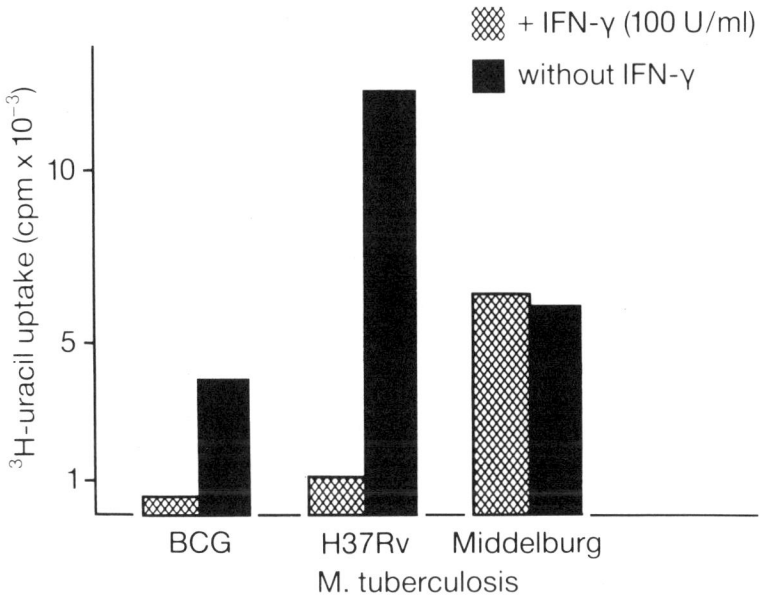

Figure 8-2. Growth Inhibition of Mycobacteria by r-IFN-γ Activated BMMØ. BMMØ were stimulated with r-IFN-γ or remained untreated. Afterwards BMMØ were infected with viable organisms of *M. bovis* BCG, *M. tuberculosis* H37Rv, or *M. tuberculosis* Middelburg. Mycobacterial growth inhibition was determined by ³H-uracil uptake as described in Reference 17. Percent inhibition=(1-³H-uracil uptake after culture with r-IFN-γ- activated BMMØ/ ³H-uracil uptake after culture with nonactivated BMMØ x 100. Data reproduced with permission from reference number 17.

Table 8-3. Effect of Recombinant Interleukins on Growth Inhibition of *M. bovis* and Secretion of Superoxide Anion (0 ⁻₂) by BMMØ

Lymphokine	Growth inhibition of *M. bovis*·	Secretion of superoxide anion·
r-IFN-γ	+++	+++
r-IL-2	-	-
r-IL-3	-	n.d.
r-IL-4	-	+
r-IL-5	-	+
r-IL-6	-	+
r-GM-CSF	-	++
r-IFN-α/β	-	+
r-TNF-α	-	+

·BMMØ were incubated with lymphokines for 24 hours and subsequently infected with live *M. bovis*. Growth inhibition of *M. bovis* by BMMØ was measured by the ³H-uracil incorporation method[17]
ᵇSecretion of superoxide anion (0 ⁻₂) was assessed by lucigenin-dependent chemiluminescence with phorbol myristate acetate as triggering signal.
n.d. = not done
+ = significant growth inhibition of 0 ⁻₂
- = no growth inhibition or 0 ⁻₂ production

The B cell-stimulatory factors, IL-4 and IL-6, induced marked inhibition of mycobacterial growth (Table 8-4). A similar result was obtained when BMMØ were infected with a temperature-sensitive strain of *L. monocytogenes* (Table 8-5).[19]

Originally, IL-4, IL-5, and IL-6 were thought to act only on B cells, but it has become evident that these factors are pleiotropic. In addition, each factor mediates multiple effects on a single target cell population.[20] Interleukin-4 was primarily defined to act as a B cell growth factor which induces entry of resting B cells into cell cycle S-phase after stimulation with anti-immunoglobulin antibodies. Furthermore, IL-4 increases IgE antibody production by activating murine B cells, stimulates proliferation of mast cells and T cells, and enhances murine peritoneal macrophages for increased tumor cytotoxicity and Ia antigen expression.[21] McInnes and Rennick showed that IL-4 induces formation of multinucleated giant cells in vitro.[22] Multinucleated giant cells are formed by the fusion of macrophages and are prominent in granulomas formed in response to tubercle

Table 8-4. Effect of Interleukins on the Tuberculostatic Activity of Infected BMMØ.

Interleukin	Concentration (U/ml)	Inhibition (%)
IFN-γ	50	40
	500	50
IL-4	50	37
	500	80
IL-6	50	38
	500	67

BMMØ were infected with viable *M. bovis* organisms. After removal of extracellular bacteria, interleukins were added for 40 hours. Viability of mycobacteria was obtained by ³H-uracil uptake.[17] Percent inhibition was calculated as indicated in Table 8-2.

bacilli. Interleukin-5 is a growth as well as differentiation factor for B cells. In addition, it stimulates differentiation of bone marrow cells into eosinophils, increases antigen-specific antibody response by B cells from antigen-primed mice, and induces the differentiation of thymocytes into cytolytic T cells.[20,21] Interleukin-6 is produced by a variety of cells including T cells, fibroblasts, endothelial cells and monocytes/macrophages. It has been shown to stimulate B cells at late developmental stages. Interleukin-6 also induces T cell growth and differentiation, is involved in the acute-phase response of hepatocytes, and activates hematopoietic stem cells.[20] Recent, reports indicate elevated levels of IL-6 in the body fluids of patients with local acute bacterial infections.[23]

Our data show that the B cell stimulatory factors IL-4 and IL-6 are highly potent in activating antimycobacterial and antilisterial functions in already infected BMMØ. These findings suggest that macrophage activation by B cell stimulatory factors depends on a second stimulus provided by live mycobacteria or listeriae.

Table 8-5. Effect of Interleukins on the Antilisterial Activity of Infected BMMØ

Interleukin	Concentration (U/ml)	Inhibition (%)
IFN-γ	50	26
	500	24
IL-4	50	86
	500	92
IL-6	50	31
	500	64

BMMØ were infected with a temperature-sensitive strain of *L. monocytogenes*. After removal of extracellular bacteria, interleukins were added for 16 hours. Viability of listeriae was determined by ³H-uracil uptake.[17] Percent inhibition was calculated as indicated in Table 8-2.

Mechanisms Involved in Tuberculostasis by IFN-γ Activated Bone Marrow Derived Macrophages

Mononuclear phagocytes can use both oxygen-dependent and -independent mechanisms for intracellular killing of microbial pathogens.[24] During and after phagocytosis of bacteria, reactive oxygen metabolites (superoxide anion, hydrogen peroxide, hydroxyl radicals, and singlet oxygen) are released into the phagocytic vacuoles, where they cause bacterial destruction. To test the involvement of reactive oxygen intermediates in mycobacterial growth inhibition by r-IFN-γ-activated BMMØ, various scavengers of reactive oxygen metabolites were employed:[25] catalase as a scavenger of hydrogen peroxide; superoxide dismutase as a scavenger of superoxide anion; histidine and diazabicyclooctane as scavengers of singlet oxygen radicals; and mannitol and tetramethylurea as scavengers of hydroxyl radicals. As shown in Table 8-6, none of these scavengers was able to reverse antimycobacterial macrophage functions. In addition, we found that phagocytosis of *M. bovis* by activated BMMØ fails to trigger an oxidative burst.[17]

An oxygen-independent mechanism would be the induction of phagosome-lysosome fusion and exposure of bacteria to lysosomal enzymes. To investigate this possibility, BMMØ were infected with *M. bovis* in the

Table 8-6. Effect of Scavengers of Reactive Oxygen Metabolites on the GrowthInhibition of *M. bovis* by IFN-γ-Stimulated BMMø

Scavengers	³H-uracil Uptake (cpm)	Inhibition (%)
Catalase (mg/ml)		
0.1	7,828	79
0.01	8,085	78
Superoxide dismutase (U/ml)		
15	6,854	82
1.5	8,083	78
0.15	8,674	77
Histidine (mg/ml)		
10	3,264	91
1	11,243	70
0.1	11,011	70
Diazabicylooctane (mg/ml)		
1	5,572	85
0.1	9,152	75
0.01	10,082	73
Mannitol (mg/ml)		
1	9,423	75
0.1	8,658	77
0.01	8,004	79
Tetramethylurea (mg/ml)		
1	5,551	85
0.1	6,362	83
0.01	7,336	80

IFN-γ-activated BMMø were infected with *M. bovis* in the presence of the scavengers. ³H-uracil uptake was measured after 4 days of incubation.[25] Percent inhibition of mycobacterial growth was calculated as indicated in Table 8-2. Data reproduced with permission from Flesch and Kaufmann.[25]

presence of agents which are known to enhance phagosome-lysosome fusion.[25] As shown in Table 8-7, the lipophilic tertiary amines chloroquine, tetracaine, and tributylamine induced growth inhibition of *M. bovis* by presence of agents which are known to enhance phagosome-lysosome fusion.[25] As shown in Table 8-7, the lipophilic tertiary amines chloroquine, tetracaine, and tributylamine induced growth inhibition of *M. bovis* by BMMØ by more than 70%. Taken together, these results argue against the involvement of an oxygen-dependent tuberculostatic mechanism but favor the notion that phagosome-lysosome fusion may be induced in IFN-γ-stimulated BMMØ.

Discussion

The immune response to the intracellular bacterium *L. monocytogenes* and *M. tuberculosis/M. bovis* requires a fine-tuned interaction between helper and cytolytic T cells and mononuclear phagocytes. Figure 8-3 summarizes the current view of acquired resistance. A major effector step is the activation of mononuclear phagocytes by lymphokines produced by antigen-specific T lymphocytes. In various experimental systems, evidence has been provided that IFN-γ is an important macrophage-activating factor in the mouse system. In human monocytes, IFN-γ fails to directly activate mycobacterial growth inhibition.[26] However, IFN-γ treatment of human monocytes activates the enzyme 25-hydroxylase which converts the circulating 25-hydroxyvitamin D3 to 1,25-dihydroxyvitamin D3.[27] 1,25-dihydroxyvitamin D3 has been shown to stimulate multiple macrophage functions including tuberculostasis.[26,27,28] Thus, IFN-γ could exert its antimycobacterial effects indirectly by inducing the synthesis of 1,25-dihydroxyvitamin D3 at the site of mycobacterial growth, which then could activate tuberculostatic macrophage functions locally.

By using murine BMMØ we could demonstrate that IFN-γ is capable of activating antimycobacterial capacity, although a possible contribution of the B cell-stimulatory factors, IL-4 and IL-6, cannot be excluded.[17] Concerning the mechanism of tuberculostasis, evidence has been provided that phagosome-lysosome fusion and exposure of bacteria to lysosomal enzymes, rather than reactive oxygen intermediates, are involved.[25] Production of IFN-γ is not restricted to MHC class II-restricted CD4 T cells, but can also be accomplished by MHC class I-restricted CD8 T cells which have a broader target spectrum. Activation of mononuclear phagocytes can also be harmful for the host. Secretion of a variety of mediators, including reactive oxygen intermediates, proteases, and tumor necrosis factor-alpha, leads to destruction of the surrounding tissue.[2]

In cases where mononuclear phagocytes within a granuloma fail to

Table 8-7. Effect of Chloroquine, Tetracaine, and Tributylamine on Anti-Mycobacterial Activity of Unstimulated BMMØ

Compound	^{3}H-uracil uptake (cpm)	Inhibition (%)
-	27,300	-
Chloroquine (5mg/ml)	7,300	73
Tetracaine (1mg/ml)	15,200	44
Tributylamine (100 mg/ml)	15,800	42

Unstimulated BMMØ were infected with *M. bovis* in the presence of the compounds indicated. Growth inhibition of *M. bovis* was determined by ^{3}H-uracil uptake.[25] Data reproduced with permission from reference 25.

eliminate intracellular pathogens, lysis of infected cells by CD8 T cells may gain importance.[14] In the mouse system, CD8 T-cell clones with specificity for *M. tuberculosis* or *L. monocytogenes*, have been established that lyse target cells primed with the appropriate antigen but do not lyse unprimed targets.[9,10,13] Lysis of BMMØ infected with viable *M. bovis* by specific CD8 T cells is paralleled by mycobacterial growth inhibition.[13] Discharge into the hypoxic necrotic granulomatous center may be harmful for the bacteria and directly leads to growth inhibition. In addition, microbial transmission from a protective niche to an aggressive environment may occur. In this way bacteria could become accessible to humoral defense mechanisms and to phagocytosis by activated mononuclear phagocytes, which finally leads to the elimination of the pathogens. Lysis of infected host cells may also cause detrimental effects like microbial discharge from the granuloma and dissemination over the body and even to other individuals. Another harmful effect of cell lysis is tissue destruction. Schwann cells provide a major habitat for *M. leprae* and nerve damage represents a major pathomechanism in leprosy.[29] In such a situation, lysis of Schwann cells by cytolytic T cells could contribute to the pathogenesis of leprosy. Thus, in antibacterial immunity, T cells can cause both detrimental and beneficial sequelae and hence represent a double-edged sword.

In summary, acquired resistance against intracellular bacteria depends on specific T lymphocytes and mononuclear phagocytes. Several *in vitro* systems have been established to study the relative contributions of helper and cytolytic T cells, as well as mononuclear phagocytes, to host resistance against mycobacteria and listeriae. It was found that CD4 and CD8 T cells are both involved in the immune response against these pathogens. After appropriate stimulation, both CD4 and CD8 T lymphocytes produce interferon-γ which is capable of activating tuberculostatic capacities in macrophages. In addition, CD8 T cells possess an antigen-specific cytolytic potential. Lysis of infected macrophages could contribute to myco-

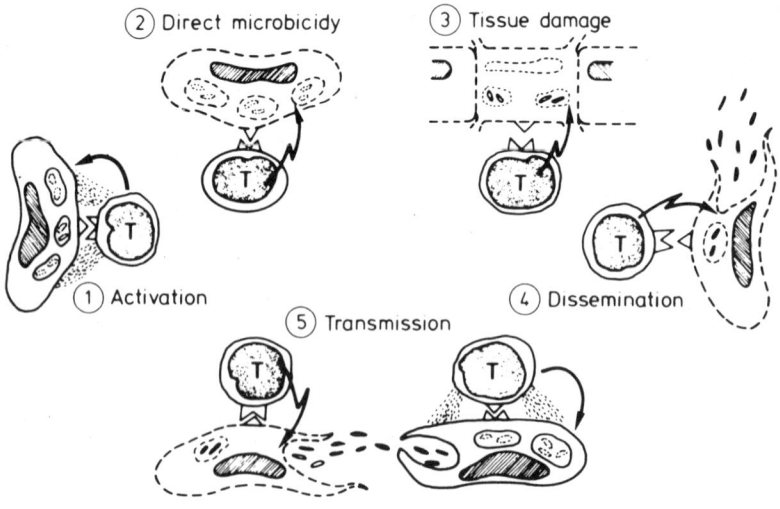

Figure 8-3. A Model of T-cell Functions in Antimicrobial Resistance. 1) T cells activate antibmicrobial macrophage functions via interleukins. Although this step is primarily beneficial, activated macrophages also secrete various compounds that may harm surrounding tissue. 2) Lysis of infected host cells affects intracellular microbes more or less directly. 3) Lysis of infected host cells leads to tissue destruction. 4) Lysis of infected host cells allows microbial dissemination. 5) Coordinated lysis of infected host cells and subseuqent activation of potent phagocytes allows microbial transmission from a protective to an aggressive surrounding.[14]

bacterial growth inhibition but may also have detrimental consequences for the host.

Acknowledgments

Financial support for this work was provided to S.H.E.K. from the United National Development Program and the World Health Organization (WHO) Special Program for Research and Training in Tropical Diseases; the WHO as part of its Program for Vaccine Development, and the A. Krupp award for young professors. The secretarial help of R. Mahmoudi is gratefully acknowledged.

References

1. Moulder JW. Comparative biology of intracellular parasitism. *Microbiol Rev* 1985;49:298-337.
2. Kaufmann SHE. Immunity against intracellular bacteria: biological effector functions and antigen specificity of T lymphocytes. *Curr Top Microbiol Immunol* 1988;138:141-176.
3. Kaufmann SHE. Listeriosis: new findings, current concern. *Microbial Pathogen* 1988;5:225-231.
4. Schlossberg D (ed). *Clinical topics in infectious disease. Tuberculosis.* New York, NY: Springer Verlag, 1988.
5. Mosmann TR, Coffman RL. Two types of mouse helper T-cell clones. Implications for immune regulation. *Immunol Today* 1987;8:223-227.
6. Kaufmann SHE, Simon MM, Hahn H. Specific Lyt123 T cells are involved in protection against *L.monocytogenes* and in delayed-type hypersensitivity to listerial antigen. *J Exp Med* 1979;150:1033-1038.
7. Kaufmann SHE. Acquired resistance to facultative intracellular bacteria: relationship between persistance, crossreactivity at the T-cell level, and capacity to stimulate cellular immunity to different *Listeria* strains. *Infect Immun* 1984;45:234-241.
8. Kiderlen AF, Kaufmann SHE, Lohmann-Matthes ML. Protection of mice against the intracellular bacterium *L.monocytogenes* by recombinant immune interferon. *Eur J Immunol* 1984;14:964-967.
9. Kaufmann SHE, Hug E, DeLibero G. *Listeria monocytogenes*-reactive T lymphocyte clones with cytolytic activity against infected target cells. *J Exp Med* 1986;164:363-368.
10. DeLibero G, Kaufmann SHE. Antigen-specific Lyt2⁺ cytolytic T lymphocytes from mice infected with the intracellular bacterium *Listeria monocytogenes*. *J Immunol* 1986;137:2688-2694.
11. Müller I, Cobbold SP, Waldmann H, Kaufmann SHE. Impaired resistance against *Mycobacterium tuberculosis* infection after selective in-vivo depletion of L3T4⁺ and Lyt2⁺ T cells. *Infect Immun* 1987;55:2037-2041.
12. Kaufmann SHE, Flesch I. Function and antigen recognition pattern of L3T4⁺ T-cell clones from *Mycobacterium tuberculosis*-immune mice. *Infect Immun* 1986;54:291-296.
13. DeLibero G, Flesch I, Kaufmann SHE. Mycobacteria-reactive Lyt-2+ T-cell lines. *Eur J Immunol* 1988;18:59-66.
14. Kaufmann SHE. CD8 T lymphocytes in intracellular microbial infections. *Immunol Today* 1988;9:168-173.
15. Adams DO, Hamilton TA. The cell biology of macrophage activation. *Annu Rev*

Immunol 1984;2:283-318.

16. Cohn ZA. The activation of mononuclear phagocytes: fact, fancy, and future. *J Immunol* 1978;121:813-815.

17. Flesch I, Kaufmann SHE. Mycobacterial growth inhibition by interferon activated bone marrow macrophages and differential susceptibility among strains of *Mycobacterium tuberculosis*. *J Immunol* 1987;138:4408-4413.

18. Kaufmann SHE, Flesch I. The role of T cell-macrophage interactions in tuberculosis. *Springer Seminars Immunopathol* 1988;10:337-358.

19. Kaufmann SHE, Flesch IEA. Cell-mediated immunity, immunodeficiency and microbial infections. In: Jackson GG, Schlumberger HD, Zeiler HJ, eds.*Perspectives in Antiinfective Therapy* Braunschweig/Wiesbaden: F. Vieweg, 1989;165-173

20. O'Garra A, Umland S, DeFrance T, Christiansen J. "B-cell factors" are pleiotropic. *Immunol Today* 1988;9:45-54.

21. Yokota T, Arai N, DeVries J, Spits H, Banchereau J, Zlotnik A, Rennick D, Howard M, Takebe Y, Miyatake S, Lee F, Arai KI. Molecular biology of interleukin 4 and interleukin 5 genes and biology of their products that stimulate B cells, T cells and hemopoietic cells. *Immunol Rev* 1988;102:137-187.

22. McInnes A, Rennick DM. Interleukin 4 induces cultured monocytes/ macrophages to form giant multinucleated cells. *J Exp Med* 1988;167:598-611.

23. Helfgott DC, Tatter SB, Santhanam U, Clarick RH, Bhardwaj N, May LT, Sehgal PB. Multiple forms of IFN-β_2/IL-6 in serum and body fluids during acute bacterial infection. *J Immunol* 1989; 142: 948-953.

24. Klebanoff SJ, Hamon CB. Antimicrobial systems of mononuclear phagocytes. In: van Furth R, ed.*Mononuclear Phagocytes in Immunity, Infection and Pathology.* Blackwell, 1975;507-529.

25. Flesch IEA, Kaufmann SHE. Attempts to characterize the mechanisms involved in mycobacterial growth inhibition by interferon-activated bone marrow macrophages. *Infect Immun* 1988;56:1464-1469.

26. Crowle AJ, Ross EJ, May MH. Inhibition by 1,25(OH^2)-vitamin D3 of the multiplication of virulent tubercle bacilli in cultured human macrophages. *Infect Immun* 1987;55:2945-2950.

27. Reichel H, Koeffler HP, Tobler A, Norman AW. 1-25-dihydroxyvitamin D3 inhibits interferon synthesis by normal human peripheral blood lymphocytes. *Proc Natl Acad Sci USA* 1987;84:3385-3389.

28. Rook GAW, Steele J, Fraher L, Barker S, O'Riordan, KR. Vitamin D3, gamma interferon, and control of proliferation of *Mycobacterium tuberculosis* by human monocytes. *Immunology* 1986;57:159-163.

29. Steinhoff U, Kaufmann SHE. Specific lysis by CD8 T cells of Schwann cells expressing *Mycobacterium leprae* antigens. *Eur J Immunol* 1988;18:969-972.

Chapter Nine

Mechanisms of Protective Immunity Against *Brucella abortus* in the Mouse Model System of Infection *Alexander J. Winter*

An important objective of current research on *B. abortus* is the development of an alternative vaccine to Strain 19. Such a vaccine should, ideally, induce a level of protection equal to or greater than that provided by Strain 19. At the same time it should be free of the disadvantages attendant upon the use of Strain 19, particularly the capacity of Strain 19 to induce disease in humans and cattle, and to produce antibody responses which confound the interpretation of serodiagnostic tests.[1]

The successful development of a subunit vaccine, or an appropriately altered living vaccine, against a facultative intracellular parasite represents a formidable task and will, in the case of *B. abortus*, require an improved understanding of the protective antigens of the organism, the pathogenesis of the disease, and the nature of protective immunity. The mouse has been widely used as a model system to investigate brucellosis, and reports to date have provided clear evidence that both humoral[2-9] and cell mediated immune (CMI) responses[7,10-13] participate in protection. Work toward these objectives conducted in our laboratory with the mouse model system during the past several years has been directed primarily at determining the participation in CMI of the CD4 and CD8 subsets of T cells, defining the limits of protection which can be bestowed by antibody, and investigating the basis of persistent infections produced by virulent strains of *B. abortus*.

Our studies have demonstrated that protective immunity against *B. abortus* in mice is due to combined effects of antibodies and of CMI responses mediated by T cells of both CD4 (L3T4) and CD8 (Lyt2) subsets.[14] An earlier report on murine brucellosis by Cheers and her coworkers[10] had shown that the Lyt2 cell was involved in protective immunity, but the role of the L3T4 cell remained unresolved due to the unavailability at that time of an L3T4-specific MAb. In defining the role of L3T4 cells in CMI by cell transfer experiments, it was of particular importance to insure that the protective effect of these cells was not attributable to their function as helper cells for antibody formation. For this reason B cells in the transferred populations were depleted as extensively as possible and antibody responses were tested in recipient mice. The fact that antibody responses in recipient animals never exceeded, and were in most experiments significantly below those of control groups[14] provides compelling evidence that protection was a consequence of CMI responses.

The biological functions of CD4 and CD8 cells, which are responsible for protective CMI against *B. abortus,* have yet to be defined, as do the respective roles of the Th1 and Th2 subsets of CD4 cells.[15-17] Our data suggest that the protective effects of antibodies, CD4 cells, and CD8 cells were largely independent of each other, although such an interpretation remains speculative. Interactive effects of antibodies and T cells, suggested by significantly better protection by both components than by either one alone, were demonstrable only when transfers were made before challenge infection.[14] Additive, nonadditive, and even antagonistic effects of *B. abortus* immune cells and serum have also been reported in passive transfer experiments in mice by Plommet et al.[11]

Significantly better protection was provided by immune serum given before, rather than after, challenge[14,18] which indicates that the protective function of the antibody against *B. abortus* is much more effective if antibodies are present in the bloodstream and tissues prior to exposure to the organism. In our experiments this difference in the magnitude of protection in the spleen could not be accounted for by increased sequestration of brucellae in the liver.[4]

The independent protective effects of antibody, better manifested if antibody was present prior to infection, led us to test whether antibodies alone might suffice to prevent infection. Our results provide strong evidence that this can occur, but only under conditions of restricted numbers of challenge organisms.[19] The isotype, affinity, and perhaps the fine specificity of the antibody appear also to constitute important limitations in the level of protection achieved. These data demonstrate the potential importance of antibodies in the immunoprophylaxis of brucellosis and, if found to be applicable to cattle, would argue strongly for the incorporation of an epitope of the O polysaccharide into subcellular vaccines to achieve maximal protection.

Orme demonstrated in murine infections with *Mycobacterium tuberculosis* that protection mediated by T cells rose as early as 5 days p.i. In contrast, protective T cells could not be demonstrated before 4 weeks p.i. in mice infected with *B. abortus*.[14] It may be inferred from mixing experiments with spleen cells from donors taken at 3 and 6 weeks post infection (p.i.)[14] that there was a relative absence of protective T cells for the first 3 weeks p.i. rather than a failure to demonstrate them due to the presence of suppressor cells.[21] At 4 and 6 weeks p.i. levels of protection provided against Strain 19 by spleen equivalent proportions of L3T4 and Lyt-2 cells were very similar,[14] whereas with *M. tuberculosis* protective activity was expressed predominantly by L3T4 cells during the first 4 months p.i.[20] We do not exclude the possibility that proportions of protective T cells may be altered at later periods after *B. abortus* infection, which may account for the loss of a majority of protective activity at 3 months p.i. following removal of Lyt-2 cells.[10]

In comparative studies of Strains 19 and 2308, a difference noted consistently was the greater refractoriness of Strain 2308 to the protective effects of antiserum.[18] This finding, together with previous reports[21-26] and our own data,[14,18,19,27,28] form the bases of a working hypothesis[27] to explain the capacity of virulent strains of *B. abortus* to produce persistent infections. In some respects this hypothesis is in accord with that proposed by Cheers.[22] It is proposed that an essential property of a virulent strain of *B. abortus* is its ability to survive in activated macrophages even though opsonized with IgG antibodies. Such survival may be minimized or overcome if the macrophages are fully activated at the time of infection,[28,29] or if the infecting organisms are in low numbers and have been opsonized by a high affinity antibody of appropriate IgG isotype.[19] In contrast, Strain 19 opsonized with IgG antibodies would be readily killed by activated macrophages.

On the basis of this hypothesis, the early stages of splenic infection by Strains 19 and 2308 would be essentially the same.[27] Large numbers of phagocytes, predominantly monocytes, would infiltrate the spleen in response to colony stimulating factors[25] induced by direct or indirect effects of bacterial LPS and outer membrane proteins.[30-33] Phagocytosis would occur in the absence of antibodies, perhaps facilitated by C3b.[34] The macrophages, although activated by LPS,[35-37] would not attain a sufficient state of activation to kill *B. abortus*, even though killing of *L. monocytogenes* was markedly increased.[14,28] The depletion of periarteriolar lymphoid tissue which occurs during the first 3 weeks p.i.[27] would delay the induction of an immune response within the spleen.[14] The direct cause of the lymphoid depletion is unknown, but it may have been a consequence of the high concentrations of brucellae and of activated macrophages within that organ.[14,28] An association of nonspecific immunosuppression with high bacterial numbers and high levels of macrophage activation has been noted in other infections.[38]

After the second week of infection, with the appearance of antibody, Strain 19 infection would come under rapid control, because newly migrated macrophages which ingested antibody opsonized bacteria would attain a brucellacidal state. It is observed that brucellacidal macrophages express relatively intense non-specific esterase (NSE) staining,[27,39-41] although no causal relationship is implied or required. The decrease in numbers of brucellae and of activated macrophages in the spleen would be followed by a resurgence of immune[14] and inflammatory[27] responses which would contribute importantly to the elimination of the organism.

Virulent Strain 2308, on the other hand, would continue to survive in activated macrophages even though opsonized. This would result in a steady state of infection, with continued depletion of lymphoid tissue in the spleen.[27] Immune responses which occur in Strain 2038 infected mice during this period of time would probably take place in less intensely infected lymphoid tissue.[28] Recovery from protection would be much more protracted and may be dependent upon the formation of antibodies of high affinity and of the required isotype, or of immune T cells with appropriate effector functions, such as lysis of *Brucella* infected host cells.[42]

Finally, it is noteworthy that, in contrast to the effects of immune serum, immune cells derived from Strain 19 or 2308-infected donors provided better protection against challenge with the homologous strain.[18] There may be several explanations for this finding but one possibility is that antigenic differences exist between Strains 19 and 2308 in T cell epitopes essential for the induction of protective immunity. If this were so it would constitute an important limitation not previously recognized on the efficacy of Strain 19 as a vaccine for cattle. The identification of the antigens of *B. abortus* are responsible for the induction of protective T cells is crucial for the development of a subcellular vaccine and represents a principal objective of research currently underway in our laboratory.

SUMMARY

Experiments have been performed in the mouse model of infection with *Brucella abortus* to elucidate the functions of antibodies and CMI responses in protective immunity and to investigate the basis of persistent infections produced by virulent strains. Passive transfer experiments demonstrated that in response to infection with attenuated *B. abortus* Strain 19, protective antibodies were present 3 weeks post infection (p.i.) while T cells mediating CMI could not be detected until 4 weeks p.i. Both CD4 (L3T4 positive) and CD8 (Lyt-2 positive) T cells contributed to protective CMI responses at equivalent levels. The data suggest that protection was mediated by independent as well as interactive effects of antibodies and immune T cells of the two subsets. Antibodies alone were capable of preventing the establishment of infection with virulent *B. abortus* Strain 2308 in a majority of animals, provided that low challenge doses were used and opsonization was performed with a high-affinity IgG2a monoclonal antibody specific for the O polysaccharide. In comparative analyses of infections produced by Strains 19 and 2308, it was demonstrated that Strain 2308 was significantly more refractory to the protective effects of antibodies, whether the antibodies were derived from donors infected with Strain 19 or 2308. On the other hand, protection provided by immune T cells was better against the homologous Strain of *B. abortus*. Splenic infection by both strains caused acute as well as granulomatous responses, and a depletion of lymphoid tissue which was most severe at 3 weeks p.i. Thereafter in mice infected with Strain 19 there occurred a rapid resurgence of lymphoid hyperplasia, a decrease in numbers of granulomas, and an increased intensity of the inflammatory response, accompanied by a rapid decrease in bacterial numbers. In contrast, bacterial counts of mice infected with Strain 2308 remained high, granulomas persisted, and lymphoid hyperplasia resumed at a markedly slower rate. Numbers of macrophages intensely stained with NSE were significantly higher in spleens of Strain 19 infected mice at 3 weeks p.i. and thereafter. It is hypothesized that the intensity of NSE staining may be directly related to the manifestation of brucellacidal activity, and that the divergent patterns of infection and inflammation manifested by the 2 strains after 2 weeks p.i. may result from the differential capacities of antibody opsonized Strain 19 and Strain 2308 to survive in activated macrophages.

Acknowledgments

I acknowledge gratefully the following individuals who contributed to the work reported in this paper: L. G. Adams, L. N. Araya, J. T. Douglas, J. R. Duncan, P. H. Elzer, F. M. Enright, G. E. Rowe, and C. G. Santisteban. I thank T. Botts, N. T. Caveney, and K. Clark for technical assistance.

This work was supported in part by U.S. Department of Agriculture Competitive Grant 85-CRCR-1-1859 and National Institutes of Health Grant 5001AI25935.

References

1. Subcommittee on Brucellosis Research: Brucellosis research: an evaluation. Report of the Subcommittee on Brucellosis Research, National Academy of Sciences, Washington, DC, National Academy Press, 1977.
2. Sulitzeanu D. Passive protection experiments with *Brucella* antisera. *J Hyg* 1955;53:133-142.
3. Pardon P. Resistance against a subcutaneous *Brucella* challenge in mice immunized with living or dead *Brucella* or by transfer of immune serum. *Ann Immunol* (Paris) 1977;128C:1025-1037.
4. Bascoul S, Cannat A, Huguet M, Serre A. Studies on the immune protection to murine experimental brucellosis conferred by *Brucella* fractions. I. Positive role of immune serum. *Immunology* 1978;35:213-221.
5. Madraso ED, Cheers C. Polyadenylic acid-polyuridylic acid (poly A:U) and experimental murine brucellosis. II. Macrophages as target cells of poly A:U in experimental brucellosis. *Immunology* 1978;35:77-84.
6. Plommet M, Plommet A-M. Immune serum-mediated effects on brucellosis evolution in mice. *Infect Immun* 1983;41:97-105.
7. Montaraz JA, Winter AJ. Comparison of living and nonliving vaccines for *Brucella abortus* in BALB/c mice. *Infect Immun* 1986;53:245-251.
8. Montaraz JA, Winter AJ, Hunter DM, Sowa BA, Wu AM, Adams LG. Protection

against *Brucella abortus* in mice with O-polysaccharide-specific monoclonal antibodies. *Infect Immun* 1986;51:961-963.

9. Limet J, Plommet A-M, Dubray G, Plommet M. Immunity conferred upon mice by anti-LPS monoclonal antibodies in murine brucellosis. *Ann Inst Pasteur Immunol* 1987;138:417-424.

10. Pavlov H, Hogarth M, McKenzie IFC, Cheers C. *In vivo* and *in vitro* effects of monoclonal antibody to Ly antigens on immunity to infection. *Cell Immunol* 1982;71:127-138.

11. Plommet M, Hue I, Plommet A-M. L'immunite anti-*brucella* transferee par serum immun et l'immunite transferee par les lymphocytes spleniques ne s'additionnent pas. *Ann Rech Vet* 1986;16:169-175.

12. Plommet M, Plommet A-M. Anti-brucella cell-mediated immunity in mice vaccinated with a cell-wall fraction. *Ann Rech Vet* 1987;18:429-437.

13. Bosseray N, Plommet M. Serum- and cell-mediated immune protection of mouse placenta and fetus against a *Brucella abortus* challenge: Expression of barrier effect of placenta. *Placenta* 1988;9:65-79.

14. Araya LN, Elzer PH, Rowe GE, Enright FM, Winter AJ. Temporal development of protective cell-mediated and humoral immunity in BALB/c mice infected with *Brucella abortus*. *J Immunol* 1989;142:3330-3337.

15. Mosmann TR, Cherwinski H, Bond MW, Giedlin MA, Coffman RL. Two types of murine helper T cell clone. I. Definition according to profiles of lymphokine activities and secreted proteins. *J Immunol* 1986;136:2348-2857.

16. Cher DJ, Mosmann TR. Two types of murine helper T cell clone. II. Delayed-type hypersensitivity is mediated by TH1 clones. *J Immunol* 1987;138:3688-3694.

17. Cherwinski HM, Schumacher JH, Brown KD, Mosmann TR. Two types of mouse helper T cell clone III. Further differences in lymphokine synthesis between Th1 and Th2 clones revealed by RNA hybridization, functionally monospecific bioassays and monoclonal antibodies. *J Exp Med* 1987;166:1229-1233.

18. Araya LN, Winter AJ. Comparative protection of mice against virulent and attenuated strains of *Brucella abortus* by passive transfer of immune T cells or serum. *Infect Immun* 1990; In press.

19. Winter AJ, Duncan JR, Santisteban CG, Douglas JT, Adams LG: Capacity of passively administered antibody to prevent the establishment of *Brucella* abortus infection in mice. *Infect Immun* 1989;57:3438-3444.

20. Orme IM. The kinetics of emergence and loss of mediator T lymphocytes acquired in response to infection with *Mycobacterium tuberculosis*. *J Immunol* 1987;138:293-298.

21. Riglar C, Cheers C. Macrophage activation during experimental murine brucellosis II. Inhibition of in vitro lymphocyte proliferation by *Brucella*-activated macrophages. *Cell Immunol* 1980;49:154-167.

22. Cheers C. Pathogenesis and cellular immunity in experimental murine brucellosis. *Develop Biol Stand* 1983;56:237-246.

23. Cheers C, Pagram F. Macrophage activation during experimental murine brucellosis: a basis for chronic infection. *Infect Immun* 1979;23:197-205.

24. Frenchick PJ, Markham JF, Cochrane AH: Inhibition of phagosome-lysosome fusion in macrophages by soluble extracts of virulent *Brucella abortus*. *Am J Vet Res* 1985;46:332-335.

25. Cheers C, Young AM. Serum colony stimulating activity and colony forming cells in murine brucellosis: relationship to immunopathology. *Micro Path* 1987;3:185-194.

26. Cheers C, Pavlov H, Riglar C, Madraso E. Macrophage activation during experimental murine brucellosis. III. Do macrophages exert feedback control during brucellosis? *Cell Immunol* 1980;49:168-177.

27. Enright FM, Araya LN, Elzer PH, Rowe GE, Winter AJ. Comparative histopathol-

ogy in BALB/c mice infected with virulent and attenuated strains of *Brucella abortus*. Submitted for publication.

28. Elzer PH, Rowe GE, Enright FM, Winter AJ. Effects of gamma radiation and azathioprine on the course of *Brucella abortus* infection in BALB/c mice. Submitted for publication.

29. Cheers C, Waller R. Activated macrophages in congenitally athymic "nude" mice and in lethally irradiated mice. *J Immunol* 1975;115:844-847.

30. Bjornson BH, Agura E, Harvey JM, Johns M, Andrews RG, McCabe WR: Endotoxin-associated protein: a potent stimulus for human granulocytopoietic activity which may be accessory cell independent. *Infect Immun* 1988; 56:1602-1607.

31. Cline MJ, Rothman B, Golde DW. Effect of endotoxin on the production of colony stimulating factor by human monocytes and macrophages. *J Cell Physiol* 1974;84:193-196.

32. Eaves AC, Bruce WR: In vitro production of colony stimulating activity. I. Exposure of mouse peritoneal cells to endotoxin. *Cell Tissue Kinet* 1975;7:19-30.

33. Ruscetti FW, Chervenick PA. Release of colony-stimulating factor from monocytes by endotoxin and polyinosinic-polycytidylic acid. *J Lab Clin Med* 1974;83:64-72.

34. Corbeil LB, Blau K, Inzana TI, et al. Killing of *Brucella abortus* by bovine serum. *Infect Immun* 1988;56:3251-3261.

35. Johnston RB Jr, Godzik CA, Cohn ZA: Increased superoxide anion production by immunologically activated and chemically elicited macrophages. *J Exp Med* 1978;148:115-127.

36. Pabst MJ, Johnston RB Jr. Increased production of superoxide anion by macrophages exposed *in vitro* to muramyl dipeptide or lipopolysaccharide. *J Exp Med* 1980;151:101-114.

37. Brozna JP, Hauff NF, Phillips WA, Johnston RB Jr. Activation of the respiratory burst in macrophages: Phosphorylation specifically associated with Fc receptor-mediated stimulation. *J Immunol* 1988;141:1642-1647.

38. Appelberg R, Soares R, Ferreira P, Silva MT. Induction of non-specific immunosuppression in mice by mycobacterial infections and its relationship to macrophage activation. *Scand J Immunol* 1989;30:165-174.

39. Rodgers KE, Imamura T, Devens BH. Investigations into the mechanism of immunosuppression caused by acute treatment of O,O,S-Trimethyl phosphorothioate. I. Characterization of the immune cell population affected. *Immunopharmacology* 1985;10:171-180.

40. Rodgers KE, Imamura T, Devens BH. Investigations into the mechanism of immunosuppression caused by acute treatment with O,O,S-Trimethyl phosphorothioate. II. Effect on the ability of murine macrophages to present antigen. *Immunopharmacology* 1985;10:181-189.

41. Wehle K, Pfitzer P. Nonspecific esterase activity of human alveolar macrophages in routine cytology. *Acta Cytologica* 1988;32:153-158.

42. Kaufmann SHE. Possible role of helper and cytolytic T lymphocytes in antibacterial defense: Conclusions based on a murine model of listeriosis. *Rev Infect Dis* 1987;9:S650-S659.

Chapter Ten

Natural Resistance to
Bovine Brucellosis

Joe W. Templeton and L. Garry Adams

Host response to infectious disease is variable and complex. Studies of the genetic control of host resistance to infectious diseases, primarily in the mouse, clearly demonstrated that the mode of inheritance of this host resistance was polygenic. Although early workers in this area of genetically controlled (natural) resistance to infectious diseases predicted that it would be theoretically possible to breed naturally resistant livestock, it has been largely ignored as a component for control of infectious disease in livestock.[1] This is due mainly to the perception that since the genetic control of natural resistance is polygenic and the host immune response is complex, the mechanisms of disease resistance were too complicated to be seriously considered as a part of a program for control or eradication of infectious disease. Antibiotics and vaccines appeared to offer a simpler solution for control or eradication of infectious diseases. This perception persisted even with the repeated observation of cattle and pigs to brucellosis that were naturally resistant (R) and the slow progress in the bovine brucellosis eradication program.

With the definitive gene mapping of the first described immune response genes in 1965,[2] studies concerning the role of genetic control of resistance to infectious diseases in mice were pursued and the phenomenon became well established. Although most of the information accumulated has concerned gene control of immune mechanisms involved in resistance to infectious diseases, there have been studies demonstrating genetic control of non-immune mechanisms of resistance/susceptibility to infectious disease.[3,4] Genetic susceptibility (S) to infectious disease has been primarily studied in mice and to a much lesser extent in humans.[5] Studies of resistance/susceptibility in mice have shown that genetically controlled disease resistance is a polygenic trait;[6] however, single genes have been observed to have a major effect on immune mediated resistance in mice in a wide range of infectious diseases. For example, single gene effects on resistance/susceptibility between two strains of mice (A and C57BL/6) have been reported for 25 different parasites, eight different bacteria, seven viruses, and three fungi.[7]

The role of macrophages in resisting infectious diseases has been shown to be under control of a single gene or gene complex for four infectious organisms: *Mycobacterium lepraemurium* (*Bcg*),[8] *Salmonella typhimurium* (*Ity*),[9] *Leishmania donovani* (*Lsh*),[10] and *Mycobacterium bovis* (*Bcg*).[11] The gene(s) controlling resistance to all four of these infectious organisms have been mapped to chromosome 1 and could possibly be the same gene.[8]

Obviously, this gene or cluster of closely linked genes on chromosome 1 is very important in resistance to these four organisms, but interaction with genes on other chromosomes has also been shown to be important for two of the diseases. Susceptibility to *Salmonella typhimurium* has been shown to be regulated by two genes - the Ity^r on chromosome 1 and the Lps^d on chromosome 4.[12] Susceptibility to *Leishmania donovani* is regulated by two genes - *Lsh* on chromosome 1 and *H-2* on chromosome 17. Apparently, the Lsh^r gene provides immediate resistance for the first 15 days of infection but *H-2* linked genes are crucial for long term resistance.[13]

Studies of genetic control of resistance to Brucellae infections have been done in mice, rabbits, and swine. Ho and Cheers[14] reported that resistance to *B. abortus* Strain 19 infection is under polygenic control in BALB/c mice. Manresa[15] reported that resistance to brucellosis is controlled by a single dominant allele in rabbits.

In swine a series of studies of genetic control of resistance to *B. suis* were conducted by Cameron and colleagues.[16,17] In the first experiments, two sows and a boar that did not develop antibody titers when exposed to *B. suis* were saved for breeding. These swine were classified as naturally resistant (R) to brucellosis. The progeny of these three apparent R swine were challenge-infected and their antibody titers to *B. suis* were compared to control groups of unselected pigs that were challenge-infected. Of of the progeny from the R swine, 73% (24 of 33) were R to the challenge infection as compared to only 9% R (3 of 24) progeny in the control. In subsequent breeding - challenge infection studies R X R matings produced 128 progeny - 76.6% were R, 22.6% were of uncertain status, and 0.8% were susceptible (S). It is remarkable that, in one generation of mass election, resistance to *B. suis* could be increased by approximately 54% over unselected controls. Obviously very few genes are involved in controlling resistance to *B. suis* in swine.

In cattle, we have observed that the frequency of natural resistance is approximately 18% (19 out of 105) (See Table 10-1) in a group of cross-bred cattle (*Bos taurus* X *Bos indicus*). Breeding animals (founders) were selected from the 105 unvaccinated challenged animals shown in Table 10-1. The cattle were non-vaccinated and immunologically naive to *B. abortus* Strain 2308 (S2308). Non-exposure to *B. abortus* was confirmed on at least three separate occasions in an eight month period prior to challenge by card, rivanol, complement fixation, enzyme-linked immunosorbent assay (ELISA), and hemolysis-in-gel tests.[18]

Table 10-1. Frequency of Natural Resistance to Brucellosis in Cows
Challenged *via* the Conjunctiva with 10^7 CFUs of S2308 *B. abortus*

Number challenged	Number resistant
105	19 (18%)

*Unvaccinated first-calf heifers challenged midgestation

The cattle were challenged by conjunctival administration of 1×10^7 colony-forming units (CFU) of live *B. abortus* S2308 during mid-gestation of their first pregnancy. The resistant cattle (n=12), retrospectively classified, developed low transient serologic titers; did not abort; and cultures of the post partum uterus, lacteal secretions, and calf meconium were negative for *Brucella*. Susceptible infected cows (n=12) developed high titers, did abort, and *Brucella* was isolated from lacteal secretions, uterus, placenta, or fetuses.[18]

These 24 cross-bred cattle were assembled for breeding studies to determine the mode of inheritance of the resistance and susceptibilty to the *Brucella* challenge. *Bos taurus* bulls were challenged in the same manner as the cows, and their semen was cultured for presence of *B. abortus* 6 weeks and 6 months post challenge. A bull (#86) was selected as a herd sire. His semen sample was culture negative. This, taken with a low transient antibody titer in the above mentioned brucellosis serology tests, was the basis for classifying the bull as resistant to brucellosis.

The antibody response to *B. abortus* is different in R and S cows. The *B. abortus* antibody response in R cows was short lived, low titered, and primarily IgM. The *B. abortus* antibody response of the S cows was long lived, high titered, and was both IgM and IgG.[18] Nine of the 12 R cows were challenge infected at mid-gestation a second time by conjunctival instillation of 10^7 CFUs of *B. abortus* S2308. None of the cows had interrupted pregnancies and the antibody response profile was similar to the antibody response profile of the first challenge infection. The tissues collected at parturition from cows and calves were culture negative for *Brucella*, further confirming their solid resistance to challenge.

The first study attempted to characterize the mode of inheritance of the resistant phenotype of the bull (#86) that was selected as the herd sire for our genetic studies following challenge of a group of bulls. Bull 86 was bred to 10 cows that had been vaccinated by S19 *B. abortus* and were not protected when challenged as stated above. Of the 10 offspring challenged, four were R and six were S (See Table 10-2). From these data we could determine that the bull was heterozygous, and we would model a mode of inheritance of monogenic inheritance of the brucellosis R phenotype in the herd of R and S cows.

Table 10-2. Results of Challenging* Unvaccinated Progeny from Bull #86 (Resistant) Mated to S19 Vaccine Failure Cows

Number resistant	Number susceptible
4	6

*Challenged intraconjunctivally with 10^7 CFUs S2308 at midgestation

We have challenge infected 28 progeny from R x S matings; 11 were R and 17 were S. We have challenge infected 15 progeny from R x R mating, and 9 were R and 6 were S (See Table 10-3). In these breeding studies, there was an increase in the frequency of resistant animals from 18% in random breedings to 39% in matings of R males to S females, and to 60% in matings of R males to R females. This doubling and trebling of the number of resistant animals in one generation of selective breeding is strong evidence for genetic determination of natural resistance to bovine brucellosis. The data from Table 10-3 are consistent with segregation of a single dominant allele controlling resistance to bovine brucellosis. A simple Mendelian recessive allele controlling the resistant phenotype is rejected by the observation that S phenotypes were observed in the R X R matings (See Table 10-3). However the characterization of the R and S founder population's immune response to *Brucella* by *in vitro* methods makes it more likely that more than one gene is controlling resistance to brucellosis in our small population.

We have further shown that there is a significant difference between the IgG2a A1 and A2 allotype response profile of R and S founders. Twenty- one of the founders (9 R and 12 S) are heterozygous for the IgG 2a allotypes-A1 and A2. Prior to challenge with *B. abortus* the ratio of expression of A1/A2 is approximately 50:50. Eight weeks after challenge there is a significant difference in the allotype response of the R and S cattle to *Brucella* LPS measured in an ELISA using monoclonal antibodies that differentiate between IgG2A-AI and A2 allotypes.[19] Most R cattle do not preferentially express one allotype (although 3 of 9 preferentially expressed the anti-LPS antibodies entirely as A2), whereas 9 of 12 of the S cattle preferentially expressed anti-LPS as A1 allotype (80 to 100% anti-LPS was A1 allotype).

We have shown that there is a difference between the ability of mononuclear phagocytic cells (Møs) of R and S founders to control replication of *B. abortus* in vitro.[20,21] The R cows can control the *in vitro* replication of *B. abortus* significantly better than S cows. Additionally, we have shown that mammary macrophages and peripheral blood monocytes both are different before challenge exposure in the ability to control replication of *B. abortus in vitro* in R and S cows.[21] Although the monocyte

Table 10-3. Heritability of Resistance to Bovine Brucellosis

Sire	Dam	Offspring Phenotype	Observed	Expectent*	$\chi 2$
R(#86)	S	R	11	14	1.29
(R/r)	(r/r)	S	17	14	(p=0.26)
R(#86)	R	R	9	11	1.80
(R/r)	(R/r;R/R)	S	6	3	(p=0.18)

*assuming segregation of a single dominant gene for resistance

replication of B. abortus in vitro.[20,21] The R cows can control the in vitro replication of B. abortus significantly better than S cows. Additionally, we have shown that mammary macrophages and peripheral blood monocytes both are different before challenge exposure in the ability to control replication of B. abortus in vitro in R and S cows.[21] Although the monocytes are not as efficient as the mammary macrophages in controlling replication of B. abortus in vitro, the direction is the same in the R and the S groups, even if the magnitude is different. These data are interpreted to mean the ability of Møs to control replication of B. abortus in vitro prior to exposure is an innate trait. Finally, we have begun preliminary investigation of the range of intracellular pathogens that could be controlled by Møs from R cows that control B. abortus replication in vitro. We studied the control of Salmonella typhimurium and S. dublin replication in vitro, and our preliminary results indicate that these organisms are also differentially controlled. The Brucella R cows are significantly better at controlling the replication of both Salmonella species in vitro. We interpret these data as indicating that the innate ability of Møs to control replication of intracellular pathogens is broad based and this innate Mø function may be a central mechanism of natural disease resistance for multiple intracellular pathogens.

Summary

It has been shown clearly that the vaccination of cows with Strain 19 B. abortus does not always elicit protection to subsequent challenge infection in all cows.[22,23] In fact, 20 to 30% of the cows failed to achieve protection by S19 vaccination in these trials. In spite of the clear demonstration in the 1930s and early 1940s by Cameron, Gregory, and Hughes[16,17] that pigs had a genetically controlled natural resistance to B. suis, the potential of natural resistance in controlling brucellosis has been largely ignored. If gene components of natural resistance to brucellosis in cattle can be identified, then the possibility of modulating these genes to improve the frequency of natural resistance by utilizing artificial insemination and embryo transfer to propagate a genotype conferring resistance is a realistic goal.

References

1. Hutt, FB. Genetic resistance to disease in domestic animals. Ithaca, NY: Comstock Publishing Associates, 1958.
2. McDevitt HO, Sela M. Genetic control of the antibody response. I. Demonstration of determinant-specific differences in the response to synthetic polypeptide antigens in two strains of inbred mice. *J Exp Med* 1965;122:517.
3. Mourant AE, Kopec AC, Domaniervska-Sobczak K. Blood Groups and Diseases. *Oxford University Press, New York* 1977;328.
4. Miller LH, Mason SJ, Clyde DF, McGinniss MH. The resistance factor to *Plasmodium vivax* in blacks. The Duffy-blood group genotype, Fy/Fy. *N Eng J Med* 1976;295:302-304.
5. Dausset J, Svejgard A. HLA and Disease. *Williams and Wilkins, Baltimore, Md* 1977;316.
6. Rosenstreich DL, Weinblatt AC, O'Brien AD. Genetic control of resistance to infection in mice. *CRC Crit Rev Immunol* 1982;3:263.
7. Nesbitt MN, Skamene E. Recombinant inbred mouse strains derived from A/J and C57BL/6J: A tool for the study of genetic mechanisms in host resistance to infection and malignancy. *J Leukocyte Biol* 1984;36:357-364
8. Brown *lepraemurium* follows the *Ity/Lsh* pattern. *Immunology* 1982;47:149-156.
9. Plant J, Glynn AA. Locating salmonella resistance gene on mouse Chromosome 1. *Clin Exp Immunol* 1979;37:1-6.
10. Bradley DJ, Taylor BA, Blackwell J, Evans EP, Freeman J. Regulation of *Leishmania* populations within the host. III. Mapping of the locus controlling susceptibility to visceral leishmaniasis in the mouse. *Clin Exp Immuno* 1979;37:7-14.
11. Gros P, Skamene E, Forget A. Genetic control of natural resistance to *Mycobacterium bovis* in mice. *J Immunol* 1981;127(6):2417-2422.
12 Blackwell J, Freeman J, Bradley D. Influence of H-2 complex on acquired resistance to *Leishmania donovani* infection in mice. *Nature* 1980;283:72-74.
13. O'Brien AD, Rosenstreich DL, Scher I, Campbell GH, MacDermott RP, Formal SB. Genetic control of susceptibility to *Salmonella typhimurium* in mice: Role of the LPS gene. *J Immunol* 1980;124(1):20-24.
14. Ho ML, Cheers C. Resistance and susceptibility of mice to bacterial infection. IV. Genetic and cellular basis of resistance to chronic infection with *Brucella abortus*. *J Infect Dis* 1982;146:381-387.
15. Manresa M, Laguna PI. Inheritance of resistance and susceptibility to infectious abortion. *J Infect Dis* 1932;51:30-71.
16 Cameron HS, Hughes EH, Gregory PW. Genetic resistance to brucellosis in swine. *J Anim Sci* 1942;1:106-110.
17 Cameron HS, Gregory PW, Hughes EH. Inherited resistance to brucellosis in inbred Berkshire swine. *Am J Vet Res* 1943;3-4:387-389.
18. Harmon BG, Templeton JW, Crawford RP, Heck FC, Williams JD, Adams LG. Macrophage function and immune response of *Brucella abortus* naturally resistant and susceptible cattle. In:*Genetic Control of Host Resistance to Infection and*

Malignancy. Adam R. Lis, Inc., 1985;345-354.

19. Estes DM, JW Templeton, LG Adams. Murine Monoclonal Antibodies to the Bovine Immunoglobulin G2a Allotypes- A1 and A2. *Animal Genetics*, Accepted 1990.

20. Harmon BG, Adams LG, Templeton JW, Smith III, R. Mammary gland macrophage function in *Brucella abortus* infected and challenge resistant cows. *Am J Vet Res*, 1989 50(4):459-465.

21. Price RE, JW Templeton, R Smith III, L G Adams. The relationship between natural resistance to bovine brucellosis and the ability of bovine mononuclear phagocytes to control replication of *Brucella abortus* in vitro. Submitted, *Infect Immun*, April 1990 (In Press).

22. Deyoe BL, Dorsey TA, Meredith KB, Garrett L. Effect of reduced dosages of *Brucella abortus* Strain 19 in cattle vaccinated as yearlings. *Proc Annu Meet US Anim Health Assoc* 1979;83:92-104.

23. Garcia-Carillo C. Comparison of *B. melitensis* Rev. 1 and *B. abortus* Strain 19 as a vaccine against brucellosis in cattle. *Zentralbl Veterinarmed [B]* 1980;27:131-138.

Chapter Eleven

Phagocyte Function in Resistance to Brucellosis

Peter C. Canning

Relevance of Phagocytes to Brucellosis

Brucella abortus is characterized as a facultative intracellular parasite capable of surviving within phagocytic cells. Phagocytic cells in general and neutrophils in particular play an important role as a "first line" of defense against infection by bacterial pathogens.

Approximately 35% of outbred cattle have been shown to possess natural resistance to virulent strains of *B. abortus*.[1] Additional evidence for the significant contribution of phagocytes to resistance from *Brucella*-induced disease is derived from recent studies which have attempted to identify immunologic differences between cattle which were naturally resistant or susceptible to *B. abortus* infection.[2] One of the primary functional differences noted between the populations of animals was the enhanced brucellacidal activity of mammary gland macrophages from the naturally resistant cattle.

The ability of *B. abortus* to evade the antimicrobial activities of phagocytes in susceptible animals plays a pivotal role in the pathogenesis of the infection. Following infection, the bacteria are rapidly ingested by neutrophils in the tissues. These cells facilitate the spread of the microbes through two distinct mechanisms. First, once ingested, the bacteria are located within an environment which protects them from the bactericidal activities of antibody and complement. Second, the phagocytes serve as vectors for transporting the *B. abortus* to regional lymph nodes where bacterial multiplication occurs, leading to systemic disease.

Smooth strains of the organism exhibit increased resistance to the brucellacidal activities of phagocytes when compared to rough strains of the bacteria. *Brucella abortus* opsonized with specific antibodies are efficiently ingested by both neutrophils and macrophages and this activity is associated with induction of the phagocyte's oxidative metabolic burst. Degranulation and the subsequent release of lysosomal enzymes by bovine neutrophils are suppressed in the presence of either viable or killed

B. abortus. Brucella abortus is susceptible to killing by products of the myeloperoxidase-H_2O_2-halide antibacterial system of neutrophils if the system is allowed to function normally. These results suggest inhibition of degranulation is an important factor in the intracellular survival of the bacteria. 5'-guanosine monophosphate and adenine are associated with the surface of virulent *B. abortus* and these materials have been shown to inhibit neutrophil primary granule release and the activity of the myeloperoxidase-H_2O_2-halide antibacterial system. The identification of specific defects in phagocyte function and the *B. abortus* components responsible for them provides researchers with a biological target on which to focus efforts for developing prophylactic or therapeutic methods of intervention which may lead to enhanced resistance to *Brucella*-induced disease.

The Phagocytic Process

The phagocytic process can be separated into five distinct events: 1) migration, 2) ingestion, 3) oxidative metabolic burst, 4) degranulation, and 5) killing.

Phagocytes emigrate from blood vessels through a complex series of processes collectively referred to as diapedesis. Migration of phagocytic cells toward a site of infection can be either random (chemokinesis) or directed (chemotaxis). A wide variety of materials can serve as chemotactic factors: bacterial proteins, complement components (C3a and C5a), components of the kinin system, and bacterial endotoxins.

Once the phagocyte reaches the site of infection, engulfment of the invading microorganisms occurs in a two-step process involving attachment of the organism to the phagocyte membrane and subsequent internalization of the particle. Although some particles can be ingested without prior opsonization, most bacteria must be coated with opsonizing proteins such as antibody (IgG or IgM) or complement (C3b) for optimal attachment and engulfment.[3]

Concomitant with ingestion, there is a dramatic increase in the metabolic activity of the phagocytes. This respiratory burst involves a series of enzymatic reactions responsible for the conversion of oxygen to active metabolites which exhibit potent microbicidal activities. These metabolites include: superoxide anion, singlet oxygen, hydroxyl radicals, and hydrogen peroxide.

The fourth step involved in the phagocytic process is that of degranulation which leads to the destruction of ingested bacteria through the microbicidal activities of the enzymes and proteins contained within cytoplasmic granules. Degranulation occurs simultaneously with the respiratory burst following stimulation of the phagocyte.[4,5]

The final step in the bacterial-phagocyte interaction involves destruction of the ingested organism by the products of the respiratory burst and degranulation. The microbicidal activities of all phagocytic cells can be divided into two broad categories: the oxygen-dependent reactions and the oxygen-independent reactions.

The myeloperoxidase-hydrogen peroxide-halide (MPO-H_2O_2-halide) system is the primary oxidative antibacterial system of neutrophils.[4,7] The components required for a functional MPO-H_2O_2-halide system include myeloperoxidase from primary cytoplasmic granules, H_2O_2 from the respiratory burst, and halide anions such as Cl^- or I^-.[7] The microbicidal activity of the MPO-H_2O_2-halide reaction results from the binding of halogen ions to tyrosine or histidine residues on microbial proteins.[7]

Phagocytes have also been shown to possess limited bactericidal capabilities under anaerobic conditions, suggesting the presence of non-oxidative killing mechanisms.[8] These mechanisms include the acid environment inside the phagolysosome and the presence of iron-binding proteins such as lactoferrin. Additional granule constituents such as lysozyme and cationic proteins exert direct degradative activity against bacterial cell surface components and interfere with microbial protein synthesis.[4,9]

Bacterial pathogens have evolved to possess mechanisms for avoiding or resisting each step in the phagocytic response to infection. Table 11-1 presents a brief summary of these mechanisms and provides examples of various bacteria that use them.

Intracellular Survival of *Brucella abortus*

Early studies of the interactions between *B. abortus* and bovine phagocytic cells compared the ability of virulent and attenuated strains of the organism grown under various conditions to survive within mixed populations of white blood cells. Smith and Fitzgeorge evaluated the relative susceptibilities of virulent and avirulent strains of *B. abortus* to the bactericidal activities of bovine buffy coat cells.[21] The virulent strain (544) exhibited greater resistance to intracellular killing than did the avirulent strain (45/0). These studies also indicated that *B. abortus* (Strain 544) isolated from infected bovine placenta resisted killing better than the same strain grown *in vitro*. Smith and Fitzgeorge extended their studies to examine the contribution of *B. abortus* cell wall extracts to the intracellular survival of the bacteria. Hughes Press cell wall preparations of *B. abortus* (Strain 544) grown *in vivo* enhanced the survival of attenuated *B. abortus* within buffy coat cells. Cell wall preparations from the same organism grown *in vitro* did not enhance the ability of *B. abortus* (45/0) to survive intracellularly. The enhancing effect of the cell wall preparations was neutralized in the presence of specific antiserum. These findings provided preliminary evidence that cell wall components contribute to the ability of

Table 11-1. Examples of Mechanisms Used by Pathogenic Bacteria to Escape Destruction by Phagocytic Cells

Mechanism	Bacteria (Reference)
Inhibits chemotaxis through deficient complement activation	*N. gonorrheae* (10); *P. aeruginosa* (11)

Inhibits attachment
  Polysaccharide capsules
  Proteinaceous capsules
	S. pneumoniae (12); *K. pneumoniae* (13) *E. coli* (14); *B. anthracis* (15)

Inhibits ingestion	*Mycoplasma sp.* (16); *N. gonorrheae* (17)
Inhibits, fails to stimulate oxidative burst	*S. typhi* (18)
Inhibits degranulation	*M. tuberculosis* (19); *H. somnnus* (20)

B. abortus to resist intracellular killing.

Further studies by Fitzgeorge and Smith indicated *B. abortus* (Strain 544) grown in medium containing 20% bovine allantoic fluids possessed an enhanced ability to survive within bovine buffy coat cells compared with bacteria grown in unsupplemented medium.[22] In addition, cell wall preparations from organisms grown in supplemented medium enhanced the ability of attenuated strains of *B. abortus* to survive within bovine buffy coat cells. However, this material was still less effective in enhancing survival than cell wall preparations from organisms grown *in vivo*.

Kreutzer et al.[23] investigated the bactericidal activity of guinea pig and human neutrophils against smooth (45/0) and rough (45/20) strains of *B. abortus*. Guinea pig phagocytes exhibited no killing of the smooth strain and only limited killing of rough organisms. Human neutrophils were more effective in killing both strains of *B. abortus*, but the *B. abortus* were killed less effectively than control preparations of *Staphylococcus aureus*.

Further studies by Riley and Robertson and Robertson et al. compared the brucellacidal activities of bovine and human neutrophils.[24, 25] Bovine neutrophils were found to be significantly more bactericidal than human cells against smooth Strain 45/0, whereas there was no difference in the bactericidal activity of the two species' neutrophils against rough Strain 45/20 *B. abortus*.

Similar results were obtained in a recent study that compared the ability of smooth (Strain 2308) and rough (Strain 45/20) *B. abortus* to survive within bovine mammary gland macrophages.[26] Intracellular survival rates for the smooth strain were significantly higher than for those of the rough strain.

Effects of *Brucella abortus* On Specific Phagocyte Functions

As stated previously, intracellular destruction of organisms such as *B. abortus* by phagocytic cells is dependent upon numerous discrete mechanisms which are susceptible to alteration by bacterial pathogens. The ability of *B. abortus* to manipulate these various activities has been intensively studied.

Effects on ingestion

Numerous studies have evaluated the ability of various strains of *B. abortus* to resist ingestion by neutrophils and macrophages. In addition, the requirement for opsonization as a prerequisite for the uptake of bacteria has been investigated.

Kreutzer et al. evaluated the interactions between guinea pig and human neutrophils and smooth (45/0) or rough (45/20) strains of *B. abortus*.[23] Both smooth and rough *B. abortus* were readily ingested by human and guinea pig neutrophils as measured by uptake of radiolabelled bacteria treated with heat-inactivated homologous serum.

Further studies by Riley and Robertson and Robertson et al. compared the ability of bovine and human neutrophils to ingest smooth (45/0) and rough (45/20) strains of *B. abortus*.[24,25] Similar to the previous studies, both strains of the bacteria were readily ingested by human and bovine cells.

The ability of *B. abortus* to alter normal neutrophil phagocytic activity was investigated by determining the effects of whole and fractionated preparations of virulent *B. abortus* (Strain 2308) upon the ability of bovine neutrophils to ingest radiolabelled *S. aureus*.[27] The results of these studies indicated this strain of *B. abortus* does not produce any substances which inhibit the phagocytic activity of bovine neutrophils.

Studies of the interactions between bovine mammary gland macrophages and smooth (2308) or rough (45/20) strains of *B. abortus* suggested both strains were readily ingested if opsonized with either complement or specific antibody.[26] The results of this study were in agreement with those of Young et al. which indicated appreciable ingestion of virulent (Strain 296) and attenuated (1119) strains of *B. abortus* by human neutrophils required prior opsonization of the bacteria with either complement or specific antibodies.[28]

Collectively these studies provide substantial evidence that B. abortus does not evade destruction by phagocytic cells through evasion of the ingestion process.

Effects on the Respiratory Burst

The pivotal role of the oxidative metabolic burst in the antibacterial processes of phagocytic cells has prompted investigation of the effects of B. abortus upon phagocyte oxidative metabolism.

Initial studies of the effects of B. abortus on the respiratory burst of bovine neutrophils indicated ingestion of non-opsonized B. abortus (Strain 544) did not induce the production of O_2^- as measured by quantitative nitroblue tetrazolium dye reduction.[29] Subsequent experiments indicated ingestion of smooth or rough strains of B. abortus did not appear to stimulate hexose monophosphate shunt activity by human neutrophils (measured as glucose oxidation).[23] Based upon the results of these studies, it was hypothesized that a lack of stimulation of the oxidative metabolic burst compromises the bactericidal capability of the neutrophil resulting in enhanced intracellular survival of B. abortus. However, it is important to note the bacteria used in these studies were either not exposed to serum or were treated with heat-inactivated normal bovine serum. Heat-inactivated normal bovine serum would possess marginal opsonic activity due to a lack of specific antibodies and active complement components.

To further investigate the relationship between the metabolic oxidative burst and intracellular survival of B. abortus, the effects of whole or fractionated B. abortus (Strain 2308) on the ability of bovine neutrophils to produce O_2^- in response to stimulation with opsonized zymosan particles were examined.[27] Neither whole heat-killed bacteria nor fractions of B. abortus inhibited production of O_2^- by stimulated phagocytes, suggesting that the bacteria does not actively suppress metabolic oxidative burst activity.

Additional studies were performed to determine if different opsonins (C3b or antibody) altered the oxidative metabolic response of bovine neutrophils to ingestion of virulent B. abortus (Strain 2308).[30] Bacteria exposed to fresh serum containing anti-B. abortus antibody, heat-inactivated anti-B. abortus serum (presumably free of complement activity), or fresh normal bovine serum (presumably free of anti-B. abortus antibody), were evaluated for their ability to stimulate an oxidative response. Brucella exposed to either fresh antiserum or heat-inactivated antiserum was capable of stimulating significant levels of both O_2^- production and MPO-H_2O_2-halide activity. In contrast, non-opsonized B. abortus and bacteria treated with normal bovine sera failed to stimulate either O_2^- production or iodination activity, confirming the findings of previous investigators.[23, 29]

Studies of the interactions between *B. abortus* and mammary macrophages have also indicated prior opsonization is required for *B. abortus* to stimulate an oxidative metabolic burst by mammary macrophages.[26]

Collectively, the results of these studies suggest *B. abortus* induces oxidative metabolism in bovine neutrophils and macrophages; however, the stimulation is dependent upon the presence of bacterial-associated opsonins. Bacteria invading an animal would most likely be opsonized with both antibody and complement prior to ingestion, therefore it would not appear that failure to stimulate oxidative metabolism contributes to the intracellular survival of the bacteria as previously hypothesized.[23, 29]

Effects on Degranulation and Oxidative or Non-oxidative Killing

Early investigations of the effects of various preparations of *B. abortus* on degranulation activity by phagocytic cells primarily focused on qualitative and quantitative procedures for measuring the relative amounts of degranulation activity in the presence of either smooth or rough strains of the bacteria. In addition, the relative resistance of various strains of *B. abortus* to the degradative activities of the enzymes contained within the cytoplasmic granules were compared.

As a part of studies to determine the interactions between *B. abortus* and human or bovine neutrophils, Riley and Robertson and Robertson et al. examined the effects of smooth and rough strains of *B. abortus* on primary and secondary granule degranulation.[24, 25] The amount of degranulation (determined by electron microscopy) in both species' neutrophils incubated with smooth (Strain 45/0) *B. abortus* was significantly reduced in comparison to control preparations involving the extracellular organism *Staphylococcus epidermidis*. Quantitative evidence of decreased degranulation was obtained by measuring the amounts of granule enzymes released into the extracellular environment and by isolating intact granules from infected cells by sucrose density gradient centrifugation. The results of these studies indicated neutrophils incubated with *B. abortus* released significantly less myeloperoxidase than did cells incubated with *S. epidermidis*. Lactoferrin release was not appreciably different between cells incubated with *B. abortus* and cells incubated with *S. epidermidis*. Results of the granule isolation studies indicated that both primary and secondary granule degranulation was suppressed in neutrophils that had ingested *B. abortus*. The amounts of primary and secondary granule release were not significantly different between neutrophils incubated with Strain 45/0 and neutrophils incubated with Strain 45/20. In addition, exposure of human neutrophils to glutaraldehyde-killed 45/0 cells also resulted in decreased release of primary and secondary granules, indicating viable organisms were not required to inhibit degranulation.

Indirect evidence for inhibition of degranulation by *B. abortus* was obtained from studies of the effects of live or heat-killed *B. abortus* (Strain 2308) upon the iodination activity (a measure of MPO-H_2O_2-halide activity) of bovine neutrophils.[27] The results of these studies indicated protein iodination by neutrophils was significantly suppressed in the presence of either viable or killed bacteria.

Granule lysates from guinea pig and human neutrophils were not brucellacidal unless they were supplemented with H_2O_2 and either Cl^- or I^-.[23] Both smooth and rough strains of *B. abortus* were susceptible to *in vitro* killing by the MPO-H_2O_2-halide mixtures.

Strain 45/0 was more resistant to oxygen-dependent killing than Strain 45/20. Comparisons of the cell envelope components of smooth and rough strains of *B. abortus* by biochemical and ultrastructural analysis indicated that the cell walls of Strain 45/0 were markedly more resistant to digestion by hydrolytic enzymes than cell walls from strain 45/20. Based on these studies, it was hypothesized that a phenol-soluble lipopolysaccharide from the cell surface of the smooth strain might be responsible for enhancing the intracellular survival of *Brucella*.[31]

Neither smooth nor rough organisms were susceptible to destruction by oxygen-independent killing mechanisms using concentrations of granule extracts which resulted in killing of rough mutants of *Salmonella typhimurium*.[32] Thus, it appears non-oxidative killing mechanisms do not contribute appreciably to the destruction of *B. abortus* by phagocytic cells.

The results of these studies suggest both virulent and avirulent *B. abortus* are susceptible to the oxidative killing mechanisms of phagocytic cells if the antimicrobial system is allowed to function normally (ie. degranulation is not altered). It is also reasonable to conclude that the ability of *B. abortus* to inhibit degranulation significantly compromises the oxidative killing capacity of the phagocytes, resulting in enhanced intracellular survival of the bacteria.

Isolation and Characterization of *Brucella abortus* Components that Inhibit Phagocyte Function

Recently, studies evaluating the interactions between *Brucella* and phagocytic cells have focused on the identification and characterization of *B. abortus* components responsible for inhibition of bovine neutrophil function.

Using the iodination reaction as a quantitative measure of MPO-H_2O_2-halide antibacterial activity, the effects of whole and fractionated *B. abortus* (Strain 2308) on neutrophil MPO-H_2O_2-halide activity were determined.[27] Iodination activity was significantly inhibited in the presence of crude supernatants from heat-killed bacteria, but not preparations of washed heat-killed cells. Transmission electron microscopic examination of negatively stained preparations of heat-killed *B. abortus* indicated the bacteria remained intact through the heating process. These results suggested the components responsible for the inhibition of MPO-H_2O_2-halide activity were released from the exterior of the bacteria by heating.

A crude estimation of the molecular weight of the active components contained within the crude supernatant was obtained by molecular filtration using 1,000-dalton cutoff membrane filters. The iodination inhibitory activity was associated with the filtrate, suggesting the inhibitory components had molecular weights of <1,000 daltons. Preliminary physical characterization of the <1,000-dalton fraction indicated neither autoclaving nor treatment with acid or base destroyed the inhibitory activity of the fraction on neutrophil iodination.

Subsequent studies by Bertram et al.[33] used transmission electron microscopy and morphometric analysis to determine the relative amounts of primary versus secondary granule degranulation induced by opsonized zymosan in the presence and absence of the <1,000-dalton fraction. This material preferentially inhibited degranulation of peroxidase positive (primary) granules and induced limited inhibition of peroxidase negative (secondary) granule release. In addition, inhibition of protein iodination by the <1,000-dalton fraction was highly correlated with inhibition of primary granule release, but was not correlated with secondary granule release. These results suggested the <1,000-dalton fraction contained components capable of inhibiting release of myeloperoxidase through suppression of primary granule degranulation by bovine neutrophils.

Isolation of the inhibitory components contained within the <1,000-dalton fraction was achieved through the use of reverse phase high performance liquid chromatography (HPLC). The results of these experiments indicated the iodination inhibitory activity was contained within two purified fractions designated 3b and 10.

Chemical characterization of fractions 3b and 10 revealed neither fraction contained detectable amounts of protein or lipid. Fraction 3b exhibited a small amount of carbohydrate in contrast with fraction 10 which contained no detectable amount. Both fractions exhibited maximal absorbance of ultraviolet light at 260 nm. Collectively, these results suggested the inhibitory components possessed chemical properties consistent with those associated with nucleotides or nucleotide-like substances.

Riches et al.[34] reported that lysosomal enzyme secretion by murine macrophages is inhibited in the presence of purine nucleosides. Corbel and Brewer[35] had previously shown that supernatant fluids from continuous cultures of *Brucella* contain up to 100 mg of soluble RNA/liter.

These studies prompted investigations to determine if the *B. abortus* components associated with the inhibition of neutrophil degranulation were nucleotides or bases and, if so, to determine their identity.[34] Comparisons between fractions 3b and 10 and authentic samples of nucleotides and bases were performed by reverse-phase HPLC and normal-phase thin layer chromatography. The results of the HPLC analyses indicated fraction 3b coeluted with 5'-guanosine monophosphate (GMP) and fraction 10 coeluted with adenine. These results were confirmed by the thin layer chromatography.

Various concentrations of adenine, GMP, and *B. abortus* fractions 3b and 10 were evaluated for their ability to suppress iodination by bovine neutrophils. All of these materials exhibited dose-dependent inhibition of iodination. Further, the shape of the titration curves for fraction 3b and GMP were similar, as were the curves for fraction 10 and adenine.

Analysis of culture supernatants from live *B. abortus* indicated both GMP and adenine are produced by viable *Brucella*, however, they are not produced by extracellular organisms such as *S. epidermidis*.

The results of these studies indicate that one of the mechanisms by which *B. abortus* may escape intracellular killing by bovine neutrophils is through the production of GMP and adenine which are associated with the bacterial surface. These materials suppress the MPO-H_2O_2-halide antibacterial system of neutrophils by inhibiting release of myeloperoxidase from primary granules.

Alteration of *Brucella*-Phagocyte Interactions by Immunomodulators

If suppression of the MPO-H_2O_2-halide activity of neutrophils plays a significant role in the survival of *B. abortus*, it seems plausible that reversal of this inhibition by an immunomodulator would enhance neutrophil brucellacidal activity.

Recombinant bovine interferon-γ (IFN-γ) has been shown to influence a variety of *in vitro* neutrophil functions including opsonized zymosan-induced superoxide anion production and iodination activity.[37] The effects of *in vitro* and *in vivo* activation of neutrophils with IFN-γ on the interactions of bovine phagocytes and *B. abortus* have been investigated.[37] Both *in vitro* and *in vivo* activation of neutrophils with IFN-γ resulted in an improved iodination response by phagocytes in the presence of either GMP and adenine or *B. abortus*.

As expected, bactericidal assays involving normal neutrophils indicated *B. abortus* was capable of resisting killing by phagocytes. Results of studies to determine the effects of IFN-γ on the brucellacidal activity of neutrophils indicated pretreatment with IFN-γ for two hours resulted in a modest, but statistically significant enhancement of the ability of phagocytes to kill *B. abortus*. Temporal studies performed to evaluate the kinetics of the phagocyte-mediated killing of *B. abortus* indicated the enhancement of killing was most notable during the first 30 minutes following the addition of the bacteria. The differences in killing potential between normal and IFN-γ-activated neutrophils decreased at 60 and 120 minutes post-exposure.

Treatment of animals with IFN-γ also resulted in slightly improved brucellacidal activity of phagocytes in a dose- and time-dependent manner. Neutrophils from animals treated with a single dose of 0.5 mg of IFN-γ exhibited small but significant increases in their ability to kill *B. abortus* within 24 hours of treatment. The magnitude of the enhancement of killing was greatest during the first 30 minutes following the addition of the bacteria to the reaction mixture, similar to the *in vitro* studies. These results suggest IFN-γ-activation of neutrophils may change the kinetics of the antibacterial activity of the phagocytes by increasing the early antibacterial capacity of the neutrophil, resulting in an overall enhanced bactericidal potential. The enhanced brucellacidal activity of neutrophils was positively correlated with enhancement of iodination by neutrophils from IFN-γ-treated cattle.

While neutrophils exposed to IFN-γ displayed an increased ability to kill *B. abortus*, it should be noted that a significant number of the bacteria survived exposure to the phagocytes for 90 to 120 minutes forcing one to question the biological significance of the increased killing potential. However, these data suggest there is an association between the ability of IFN-γ to enhance the brucellacidal activity of bovine neutrophils and its ability to reverse suppression of neutrophil function by bacterial virulence factors.

References

1. Harmon BG, Adams LG, Templeton JW, et al. Macrophage function in mammary glands of *Brucella abortus*-infected cows and cows that resisted infection after inoculation of *Brucella abortus*. *Am J Vet Res* 1989;50:459-465.
2. Harmon BG, Templeton JW, Crawford FC, et al. Macrophage function and immune response of naturally resistant and susceptible cattle to *Brucella abortus*. In: Skamene E, ed. *Genetic control of host resistance to infection and malignancy*. New York: Alan R. Liss Inc,1985;345-354.
3. Densen P, Mandell GL. Granulocytic phagocytes. In: Mandell GL, Douglas RG, Bennett JE, eds. *Principles and practice of infectious diseases*. New York: John Wiley and Sons, 1979;63-82.
4. Goldstein IM, Kaplan HB,Radin A, et al. Independent effects of IgG and complement upon human PMN leukocyte function. *J Immunol* 1976;117:1282-1287.
5. Henson PM, Oades ZG. Stimulation of human neutrophils by soluble and insoluble Immunoglobulin aggregates. *J Clin Invest* 1975;56:1053-1061.
6. Klebanoff SJ. Antimicrobial mechanisms in neutrophilic PMN leukocytes. *Sem Hematol* 1975;12:117-142.
7. Klebanoff S J. Iodination of bacteria: A bactericidal mechanism. *J Exp Med* 1967;126:1063-1078.

8. Mandell GL. Bactericidal activity of aerobic and anaerobic polymorphonuclear neutrophils. *Infect Immun* 1974;9:337-341.

9. Odeburg H, Olsson I. Antibacterial activity of cationic proteins of human granulocytes. *J Clin Invest* 1975;56:1118-1124.

10. Densen P, MacKeen L, Clark RA. Gonococci causing uncomplicated gonorrhea of disseminated gonococcal infection differ in stimulation of neutrophil chemotaxis [abstract no. 4]. In: *Proceedings* of the 11th International Congress of Chemotherapy and the 19th Interscience Conference on Antimicrobial Agents and Chemotherapy. Washington DC, American Society for Microbiology, 1979.

11. Schultz DR, Miller KD. Elastase of *Pseudomonas aeruginosa* : Inactivation of complement components and complement derived chemotactic and phagocytic factors. *Infect Immun* 1974;10:128-135.

12. Foley MJ, Wood WB. Studies on the pathogenicity of group A streptococci. II. The antiphagocytic effects of M protein and the capsular gel. *J Exp Med* 1959;110:617-628.

13. Smith MR, Wood WB. Studies on the mechanism of recovery in pneumonia due to Friedlander's bacillus. III. The role of "surface phagocytosis" in the destruction of the microorganisms in the lung. *J Exp Med* 1947;86:257-266.

14. Howard CJ, Glynn AA. The virulence for mice of strains of *Escherichia coli* related to the effects of K antigens on their resistance to phagocytosis and killing by complement. *Immunology* 1971;20:767-777.

15. Keppie J, Harris-Smith PW, Smith H. The chemical basis of the virulence of *Bacillus anthracis*. IX. Its agressions and their mode of action. *Br J Exp Pathol* 1963;44:446-453.

16. Zucker-Franklin D, Davidson M, Thomas L. The interaction of mycoplasmas with mammalian cells. I. HeLa cells, neutrophils and eosinophils. *J Exp Med* 1966;124:521-532.

17. Watt PJ. The fate of gonococci in polymorphonuclear leukocytes. *J Med Microbiol* 1970;3:501-509.

18. Kossack RE, Schadelin J, Guerrant RL, et al. Diminished neutrophil oxidative metabolism following phagocytosis of virulent *Salmonella typhi* [abstract]. *Clin Res* 1978;26:28A.

19. Goren MB, D'Arcy-Hart P, Young MR, et al. Prevention of phagosome-lysosome fusion in cultured macrophages by sulfatides of *Mycobacterium tuberculosis*. *Proc Nat Acad Sci U S A* 1976;73:2510-2514.

20. Chiang YW, Kaeberle ML, Roth JA. Identification of suppressive components in *Haemophilus somnus* fractions which inhibit bovine polymorphonuclear leukocyte function. *Infect Immun* 1986;52:792-797.

21. Smith H, Fitzgeorge RB. The chemical basis of the virulence of *Brucella abortus*. V. The basis of intracellular survival and growth in bovine phagocytes. *Br J Exp Pathol* 1964; 45:174-186.

22. Fitzgeorge RB, Smith H. The chemical basis of the virulence of *Brucella abortus*. VII. The production *in vitro* of organisms with an enhanced capacity to survive intracellu-larly in bovine phagocytes. *Br J Exp Pathol* 1966;47:558-562.

23. Kreutzer DL, Dreyfus LA, Robertson DC. Interactions of polymorphonuclear leukocytes with smooth and rough strains of *Brucella abortus*. *Infect Immun* 1979;23:737-742.

24. Riley LK, Robertson DC. Ingestion and intracellular survival of *Brucella abortus* in human and bovine polymorphonuclear leukocytes. *Infect Immun* 1984;46:224-230.

25. Robertson DC, Riley LK, Kreutzer DL, et al. Intracellular survival of smooth and rough strains of *Brucella*. In: Schlessinger D, ed. *Microbiology 1979*. Washington DC, American Society for Microbiology, 1979;150-153.

26. Harmon BG, Adams LG, Frey M. Survival of rough and smooth strains of *Brucella*

abortus in bovine mammary gland macrophages. *Am J Vet Res* 1988;49:1092-1097.

27. Canning PC, Roth JA, Tabatabai LB, et al. Isolation of components of *Brucella abortus* responsible for inhibition of function in bovine neutrophils. *J Infect Dis* 1985;152:913-921.

28. Young EJ, Borchert M, Kreutzer FL, et al. Phagocytosis and killing of *Brucella* by human polymorphonuclear leukocytes. *J Infect Dis* 1985;152:682-690.

29. Morris JA. The interaction of *Brucella abortus* 544 and neutrophil polymorphonuclear leucocytes. *Ann Sclavo* 1977;19:143-150.

30. Canning PC, Deyoe BL, Roth JA. Opsonin-dependent stimulation of bovine neutrophil oxidative metabolism by *Brucella abortus*. *Am J Vet Res* 1988;49:160-163.

31. Kreutzer DL, Robertson DC. Surface macromolecules and virulence in intracellular parasitism: Comparison of cell envelope components of smooth and rough strains of *Brucella abortus*. *Infect Immun* 1979;23:819-828.

32. Riley LK, Robertson DC. Brucellacidal activity of human and bovine polymorphonuclear leukocyte granule extracts against smooth and rough strains of *Brucella abortus*. *Infect Immun* 1984;46:231-236.

33. Bertram TA, Canning PC, Roth JA. Preferential inhibition of primary granule release from bovine neutrophils by a *Brucella abortus* extract. *Infect Immun* 1986;52:285-292.

34. Riches DW, Watkins JL, Henson PM, et al. Regulation of macrophage lysosomal secretion by adenosine, adenosine phosphate esters, and related structural analogues of adenosine. *J Leuk Biol* 1985;37:545-557.

35. Corbel MJ, Brewer RA. Isolation and properties of an RNA fraction present in *Brucella* culture supernatants. *J Hyg* London, 1980;84:223-236.

36. Canning PC, Roth JA, Deyoe BL. Release of 5'-guanosine monophosphate and adenine by *Brucella abortus* and their role in the intracellular survival of the bacteria. *J Infect Dis* 1986;154:464-470.

37. Canning PC, Roth JA. Effect of *in vitro* and *in vivo* administration of recombinant bovine interferon-γ on bovine neutrophil responses to *Brucella abortus*. *Vet Immunol Immunopath* 1989;20:119-133.

Chapter Twelve

T Lymphocyte-Mediated Mechanisms of Acquired Protective Immunity Against Brucellosis in Cattle

Roger Smith III

Since the early experiments of Mackaness and others, immunity to facultative intracellular bacteria has been assumed to be primarily T-lymphocyte-mediated, with activated macrophages carrying out the effector functions of phagocytosis and killing of organisms.[1-5] While it appears that this paradigm has held up well over the years, new mechanisms of cell-mediated immunity to intracellular bacteria have been proposed,[6,9] and the role of lymphokines in mediating resistance has received greater attention.[7,8,10] In brucellosis, most of the traditional concepts for the role of cell-mediated immunity have persisted, but are tempered by an awareness of the important contribution that antibodies make toward host resistance to brucellosis.[5,11-13] Because many of the experimental manipulations that are possible in laboratory animals are not practical in cattle, the relative roles of cellular and humoral immunity have not been clearly delineated. Further, the relevant mechanisms by which bovine T-lymphocytes contribute to immunity to brucellosis are not as clear as in other disease models in rodents.

This review will focus on two important issues regarding T-lymphocyte-mediated immunity to brucellosis in cattle: the mechanisms by which cellular immunity develops and the relevance of those mechanisms to host resistance. Three general categories of cellular mechanisms will be considered in this review: 1) antigen presentation to *Brucella*-reactive T lymphocytes, 2) specificity of *Brucella*-reactive T lymphocytes, and 3) functional capacity of the *Brucella*-reactive T lymphocytes. The relevance of T lymphocyte-mediated mechanisms in cattle has been more difficult to evaluate, and two approaches to the question will be considered: the correlation of immunity to brucellosis with T-lymphocyte reactivity in experimentally vaccinated animals and its correlation with T-lymphocyte reactivity in naturally resistant animals.

Measures of T Lymphocyte Reactivity in Bovine Brucellosis

Three assays of cellular immunity have been applied to the study of brucellosis in cattle: dermal hypersensitivity, lymphocyte proliferation (blastogenesis, lymphocyte transformation), and mononuclear leukocyte migration inhibition. At best, these assays measure only a single aspect of cellular immunity, and the *in vitro* lymphocyte proliferation assay is the most removed from *in vivo* mechanisms of immunity. Still, these tests are the most commonly used in cattle for the study of brucellosis and are used in many other infectious diseases of cattle and other species.

Lymphocyte proliferation is a direct measurement of the ability of an antigen-specific clone to expand in response to appropriately presented antigen. As such, it is dependent on both the antigen-presenting capacity of the monocyte or macrophage and on the specificity and responsiveness of the T lymphocytes in the culture. Migration inhibition probably measures one aspect of the *in vivo* response measured by dermal hypersensitivity reactions. In dermal hypersensitivity, macrophages are recruited by attractant(s) and migration inhibition factor(s) (MIF) and activated by various macrophage activation factors (MAF), one of which is interferon-γ (IFNγ). The first published report regarding T lymphocyte-mediated cytotoxic activity on infected macrophages appears in this Symposium (Likos-Burkhart and Wyckoff, this volume). There are no reports on the production of lymphokines (other than interleukin–2) or on the ability of T-lymphocytes to regulate immunoglobulin secretion by B lymphocytes in bovine brucellosis.

Presentation of *Brucella* Antigens to Bovine T Lymphocytes

Identity of the Antigen-Presenting Cells for *Brucella*

Macrophages serve as a reservoir for *Brucella* organisms in chronic brucellosis[11] and have been identified as an antigen-presenting cell type for induction of T–lymphocyte activation.[14] In a lymphocyte proliferation assay, plastic-adherent cells (97-98% esterase-positive) were required for presentation of *Brucella* antigens to a T lymphocyte-enriched (71-79% CD2$^+$) population.[14] In other antigen systems, B lymphocytes are important antigen-presenting cells, especially for presentation of their cognate antigen.[15] Some have presented evidence that B lymphocytes are absolutely required for antigen presentation in primary immune responses.[16,17] The role of the B cell in presenting *Brucella* antigens has not been studied in any animal system. In view of the dominant response to the *Brucella* "O"-polysaccharide by bovine B lymphocytes,[11] it would be especially interesting to determine their role in presenting antigens to bovine T lymphocytes. If B lymphocytes are important antigen-presenting cells in bovine brucellosis, one might predict that the T lymphocyte response might be skewed to react with those proteins covalently linked to *Brucella* lipopolysaccharide (LPS).[18]

Antigen Uptake and Processing

To study the mechanisms of antigen presentation, Splitter and Everlith pulsed adherent cells with acetone-killed *B. abortus* overnight, then trypsinized and washed the adherent cells to remove extracellular bacterial organisms from the cell surface.[14] The trypsinized adherent cells were effective in presenting *B. abortus* to sensitized T lymphocytes. These results indicated that antigen uptake and processing by the adherent cells had occurred during the overnight incubation period, and that the processed antigen was sufficient for activation of *Brucella*-specific T lymphocytes. Possible roles in antigen-presentation of acidification of intracellular compartments and of proteolytic digestion have not been investigated for *Brucella* antigens.

Class II Major Histocompatibility Complex

In the previous study, involvement of major histocompatibility complex (MHC) class II molecules in the presentation of *B. abortus* antigens was studied by including a monoclonal antibody (MAb) specific for class II molecules in the culture of adherent cells with T lymphocytes.[14] The absence of a proliferative response in the presence of the class II-specific MAb provided evidence that sterically covering up the class II molecule was sufficient to prevent T-lymphocyte recognition of *Brucella* antigens physically bound to the class II molecule.[19-21]

Interleukin-1

In addition to physically presenting antigen to T lymphocytes, antigen-presenting cells may provide accessory functions necessary for the activation of T lymphocytes.[21,22] Interleukin-1 (IL–1) is generally regarded as the most important of the accessory functions provided by antigen-presenting cells.[21,22] Involvement of IL–1 in the response of bovine T lymphocytes to *Brucella* was demonstrated in an interesting series of experiments by Splitter and Everlith.[23] These investigators found that incubation of adherent cells and T lymphocytes with *B. abortus* and IFNγ reduced the proliferative response. The reduced response could not be attributed to an alteration of class II molecule expression induced by IFNγ, because IFNγ actually increased the density of class II molecules expressed by the adherent cells. Instead, the reduced response was correlated with a reduced expression of the membrane form of IL–1 by the adherent cells. Interestingly, the secreted form of IL–1 was not affected by IFNγ, and the addition of exogenous recombinant bovine IL–1β did not restore the response. These data indicated that the membrane form of IL–1 is likely important for T-lymphocyte activation; unfortunately, MAbs to bovine IL–1 are not available to test this hypothesis more directly.

An extremely interesting finding in these studies was the interaction of *B. abortus* "O"-polysaccharide with IFNγ in suppressing T lymphocyte activation.[23] Thus, only the smooth Strain 1119 synergized with IFNγ to reduce membrane IL–1 expression; the rough Strain 45/20, with IFNγ, did not reduce T-lymphocyte proliferation. Furthermore, the timing of addition of *B. abortus* Strain 1119 and IFNγ to the adherent cells was important. Addition of *B. abortus* and IFNγ after overnight incubation of the adherent cells, or after 7 days incubation, did not reduce the T lymphocyte response. It was not determined whether the lack of effect at these time points was due to differences in the differentiation state of the adherent cells or to the participation of nonadherent cells in the suppressive mechanism.

In view of these studies by Splitter and Everlith, several interesting questions are provoked regarding the processing of *Brucella* antigens by macrophages. If IFNγ is produced by T lymphocytes responding to *Brucella* (which has not yet been demonstrated), then do these T lymphocytes down-regulate the immune response during an ongoing infection, and if so, are these T lymphocytes responsible for the chronicity of the infection with smooth strains of *Brucella*? What, if any, is the role of other biochemical forms of the "O"-polysaccharide in altering the presentation of antigens?

Specificity of Bovine T Lymphocytes Reactive with *Brucella*

There are two inherent aspects to the question of T-lymphocyte specificity: the ability of the antigen-presenting cells to present the antigen and the ability of the T lymphocyte antigen receptor to recognize the antigen as presented. In any study of T lymphocyte specificity, failure to identify a response may be due to either a failure of macrophages to present antigen or a failure of the T lymphocyte to respond.[23] In the following discussion, this point is not explicitly repeated, but must be kept in mind when interpreting results.

Species Specificity

Using both long-term cultured T lymphocytes and fresh peripheral blood mononuclear cells as responders in proliferative assays, we have observed a difference in responsiveness to different species of *Brucella*.[24] In these experiments, unvaccinated heifers were challenged with *B. abortus* Strain 2308 at mid-gestation. Lymphocytes were later assayed for responsiveness to equal numbers of irradiated organisms from four species of *Brucella*: *B. abortus* (Strain 2308, Strain 19, and rough Strain RB51), *B. canis* (Strain RM666), *B. suis* (Strain 1330), and *B. melitensis* (Strain 16M). Some, but not all, of the cows clearly responded with a greater degree of proliferation to *B. abortus* than to *B. suis*, *B. melitensis*, or both. Generally, responses to *B. canis* were equivalent to those to *B. abortus*. To compare responses of a single cow in multiple assays, and to compare the responses between cows, data were normalized to express the responses to *B. suis* and *B. melitensis* as a fraction of the response to *B. abortus* in each assay. With this transformation, it was observed that the relative responsiveness to *B. suis* and *B. melitensis* was stable for most cows over different assays and sampling dates, suggesting that the differences in lymphocyte reactivity reflected inherent differences in reactivity of the cows. No correlation was observed between the differences in reactivity and MHC class I alleles. What is not clear, though, is whether these differences are due to altered repertoires of T lymphocyte receptors for *Brucella* antigens in association with MHC class II molecules or to differences in the presentation of antigens to the T lymphocytes by macrophages in the cultures.

Kaneene and colleagues have also reported lower proliferative responses to *B. melitensis* than to *B. abortus*, although that comparison was not the primary purpose of their studies.[25,26] In the first report, using cold saline extracts of rough strains of *B. abortus* (Strain 45/20) and *B. melitensis*, the authors observed at least three cows for which the response to the *B. abortus* extract was approximately twice that to the *B. melitensis* extract.[25] Additionally, in part B of their study, the average stimulation index to the *B. abortus* extract was almost twice that to the *B. melitensis* extract. In the second report, the responses of cows vaccinated once or twice with *B. melitensis* Strain H-38, or left unvaccinated were compared.[26] Two antigen preparations were used for proliferative assays: *B. abortus* soluble antigen (BASA) and BMPA, a cold saline extract of *B. melitensis* (rough) Strain B115. The unexpected result was that the *B. abortus* antigen BASA induced a higher level of response in these heifers than did the *B. melitensis* antigen BMPA, in spite of the fact that the lymphocytes had been primed to a strain of *B. melitensis*. However, all assays were performed after challenge with *B. abortus* Strain 2308, and the two antigen preparations in the proliferation assays were not comparable in terms of their preparation or their final concentration.

Molecular Specificity

There are two general approaches to the study of molecular specificity of T lymphocytes in brucellosis. The first is to immunize cattle with a mixture of *Brucella* antigens (as in vaccination with Strain 19, experimental challenge, or natural infections), then to test for lymphocyte reactivity with more purified fractions of the bacterium. This approach addresses the question of which antigens of *Brucella* activate T lymphocytes when the whole, replicating organism is presented. Theoretically, the dominant antigens of *Brucella* activate most of the responding lymphocytes, and less immunogenic molecules activate fewer lymphocytes.

The second approach is to immunize cattle with more purified antigens of *Brucella* and to test for lymphocyte reactivity with either the immunizing antigen or whole *Brucella* organisms. This approach addresses the question of which antigens of *Brucella* are sufficient to activate T lymphocytes *in vivo*.

The two approaches are not equivalent and may yield very different answers. Thus, an antigen that is not stimulatory when presented as part of a whole organism (first approach) may be stimulatory when separated from more dominant antigens and presented alone (second approach). Alternatively, dominant antigens that are stimulatory when presented as part of a whole organism (first approach) may require linkage to lipid moieties in the organisms or the presence of bacterial peptidoglycan to stimulate T lymphocytes. Thus, presentation without such linkages may not be successful in stimulating a T lymphocyte response.

Further considerations on the stimulatory capacity of *Brucella* antigens would be the presentation of the antigen as part of a replicating organism, or in a non-replicating form, and the selection of adjuvants for use with non-replicating immunogens. To date, presentation of *Brucella* antigens in replicating organisms has been exclusively as a strain of *Brucella* species, although the cloning of *Brucella* antigens into viral or bacterial vectors will soon permit the immunization with isolated *Brucella* antigens in a novel replicating form.

Immunization with Whole Organism, Testing with Specific Antigen

During the 1970's, three groups fractionated *Brucella* organisms and tested the activity of selected fractions in assays of T lymphocyte reactivity.[27-29] Bhongbhibhat, Elberg, and Chen studied the allergenic activity of saline-extracted antigens of *B. melitensis* in dermal hypersensitivity.[27] The PII fraction, containing 67-74% protein with an approximate molecular weight of 30,000, was most allergenic. At least three major bands were identified by polyacrylamide electrophoresis of the PII fraction, and all contained some allergenic activity in guinea pigs. Pronase treatment of the PII allergen destroyed its allergenicity, implying that the active moiety was a protein. Cunningham et al. used a modification of the antigen-enrichment scheme of Bhongbhibhat, Elberg, and Chen.[29]

A chief modification that increased sensitivity and specificity without inducing reactivity on repeated testing was to remove high molecular weight material by ultrafiltration using a hollow fiber concentrator with a 100,000 molecular weight cut-off. Kaneene et al. used fractions of column chromatographed BASA as antigens in proliferative assays to study the molecular specificity of the T lymphocyte response.[28] Molecular weight determinations were not given, but the apparently higher molecular weight fractions (PI and PII) were more stimulatory than the low molecular weight peak PIII.

Similar reports over the past six years have been characterized by more careful fractionation procedures, more precise identification of the molecular species being used, and better characterization of the bovine responses. The results of reports from the laboratories of Winter and Splitter can be briefly summarized as follows: 1) T lymphocyte-stimulating antigens of B. abortus are found in peptide species of a broad spectrum of molecular weights and 2) at least two of the T lymphocyte-stimulating antigens are the group 2 (porin) and group 3 proteins.

Baldwin, Antczak, and Winter used group 2 (porin) proteins and BASA in proliferative assays to assess the response of cattle lymphocytes to experimental infection with B. abortus Strain 2308 or Strain 19 vaccination.[30] The antigen designated as group 2 (porin) derived from rough Strain 45/20 induced less than 13% false positive reactions and was effective at eliciting responses in lymphocytes from infected cows. However, infected open heifers were less reactive in the assay than infected pregnant heifers. The crude BASA preparation from Strain 1119 induced higher levels of reactivity, but reactivity was also noted in about 50% of unexposed heifers.

Baldwin, Verstreate, and Winter used group 2 (porins) and group 3 outer membrane proteins in proliferative assays to assess the response of cattle lymphocytes to experimental infection with B. abortus Strain 2308 or Strain 19 vaccination.[31] The antigen designated as group 2 (porin) derived from rough Strain 45/20 contained less than 1.5% lipopolysaccharide (w:w) and was the best antigen preparation found in this study for stimulation of specific responses in vitro. The crude BASA preparation from Strain 1119 induced higher levels of reactivity, but reactivity was also noted in unexposed heifers.

The reactivity of unimmunized cattle to Strain 1119 BASA could not be attributed to reactivity with Brucella LPS, because the same investigators found that preparations enriched for LPS (fraction f5p) were not mitogenic for bovine lymphocytes.[32] The f5p fraction of Strain 1119 was titrated according to protein concentration and used to stimulate lymphocytes of cattle that had been previously vaccinated with Strain 19.[32] This preparation was stimulatory in 2 of 3 cows in one experiment and stimulated an average ∆(cpm) of 10-15,000 in seven other vaccinated heifers. Whether the reactivity was due to direct activity of bovine T lymphocytes with *Brucella* LPS or to contaminating protein, especially proteins covalently bound to LPS, was not clear in these experiments.

Brooks-Alder and Splitter separated membrane proteins of *B. abortus* Strain 19 by polyacrylamide gel electrophoresis and blotted the antigens to nitrocellulose.[33] Three fractions, of high (>45,000), medium (25–45,000), and low (<25,000) molecular weight, were used in lymphocyte proliferative assays. Lymphocytes were taken from Strain 19–vaccinated animals. The design of the experiments was to prime lymphocytes *in vitro* on *Brucella* antigens of one fraction, then restimulate the primed lymphocytes with each of the three fractions in a thymidine-uptake assay. Their results indicated that the priming of lymphocytes was specific and that all three fractions contained antigens that could stimulate bovine T lymphocytes. The specificity of the lymphocytes for antigens to which they had been primed *in vitro* indicated that LPS, which was present in all three fractions, was not the stimulatory antigen.

Because T lymphocytes recognize processed antigens, it is not necessary that T lymphocyte-stimulating antigens be normally accessible in intact organisms. Thus, cytoplasmic or periplasmic proteins of *Brucella* might also be stimulatory for T lymphocytes. In a preliminary test of this hypothesis, we separated cell envelope and cytoplasmic fractions of *B. abortus* rough Strain RB51, using sonication in a hypotonic solution and differential sonication.[34] When tested for their ability to stimulate long-term cultures of oligoclonal T-lymphocyte lines, both fractions were stimulatory (See Figure 12-1). In all cases, the cell envelope preparation was more stimulatory on a weight basis, and in some cell lines, virtually no reactivity to cytoplasmic fractions was observed. For other cell lines, however, responses to cytoplasmic proteins were almost equivalent to those to cell envelopes. The differences may be more reflective of the relative ability of macrophages to ingest and process particulate (cell envelopes) and soluble (cytoplasmic) antigens than of the representation of antigen-reactive T lymphocytes in these cultures.

Immunization with Specific Antigen

In a long series of experiments, Winter and his colleagues have used various preparations of outer membranes, cell envelopes, outer membrane proteins, and peptidoglycan to immunize cattle.[35-37] Immunization of four cows with 5 mg or 25 mg of proteins extracted from the outer membrane of Strain 45/20 induced responses that could be measured by *in vitro* lymphocyte proliferative assays.[35] In a larger group of animals, similar responses could be observed in cows immunized with outer membrane proteins,

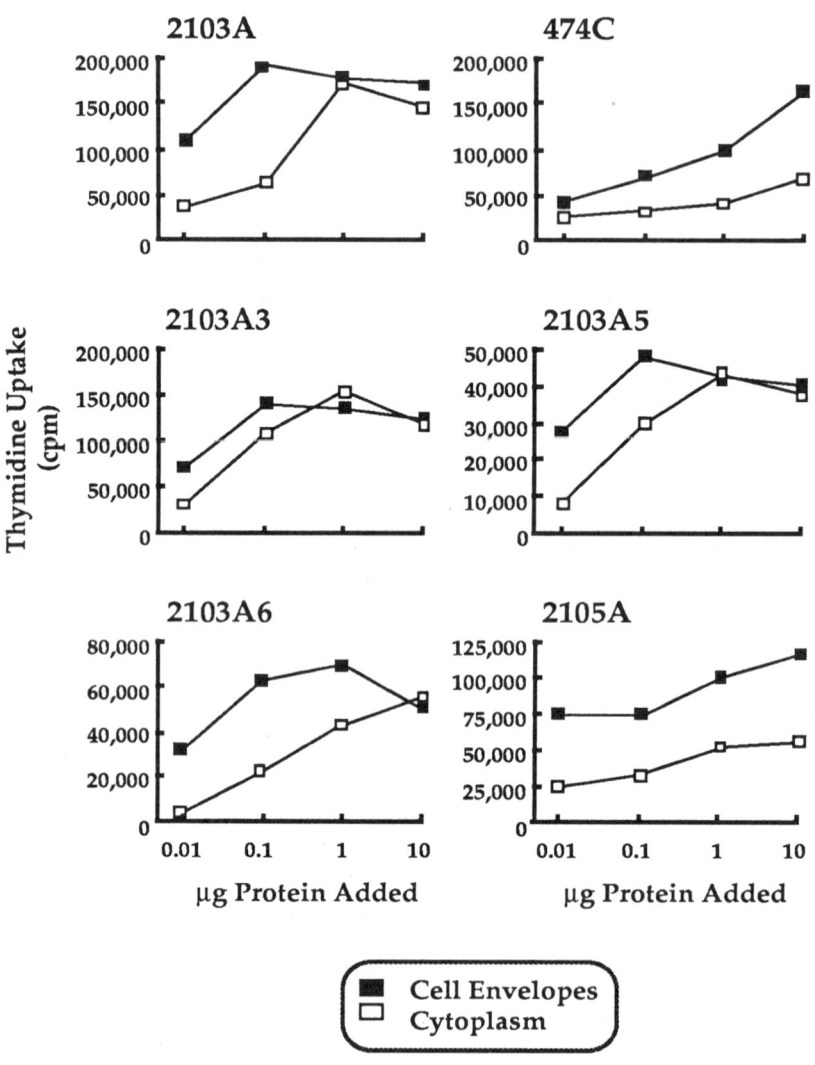

Figure 12-1. Proliferative Response of Bovine T–Lymphocyte Lines to Cell Envelope and Cytoplasmic Fractions of *B. abortus* Strain RB51.

outer membranes, or whole cells. The responses measured in these animals, however, were secondary responses in that all had been calfhood vaccinated with Strain 19.[35]

Winter and Rowe immunized cattle with cell envelopes, outer membrane proteins, or peptidoglycan from *B. abortus* Strain 2308 and measured proliferative responses and dermal hypersensitivity reactions to group 2 (porin) and group 3 outer membrane proteins.[37] All but one experimental group received antigen in an adjuvant of trehalose dimycolate and muramyl dipeptide in squalene and spermidine. Proliferative responses were detected in 1 of 2 cows immunized with cell envelopes, in 2 of 3 cows immunized with outer membrane proteins, in 3 of 3 cows immunized with peptidoglycan and adjuvant, and in 1 of 3 cows immunized with peptidoglycan alone. Dermal hypersensitivity tests did not correlate with in vitro lymphocyte proliferative responses in 3 of the heifers, but the overall results for the experimental groups was comparable. The conclusion of this and a second experiment comparing vaccination with either cell envelopes or peptidoglycan, both in adjuvant, was that the cell-mediated immune response was indistinguishable in duration and magnitude.

Confer et al.[38] studied the response of cattle to salt extractable proteins (CSP) originally described by Tabatabai and Deyoe.[39,40] In their experiments, cattle were either vaccinated with CSP in Freund's complete adjuvant or with derivatized CSP (dCSP). Derivatized CSP was prepared by chemical modification with dodecanoyl anhydride.[40] For both preparations, the immunization schedule included two inoculations at 6 week intervals in Freund's complete adjuvant. Five experimental groups were included: 1) Freund's complete adjuvant in saline, 2) two doses of CSP, 3) two doses of dCSP, 4) CSP followed by dCSP, and 5) dCSP followed by CSP. Using heat-killed Strain 1119 antigen, lymphocyte proliferative assays were performed on five cows from each group at 2-week intervals starting 4 weeks after the initial vaccination. Only at week 4 (prior to the booster inoculation) were the responses significantly greater in the vaccinated cattle than in the control group. At other time points, there were sporadic increases in one group or another, but no consistent increase in lymphocyte reactivity. Responses measured with BASA as antigen were inconsistent, and there were frequent responses measured in the unimmunized control group.

Previous experiments were confounded by the presence of *Brucella* LPS in all protein preparations. In two separate experiments, we tested for immunogenicity of five preparations of subcellular antigens of *B. abortus* in cattle. In the first experiment, four separate molecular preparations were emulsified in an adjuvant and administered to cows in two injections at an interval of 60 days (See Table 12-1). The first three of these preparations were completely free of *Brucella* LPS. *In vitro* lymphocyte proliferation responses were measured using whole cell, irradiated Strain 2308 as

Table 12-1. Frequency of Cattle Responding to Subcellular Immunogens of *B. abortus.*

In vivo Immunogen	*In vivo* Antigen: S2308		
	Pos.	Neg.	Fisher's Test*
Adjuvant	0	14	—
Strain 19	8	4	p = 0.0003
Fusion Products 7.5 kDa Baomp I Baomp IIB1 Baomp III1	2	14	p = 0.4851
Proteins Baomp I Baomp IIB1 Baomp III1	4	12	p = 0.1029
Proteins 7.5 kDa 8.8 kDa	4	10	p = 0.0978
Strain 2308 LPS (17% Protein)	5	5	p = 0.0059

* $df = 1$ $\alpha = (0.05 \div 5) = 0.01$

antigen. The first preparation consisted of a combination of β–galactosidase fusion products (7.5 kDa protein, Baomp I, Baomp IIB1, and Baomp III1) purified from *E. coli* by affinity chromatography. Two of 16 cattle responded to this preparation, but this number was not significantly different from the number of unimmunized (adjuvant only) cattle with measurable responses (0 of 14). The second preparation was a combination of proteins (Baomp I, Baomp IIB1, and Baomp III1) that were eluted from sodium dodecylsulphate-polyacrylamide gel electrophoresis (SDS-PAGE) of rough-Strain RB51. This highly purified preparation (lacking *Brucella* LPS because rough LPS does not migrate in this part of the gel) stimulated detectable responses in 4 of 16 cows, but this also was not significantly different from the unimmunized group. The third preparation was a combination of two low molecular weight proteins (7.5 kDa and 8.8 kDa) that were eluted from SDS-PAGE of the smooth Strain 2308. This preparation also stimulated detectable responses in a small percentage of animals (4 of 14), but was not significantly different from unimmunized animals. In the fourth group, detectable responses were measured in 5 of 10 cows. These received an LPS fraction from strain 1119.3 containing approximately 17% protein by weight.[41] The response of this group was significantly different from the unimmunized group, and not significantly different from the frequency of responses to Strain 19 vaccination (p = 0.6656).

The results of this first experiment suggested the possibility that highly purified products might stimulate responses in a subset of animals, but not in a sufficiently large number that would make them feasible to use as vaccines. Similarly, one antigenic preparation, the LPS containing 17% protein, stimulated lymphocyte responsiveness in a substantial proportion of cattle. Thus, it appeared that either the LPS itself was immunogenic or that its associated protein was immunogenic. Failure to observe substantial responsiveness in cows vaccinated with the other preparations, some of which included LPS-associated proteins, may have been due to lack of responsive lymphocytes or inadequate dosage. Alternatively, the LPS may have facilitated responsiveness by acting as an adjuvant or by facilitating presentation of the associated *Brucella* antigens by macrophages.

A second experiment was designed to test the responses of cows to cell envelope preparations of the rough mutant Strain M106, derived by Tn5 mutagenesis of Strain 2308.[42] The cell envelope preparation was, therefore, similar to one used by Winter et al.[35-37] except that Winter's cell envelopes were prepared by detergent extraction and ours by sonication. Further, the strain used as sources of cell envelopes differed, in that Winter's group used rough Strain 45/20 which occasionally includes organisms expressing smooth LPS and reverts to smooth form, and we used the transposon mutant Strain M106 which is a stable mutant of Strain 2308. In this experiment, two antigens were used to measure *in vitro* responsiveness (Table 12-2). The first was whole cell, irradiated Strain 2308, and the second was a cell envelope preparation similar to the one used for immunization, but derived from the rough Strain RB51. With either antigen *in vitro*, a substantial number of cows immunized with cell envelopes gave detectable responses: 16 of 23 with Strain 2308 antigen (p = 0.0004) and 15 of 23 with cell envelope antigen (p < 0.0001).

Responses were also measured in the group immunized with Strain 19, but an interesting difference emerged. When whole cell Strain 2308 organisms were used as antigen, responses were detected in 16 of 24 cows, but when cell envelope preparations were used, responses were detected in only 7 of the 24 cows. Similarly, in the 7 cows with detectable responses to cell envelopes, the magnitude of the response, measured as D (cpm) was less than that to Strain 2308 cells. The correlation of responsiveness to

Table 12-2. Frequency of Cattle Responding to Cell Envelopes of
B. abortus.

In Vivo Immunogen	In Vitro Antigen: S2308		
	Pos.	Neg.	Fisher's Test*
Adjuvant	4	20	—
Strain 19	16	5	p = 0.0010
M106 Cell Envelopes	16	5	p = 0.0004

In Vivo Immunogen	In Vitro Antigen: Cell Envelopes		
	Pos.	Neg.	Fisher's Test*
Adjuvant	0	24	—
Strain 19	7	17	p = 0.0094
M106 Cell Envelopes (17% Protein)	15	8	p < 0.0001

* df = 1 $\alpha = (0.05 \div 2) = 0.025$

whole cell Strain 2308 and to cell envelopes in these two groups of
immunized cows is depicted in Figure 12-2. In cows immunized with cell
envelopes, the relative magnitude of the in vitro response to cell envelopes
was approximately 87% of that to Strain 2308 organisms. By contrast, the
relative magnitude was only 28% in cows immunized with Strain 19. The
differences in the apparent specificity of the responses in these two groups
could be attributed to any of the three major differences in the immunogens used: live Strain 19 versus nonviable cell envelopes, presence of
"O"–polysaccharide in Strain 19 versus its absence in the cell envelopes,
or the presence of cytoplasmic antigens in Strain 19 versus their absence in
the cell envelopes. From the design of these experiments, it was not
possible to distinguish these alternatives.

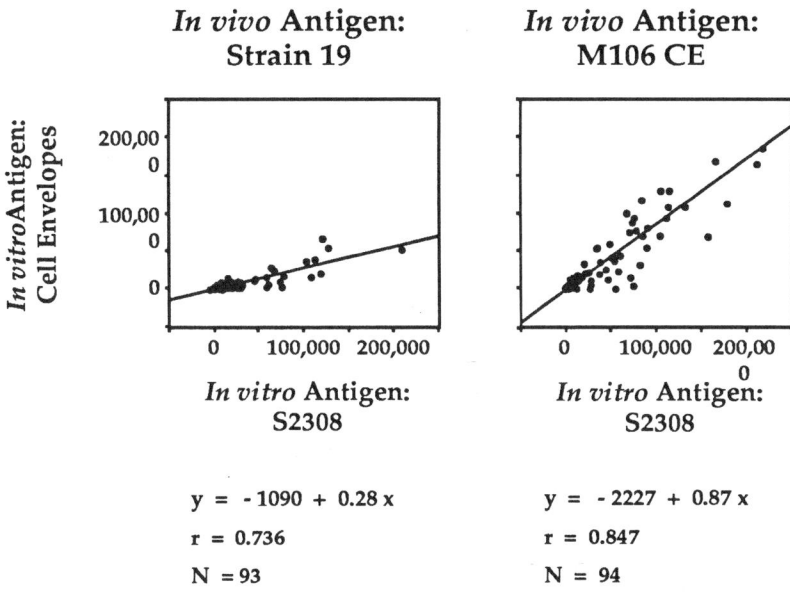

Figure 12-2. Proliferation Response of Bovine T-Lymphocytes to *B. abortus* Strain 2308 Whole Organisms Versus Cell Envelopes of *B. abortus* Strain RB51. Cows were immunized with either Strain 19 or cell envelopes of *B. abortus* Strain M106 and assayed for reactivity to the two antigens in proliferative assays. Each point represents a single assay on a single cow. Slopes of the regression lines, correlation coefficients, and number of observations are given.

Based on our experiments and those of others using relatively pure immunogens of *B. abortus*, several conclusions might be drawn. First, there were fewer responder cows when isolated proteins, or combinations of proteins, were used as imunogens. Second, three preparations have stimulated responsiveness in a substantial number of cows: Strain 19, the LPS preparation from either rough or smooth strains of *B. abortus*. Third, the form of the immunogen may significantly alter the apparent specificity of the lymphocyte response.

Functional Activity of Bovine T Lymphocytes in Bovine Brucellosis

Three types of evidence can be used to determine the functional capacity of T lymphocytes: surface phenotype, lymphokine secretion, and activity in direct assays of function. Few studies have addressed these questions regarding T lymphocytes of cattle.

Surface Phenotypes

One indication of T-lymphocyte function is the surface phenotype of the cells. Although the surface phenotype is more directly related to the MHC class that restricts antigen recognition, there are some generalities that can be made regarding the correlation of phenotype and function. CD4+ T lymphocytes generally are involved in providing help for B–cell activation, proliferation, and differentiation. CD8+ T lymphocytes are generally involved in cytotoxic and suppressive functions. We have generated long-term cultures of bovine T lymphocytes that are reactive with *B. abortus*.[43] These cultures were initiated and maintained without the addition of exogenous growth factors so as to bias the selection toward cells that produce their own growth factors. Most of the mixed cultures were nearly 100% CD4+, but some cultures were found that included a substantial proportion of T lymphocytes (CD2+) expressing neither CD4 nor CD8. Presumably the CD4+ cells in these long-term cultures are comparable to those involved in dermal hypersensitivity reactions, macrophage migration inhibition and activation, B–lymphocyte activation or differentiation, or some combination of these activities, attributed to CD4+ cells in other species.[21] The CD4-CD8- T lymphocytes are interestingly similar to cells reported in human and murine T cell populations expressing the γ/δ T-cell antigen receptor.[44-47]

whole

Lymphokines Secreted

Only a single report has assayed any lymphokine secreted in T-lymphocyte reactions to *Brucella*. Splitter and Everlith demonstrated that T lymphocytes responding to *Brucella*-pulsed adherent cells produce IL-2, as measured by the ability to support proliferation of long-term cultures of T lymphocytes generated in a mixed lymphocyte culture.[14]

Functional Assays

Migration Inhibition

An assay for detection of migration inhibition factor(s) (MIF) was developed using BASA as antigen and measuring migration of mononuclear leukocytes in agarose.[48] The report examined the optimal concentration of antigen, cell density, and duration for the assay. Animals vaccinated with Strain 19 and unvaccinated animals were used as donors of leukocytes to demonstrate specificity of the assay.

The leukocyte migration inhibition assay was used to measure responses of vaccinated and unvaccinated heifers to experimental challenge with Strain 2308.[49] All heifers demonstrated increased migration inhibition after challenge, but, interestingly, the vaccinated heifers were significantly lower in their responses than the unvaccinated heifers.

Dermal Hypersensitivity

Several groups have studied dermal hypersensitivity as a possible adjunct test for diagnosis of bovine brucellosis.[27,29,50-56] Antigen preparations have varied somewhat among the studies and have included heat-killed organisms, sonic extracts, and chemical extracts (for example abortin, melitin, brucellergen, brucellin, BPA, and BASA). The presence of positive reactions in infected, but not in unexposed, animals suggested that a delayed-type hypersensitivity response had occurred. Currently, these reactions are thought to be mediated by a subset of T lymphocytes secreting a wide variety of lymphokines, including IL-2, IFNγ, certain CSFs, TNFα and/or TNFβ, and other lymphokines that have not been well-characterized (MIF, other MAFs, fusion factors, etc).

Cytolytic Activity

Kaufmann has identified cytolytic T lymphocytes in mice infected with *Mycobacterium* and has suggested a role for such cells in the clearance of facultative intracellular parasites.[7,8] Although the importance of cell lysis in clearance of facultative intracellular organisms seems less compelling than for obligate intracellular parasites, the possibility remains that release of viable organisms from inefficient phagocytes by cell lysis might permit their uptake and killing by more efficient cells. Only recently was such cytolytic activity identified in cattle against *Brucella* (Likos-Burkhart and Wyckoff, this volume). The CD4·CD8· cells we have identified in some of our T-lymphocyte cultures may be candidates for such cytolytic cells.

Relevance of T Lymphocytes to Protective Immunity in Bovine Brucellosis

A major, or at least underlying, aim of most research on cellular immunity to *B. abortus* has been to assess its relevance for resistance to infection. Such an assessment is extremely difficult to make in cattle, and somewhat easier to make in laboratory mice. Studies in mice have demonstrated that pre-existing antibodies to *Brucella* "O"–polysaccharide were effective in reducing the bacterial load after challenge.[57-59] Adoptive transfer of immune lymphocytes have given conflicting results. Cheers and colleagues were able to transfer a degree of protection and showed that the protective subset was the CD8· (Ly1·2·) T lymphocytes.[60] Winter and colleagues, however, were unable to transfer protection consistently with lymphocytes.[61] Differences between these observations may be due to choice of strain of mice, timing of the recovery of immune lymphocytes for transfer, timing of the transfer, and dose and virulence of the challenging organism.

Such transfer studies are not possible with large animals, and investigators have instead attempted to correlate the presence or absence of a particular immune response modality to resistance or susceptibility to brucellosis. No such correlation has been made in bovine brucellosis. After experimental infection, most animals respond in various measures of cellular immunity, regardless of whether they resist or succumb to infection. In fact, susceptible animals generally tend to have quantitatively higher and more prolonged immune responses than do recovering animals.[62] This difference is probably due to the quantity and persistence of the antigen in infected animals.

A second approach is to vaccinate animals for brucellosis and attempt to predict resistance based on measures of immune responsiveness to the vaccine. Several groups have taken this approach, and these are discussed below. We have used both this approach and an alternative approach based on the observation that approximately 20% of unimmunized cows are naturally resistant to a standard challenge with *B. abortus*.[62] These studies are relevant to our understanding of acquired immunity to brucellosis, in that they are likely to direct us to those immune functions that are important for protective immunity and that may be enhanced by specific immunization.

Studies in Vaccinated Animals

Kaneene and colleagues, in a series of reports, found low levels of responsiveness in vaccinated cows when their lymphocytes were assayed *in vitro* for proliferative responses to BASA.[63] Others, however have not detected such low responses in vaccinated cattle.[30,64]

In two separate reports on vaccination and challenge experiments, Confer and colleagues measured lymphocyte proliferative assays following vaccination, challenge, or both.[38,65] In the first report, two doses of Strain 19 were compared as vaccines, and lymphocyte proliferation was assessed after challenge.[65] Vaccinated animals demonstrated higher responses on days 2 and 9 post-challenge in one experiment. But in the second experiment, vaccinated animals displayed higher responses 28 days post-challenge. In both experiments, the magnitude of the proliferative response was not associated with resistance to abortion or with culture results.

In the second report, CSP and dCSP were used as immunogens in Freund's complete adjuvant, and lymphocyte proliferative responses to heat-killed *B. abortus* and to BASA were measured after immunization.[38] The responses to BASA did not differ between heifers that aborted and those that did not. However, the response to the heat-killed antigen was significantly lower in heifers that subsequently aborted than in those that did not.

In our experiment using subcellular fractions of *B. abortus* as immunogens (Table 12-1), the cows were challenged with a virulent strain of *B. abortus* at mid-gestation to test for the presence of protective immunity by culture of maternal and fetal tissues. The cows were classified according to the frequency of positive proliferative responses after immunization, but before challenge. For the purpose of analyzing the correlation of positive proliferative responses with protection from challenge, cows that received adjuvant only were not considered, and all other groups were combined (See Table 12-3). There was a significant correlation between frequency of positive CMI responses and protection from infection: χ^2 = 9.030 (p < 0.05). Of those cows that responded in fewer than 25% of the proliferative assays, only 6 of 28 (21%) were protected. In a large series of such experiments, we have observed that approximately 20% of unimmunized cows are naturally resistant to brucellosis.[62] Thus, the immunized cows that were unresponsive in the proliferative assay were indistinguishable from unimmunized cattle in their level of protection. By contrast, those cows responding in greater than 50% of the proliferative assays were more likely to be protected (4 of 6). Although the number of animals was small in this experiment, there was presumptive evidence for a relationship, and a statistically significant correlation, between positive proliferative responses and protection from experimental challenge.

Table 12-3. Relationship of Lymphocyte Responsiveness to Protection
Against Brucellosis

Frequency of Positive Responses	Culture Negative	Culture Positive
0 - 25%	6	22
25 - 50%	0	5
50 - 75%	2	2
75-100%	2	0
	10	29

$$\chi^2 = 9.030 \ (df = 3) \qquad\qquad p < 0.05$$

Studies in Genetically Resistant Animals

An alternative approach to the question of the relationship between lymphocyte responsiveness and protection from challenge is to study responses in cattle that are naturally resistant or susceptible to brucellosis. A confounding factor in understanding protective immunity in brucellosis is the presence of chronic infection in cattle that are producing high levels of serum antibodies and display positive proliferative responses *in vitro*. Our strategy was to look for qualitative, rather than quantitative, differences in the responses of these two groups of cattle. The difference in reactivity of lymphocytes from different cows to other species of *Brucella* provided an opportunity to study the correlation of this difference in the apparent specificity of lymphocytes with resistance to brucellosis.

In a study of 20 cows (8 resistant and 12 susceptible), the lymphocyte proliferative responses to *B. abortus*, *B. suis*, and *B. melitensis* were determined, and responses to the latter two species were expressed as a percentage of the response to *B. abortus* (See Figure 12-3). The degree of relative cross-reactivity with *B. suis* was less than 70% in all of the assays of resistant cows, with a median value of approximately 20%. For susceptible cows, the range was much greater, with a median value of approximately 60%. The same pattern held for cross-reactivity with *B. melitensis*, in that the level of cross-reactivity in resistant cows was restricted to less

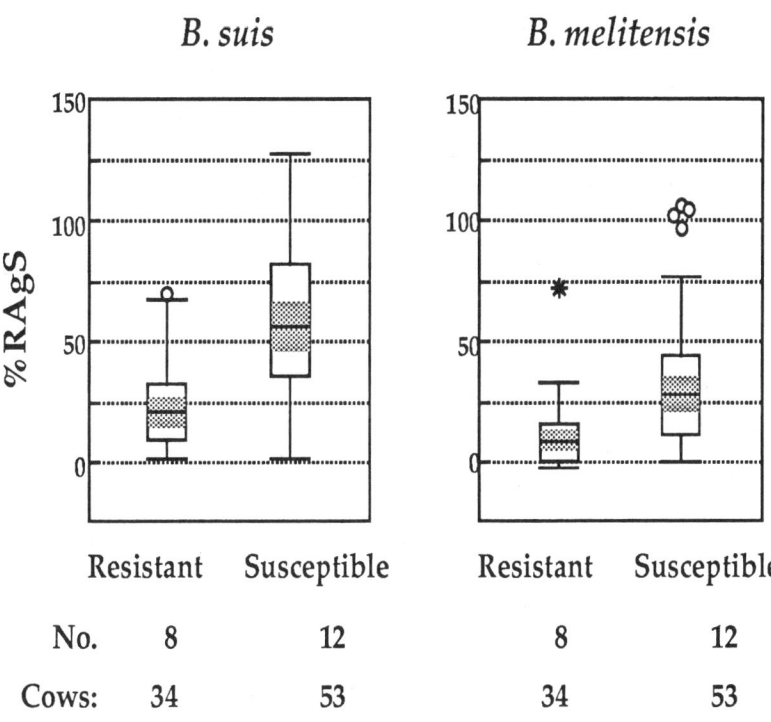

Figure 12-3. Relative Responsiveness of Bovine T–LymphocyteLines and T Lymphocytes to *B. suis* or *B. melitensis* after Experimental Challenge with *B. abortus* Strain 2308. Resistant cows and their calves were culture negative for *B. abortus* after challenge, but *B. abortus* was cultured from susceptible cows and their calves. Data are expressed as the percent relative antigenic stimulation (%RAgS), which is a percentage of the response to *B. abortus* Strain 2308 in the same assay. In the box plots presented, the median is indicated by the single horizontal line and the 25th and 75th percentiles (interquartile difference) by the extent of the box. The vertical lines indicate the extent of the outlier cutoffs determined by the method of Tukey and colleagues.[68] The 95% confidence interval is indicated by the shaded area.

mately 60%. The same pattern held for cross-reactivity with B. *melitensis,* in that the level of cross-reactivity in resistant cows was restricted to less than 35% (median = 12%), with a broader range for susceptible cows (median = 30%). Thus, resistant cows had lymphocytes that displayed very limited cross-reactivity with these other species, while susceptible cows had lymphocytes with a wide range of cross-reactivity. Most of the susceptible cows, however, had higher levels of cross-reactivity than even the most cross-reactive lymphocytes from resistant cows. The lack of overlap of the 95% confidence intervals for the two groups in responses to either B. *suis* or B. *melitensis* indicated a statistically significant difference between the two groups.

The conclusion that differences in reactivity to B. *abortus,* B. *suis,* and B. *melitensis* correlates with resistance and susceptibility raises important questions of causality. Is this a difference in the T-cell receptors expressed in these cows, or in the antigen-presenting capacity of their macrophages? Does the difference observed contribute to resistance, or is it a consequence of resistance? At least four possible explanations can be envisioned. First, cross-reactive lymphocytes appear as a result of chronic antigenic stimulation late in infection, generally after the resistant cow has cleared the organism. Second, the cross-reactive lymphocytes may appear early in infection, but there continued presence depends on chronic antigenic stimulation. Third, the difference in cross-reactivity may reflect an apparent difference in T-lymphocyte specificity caused by differences in the processing and presentation of antigens by the macrophages. Finally, there may be a real difference in the repertoire of T-cell receptors between resistant and susceptible cows, and that difference may contribute directly to the relative degree of resistance of the cows.

Of the four possibilities, only the first two are mutually exclusive, and these can be differentiated by studies on the kinetics of appearance of cross-reactive lymphocytes after experimental challenge. Such studies are now being planned. The other two possibilities are not necessarily mutually exclusive, with each other or with either of the first two alternatives. The third alternative, that macrophage processing and presentation of antigen is responsible for the differences observed between resistant and susceptible cows, is an interesting one in view of the known differences in macrophages between the two groups. The higher level of killing and the higher respiratory burst observed in macrophages from resistant cows may be related to such issues as efficiency of antigen presentation, as well. Especially interesting is the reported differences in antigen presentation in macrophages from mice resistant and susceptible to multiple facultative intracellular parasites by virtue of polymorphism at the *Bcg* locus on chromosome 1.[66,67] Experiments are now being designed to compare the relative efficiency of antigen presentation by macrophages in these two groups of cows.

Conclusions and Questions

Figure 12-4. summarizes our state of understanding of the T-lymphocyte response to *Brucella*.

Antigen Presentation

It has been demonstrated that MHC class II molecules and IL-1 participate in presentation of *Brucella* antigens to bovine T lymphocytes and that the form of the *Brucella* antigen—smooth versus rough strains—alters antigen presentation. In light of these observations, the contribution of antigen presentation to the ultimate specificity and function of T lymphocytes needs to be addressed. In cattle that are naturally resistant or susceptible to brucellosis, differences in macrophage activation have been identified.[62] These differences in macrophage activity need to be studied to determine whether a similar difference occurs for efficiency of antigen presentation.

Specificity

Subcellular fractions of *Brucella* cells generally stimulate lymphocytes in only a fraction of cows. Thus far, several effective subcellular fractions have been identified. These include: 1) LPS and associated proteins, 2) cell envelopes of rough mutants, and 3) Baomp II and III preparations (that include LPS). As noted above, the form in which the antigen is given to the cow may alter the lymphocyte specificity, and this may reflect alterations in presentation of *Brucella* antigens. A major gap in our knowledge about the specificity of T lymphocytes reacting to *Brucella* is whether some antigens stimulate protective responses and others non-protective or even suppressive responses.

Function

In vitro and *in vivo* assays have demonstrated that macrophage migration inhibition and dermal hypersensitivity result from immunization with *Brucella*, but other studies of function have not been studied. In this symposium, there was a report of cytolytic T lymphocytes. These need to be characterized more fully and their specific role in protective immunity to brucellosis needs to be determined.

At least two other major areas of T-lymphocyte function deserve

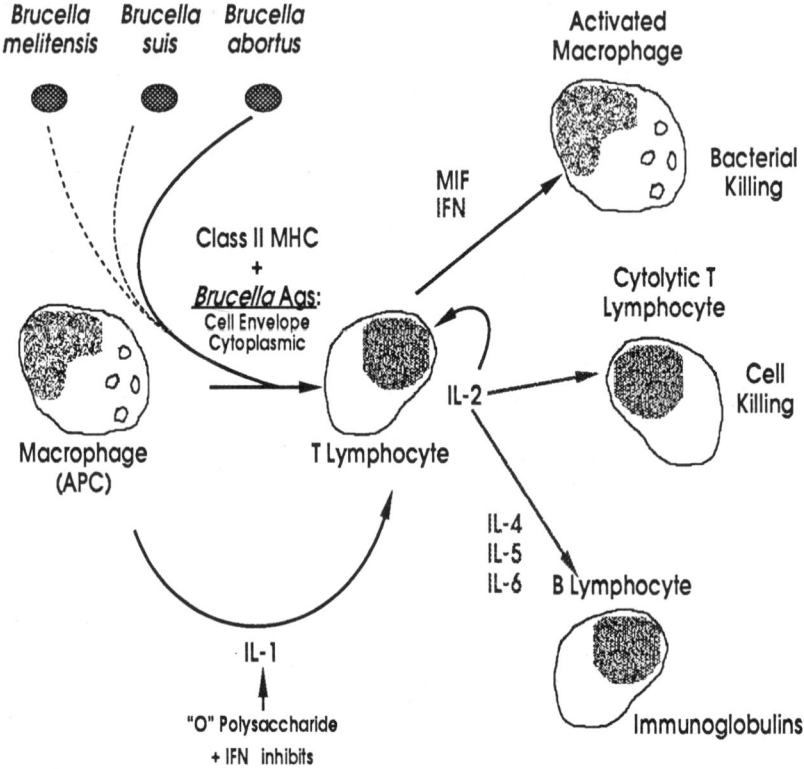

Figure 12-4. Cellular Interactions Leading to the Induction and Expression of T-Lymphocyte Activity in Bovine Brucellosis. Shaded arrows indicate mechanisms that have not been studied or demonstrated in bovine responses to B. abortus.

attention (See Figure 12-4.). First, a study of patterns of lymphokine secretion in *Brucella*-specific T lymphocytes should be undertaken. Second, there needs to be a better understanding of the interactions between bovine T and B lymphocytes in generating humoral responses to *Brucella*, especially in regard to isotype-switching mechanisms.

Relevance of Lymphocytes to Protective Immunity

Although definitive studies of the importance of T lymphocytes are difficult in large farm animals, we have provided evidence, derived from vaccinated cows and from naturally resistant cows, that points to a contributing role of cellular immunity in protection from brucellosis. Based on our preliminary results, continued studies on the relevance of vaccine-induced lymphocyte reactivity to *Brucella* to protective immunity are warranted. It will be especially important to correlate the specificity and functions of T–lymphocytes induced by vaccination to subsequent protection from challenge. In cows genetically resistant to brucellosis, there is a need for further studies to sort out the relative contributions of macrophage activity and T–lymphocyte cross-reactivity to one another and to protective immunity.

References

1. Mackaness GB. Cellular resistance to infection. *J Exp Med* 1962;116:381-406.
2. Mackaness GB. The immunological basis of acquired cellular resistance. *J Exp Med* 1964;120:105-120.
3. Mackaness GB. The influence of immunologically committed lymphoid cells on macrophage activity in vivo. *J Exp Med* 1969;129:973-992.
4. Lane FC, Unanue ER. Requirement of thymus (T) lymphocytes for resistance to listeriosis. *J Exp Med* 1972;135:1104-1112.
5. Collins FM, Campbell SG. Immunity to intracellular bacteria. *Vet Immunol Immunopathol* 1982;3:5-66.
6. Campbell PA. Are inflammatory phagocytes responsible for resistance to facultative intracellular bacteria? *Immunol Today* 1986;7:70-72.
7. Kaufmann SHE. CD8+ T lymphocytes in intracellular microbial infections. *Immunol Today* 1988;9:168-174.
8. Kaufmann SHE. Immunity to bacteria and fungi. *Curr Opinion Immunol* 1989;1:431-440.
9. Janis EM, Kaufmann SHE, Schwartz RH, et al. Acitvation of γδ T cells in the primary immune response to *Mycobacterium tuberculosis*. *Science* 1989;244:713-716.
10. Dijkmans R, Billiau A. Interferon γ: a master key in the immune system. *Curr Opinion Immunol* 1989;1:269-274.
11. Alausa, OK, Corbel, MJ, Elberg, SS, et al. *Report of the Joint FAO/WHO Expert Committee on Brucellosis*. 6th ed. Geneva:World Health Organization, 1986.
12. Schultz RD. The role of cell-mediated immunity in infectious diseases of cattle. *Adv Exp Biol Med* 1981;137:57-90.

13. Winter AJ. Discussions on *Brucella abortus*. *Ann Inst Pasteur (Microbiol)* 1987;138:135-137.

14. Splitter GA, Everlith KM. Collaboration of bovine T lymphocytes and macrophages in T-lymphocyte response to *Brucella abortus*. *Infect Immun* 1986;51:776-783.

15. Chestnut RW, Grey HM. Antigen presenting cells and mechanisms of antigen presentation. *CRC Crit Rev Immunol* 1985;5:263.

16. Janeway CA Jr, Ron J, Katz ME. The B cell is the initiating antigen-presenting cell in peripheral lymph nodes. *J Immunol* 1989;138:1051-1055.

17. Ron Y, Sprent J. T cell priming in vivo: a major role for B cells in presenting antigen to T cells in lymph nodes. *J Immunol* 1987;138:2848-2856.

18. Perera VY, Winter AJ, Ganem B. Evidence for covalent bonding of native hapten-protein complexes to smooth lipopolysaccharide of *Brucella abortus*. *FEMS Microbiol Lett* 1984;21:263-266.

19. Schwartz RH. T-lymphocyte recognition of antigen in association with gene products of the major histocompatibility complex. *Ann Rev Immunol* 1985;3:237-261.

20. Brown JH, Jardetzky T, Saper MA, et al. A hypothetical model of the foreign antigen binding site of class II histocompatibility molecules. *Nature* 1988;332:845-850.

21. Stobo JD. Lymphocytes: development and function. In: Gallin JI, Goldstein IM, Snyderman R, eds. *Inflammation: Basic Principles and Clinical Correlates*. New York:Raven Press, Ltd., 1988;599-612.

22. Dinarello CA. Cytokines: interleukin-1 and tumor necrosis factor (cachectin). In: Gallin JI, Goldstein IM, Snyderman R, eds. *Inflammation: Basic Principles and Clinical Correlates*. New York:Raven Press,Ltd., 1988;195-208.

23. Splitter GA, Everlith KM. *Brucella abortus* regulates bovine macrophages-T cell interaction by major histocompatibility complex class II and interleukin-1 expression. *Infect Immun* 1989;57:1151-1157.

24. Smith R III, Kapatsa JC, Sherwood SJ, et al. Differential reactivity of bovine lymphocytes to species of *Brucella*. *Am J Vet Res* 1989;in press.

25. Kaneene JMB, Anderson RK, Johnson DW, et al. *Brucella* antigen preparations for in vitro lymphocyte immunostimulation assays in bovine brucellosis. *Infect Immun* 1978;22:486-491.

26. Kaneene JMB, Anderson RK, Johnson DW, et al. Cell-mediated immune responses in cattle vaccinated with killed *Brucella melitensis* strain H-38 vaccine or infected with viable *Brucella abortus* strain 2308 organisms, or both. *Am J Vet Res* 1979;40:40-47.

27. Bhongbhibhat N, Elberg S, Chen TH. Characterization of *Brucella* skin-test antigens. *J Infect Dis* 1970;122:70-82.

28. Kaneene JMB, Muscoplat CC, Angus RD, et al. Specific in-vitro lymphocyte immunostimulation activities of *Brucella abortus* fractions obtained by column chromatography. *Comp Immunol Microbiol Infect Dis* 1979;2:9-21.

29. Cunningham B, Miler JJ, Dolan L, et al. Immunological characteristics in cattle of allergens derived from smooth *Brucella abortus* S99. *Vet Rec* 1980;107:369-375.

30. Baldwin CL, Antczak DF, Winter AJ. Evaluation of lymphocyte blastogenesis for diagnosis of bovine brucellosis. *Dev Biol Stand* 1984;56:357-370.

31. Baldwin CL, Verstreate DR, Winter AJ. Immune response of cattle to *Brucella abortus* outer membrane proteins measured by lymphocyte blastogenesis. *Vet Immunol Immunopathol* 1985;9:383-396.

32. Baldwin CL, Winter AJ. Blastogenic response of bovine lymphocytes to *Brucella abortus* lipopolysaccharide. *Infect Immun* 1985;47:570-572.

33. Brooks-Alder B, Splitter GA. Determination of bovine lymphocyte responses to extracted proteins of *Brucella abortus* by using protein immunoblotting. *Infect*

Immun 1988;56:2581-2586.

34. Sowa BA, Kelly KA, Frey M, et al. Partial N-terminal sequences of intact and CNBr fragments of SDS-soluble and peptidoglycan-bound *B. abortus* outer membrane proteins reveal post-translational additions to the porin gene product. *Vet Microbiol* 1990 ; submitted.

35. Winter AJ, Verstreate DR, Hall CE, et al. Immune response to porin in cattle immunized with whole cell, outer membrane, and outer membrane protein antigens of *Brucella abortus* combined with trehalose dimycolate and muramyl dipeptide adjuvants. *Infect Immun* 1983;42:1159-1167.

36. Winter AJ, Hall CE, Jacobson RH, et al. Effect of pregnancy on the immune response of cattle to a *Brucella* vaccine. *J Reprod Immunol* 1986;9:313-325.

37 Winter AJ, Rowe GE. Comparative immune responses to native cell envelope antigens and the hot sodium dodecyl sulfate insoluble fraction (PG) of *Brucella abortus* in cattle and mice. *Vet Immunol Immunopathol* 1988;18:149-163.

38. Confer AW, Tabatabai LB, Deyoe BL, et al. Vaccination of cattle with chemically modified and unmodified salt-extractable proteins from *Brucella abortus*. *Vet Microbiol* 1987;15:325-339.

39. Tabatabai LB, Deyoe BL. Characterization of salt-extractable protein antigens from *Brucella abortus* by crossed immunoelectrophoresis and isoelectric focusing. *Vet Microbiol* 1984;9:549-560.

40. Tabatabai LB, Deyoe BL. Biochemical and biological properties of soluble protein preparations from *Brucella abortus*. *Dev Biol Stand* 1984;56:199-211.

41. Wu AM, Adams LG, Pugh R. Immunochemical and partial chemical characterization of fractions of membrane-bound smooth lipopolysaccharide-protein complex from *Brucella abortus*. *Mol Cell Biochem* 1987;75:93-102.

42. Ficht T.A. Tn5 mutagenesis of *B. abortus*. (Unpublished).

43. Smith R III, Kapatsa JC, Rosenbaum BA, et al. Bovine T-lymphocyte lines reactive with *Brucella abortus*. *Am J Vet Res* 1989;in press.

44. Lanier LL, Ruitenberg JJ, Phillips JH. Human CD3⁺ T lymphocytes that express neither CD4 nor CD8 antigens. *J Exp Med* 1986;136:339-344.

45. Bank I, DePinho RA, Brenner MB, et al. A functional T3 molecule associated with a novel heterodimer on the surface of immature human thymocytes. *Nature* 1986;322:179-181.

46. Lanier LL, Le AM, Cwirla S, et al. Antigenic, functional, and molecular genetic studies of human natural killer cells and cytotoxic T lymphocytes not restricted by the major histocompatibility complex. *Fed Proc* 1986;45:2823-2828.

47. Janeway CA Jr, Jones B, Hayday A. Specificity and function of T cells bearing γδ receptors. *Immunol Today* 1988;9:73-76.

48. Azadegan A, Kaneene JMB, Muscoplat CC, et al. Development of a migration inhibitory factor assay under agarose of bovine mononuclear leukocytes, using an antigen of *Brucella abortus*. *Am J Vet Res* 1981;42:122-125.

49. Dorsey TA, Deyoe BL. Leukocyte migration-inhibition responses of nonvaccinated and vaccinated heifers to experimental infection with *Brucella abortus*. *Am J Vet Res* 1982;43:548-550.

50. Olitzki, A. *Immunological Methods in Brucellosis Research. II. In Vivo Procedures.* New York:S. Karger, 1970.

51. Klesius PH, Kramer TT, Swann AI, et al. Cell-mediated immune response after *Brucella abortus* S19 vaccination. *Am J Vet Res* 1978;39:883-886.

52. Rossi CR, Kiesel GK, Kramer TT, et al. Cell-mediated and humoral immune response of cattle to *Brucella abortus*, Mycobacterium bovis, and tetanus toxoid: evaluation of immunization and assay techniques. *Am J Vet Res* 1978;39:1738-1741.

53. Rossi CR, Kiesel GK, Hudson RS. Kinetics of detection of blastogenic responses of neonatal calves immunized in utero with tetanus toxoid, killed *Mycobacterium bovis*, and killed *Brucella abortus*. *Am J Vet Res* 1979;40:576-579.

54. Nicoletti P. The use of a *Brucella* protein antigen in dermal hypersensitivity as an adjunct method to diagnose bovine brucellosis. *Vet Immunol Immunopathol* 1983;5:27-31.

55. Chukwu CC. Comparison of the brucellin skin test with the lymphocyte transformation test in bovine brucellosis. *J Hyg ,Camb* 1986;96:403-413.

56. Chukwu CC. Differentation of *Brucella abortus* and *Yersinia enterocolitica* serotype O:9 infections in cattle: the use of specific lymphocyte transformation and brucellin skin tests. *Vet Q* 1987;9:134-142.

57. Montaraz JA, Winter AJ, Hunter DM, et al. Protection against *Brucella abortus* in mice with O-polysaccharide- specific monoclonal antibodies. *Infect Immun* 1986;51:961-963.

58. Plommet M. Brucellosis and immunity: humoral and cellular components in mice. *Ann Inst Pasteur (Microbiol)* 1987;138:105-110.

59. Limet J, Plommet A, Dubray G, et al. Immunity conferred upon mice by anti-LPS monoclonal antibodies in murine brucellosis. *Ann Inst Pasteur (Immunol)* 1987;138:417-424.

60. Pavlov H, Hogarth M, McKenzie IFC, et al. In vivo and in vitro effects of monoclonal antibody to Ly antigens on immunity to infection. *Cell Immunol* 1982;71:127-138.

61. Montaraz JA, Winter AJ. Comparison of living and nonliving vaccines for *Brucella abortus* in BALB/c mice. *Infect Immun* 1986;53:245-251.

62. Harmon BG, Templeton JW, Crawford RP, et al. Macrophage function and immune response of naturally resistant and susceptible cattle to *Brucella abortus*. In: Skamene E, ed. *Genetic Control of Host Resistance to Infection and Malignancy*. New York:Alan R. Liss, Inc., 1985;345-354.

63. Kaneene JMB, Johnson DW, Anderson RK, et al. Specific lymphocyte stimulation in cattle naturally infected with strains of *Brucella abortus* and cattle vaccinated with *Brucella abortus* Strain 19. *Am J Vet Res* 1978;39:585-589.

64. Wilkinson R, Cargill C, Lee K. Humoral and cell-mediated immune responses in non-pregnant heifers following infection and vaccination with *Brucella abortus*. *Vet Immunol Immunopathol* 1988;18:379-383.

65. Confer AW, Hall SM, Faulkner CB, et al. Effects of challenge dose on the clinical and immune responses of cattle vaccinated with reduced doses of *Brucella abortus* strain 19. *Vet Microbiol* 1985;10:561-575.

66. Denis M, Forget A, Pelletier M, et al. Pleiotropic effects of the *Bcg* gene. I. Antigen presentation in genetically susceptible and resistant congenic mouse strains. *J Immunol* 1988;140:2395-2400.

67. Denis M, Buschman E, Forget A, et al. Pleiotropic effects of the *Bcg* gene. II. Genetic restriction of responses to mitogens and allogeneic targets. *J Immunol* 1988;141:3988-3993.

68. Emerson JD, Strenio J. Boxplots and batch comparison. In: Hoaglin DC, Mosteller F, Tukey JW, eds. *Understanding Robust and Exploratory Data Analysis*. New York:John Wiley & Sons, Inc., 1983;58-96.

Chapter Thirteen

Mechanisms of Self Cure in
Brucella abortus Infected Cattle

Fred M. Enright

With so much of the *B. abortus* literature dealing with persistence of the infection, does self-cure *really* occur? If it really exists, what "yardsticks" have been used to document the event? A vague and somewhat "old fashioned" topic like self-cure is stimulating for it forces one to re-examine some of the old and very basic axioms of infectious diseases. We should briefly consider how infections are directly or indirectly spread. What are special features in the spread of brucellosis? If we think about its transmission, we see that the disease can be spread by direct and indirect means; that it can be spread by cattle with clinical symptoms and by asymptomatic cattle. Brucellosis can also be transmitted either *in utero* or immediately after birth to offspring.

Looking at just these transmission factors one would wonder why every cow in the world doesn't have brucellosis. However, when the host resistance factors are considered, one realizes the host has a great deal to do with not becoming infected. The resistance factors of the host are varied and many have been specifically addressed in other presentations at this conference. Mucosal barriers, inflammatory reactions, non-specific and immune directed phagocytosis, and specific humoral and cellular immune responses are all involved in host resistance. Lewis Thomas[1] suggests that our obsession with disease often results in our failure to appreciate the natural order or balance in the biological events associated with the interactions of different organisms. He points out that more often than not cooperative arrangements between microbes and higher phyla usually result in mutually beneficial circumstances. Non-cooperative relationships or diseases represent unusual exceptions in this scheme. While no examples of beneficial events are known to be associated with *B. abortus* infection, we recognize that other than the fetal wastage associated with initial infections, the *B. abortus*-bovine relationship is largely an uneventful one.

Let's examine self-cure from several different perspectives. We will briefly consider the earlier literature on "ceased" reactors. These observations will be considered in light of what we listened to today concerning innately resistant cattle. We will also examine data on the preferential replication of *B. abortus* within host tissues and the unique sensitivity of ruminant fetuses to *Brucella* infections. Finally, I would like to discuss the natural course of brucellosis in several herds of cattle raised in the marshes of southwest Louisiana.

The literature concerning the pathogenesis of bovine brucellosis is dominated by findings related to the persistence of infections in the host's tissues. In lectures to students and presentations to learned groups, how often have we *all* stated that brucellosis is a chronic bacterial disease; that infected cattle remain infected for life; that though most cows only abort once, most remain chronic carriers shedding the bacteria in milk and in reproductive tract discharges following an apparently normal subsequent calving.[2,3] How true are these statements? My own experiences with both experimentally infected cattle and with naturally infected cattle would suggest that persistent shedders are the exception rather than the rule. One might even ask, are cattle that continue to abort and/or continue to shed *Brucella* normal? Are they genetically different? Are they immunologically competent?

In 1940 Beach, Irwin and Ferguson[4] reported on the significance of "ceased" reactors in the transmission of brucellosis. Ceased reactors were cattle that no longer serologically reacted to *B. abortus* antigens following variable periods of positive reactivity to these antigens. Twenty-one "ceased" reactors were mixed with 54 *Brucella* negative cattle for one or two gestational periods. During the study one "ceased" reactor experienced a transitory infection in one-quarter of the udder. Other than this animal, *B. abortus* was not recovered in any of these cattle by culture or by guinea pig inoculation. One of the 54 normal cows developed a low titer but remained culture negative.

In 1943, Hamann[5] assembled a group of reactor and suspect cattle to determine what proportion of either group would remain or become reactors over a 5 year period. Of the 58 original reactor cows, 18 became permanent non-reactors (31%). Two of the 23 suspicious cows became reactors. He concluded that "the disease is more self-limiting than heretofore recognized."

In even earlier experiments, it was demonstrated that young calves orally exposed to *B. abortus* would develop infected lymphoid tissues and slight serological responses. These infections were transitory and the young calves were able to rapidly eliminate the bacteria from their tissues after oral exposure ceased.[6,7]

A significant number of non-pregnant adult cattle are also resistant to infection with *B. abortus*. As with calves, the lymph nodes draining the initial site of invasion become colonized with the bacteria. These are able to slow the spread of infection. They generally develop transient serological reactions and many become serologically negative (ceased reactors).[8,9]

From these samplings of the bovine brucellosis literature, I think one can safely say that a significant number of cattle are able to eliminate or at least control their infections. Presumably these cattle achieve their "cured" status as a result of either their natural resistance or the combined effects of natural resistance and acquired immunity.

As discussed earlier today, there are individuals among the general population of cattle that are extremely resistant to infection with *B. abortus*. Their resistance is thought to be related to the ability of their macrophages to more effectively ingest and kill *B. abortus*.[10] Naturally resistant cattle may still be infected with *B. abortus* following exposure to very large numbers of virulent bacteria; however, these cattle may also be those most likely to eliminate their infections.

In chronic or persistent *B. abortus* infections, the bacteria remain closely associated with the host's lymphoreticular system. This statement is based on several points. First, the organisms are most frequently recovered from these host tissues. Second, the typical histological reaction associated with brucellosis is observed most frequently in these tissues. The reaction is characterized as a granulomatous inflammatory response composed of epithelioid macrophages, monocytes, and lymphocytes. Variable numbers of neutrophils and eosinophils may be present. Multinucleated giant cells are rare in these reactions.[11] The kinetics of granuloma formation and the the turnover rates of various cells within the granulomas in *B. abortus*-infected cattle have not been studied. The localization of *B. abortus* within these reactions is also poorly understood.

Very little is also known about the intracellular replication of *Brucella* within the infected macrophages. Ultrastructural studies demonstrate the bacteria within membrane-lined vacuoles within these cells. Histochemical studies have demonstrated *Brucella* antigen (intact-appearing bacteria) within scattered cells throughout these granulomatous reactions (Meador et al. 1988; Detilleux et al. 1988). Seldom are large numbers of *Brucella* found within these macrophages. It would seem that the macrophage represents a protected site that allows the bacteria to remain alive rather than a "factory" geared to allowing massive replication of the bacteria.

The infection and growth of *B. abortus* within chorionic trophoblasts of the placenta is very different from that observed in infected macrophages. First, the bacteria are most often located within the rough endoplasmic reticulum of these cells. Second, infected cells very frequently contain large numbers of bacteria. There can be little doubt that prodigious replication of *Brucella* occurs in these specialized cells. The cellular and biochemical mechanisms responsible for the growth of these bacteria and for their selection of a unique intracellular site for replication are not known.[12,13,14]

Much research on the pathogenesis of bovine brucellosis has demonstrated that pregnant cattle are most susceptible to infection. It is also generally accepted that the level of bacteremia in pregnant cattle is directly related to an increase in fetal infections and abortion.[15] Earlier explanations for the correlation suggested that the *B. abortus* preferentially localized within the pregnant uterus.[16] In a series of experiments on the pathogenesis of *B. abortus* infections in pregnant mice, preferential placental localization of the bacteria has been questioned. In these studies fewer *B. abortus* were initially present in the placental tissue than in the spleen. However, by 72 hours post-inoculation, very large numbers of *B. abortus* were present within the placenta and relatively small numbers were found in the spleen.[17]

The persistence of *Brucella* spp. within macrophages of the lymphoreticular system in chronically infected animals may be viewed as a process that isolates the bacteria from their preferential growth sites. To perpetuate *B. abortus*, the bacteria must utilize some biological trick or take advantage of some derangement of the cow's immune system to reach their preferred sites - sites where they may replicate unchecked and, when conditions are correct, escape the host.

In our laboratory, we have used relatively low doses of virulent *B. abortus* to infect bovine, ovine, and caprine fetuses. In these studies, I was most impressed with the consistency of the intervals of time between fetal infection and abortion. Less pathogenic strains of *B. abortus* resulted in prolonged intervals between infection and delivery.[18,19,20] These studies indicate how remarkably sensitive ruminant fetuses are to infection with *B. abortus*. In view of the remarkable susceptibility of ruminant fetuses to infection with *B. abortus*, we must assume that most persistently infected cattle which abort only once are capable of preventing *Brucella* spp. from reaching their gravid reproductive tract. While such cattle may not be classified as absolutely cured, they should be considered immune and functionally cured.

Finally, I would like to direct some comments toward the natural course of bovine brucellosis. Have any of you recently thought about what would happen if *B. abortus* infected cattle were left alone for 10, 15, or 20 years? There are not too many places in the world where this occurs. Thimm[21] indicates that in 1964 in three east African countries—Kenya, Tanzania and Uganda—there were 19.3 million cattle with an average *B. abortus* infection rate of 13.7%. He goes on to state that there were very uniform bovine brucellosis prevalence rates of 10 to 16% over large regions of both East and West Africa and suggested that this uniformity may be due to the highly efficient process of natural field immunization.[22]

I was able to study a number of infected herds in the coastal marshes of southwest Louisiana. In 1980 50 to 60% of the herds in this region were quarantined due to brucellosis. Many of the herds studied consisted of moderately large numbers of indigenous cattle ranged on large tracts of marsh land. In this section of Louisiana, beef production represents the principal agricultural industry for large areas of untillable marsh land. The cattle are ranged from late fall to early spring in the marshes. In the spring, the cattle are gathered and transported or driven to higher summer pastures. The cattle are counted, marked, vaccinated, and treated for parasites twice a year as they are moved into or out of the marsh. The cattlemen in this area did not vaccinate their replacement heifers for bovine brucellosis. Cattle were bred year round and market calves and a few culled cows (most died in the marsh) were removed only twice a year. Replacement heifers and bulls were generated from within the herds.

Cattle have been raised in this area in a similar fashion for approximately 100 years. In 1957 a hurricane virtually wiped out the indigenous cattle population. New herds were formed by the surviving cattlemen within a few years and it is these herds that we were able to study. In 1980 the average prevalence percent of *B. abortus* infection (based on the card agglutination test) was 8%. The five herds we closely studied had a slightly lower average prevalence of 5.4.% The prevalence percent ranged from 3.1 to 16.1. Field strain *B. abortus* was isolated from a few cattle in these herds. These herds are unique in that they had been left alone for 21 to 22 years. As one might expect the very few new cases of brucellosis in these herds were limited to 2-to 3-year-old heifers.[23] This field study serves to illustrate an example of biological balance between an infectious agent and its host. Can we consider the majority of cattle in these herds "cured?" Similar findings on "cured" cattle following experimental *B. abortus* infection are presented by (R.P. Crawford, L.G. Adams, J.D. Williams, and R.A.Dietrick, "Economic Losses Attributable to Brucellosis," this volume).

In conclusion, are-examination of the definition of "cure" is necessary. A general definition of cure is the restoration of health. In its strictest interpretation, this means that in the case of bovine brucellosis the bacteria are totally eliminated from all host tissues. A looser interpretation would suggest that the host controls the spread of the bacteria, i.e., an equilibrium is reached which results in the inability of the agent to gain access to the environment in sufficient numbers to infect new hosts. In one case, there is an absolute cure and in the other, a functional "cure" results. There is evidence that both cases occur in bovine brucellosis.

References

1. Thomas L. The lives of a cell; Notes of a biology watcher. NY. Viking Press, 1974;5-10.

2. Brinley-Morgan WJ. The diagnosis of *Brucella abortus* infection in Britain. In: RP Crawford and RJ Hidalgo (eds.), Bovine Brucellosis, an international symposium. College Station and London, Texas A&M University Press. 1977;22-19.

3. Cunningham B. A difficult disease called Brucellosis In: Crawford, RP and RJ Hidalgo (eds.), Bovine Brucellosis, an international symposium. College Station and London, Texas A&M University Press. 1977;11-20.

4. Beach BA, Irwin MR, Ferguson LC. The significance of the "ceased" reactor to Bang's disease. *J Agric Res* 1940;61(1):75-80.

5. Hamann EE. A study of Bang's disease in cattle in a large dairy herd. In: Studies in Brucellosis II: A series of 5 papers by Huddleson IF; San Clemente CL; Stahl WH; Hutchings LM and Hammn EE. Michigan State College of Agricultural Experiment Station Technical Bulletin 1943;182:79-80.

6. Barger EH, Hayes FM. The discharge of *Bacterium abortum* in the feces of calves fed milk containing the organism. *J Am Vet Med Assoc*, 1924;66:328-336.

7. Carpenter CM. *Bacterium abortum* invasion of the tissues of calves from the ingestion of infected milk. *Cornell Vet* 1924;15:16-31.

8. Huddleson IF. Brucellosis in Man and Animals. Commonwealth Fund, NY, 1943;165.

9. Cunningham B. Vaccines prepared from killed *Brucella abortus* Strain 45/20 in oil adjuvant. Proceedings, 19th World Veterinary Congress, 1971; 994-996.

10. Harmon BG, Templeton JW, Crawford RP, et al. Macrophage function and immune response of naturally resistant and susceptible cattle to *Brucella abortus*. In: Skamene E ed. *Genetic Control of Host Resistance to Infection and Malignancy*. New York: A.R. Liss Inc, 1985;345-354.

11. Thoen CO, Enright FM. *Brucella*: *In*: *Pathogenesis of Bacterial Infection in Animals*. Gyles, CL, Thoen CO eds. Ames: Iowa State University Press, 1986; Chapter 20.

12. Meador VP, Hagemoser WA, Deyoe BL. Histopathologic findings in *Brucella abortus*-infected goats. *Am J Vet Res* 1988;49: 274-280.

13. Detilleaux PG, Cheville NF, Deyoe BL. Pathogenesis of *Brucella abortus* in chicken embryos. *Vet Pathol* 1988;25:138-146.

14. Anderson TD, Cheville NF, Meador VP. Pathogensis of Placentitis in the goat inoculated with *Brucella abortus*. II. Ultrastructural studies. *Vet Pathol* 1986;23:227-239.

15. Manthei CA, Carter RW. Persistence of *Brucella abortus* infection in cattle. *Am J Vet Res* 1950;II:173-180.

16. Keppie J, Williams AE, Witt K, et al. The role of Erythritol in tissue localization of the Brucellae. *Br J Exp Pathol* 1965;46:104.

17. Bosseray N. Colonization of mouse placentas by *Brucella abortus* inoculated during pregnancy. *Br J Exp Path* 1980;61:361-368.

18. Enright FM, Walker JV, Jeffers GW, et al. Cellular and Humoral Responses of *Brucella abortus* infected bovine fetuses. *Am J Vet Res* 1984;45:424-430.

19. Enright FM, Roop III M, Schurig G. 1985. Unpublished data on fetal goats inoculated with different strains of *Brucella abortus*.

20. Gorham SL, Enright FM, Snider III TG, et al. Morphologic lesions in *B. abortus* infected ovine fetuses. *Vet Pathol* 1986;23:331-332.

21. Thimm B. General Discussion Session VI, Chairman Ray WC, Ragamey RH, Alise EC, Vallette L (eds.). *International Symposium on Brucellosis. II. Developments in Biological Standardization* Vol. 31. Basel S. Karger 1976;293.

22. Thimm B, Wundt W. The epidemilogical situation of Brucellosis in Africa. Ragamey RH, Ailse EC, Vallette L, (eds.). *International Symposium on Brucellosis. II. Developments in Biological Standardization* Vol. 31. Basel. S. Karger. 1976;201-217.

23. Enright FM, Hugh-Jones ME. Effects of reactor retention in the spread of Brucellosis in Strain 19 adult vaccinated herds. *Prevent Vet Med* 1984;2:505-514.

PART FIVE

VACCINATION AGAINST BRUCELLOSIS

Chapter Fourteen

Development of Replicating Sub-Unit Vaccines Against Bacterial Pathogens

John D. Clements

Secretory IgA (sIgA) antibodies directed against specific virulence determinants of infecting organisms play an important role in overall mucosal immunity. Secretory IgA may prevent the initial interaction of the pathogen with the mucosal surface by blocking attachment and/or colonization, may neutralize surface acting toxins, or may prevent invasion of the host cells. Parenterally administered vaccines are not effective for eliciting mucosal sIgA responses and are generally ineffective against organisms that colonize mucosal surfaces and do not invade. Orally administered vaccines, especially live attenuated vaccines, have been shown to be effective in inducing specific sIgA responses, presumably because antigen is delivered to the T and B lymphocytes of the gut associated lymphoid tissue (GALT). The primed B cells then migrate to the mesenteric lymph nodes and undergo differentiation. These B cells enter the thoracic duct, then the general circulation, and subsequently seed all of the secretory tissues of the body, including the lamina propria of the gut and respiratory tract. IgA is then produced by the mature plasma cells and is transported onto the mucosal surface where it is available to interact with invading pathogens[1,2] (Figure 14-1).

A variety of techniques, including use of live oral vaccines, have been employed to deliver antigens to the GALT in an attempt to initiate production of specific sIgA. One recent approach has been to employ avirulent derivatives of *Salmonella* as carriers for plasmids which code for virulence determinants of heterologous mucosal pathogens (recently reviewed by Clements[3]). Antigens expressed by these strains would presumably be delivered directly to the antibody-forming cells in the GALT. This has been shown to be an effective means of stimulating significant levels of specific mucosal sIgA directed against the carrier strain and the heterologous antigen, and has been shown to stimulate production of serum antibodies as well.[4]

A number of investigators have employed a variety of mutants for this purpose, including *galE* mutants, which lack the enzyme uridine diphosphate (UDP)-galactose-4-epimerase,[5-7] and *aroA* mutants, which have spe-

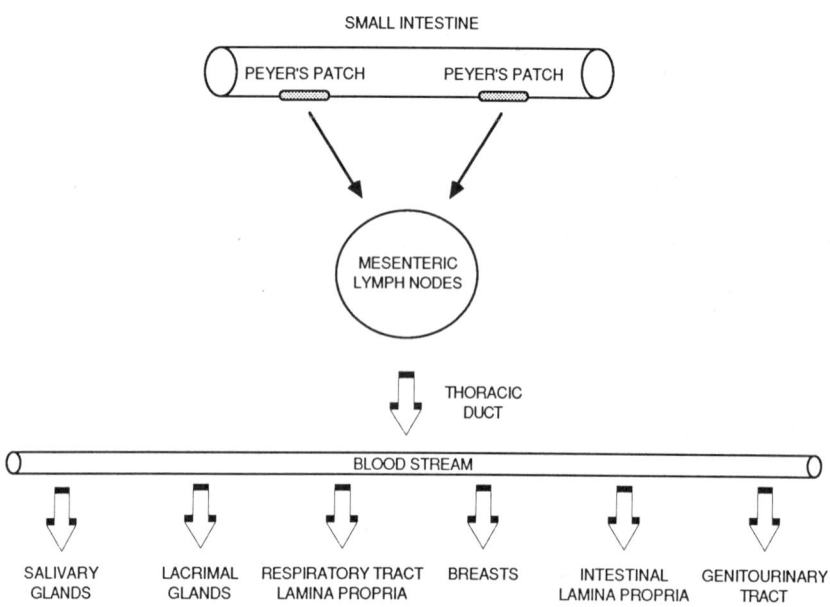

Figure 14-1. Generalized Pathway for Stimulation of Specific Mucosal Secretory IgA. From Clements (1987).

cific non-reverting deletions in the common aromatic biosynthetic pathway leading to chorismic acid.[8-12] The *galE* mutants of *Salmonella* have been used as carriers by: Formal et al.[13] who conjugally transferred the form I plasmid of *Shigella sonnei* to *S. typhi* Ty21a; Clements and El-Morshidy,[14] who utilized *S. typhi* Ty21a as a recipient for a recombinant plasmid containing the gene for production of the nontoxic B subunit of the heat-labile enterotoxin of *Escherichia coli* (LT-B); Yamamoto et al.,[15] who transferred a plasmid encoding colonization factor antigen (CFAI) and heat-stable enterotoxin from *E. coli* into *S. typhi* Ty21a; and Manning et al.,[16] who introduced molecularly cloned antigenic determinants of Inaba and Ogawa serotypes of *Vibrio cholerae* O1 lipopolysaccharide into derivatives of *S. typhi* Ty21a and an analogous *S. typhimurium* strain for experiments in mice.

The *aroA* mutants of *Salmonella* have been used as carriers by Clements et al.[4] to study mucosal and serum antibody responses to both the carrier and LT-B following oral immunization; by Dougan et al.[17] to construct an *aroA S. typhimurium* strain containing a plasmid which codes for the K88 fimbrial antigen of enterotoxigenic *E. coli*; by Maskell et al.[18] who demonstrated that mucosal anti-LT-B IgA increased following immunization with a *S. typhimurium* derivative containing a plasmid coding for production of LT-B; and by Brown et al.[19] to study antibody responses of mice to β–galactosidase (GZ) expressed in *S. typhimurium* Strain SL3261.

Attenuated mutants of *Salmonella* have also been examined as carriers for antigens of *Streptococcus mutans* in the development of a potential anticaries vaccine.[2,20,21] These researchers have constructed a number of *S. typhimurium* and *S. typhi* strains possessing various deletion mutations and capable of expressing both surface protein antigen A (Spa A) and glucosyltransferase of *S. mutans*. More recently, Sadoff et al.[22] reported the construction of a potential anti-malaria vaccine using a non-virulent *S. typhimurium* strain as a carrier for a plasmid expressing the circumsporozoite protein of *Plasmodium berghei*. Finally, Childress and Clements have investigated the use of *Salmonella* as carriers in the development of potential anti-herpes virus vaccines.[23]

A number of the efforts outlined above have been initiated in an attempt to elicit mucosal antibodies against relevant virulence determinants of enterotoxigenic *E. coli* (ETEC), principally toxins (toxoids) and colonizing factor antigens (CFAs). The remainder of this review will describe our efforts, and those of others, on the use of avirulent *Salmonella* as a carrier for ETEC antigens. Specifically, we will focus on the use of *Salmonella* as a carrier for a recombinant plasmid that codes for production of the B subunit of the heat-labile enterotoxin (LT-B) of *E. coli*. We will also address two related questions: 1) the effect of multiple genetic mutations on carrier efficacy and 2) the effect of repeated use on carrier efficacy. Finally, we will summarize the reported findings of a number of other laboratories on the development of ETEC vaccines based upon this principal.

Construction of a Potential Multivalent Live Oral Vaccine for Both Typhoid Fever and the Cholera -*E. coli* Related Diarrheas

We have constructed a potential multivalent live oral vaccine for both typhoid fever and the cholera - *E. coli* related diarrheas utilizing the galactose epimeraseless (*galE*) mutant of *S. typhi* which has been shown to be a safe, effective live oral vaccine for typhoid fever.[14] We used *S. typhi* Ty21a as a recipient for a recombinant plasmid (pJC217) containing the gene for production of the nontoxic B subunit of the heat-labile enterotoxin of *E. coli* (LT-B). This protein shares extensive sequence and immunologic homology with the B subunit of the *Vibrio cholerae* enterotoxin. The *S. typhi* derivative, Strain SE12, produced LT-B and induced a significant serum antitoxin antibody response when injected parenterally into mice and guinea pigs. We were not, however, able to test the full potential of this strain as a live oral vaccine, or of this method of antigen delivery as a means of stimulating mucosal antitoxin antibodies, due to the limited host range of *S. typhi*.

We subsequently obtained an avirulent mouse strain of *Salmonella* capable of producing an infection following oral inoculation of mice analogous to the events associated with oral inoculation of man with Ty21a. We reasoned that this may provide a suitable model for testing the theory of direct stimulation of the antibody-forming cells in the GALT with antigen as a means of stimulating significant levels of mucosal antibodies.[4] In this study, *S. dublin* Strain SL1438 *aroA* was transformed with plasmid pJC217, characterized for production of LT-B, and examined for efficacy as an oral vaccine in mice. The derivative strain, designated EL23, produced LT-B that was, by all criteria, identical to LT-B produced by *E. coli* or by *S. typhi* Strain SE12.

Effect of Primary Immunization

Initial priming studies comparing oral immunization with LT-B to oral immunization with Strain EL23 showed that immunization with LT-B produces significantly higher levels of antitoxin serum IgG (Figure 14-2A) and initially higher levels of antitoxin mucosal secretory IgA (Figure 14-2B). The differences in IgA levels were no longer significant by the fifth week. Mice receiving Strain EL23 orally also developed progressively increasing mucosal and serum antibody responses to the LPS of the vaccine strain (not shown).

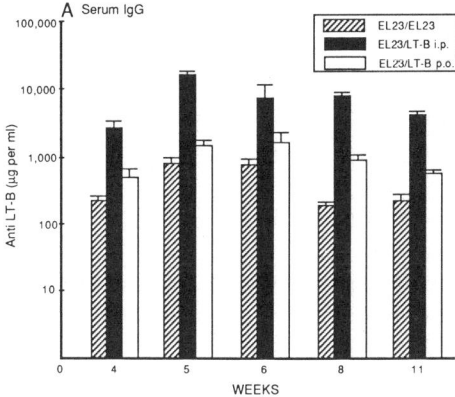

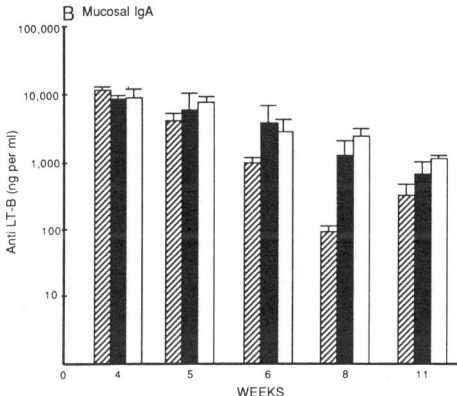

Figure 14-2. Serum IgG (A) and Mucosal IgA (B) Antitoxin Responses Following Oral Immunization with either LT-B or *S. dublin* Strain EL23. Female BALB/c mice were immunized orally with two doses containing either 64 µg of LT-B or 10^{10} CFU each of strain EL23 on days 0 and 4. Groups of animals were sacrificed at weekly intervals thereafter and analyzed for production of antibodies to LT-B. Serum and mucosal antitoxin levels were zero for control animals throughout the study. Each data point represents the mean of determinations in four to six animals. Standard error bars are shown. Mice immunized orally with LT-B developed progressively increasing levels of serum and mucosal antitoxin antibodies throughout the course of the experiment, five weeks post primary immunization. Serum and mucosal antitoxin levels for unimmunized controls were zero. From Clements et al. (1986).

Effect of Boosting

The effect of boosting mice primed orally with Strain EL23 was also investigated, and boosting i.p. with LT-B gave the highest sustained levels of antitoxin serum IgG (Figure 14-3A), while boosting i.p. or p.o. with LT-B gave equivalent mucosal antitoxin IgA responses (Figure 14-3B).

In Vitro Toxin Neutralization

The mucosal antibody response was also shown to be IgA specific and to be capable of neutralizing the biological activities of both LT and cholera toxin *in vitro* (Table 14-1).

Effect of Multiple Mutations on the Efficacy of *Salmonella* Vectors

In contrast to results obtained with *S. dublin aroA* mutants in mice, a recent study reported that human vaccine recipients receiving *S. typhi* (*aroA, purA*155, *hisG* 46) mutants[24] developed low humoral responses to the O polysaccharide of the vaccine strain.[25] It is not clear why the *S. typhi* mutants were unable to induce a humoral response; this may have been due to the presence of two non-reverting auxotrophic characters in the *S. typhi* strains, as contrasted with a single non-reverting auxotrophic character in the studies employing *S. dublin* mutants in mice, or to the single *purA* mutation not present in the oral mouse studies.

Use of *Salmonella* as a carrier for delivery of heterologous antigens in humans will likely employ an attenuated *S. typhi*, perhaps one derived as above. It was therefore of interest to determine if the failure to induce a humoral response noted above was a function of the double mutation or of either single mutation. To accomplish this, we examined three strains of *S. dublin* containing either an *aroA* mutation, a *purA* mutation, or both *aroA* and *purA* mutations for the ability to colonize, invade, persist in tissues, and evoke serum and mucosal antibody responses to the lipopolysaccharide of the parent strain following oral feeding of mice. The organisms used for this study were nalidixic acid resistant derivatives of *S. dublin* Strain SL5608 (wild type) and included *S. dublin* Strain SL7163 (*aroA*148), *S. dublin* Strain SL7165 (*purA*155), and *S. dublin* Strain SL7164 (*aroA*148, *purA*155). We below refer to these three nalidixate-resistant auxotrophic strains just as *aroA*, *purA*, and *aroA purA* instead of by their strain numbers.

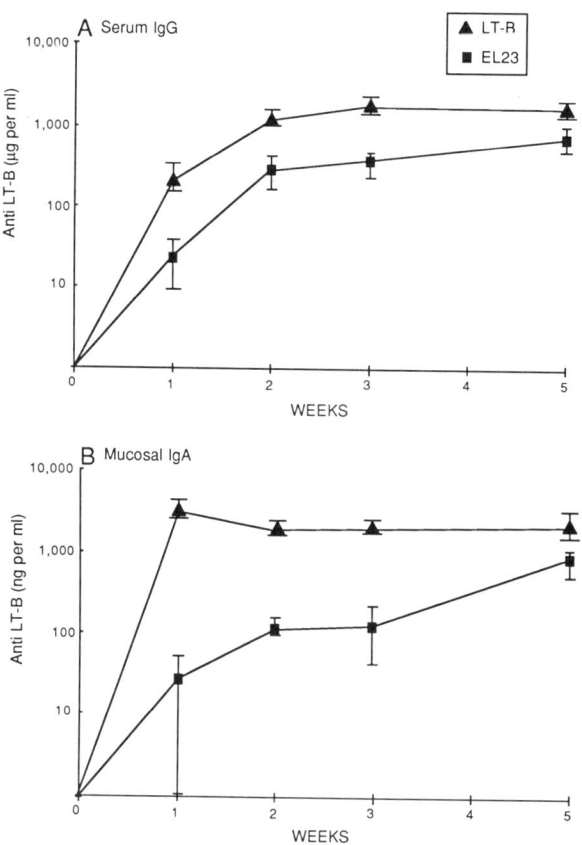

Figure 14-3. Serum (A) and Mucosal (B) Antitoxin Responses after Boosting Primed Animals with either LT-B or *S. dublin* Strain EL23. Female BALB/c mice were immunized orally with two doses containing 10^{10} CFU each of Strain EL23 on days 0 and 4. At 21 days post primary immunization, groups of animals were boosted with either 10^{10} CFU of EL23, 100 μg of LT-B given i.p., or 100 μg of LT-B given p.o. Groups of animals were sacrificed at weekly intervals thereafter and analyzed for production of antibodies to LT-B by ELISA. Values shown begin at week 4 post primary immunization (i.e., 1 week following booster immunizations). Serum and mucosal antitoxin levels were zero for control animals throughout the study. Each data point represents the mean of determinations in four to six animals. Standard error bars are shown. From Clements et al. (1986).

Table 14-1. Neutralization of Adrenal Cell Activity* of Cholera and
E. coli Enterotoxins†

Antiserum	Cholera Toxin	LT
Pooled Mucosa	128‡	256‡
Pooled Mucosa + goat antiserum against mouse IgA	6	32
Pooled Mucosa + rabbit antiserum against mouse IgG	128	256

*The adrenal cell assay was conducted using mouse Y-1 adrenal cells in
miniculture.
†Approximately 10 minimal rounding doses were used.
‡Reciprocal of highest serum dilution showing complete neutralization of
biological activity. Pooled mucosa from control animals had no effect.

Colonization, Invasion, and Persistence in Mouse Tissues

As shown in Table 14-2, there was evidence for colonization of the small
intestines, invasion, and persistence in mouse tissues only with *aroA*,
which was isolated from the small intestines, Peyer's patches, livers, and
spleens of animals up through the third day post-inoculation. Thereafter,
only the livers and, beginning at day 8 post-inoculation, the small intestines were infected. *aroA* could be isolated only from the blood of one
animal on one day (day 3 post-inoculation). Of the 20 animals immunized
in this group, *aroA* was isolated from the small intestines of nine, from the
the Peyer's patches of five, from the livers of seven, from the spleens of
two, and from the blood of one (Table 14-2).

The *purA* strain was isolated from the small intestine, liver, and blood
of only a single animal, and then only on the first day post-inoculation.
Thereafter, *purA* was not detected in any tissue throughout the 21 days of
the study. Similarly, *aroA purA* was isolated from the Peyer's patches of
a single animal at one day post-inoculation and not subsequently detected
in any tissue throughout the 21 days of the study.

Table 14- 2. Colonization, Invasion, and Persistence in Mouse Tissues

aroA	1*	3	Day 7	8	14	21	Total
small intestine	3/3	3/3	0/3	1/3	1/3	1/5	9/20
Peyer's patches	3/3	2/3	0/3	0/3	0/3	0/5	5/20
liver	2/3	1/3	1/3	1/3	1/3	1/5	7/20
spleen	1/3	1/3	0/3	0/3	0/3	0/5	2/20
blood	0/3	1/3	0/3	0/3	0/3	0/5	1/20
purA							
small intestine	1/3	0/3	0/3	0/3	0/3	0/4	1/19
Peyer's patches	0/3	0/3	0/3	0/3	0/3	0/4	0/19
liver	1/3	0/3	0/3	0/3	0/3	0/4	1/19
spleen	0/3	0/3	0/3	0/3	0/3	0/4	0/19
blood	1/3	0/3	0/3	0/3	0/3	0/4	1/19
aroA purA							
small intestine	0/3	0/3	0/3	0/3	0/3	0/4	0/19
Peyer's patches	1/3	0/3	0/3	0/3	0/3	0/4	1/19
liver	0/3	0/3	0/3	0/3	0/3	0/4	0/19
spleen	0/3	0/3	0/3	0/3	0/3	0/4	0/19
blood	0/3	0/3	0/3	0/3	0/3	0/4	0/19

*Number of specimens culture positive/number tested

Humoral Response Following Immunization with the Attenuated Mutants

A major consideration in the selection of an appropriate live vaccine or carrier organism is the ability of that organism to evoke an appropriate immunologic response. As an indicator of that response, we examined the serum immunoglobulin G (IgG) and mucosal immunoglobulin A (IgA) responses against the lipopolysaccharide (LPS) of the parent *S. dublin* Strain, SL5608. Mice immunized orally with *aroA*, *purA*, and *aroA purA* developed serum anti-LPS antibodies and maintained them throughout the course of the experiment, 5 weeks post-primary inoculation (Table 14-3). There was, however, great variability between individual animals in all groups; statistical differences between immunized groups and control

Table 14-3. Serum and Mucosal Anti-LPS Responses

IgG* (μg/ml)	Week 1	Week 2	Week 3	Week 4	Week 5
aroA	1.32±0.30	4.83±0.73	7.71±2.78	7.66±2.00	14.1±4.21
purA	0.47±0.25	0.85±0.25	2.80±1.95	0.58±0.22	2.89±2.17
aroA purA	8.05±6.6	5.35±3.31	5.00±1.44	1.32±0.91	2.37±0.82

IgA† (μg/ml)	Week 1	Week 2	Week 3	Week 4	Week 5
aroA	2.78±0.72	45.29±12.72	15.28±2.75	26.45±7.04	27.3±5.19
purA	0.57±0.19	1.41±0.17	0.40±0.19	0.17±0.07	1.36±0.85
aroA purA	1.08±0.73	0.14±0.05	0.39±0.16	0.21±0.09	0.97±0.75

*Mean ± s.e.m. as determined by ELISA. See text for details.
†Mean ± s.e.m. as determined by ELISA. See text for details.

values from unimmunized animals were not consistent at one, two, or three weeks following the primary inoculation. By the end of the fifth week (Figure14- 4A), serum anti-LPS IgG had increased from zero to 14.1 μg/ml in animals immunized with aroA, a value significantly greater than that obtained following immunization with either purA - 2.89 μg/ml, or with aroA purA - 2.37 μg/ml homologous antigens. This was also suggested by the findings of O'Callaghan et al.[26] in a study characterizing aromatic- and purine-dependent S. typhimurium for virulence, persistence, and the ability to induce protective immunity following i.v. and oral immunization of BALB/c mice. Those authors did not measure serum and mucosal antibody responses, but did demonstrate that organisms containing the single aroA deletion, given orally or intravenously, were more effective at protecting against intravenous challenge than were mutants containing either a single purA deletion or both deletions together. Our findings differed from theirs in the degree of persistence of the various mutants. In their hands, following i.v. inoculation, all three mutants persisted in livers and spleens for up to 10 weeks after infection. We immunized orally and found that only the aroA mutants were able to colonize the small intestine, invade, and persist in mouse tissues. These differences can probably be ascribed to the different routes of inoculation.

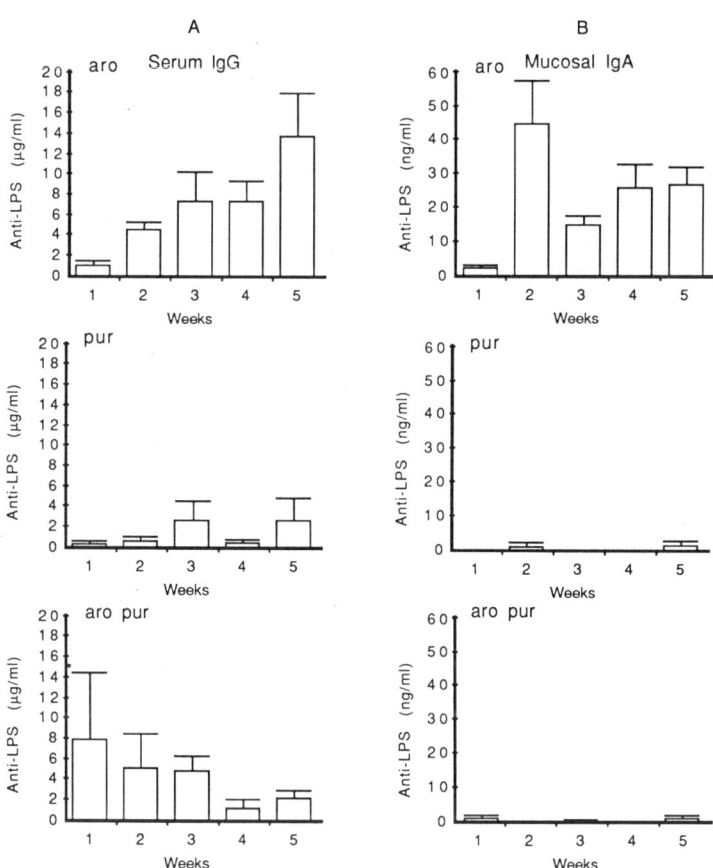

Figure 14-4. Serum (A) and Mucosal (B) Anti-LPS Responses after Oral Immunization with Three Auxotrophic Mutants of *S. dublin*. Groups of female BALB/c mice were immunized by gavage with two doses, each containing 10^{10} CFU of one or another of the three auxotrophic strains, on days 0 and 4. The strains examined were nalidixate-resistant strains SL7163 (*aroA*148), SL7165 (*purA*155), and SL7164 (*aroA*148, *purA*155). Groups of animals were sacrificed at weekly intervals and analyzed for production of antibodies to LPS of the parent strain by ELISA. Serum and mucosal anti-LPS levels were zero for control animals throughout the study. Standard error bars are shown. Of the three strains tested, only SL7163 with the single *aroA* mutation was able to evoke significant, sustained serum and mucosal antibody responses. Neither SL7165 (*purA*155) nor SL7164 (*aroA*148, *purA*155) demonstrated these characteristics.

We conclude from these results, that even though the *purA* mutation decreases the virulence of these organisms, it so attenuates the organisms as to make them unusable. These finding may be important in the selection of attenuated *S. typhi* strain for use in humans, either as an anti-typhoid live-vaccine, or as a vector for antigens of other pathogens.

Effect of Multiple Use on Carrier Efficacy

A major consideration in the proposed use of *Salmonella* as a carrier for heterologous antigens is the consequence of repeated use of the carrier. Specifically, if *Salmonella* is used as a carrier for one antigen, will it be an effective vehicle for delivery of other antigens? Does prior experience with the carrier limit the immunologic response to a heterologous antigen? We have addressed this question in a preliminary fashion by immunizing (priming) some groups of mice with a carrier (*Salmonella* SL1438), boosting with the carrier containing a heterologous antigen (LT-B), and comparing serum and mucosal responses against the antigen between groups primed with the carrier and those not primed with the carrier. As shown in Figure 14-5, the serum IgG anti-LT-B response in animals previously exposed to the carrier was reduced by approximately 60% (210 μg/ml versus 85 ug/ml) of that found in the unprimed group at two weeks after immunization with the carrier/antigen. At four weeks after immunization with the carrier/antigen, the serum IgG anti-LT-B response was further reduced to approximately 17% of that found in the unprimed group (37 μg/ml versus 224 μg/ml). Similar responses were seen for mucosal IgA. Mucosal IgA anti-LT-B responses in primed animals were reduced to 3% of levels found in unprimed animals at two weeks after immunization with the carrier/ antigen (84 μg/ml versus 101 μg/ml). At four weeks, primed levels had further decreased to less that 1% of unprimed levels (0.76 μg/ml versus 81 μg/ml). These are clearly very preliminary findings, but indicate 83% of levels found in unprimed animals at two weeks after immunization with the carrier/antigen (84 μg/ml versus 101 μg/ml). At four weeks, primed levels had further decreased to less that 1% of unprimed levels (.76 μg/ml versus 81 μg/ml). These are clearly very preliminary findings, but indicate that prior use of a carrier may indeed influence the subsequent immunological response to a second antigen delivered by the same carrier, especially on the mucosal antibody response. There are a number of unresolved questions including 1) the nature of the effect if the two strains of *Salmonella* are serologically different, 2) the temporal relationship of the priming and boosting doses, 3) the duration of the effect, and 4) the biological relevance of the reduction.

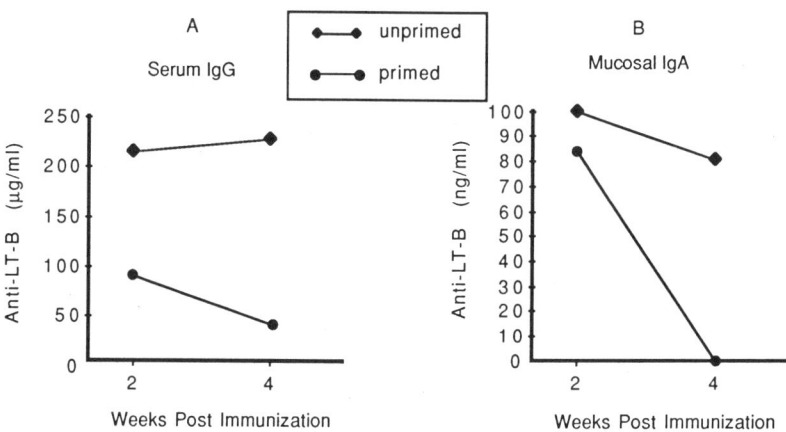

Figure 14-5. Serum (A) and Mucosal (B) Anti-LT-B Responses after Immunizing Primed and Unprimed Animals with *S. dublin* Strain EL23. Primed animals were immunized orally with two doses containing 10^{10} CFU each of strain SL1438 on days 0 and 4. At 4 weeks post primary immunization, groups of animals were boosted with 10^{10} CFU of EL23. Groups of animals were sacrificed at two and four week intervals thereafter and analyzed for production of antibodies to LT-B by ELISA. Serum and mucosal antitoxin levels were zero for control animals throughout the study. Each data point represents the mean of determinations in four to six animals.

Other Reported Efforts

There have been a number of other reported applications of this principle to the development of ETEC vaccines. Dougan et al.[17] constructed an *aroA S. typhimurium* strain containing a plasmid which codes for the K88 fimbrial antigen of enterotoxigenic *E. coli* associated with diarrheal disease in neonatal piglets. Antibodies directed against the K88 fimbrial antigen have been shown to passively protect against diarrheal disease due to enterotoxigenic organisms possessing the K88 fimbriae. Mice were immunized orally and intravenously with the derivative strain and were strongly protected against subsequent challenge with virulent *S. typhimurium*. Serum from these mice contained antibodies against the K88 fimbrial antigen as determined by Western blots. Some groups of mice were boosted intravenously with the derivative strain and serum from the reimmunized mice was able to agglutinate an *E. coli* K-12 strain expressing the antigen. Additional studies by this group[18] also demonstrated that mucosal anti-LT-B IgA increased following immunization with a *S. typhimurium* derivative containing a plasmid coding for production of LT-B. Additionally, Yamamoto et al.[15] transferred a plasmid encoding colonization factor antigen (CFAI) and heat-stable enterotoxin (ST) from *E. coli* into a streptomycin resistant isolate of *S. typhi* Ty21a. Transconjugants were shown to produce both ST and CFAI.

In summary, the use of avirulent *Salmonella* as a carrier for heterologous antigens provides the following advantages: 1) the most appropriate antigen(s) delivered by the most effective route in a manner designed to stimulate a protective mucosal and serum immune response, 2) development of a minimal number of untoward side effects, and 3) cost effectiveness. In addition to direct stimulation of the appropriate target cells in the lymphoid tissues, such a vaccine eliminates the consequences of repeated parenteral injections of endotoxin associated with many of the currently available bacterial vaccines.

References

1. Cebra JJ, Fuhrman JA, Lebman DA, London SD. Effective gut mucosal stimulation of IgA-committed B cells by antigen. In: F Brown, RM Channok, RA Lerner eds., Vaccines 86. *New approaches to immunization. Developing vaccines against parasitic, bacterial, and viral diseases*. Cold Spring Harbor: Cold Spring Harbor Laboratory, 1986;129-133.

2. Curtiss R, III. Genetic analysis of *Streptococcus mutans* virulence and prospects for an anticaries vaccine. *J Dent Res* 1986;65:1034-1045.

3. Clements JD. Use of attenuated mutants of *Salmonella* as carriers for delivery of heterologous antigens to the secretory immune system. *Pathol Immunopathol Res* 1987;6:137-146.

4. Clements JD, Lyon FL, Lowe KL, Farrand AL, El-Morshidy S. Oral immunization

of mice with attenuated *Salmonella enteritidis* containing a recombinant plasmid which codes for production of the B subunit of heat-labile *Escherichia coli* enterotoxin. *Infect Immun* 1986;53:685-692.

5. Germanier R, Fürer E. Isolation and characterization of *galE* mutant Ty21a of *Salmonella typhi*: a candidate strain for a live, oral typhoid vaccine. *J Infect Dis* 1975;131:553- 558.

6. Gilman RH, Hornick RB, Woodward WE, DuPont HL, Snyder MJ, Levine MM, Libonati JP. Evaluation of a UDP-glucose-4- epimeraseless mutant of *Salmonella typhi* as a live oral vaccine. *J Infect Dis* 1977;136:717-723.

7. Wahdan MH, Serie C, Germanier R, Lackany A, Cerisier Y, Guerin N, Sallam S, Geoffroy P, Sadek el Tantawi A, Guesry P. A controlled field trial of live oral typhoid vaccine Ty21a. *Bull WHO*1980;58:469-474.

8. Hoiseth SK, Stocker BAD. Aromatic-dependent *Salmonella typhimurium* are non-virulent and effective as live vaccines. *Nature* 1981; 291:238-239.

9. Robertsson JA, Lindberg AA, Hoiseth S, Stocker BAD. *Salmonella typhimurium* infection in calves: protection and survival of virulent challenge bacteria after immunization with live or inactivated vaccines. *Infect Immun* 1983;41:742-750.

10. Smith BP, Reina-Guerra M, Hoiseth SK, Stocker BAD, Habasha F, Johnson E, Merritt F. Aromatic-dependent *Salmonella typhimurium* as modified live vaccines for calves. *Am J Vet Res* 1984;45:59-66.

11. Smith BP, Reina-Guerra M, Stocker BAD, Hoiseth SK, Johnson E. Aromatic-dependent *Salmonella dublin* as a parenteral modified live vaccine for calves. *Am J Vet Res* 1984;45:2231-2235.

12. Stocker BAD, Hoiseth SK, Smith BP. Aromatic-dependent *Salmonella* species as live vaccines in mice and calves, Vol. 53, p. 47-54. In: International symposium on enteric infections in man and animals: standardization of immunological procedures, Dublin, Ireland, 1982. *Develop Biol Stand* 1983.

13. Formal SB, Baron LS, Kopecko DJ, Washington O, Powell C, Life CA. Construction of a potential bivalent vaccine strain: introduction of *Shigella sonnei* form I antigen genes into the *galE Salmonella typhi* Ty21a typhoid vaccine strain. *Infect Immun* 1981;34:746-750.

14. Clements JD, El-Morshidy S. Construction of a potential live oral bivalent vaccine for typhoid fever and cholera- *Escherichia coli*- related diarrheas. *Infect Immun* 1984;46:564-569.

15. Yamamoto T, Tamura Y, Yokota T. Enteroadhesion fimbriae and enterotoxin of *Escherichia coli*: genetic transfer to a streptomycin-resistant mutant of the *galE* oral-route live vaccine *Salmonella typhi* Ty21a. *Infect Immun* 1985; 50:925-928.

16. Manning PA, Heuzenroeder MW, Yeadon J, Leavesley DI, Reeves PR, Rowley D. Molecular cloning and expression in *Escherichia coli* K-12 of the O antigens of the Inaba and Ogawa serotypes of the *Vibrio cholerae* O1 lipopolysaccharides and their potential for vaccine development. *Infect Immun* 1986;53:272-277.

17. Dougan G, Sellwood R, Maskell D, Sweeney K, Liew FY, Beesley J, Hormaeche C. *In vivo* properties of a cloned K88 adherence antigen determinant. *Infect Immun* 1986; 52:344-347.

18. Maskell D, Liew FY, Sweeney K, Dougan G, Hormaeche CE. Attenuated *Salmonella typhimurium* as live oral vaccines and carriers for delivering antigens to the secretory immune system. In: F Brown, RM Channok, RA Lerner eds., Vaccines 86: *New approaches to immunization. Developing vaccines against parasitic, bacterial, and viral diseases.* Cold Spring Harbor: Cold Spring Harbor Laboratory, 1986;213-217

19. Brown A, Hormaeche CE, Demarco de Hormaeche R, Winther M, Dougan G, Maskell DJ, Stocker BAD. An attenuated *aroA Salmonella typhimurium* vaccine elicits humoral and cellular immunity to cloned β-galactosidase in mice. *J Infect Dis* 1987; 155:86-92.

20. Curtiss R III, Goldschmidt R, Kelly S, Lyons M, Michalek S, Pastian R, Stein S. Recombinant avirulent *Salmonella* for oral immunization to induce mucosal immunity to bacterial pathogens. In: H Kohler, PT LoVerde eds. *Vaccines: new concepts and developments. Proceedings* of the 10th International Convocation on Immunology. Harlow, Essex, Great Britain: Longman Scientific and Technical, 61-271;1987.

21. Curtiss R, III, Kelly SM. *Salmonella typhimurium* deletion mutants lacking adenylate cyclase and cyclic AMP receptor, protein are avirulent and immunogenic. *Infect Immun* 1987;55:3035-3043.

22. Sadoff JC, Ballou WR, Baron LS, Majarian WR, Brey RN, Hockmeyer WT, Young JF, Cryz SJ, Ou J, Lowell GH, Chulay JD. Oral *Salmonella typhimurium* vaccine expressing circumsporozoite protein protects against malaria. *Science* 1988;240:336-340.

23. Childress AM, Clements JD. Construction of a chimeric plasmid expressing glycoprotein b of herpes simplex virus type 1 and heat-labile enterotoxin of *Escherichia coli*. 88th Annual Meeting of the American Society for Microbiology, 1988:60.

24. Edwards MF, Stocker BAD. Construction of DaroA his Dpur strains of *Salmonella typhi*. *J Bacteriol* 1988;170:3991-3995.

25. Levine MM, Herrington D, Murphy J, Morris JG, Losonsky G, Tall B, Lindberg A, Svenson S, Baqar S, Edwards MF, Stocker B. Safety, infectivity, immunogenicity and *in vivo* stability of two attenuated auxotrophic mutant strains of *Salmonella typhi*, 541Ty and 543Ty, used as oral vaccines in man. *J Clin Invest* 1987;79:888-902.

26. O'Callaghan D, Maskell D, Liew FY, Easmon CSF, Dougan G. Characterization of aromatic- and purine- dependent *Salmonella typhimurium*: Attenuation, persistence, and ability to induce protective immunity in BALB/c mice. *Infect Immun* 1988;56:419-423.

Chapter Fifteen

Killed Vaccines in Cattle:
Current Situation and Prospects
Michel Plommet

Before the introduction of an oil adjuvant by Freund in 1944, attempts to develop an efficient killed vaccine against animal brucellosis had been unsuccessful. With the new concept of adjuvanticity—the capacity of bacterial constituents suspended in a water-in-oil-mixture to increase both humoral and cellular immune responses—two groups simultaneously developed two killed vaccines with the *Brucella* cell itself acting as adjuvant and specific antigen.

The rough (R), avirulent *Brucella abortus* Strain 45/20 was first intended to be a non-agglutinogenic substitute to Strain 19, but *in vivo* reversion to the virulent smooth (S) phase prompted McEwen and Samuel[1] to test the heat-killed strain in oil adjuvant. Research was then conducted to compare efficacy and serological responses in different conditions of dose, adjuvant, recall, and age at vaccination.[2,3] Several commercial brands were marketed, some of which were not really non-agglutinogenic[4,5] as a likely result of the genetic instability of the strain[2,3,6] and poor cloning of R-colonies. Two (usually) non-agglutinogenic commercial vaccines[a] more intensively studied can be considered as reference.

Vaccine H38 was, in contrast, purposely derived from formalin-killed highly virulent *B. melitensis* smooth Strain 53H38 by Renoux, on the assumption that virulence factor(s) may also be the best protective antigen(s).[7] First intended against *B. melitensis* infection in goats and sheep, it was later extended to *B. abortus* infection in cattle[8]. While several brands were marketed in Europe, only one[b] was properly studied and used in several countries. Due to a high amount of smooth-lipopolysaccharide (S-LPS) on the strain and oil adjuvant, vaccine H38 often induces an important reaction at the injection site and a high anti-LPS antibody response. After two injections, diagnostic tests may remain positive for at least two years.[9]

---

[a]Duphavac, Philips Duphar, Amsterdam. Abortox, Iffa Merieux, Lyon
[b]Aborlane, Iffa Merieux, Lyon

Efficacy of Killed Vaccines

Evaluation of efficacy

The evaluation of a vaccine proceeds along three steps: in laboratory animal(s), in natural hosts experimentally challenged, and in natural conditions. The second step which gives the most meaningful quantitative response will be considered first.

With cattle, the generally accepted method compares infection and abortion rates in groups of heifers challenged via the conjunctival route at mid-pregnancy. Challenge strain and dose are chosen to infect 90% to 100% of the control. Usually a reference vaccinated group is included to give a reference level of protection in that particular trial; with living Strain 19 (S19), protection of the heifers should be in the 50-70 range. Infection of the dams is established by bacteriological tests from specimens taken at calving and at slaughter performed usually 1 to 2 months thereafter. Instead of abortion, whose definition differs between authors, survival of the calf is easier to interpret. In addition to these, other information may also be recorded, such as index of infection, infection rate in non-pregnant heifers, serological responses. However, these data are not easily comparable between trials on a statistical basis.

Therefore, comparisons of rates (of protection and survival) between control, reference vaccine, and experimental vaccine groups lead unavoidably to poor statistical discrimination unless very large groups are available. For example, for a protection of 46% *versus* 66% in two vaccine groups with 6% in control, difference between vaccines would not be significant with 30 cows per group. As a consequence, objective efficacy of a vaccine can only be appreciated by replication of trials.

Then a second problem arises: replication in successive trials happens to be not as good as expected, sometimes in the control, more often in the reference vaccine group. For example, in one trial including two control groups of respectively 35 and 39 heifers, inoculated three months apart with 8.3 x 10^5 colony forming units (CFU) Strain 2308, infection rates were unexpectedly 100% and 56%.[10] Examples of poor protection in S19 groups are given in Table 15-1 (trials 1A, 1B, and 1C),[11,12] and 15-2 (trials D and E).[4,13] These fluctuations may result either from the challenge strain or from the host. For a particular strain, too high a dose may overcome the vaccinal immunity, which would be demonstrated against a lower dose (Table 15-1, 1B *versus* 1C).[12] Virulence of the challenge strain may also change with time[10] but, because we have not observed such change with the reference challenge strain *B. abortus* 544 (measured in the mice model) over the time, we feel that the actual immune response of the host may be the most important factor.

Table 15-1. Protection Conferred on 6 to 12-Month-Old Heifers by Strain 19 in Trials Differing by Vaccine Dose and Recall, Challenge Strain, and Dose

Vaccine Group	Heifers		Calves
	Total	Protection %*	Living
Trial 1A[11] Challenge: Strain 544 1.5 x 10^7 CFU			
Control	12	0	5
S19 9 x 10^{10} CFU	12	8	8
S19 + recall[§]	34	41[†]	27[†]
Trial 1B[12] Challenge: Strain 2308 9 x 10^6			
Control	9	22	1
S19 1 x 10^9	11	81[‡]	10[‡]
S19 1 x 10^{10}	10	30	7
Trial 1C[12] Challenge: Strain 2308 5.2 x 10^7			
Control	9	11	0
S19 1 x 10^9	10	20	2
S19 1 x 10^{10}	8	12	0

*Protection: no *Brucella* isolated from specimens taken at calving and slaughter
†Living: healthy or weak but surviving.
† and ‡ differ significantly (χ^2 test) from control at $P<0.05$ and $P<0.01$ respectively
§Recall by conjunctival route 5 x 10^9 CFU 6 months after SC primary vaccination.

After instillation on the conjunctiva of a challenge bacteria, a competition occurs between the invading bacteria and the build up by the host of a line of defense in the regional lymph nodes, by a cellular recruitment and immune response. If the response is fast enough, invading bacteria would then be intercepted locally before systemic dissemination. We have indeed observed that a recall vaccination by Strain 19, which may speed up the immune response to the infection itself at the early phase of colonization, increased consistently the protection rate (See Table 15-1, trial 1A).[11] In natural conditions of contamination, where exposure is usually not a 100% infective dose all at once but a succession of smaller contacts, each contact may recall the immunity, hence a higher overall protection. On that assumption, very subtle differences between successive experiments may lead to either high or low protection against an experimental challenge.

With these reservations in mind, I collected results of trials which compared, on a basically correct method, efficacy of vaccines H38 and 45/20 (see Table 15-2 and 15-3). It is a pity that all trials did not include a reference S19 group, or that groups of pregnant heifers were too small, but these data are quite a good illustration of experimental problems and overall results. Other results are also available, reviewed in 1968,[2] 1976[14] and 1978[3] or more recently,[15,16,17,18] that are in agreement with conclusions drawn from Tables 15-2 and 15-3.

Vaccine H38

As shown in Table 15-2, vaccine H38 was compared in two trials to vaccine S19. In the first (2D),[13] no protection of the dams was observed with either vaccine. In the second (2E),[4] protection was better than with S19 but the group was too small to be of real significance. In the other two trials, protection was observed in groups vaccinated at the age of 6 months (2F),[9] but no or only marginal protection was observed in older vaccinated groups (2F, 2G).[9] In contrast, a high level of protection of calves was observed in all groups. Thus quite a clear picture emerged: high protection of newborn calves, low protection against infection of the dams, two vaccinations more efficient than one and better response of young heifers.

Having been used extensively in France when brucellosis prevalence was high, vaccine H38 was considered by the veterinarians as very effective indeed against abortion and also against infection at the herd level, by concomitant increase of individual resistance and decrease of environmental contamination. However, being highly agglutinogenic, the vaccine was later prohibited, when test and slaughter had to be applied.

Vaccine 45/20

Data from vaccine 45/20 trials are even more difficult to interpret. There were several commercial vaccines, which differed not only by the adjuvant (commercially patented and often secret) but also by the quality of the strain. There were indeed vaccines which induced agglutininogenic responses, due to insufficient care at cloning R-colonies, even among good company batches.[34] There were also batches of vaccines which conferred no protection at all in our method control in mice, whereas others were quite good (Figure 15-1).[20]

Table 15-2. Protection Conferred on Heifers of Different Ages by One or Two Injections* of H38 Vaccine

Vaccine Group	Heifers		Calves
	Total	Protection %	Living
Trial 2D[13] Challenge: strain 544 1.5 x 10^7 CFU			
Control	11	0	5
S19 6 x 10^{10} CFU	21	0	9
H38 One at 6 month	22	0	15
Trial 2E[4] Challenge: strain 544 1.5 x 10^7			
Control	22	10	7
S19 6 x 10^{10}	17	41[†]	12[‡]
H38 Two at 6 month	8	100[‡]	6[‡]
Trial 2F[9] Challenge: strain 544 1.5 x 10^7			
Control	26	15	17
H38 One at 6 month	25	60[‡]	18
H38 Two at 6 month	26	73[‡]	23
H38 One at 30 month	25	44	17
H38 Two at 30 month	14	57[†]	12
Trial 2G[19] Challenge: strain 2308 8 x 10^5			
Control	24	0	1
H38 One at 12 month	23	22	19[‡]
H38 Two at 12 month	23	27[†]	19[‡]

*Second vaccination 2 to 3 months after the first
† and ‡ differ from control at P<0.05 andP< 0.01 respectively

Protection conferred by several vaccines 45/20 in five trials is shown in Table 15-3. Protection of the dams was erratic, near nil in cows more than 12 month-old at vaccination (3I, 3J, 3L)[5,21-23] to quite good in young heifers (3H, 3J).[4,21] Protection was however lower than with vaccine S19 as well in young as in adult heifers. Protection of the newborn calves usually compared with Strain 19 in young vaccinated heifers (3H,3J)[4,21] but was lower in older heifers (3I, 3L).[5-23]

Vaccine 45/20 does not usually induce serological responses to standard agglutination and Rose bengal plate tests, but complement fixation and Coombs tests usually become positive, with wide variations between experiments. Delayed hypersensitivity skin tests and lymphocyte trans-

Table 15-3. Protection Conferred on Heifers of Different Ages by One or Two Injections* of Several Commercial 45/20 Vaccines

Vaccine Group	Heifers		Calves
	Total	Protection %	Living
Trial 3H[4] Challenge: strain 544 1.5 x 10⁷ CFU			
Control	22	10	7
S19 6 x 10¹⁰ CFU	17	41[†]	12[†]
Ola # Two at 6 month	21	62[‡]	15[†]
Mono Two at 6 month	17	29	11
Abor Two at 6 month	12	75[‡]	10[†]
Trial 3I[5] Challenge: strain 544 1.5 x 10⁷			
Control	21	5	4
Ola Two at 30 month	25	12	16[†]
Mono Two at 30 month	17	12	7
Abor Two at 30 month	22	4	6
Trial 3J[21] Challenge: strain 544 1 x 10⁷			
Control	8	12	3
S19 4 x 10¹⁰ at 3-6 month	18	72[†]	15
Dupha Two at 3-6 month	9	55	8
Dupha Two at 14-16 month	9	22	8
Trial 3K[22] Challenge: strain VR13 1.3 x 10⁷			
Control	5	0	2
S19 3 x 10⁸	10	60	4
Dupha One at 15-24 month	10	50	5
Dupha Two at 15-24 month	5	20	3
Trial 3L[23] Challenge: strain 544 2 x 10⁸			
Control	8	0	0
S19 2.4 x 10¹⁰	6	83[‡]	4[†]
Dupha Two at 19-33 month	8	25	3
Abor Two at 19-33 month	28	35	12

*Second vaccination 1-2 months after the first
*Abbreviations refer to commercial brands
[†] and [‡] Differ from control at $P<0.05$ and $P< 0.01$ respectively

formation test remain positive, like with vaccine H38, for a very long time.

Vaccine 45/20 has been used in Great Britain, Ireland, Australia, France, and other countries. Its contribution to eradication of the disease and its usefulness in veterinary practice are debatable. Some veterinarians favored it for easiness of use (no age limitation but low efficiency in adults), in spite of erratic post vaccinal responses when used to recall a S19 primary vaccination. Others considered it to be inefficient in practice. It seems that a good 45/20 vaccine (from a reliable company) may, when used in young (6-10 months) heifers, induce a serviceable herd immunity, like H38 vaccine, by increasing basic resistance of naïve heifers and decreasing abortion rate, hence environmental contamination. But this immunity does not advantageously compare with the one induced by S19 vaccine.

Prospect: New Killed Vaccine?

Improving the old whole cell killed vaccine despite many efforts directed towards strain(s), adjuvant(s), dose, and recall(s) has been quite unsuccessful. Without a clear guide indicating what mechanisms involved in vaccinal protection should be specifically stimulated, improvement would not likely succeed. This guide is being established—though it is still far from complete—by research conducted primarily in the United States and in France. Important facts can be summarized as follows:

1. Vaccinal protection can be conveniently measured in mice. After a standard challenge, there is a vaccine dose-spleen count response relationship with killed or fraction vaccines. Thus, the protective activity of a vaccine can be expressed by the smallest protective dose (Figure 15-1).[20]
2. Protective activity of a whole cell vaccine can thus be quantitatively followed in successive fractions extracted from the bacterial cell. Two fractions extracted from *Brucella* confer protection to mice, namely S-LPS and PG.[26-27]
3. S-LPS protects mice, but not guinea pigs[28] through antibodies directed against the O-polysaccharide chain.[29-32]
4. PG, a hot sodium dodecylsulfate insoluble fraction, represents the rigid cell wall peptidoglycan structure, or sacculi, of about 4% of the total cell weight[26,33] on which three of major protein groups are closely linked.[34] Two of these proteins are similar to group 2 and 3 proteins extracted from

---

ᶜDubray G, personal communication

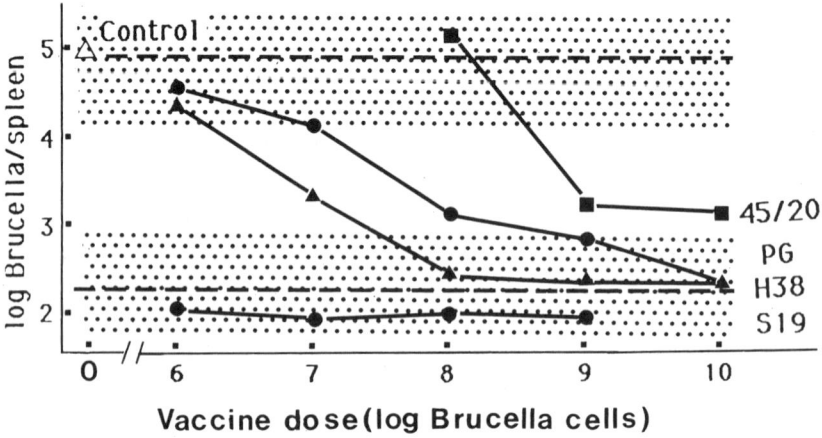

Figure 15-1. Responses of Mice to a Standard *Brucella* Challenge, Expressed by Spleen Counts 15 Days Post-Challenge. Responses to control (not vaccinated) and vaccinated with living Strain 19 taken as reference. Responses to killed vaccines (H38, 45/20) and fraction (PG) being dose dependent, the smallest protective dose can be calculated. Dose of PG fraction in equivalence of bacterial cell, with 10^9 = 10 mg. Thick line: average reference responses. Shaded grey zone: least-significant difference between two groups of six mice.[20]

the outer membrane.[35] Depending on the extraction procedure, PG may or may not contain, small amounts of S-LPS.[c] PG confers protection to mice and guinea pigs, with a dose response comparable to that of whole cell vaccine (Figure 15-1). [20,28]

5. Immunity induced by PG can be transferred to mice by immune serum, through LPS antibodies and possibly others,[29] or by splenic or lymphoid T-cells.[36] Specific antigens involved in this cellular immunity are not yet known, but are likely the two or three major proteins. Antibodies and T-cells did not behave in synergy in protective activity in the mice model.[37,38]

6. PG added to adjuvant induced in sheep a skin test-delayed hypersensitivity with itself but not with brucellin.[d] It induced in heifers positive skin and blastogenesis tests with groups 2 (porin) and 3 purified proteins.[27]

7. Purified porins extracted from the outer membrane did not induce protection in mice unless complexed with O-polysaccharide.[32]

All these facts are known and have been discussed in view of developing new killed or biotechnology-devised vaccines.[27,32,39-41] However, immune mechanisms involved in protection induced by killed vaccines in cattle are in part speculative. Transferring mechanisms demonstrated in mice, to cattle should be done very carefully.

8. In cattle, killed vaccines induce both humoral and cellular responses. Depending on the vaccine, H38 or 45/20, antibodies directed against the cell surface antigens S-LPS or R-LPS and outer membrane protein antigen, may act like opsinin at several steps: 1) intercepting the invading bacteria inside systemic reticulo-endothelial organs, in particular regional lymph nodes.[39,41,42] 2) protecting the placenta, thence the foetus from blood carried bacteria. This phenomenon is so efficient in mice[43,44] that it may explain the protection conferred by vaccines H38 and 45/20 to the newborn calf. 3) increasing phagocytosis and killing of *Brucella* by neutrophil and mononuclear cells.[45-46]

9. Cellular responses to killed vaccines have been studied *in vivo* by the delayed hypersensitivity skin-test and *in vitro* by lymphocytes transformation tests. Having however been mostly used for diagnostic purposes,[25,47] these tests have been performed with unpurified extracts or with a saline extracted protein allergen (brucellin), known to not be related to protection.[48] In these conditions, the two killed vaccines induced a strong and long lasting cellular response,[23-25] stronger in fact than vaccine S19[18,46,49] with no evidence of relationship with protection.[12,18,50,51] When purified protein antigens were used in the test, it was observed that experimental vaccine similar to 45/20 and PG with adjuvant induced important *in vivo* and *in vitro* responses.[27,52] Whether such responses are correlated with protection will be tested in the near future.[27]

---

[d]Fensterbank R, personal communication

Summary

Killed vaccines against bovine brucellosis were originally prepared with whole bacterial cells suspended in an oil adjuvant. Vaccine H38 made use of the formalin killed-highly virulent Strain *Brucella melitensis* 53 H38, which being in smooth (S) phase, induced long lasting serological responses in usual diagnostic tests. Vaccine 45/20 made use of the heat killed-low virulent rough (R) Strain *B. abortus* 45/20, which did not usually induce response to S-LPS in diagnostic tests, but induced instead antibodies against R-LPS and other surface antigens. Several commercial type 45/20 vaccines, differing by sub-strain(s) and adjuvants have been marketed. In addition to antibodies, killed vaccines induced cellular-dependent responses with *Brucella* cell extracts evidenced by delayed hypersensitivity tests *in vivo* and lymphocytes transformation tests in vitro.

Protection conferred by vaccine to cattle should ideally be assessed by comparison of infection rates between groups of heifers vaccinated or not, challenged at mid-pregnancy. A trial should include a control (not vaccinated) group, a reference vaccine (living Strain 19) group, and the tested vaccine group. Published trials did not always include the reference vaccine group and groups were often too small to give statistically valid informations *per se*. However, considering protection rates and survival of the newborn calves as indicators of protection in representative trials of the last 15 years, one may conclude that vaccines H38 and 45/20 confer protection to the dam and even more to the calf, in particular when vaccines were administered twice to 6 to 12 month-old heifers. With a few exceptions, protection was lower that conferred by Strain S19. Antigens of killed vaccines and immune mechanisms involved in protection have been studied in mice: a small fraction of the bacterial cell may induce a protection equal to that of the whole cell. The S-LPS O-polysaccharide chain, which induced an antibody-dependent immunity, and outer membrane proteins linked to the cell wall, which induced a cell mediated immunity, may be the two main active immunogens of killed vaccines. If these results were transposed to cattle, new killed vaccine containing only those active constituents may expectedly be more efficient than whole cell vaccines.

In conclusion, killed whole cell vaccines have been developed from the concept that adjuvants increasing both humoral and cellular responses may trigger those immune mechanisms involved in protection. In spite of the dominant opinion of this era that immunity against facultative intracellular bacteria can be induced only by living vaccine, killed vaccines have been shown beyond any doubt to confer protection in all tested animal species. This immunity was however equal or lower than immunity induced by living vaccines. Hence, in veterinary practice, after taking into consideration all facts for a correct choice for a control program, killed vaccines after initial success have been progressively either abandoned or prohibited as too agglutinogenic and/or of irregular efficacy.

Because immune mechanisms triggered by killed vaccines and involved in protection were unknown, no real progress was attained for 30 years. From recent research in mice, which has to be transposed to cattle, we know that only a small part of the bacterial cell is required to induce an immunity mediated by both antibodies and T-cells. We still do not know whether both arms are required to confer protection to cattle, and how to manage to induce this or these arm(s) for an efficient and long lasting immunity. It seems however that after the old killed vaccines, a new generation of vaccine extracted from the *Brucella* cell, disencumbered of all useless, possibly noxious, materials may find its way toward a specific, efficient, and stable immunity.

References

1. McEwen AD, Samuel JMcA. *Brucella abortus*: heat stable protective antigen revealed by adjuvant and present in a "rough" variant, Strain 45/20: immunisation experiments on guinea pigs. *Vet Rec* 1955;67:546-548.
2. Brinley-Morgan WJ, McDiarmid A. Adjuvant vaccines prepared from killed *Brucella abortus* Strain 45/20. *Vet Rec* 1968;83:184-189.
3. Alton GG. Recent developments in vaccination against bovine brucellosis. *Aust Vet J* 1978;54:551-557.
4. Dhennin L. Resultat de l'étude comparée de sept vaccins anti-brucelliques chez la génisse. *Bull Acad Vet France* 1973; 46:171-189.
5. Dhennin L. Expérience de Fougères. Contrôle de cinq vaccins anti-brucelliques. Primo vaccination de la vache adulte. *Bull Acad Vet France* 1974;47:340-353.
6. Chukwu CC. The instability of *Brucella abortus* Strain 45/20 and a note of significance of using an unstable rough strain in the dignosis of bovine brucellosis. *Int J Zoonose* 1985;12:120-125.
7. Renoux G, Alton G, Amarasinghe A. Etudes sur la brucellose ovine et caprine. XI. Comparaison chez la chèvre suédoise, de la valeur immunisante d'un vaccin tué en excipient irresorbable et de deux vaccins vivants. *Arch Inst Pasteur Tunis* 1957;34:3-17.
8. Renoux G, Nicolas A, Imbert R, et al. Immunisation des génisses contre l'infection par *Brucella abortus*. Comparaison de quatre vaccins. *Rev Immunol Paris* 1964;28:121-140.
9. Dhennin L. Expérience de Fougères. Immunisation de la génisse et de la vache avec 1 ou 2 doses de vaccin H-38 contre l'infection expérimentale à *Brucella abortus*. *Bull Acad Vet France* 1977;50:167-181.
10. Meyer ME, Gibbons RW. Results of using H-38 *Brucella* vaccine as a therapeutic agent in beef cattle experimentally infected with *Brucella abortus* Strain 2308. Proceedings of the eighty-second annual meeting of the United States Animal Health Association, Buffalo, NY 1978;120-132.
11. Fensterbank R, Plommet M. Vaccination against bovine brucellosis with a low dose of Strain 19 administered by the conjunctival route. IV: Comparison between two methods of vaccination. *Ann Rech Vet* 1979;10:131-139.
12. Confer AW, Hall SM, Faulkner CB, et al. Effects of challenge dose on the clinical and immune responses of cattle vaccinated with reduced doses of *Brucella abortus* 19. *Vet Microbiol* 1985;10:561-575.
13. Plommet M, Renoux G, Philippon A, et al. Brucellose bovine expérimentale.

Comparaison de l'efficacité des vaccins B19 et H-38. *Ann Rech Vet* 1970;1:189-201.

14. Ray WC. An assessment of investigations conducted in the USA on *Brucella abortus* Strain 45/20 bacterins. *Dev Biol Stand* 1976;31:335-342.

15. Worthington RW, Horwell FD, Mulders MSG, et al. An investigation of the efficacy of three *Brucella* vaccines in cattle. *J South Afr Vet Assoc* 1974;45:87-91.

16. McKeon FW. A recent trial comparing two 45/20 adjuvant *Brucella* vaccines. *Dev Biol Stand* 1976;31:343-350.

17. Hall WTK, Ludford CG, Ward WH. Infection and serological responses in cattle given 45/20 vaccine and later challenged with *Brucella abortus*. *Aust Vet J* 1976;52:409-413.

18. Woodard LF, Jasman RL. Comparative efficacy of an experimental 45/20 bacterin and a reduced dose of Strain 19 vaccine against bovine brucellosis. *Am J Vet Res* 1983;44:907-910.

19. Meyer ME, Gibbons RW. Results of trial use of H-38 vaccine for immunizing beef heifers against experimental exposure to *Brucella abortus* Strain 2308. Proceeding of the 82nd annual meeting of the US Animal Health Association, Buffalo, NY 1978; 106-119.

20. Bosseray N, Plommet AM, Plommet M. Theoretical, practical and statistical basis for a general control method of activity for anti-*brucella* vaccines. *Dev Biol Stand* 1983;56:257-270.

21. Sutherland SS, Robertson AG, Le Cras DV, et al. The effect of challenge with virulent *Brucella abortus* on beef cattle vaccinated as calves or adults with either *Brucella abortus* Strain 19 or 45/20. *Aust Vet J* 1981;57:470-473.

22. Alton GG, Corner LA, Plackett P. Vaccination of cattle against brucellosis using either a reduced dose of Strain 19 or one or two doses of 45/20 vaccine. *Aust Vet J* 1983;60:175-177.

23. Chukwu CC. Cell-mediated immunity related to challenge exposure of cattle immunized with attenuated or inactivated strains of *Brucella abortus*. *Microbios lett* 1987;34:147-158.

24. Kaneene JMB, Anderson RK, Johnson DW, et al. Cell-mediated immune responses in cattle vaccinated with killed *Brucella melitensis* Strain H-38 vaccine or infected with viable *Brucella abortus* Strain 2308 organisms, or both. *Am J Vet Res* 1979;40:40-47.

25. Chukwu CC, Cunningham B. Humoral and cell mediated immune responses in cattle after vaccination and revaccination with *Brucella abortus* killed 45/20 adjuvant vaccine. *Irish Vet J* 1986;40:62-71.

26. Dubray G, Bosseray N, Plommet M. Propriétés vaccinales de fractions de *Brucella*. *CR Acad Sci Paris* 1974;279:1805-1808.

27. Winter AJ, Rowe GE. Comparative immune responses to native cell envelope antigens and hot sodium dodecyl sulfate insoluble fraction (PG) of *Brucella abortus* in cattle and mice. *Vet Immunol Immunopathol* 1988;18:149-163.

28. Bosseray N, Plommet M, Dubray G. Immunogenic activity of a cell wall fraction extracted from *Brucella abortus* in guinea pigs. *Ann Microbiol (Inst Pasteur)* 1978;129B:571-579.

29. Plommet M, Plommet AM. Immune serum-mediated effects on Brucellosis evolution in mice. *Infect Immun* 1983;41:97-105.

30. Montaraz JA, Winter AJ, Hunter DM, et al. Protection against *Brucella abortus* in mice with O-polysaccharide-specific monoclonal antibodies. *Infect Immun* 1986;51:961-963.

31. Limet J, Plommet AM, Dubray G, et al. Immunity conferred upon mice by anti-LPS monoclonal antibodies in murine Brucellosis. *Ann Inst Pasteur/Immunol* 1987;138:417-424.

32. Winter AJ, Rowe GE, Dungan JR, et al. Effectiveness of natural and synthetic complexes of porin and O-polysaccharide as vaccines against *Brucella abortus* in mice. *Infect Immun* 1988;56:2808-2817.

33. Dubray G. Le peptidoglycan des *Brucella*: mise en évidence d'une structure à triple feuillet. *CR Acad Sci Paris* 1973;277:2281-2283.

34. Dubray G, Bezard G. Isolation of three cell-wall antigens protective in murine experimental brucellosis. *Ann Rech Vet* 1980;11:367-373.

35. Douglas JT, Rosenberg EY, Nikaido H, et al. Porins of *Brucella* species. *Infect Immun* 1984;44:16-21.

36. Plommet M, Plommet AM. Anti-*Brucella* cell-mediated immunity in micevaccinated with a cell-wall fraction. *Ann Rech Vet* 1987;18:429-437.

37. Plommet M, Hue I, Plommet AM. L'immunité anti-*Brucella* transférée par sérum immun et l'immunité transférée par les lymphocytes spléniques ne s'additionnent pas. *Ann Rech Vet* 1986;16:169-175.

38. Araya LN, Rowe GE, Elzer PH, et al. Temporal development of humoral and cell-mediated immunity in BalB/C mice infected with *Brucella abortus* Strain 19. 69th Annual Meeting of Conference of Research Workers in Animal Disease, Chicago, IL, 1988.

39. Plommet M. Brucellosis and immunity: humoral and cellular components in mice. *Ann Inst Pasteur/Microbiol* 1987;138: 105-110.

40. Plommet M, Serre A, Fensterbank R. Vaccines, vaccination in brucellosis. *Ann Inst Pasteur/Microbiol* 1987;138:117-122.

41. Winter AJ. *Brucella* and Brucellosis: an update. *Ann Inst Pasteur/Microbiol* 1987;138:135-137.

42. Plommet M, Plommet AM. Immunity to *Brucella abortus* induced in mice by popliteal lymph node restricted Strain 19 vaccination. *Ann Rech Vet* 1989;20:73-81.

43. Bosseray N. *Brucella* infection and immunity in placenta. *Ann Inst Pasteur/Microbiol* 1987;138:110-113.

44. Bosseray N, Plommet M. Serum and cell-mediated immune protection of mouse placenta and fetus against a *Brucella abortus* challenge: expression of barrier effect of placenta. *Placenta* 1988;9:65-79.

45. Canning PC, Deyoe BL, Roth JA. Opsonin-dependent stimulation of bovine neutrophil oxidative metabolism by *Brucella abortus*. *Ann J Vet Res* 1988;49:160-163.

46. Harmon BG, Adams LG, Frey M. Survival of rough and smooth strains of *Brucella abortus* in bovine mammary gland macrophages. *Am J Vet Res* 1988;49:1092-1097.

47. Kaneene JM, Nicoletti P, Anderson RK, et al. Cell-mediated immune responses in cattle adult vaccinated with *Brucella abortus* Strain 19 and in cattle infected with *Brucella abortus* field strain. *Am J Vet Res* 1979;40:1503-1509.

48. Bosseray N, Plommet M. Antagonism between two immunogens extracted from *Brucella* (cell wall peptidoglycan and lipopolysaccharide fractions) and inactivity of the brucellin allergen in immunization of the mouse. *Ann Microbiol/Inst Pasteur* 1980;131A:157-169.

49. Chukwu CC. Effect of repeated vaccination on cell-mediated immune response to *Brucella abortus* Strain 19 vaccine in cattle. *Microbios lett* 1987;34:35-41.

50. Confer AW, Tabatabai LB, Deyoe BL, et al. Vaccination of cattle with chemically modified and unmodified salt-extractable proteins from *Brucella abortus*. *Vet Microbiol* 1987; 15:325-339.

51. Sutherland SS. Immunology of bovine brucellosis. *Vet bull* 1980;50:359-368.

52. Winter AJ, Verstreate DR, Hall CE, et al. Immune response to porin in cattle immunized with whole cell, outer membrane, and outer membrane protein antigens of *Brucella abortus* combined with Trehalose dimycolate and muramyl dipeptide adjuvants. *Infect Immun* 1983;42:1159-1167.

Chapter Sixteen

An Evaluation of Reduced Dose
Brucella abortus Strain 19
Vaccination

John. D. Huber,

Victor. C. Beal, Jr.,

Richard. P. Crawford,

and L. Garry . Adams

Brucella abortus Strain 19 vaccine was introduced into the United States brucellosis program in 1941. The standard dose was approximately 5 x 10^{10} colony forming units (CFU). Beginning in 1981, some states changed to a reduced dose range of 3 x 10^{8} to 3 x 10^{9} CFU. The standard dose was entirely discontinued by January 1, 1985. The current reduced dose range is 3 x 10^{9} to 1 x 10^{10} CFU. The three objectives of reducing the dose of Strain 19 for calfhood vaccination were as follows:

1. Reduce post-vaccination serum-antibody titers.
2. Reduce other post-vaccination reactions and side-effects.
3. Raise the vaccination-eligible age to 4 through 12 months.

There is a considerable amount of discussion and agreement that objective number one has not been achieved. Solutions to the problem of post-vaccination titers frequently proposed are:

1. Lower the dose of Strain 19.
2. Lower the vaccination-eligible age.
3. Discontinue mandatory calfhood vaccination in low-incidence areas.
4. Develop improved vaccines.
5. Develop improved diagnostic tests.

There is also a concern about the protection provided by reduced dose calfhood vaccination. Whole herd or adult vaccination is frequently used as an attempt to enhance immunity in brucellosis-affected herds where calfhood vaccination has been practiced.

The purpose of this review was to summarize data produced in the last 10 years on age at inoculation and dose effects of Strain 19 on post-vaccination sero test results and infection rates with challenge strains of

Materials and Methods

Source of Data

The data were obtained from 13 sources on post-vaccination card test or rose bengal plate test (RBPT) results on 910 heifers.[1-13] Of the 910 heifers,

78 were dairy and 832 were beef types. Age and dose ranges selected for evaluation were influenced by the data available and standard methods and practices. The youngest age group represented was 20 dairy heifers ranging from 3 to 6 months at the time of vaccination.[1] At least one of three beef heifers would have been as old as 20 months and some of 10 dairy heifers were as old as 23 months.[8,13] Of the 910 vaccinated heifers, 344 were challenged with virulent *B. abortus* during their first pregnancy.[1,2,6,8-10,14] Isolation rates of the challenge strains at or following parturition were categorized by slightly different age ranges, the same vaccine dose ranges, and challenge strain dose. Of the 344 heifers challenged, some of 20 dairy heifers were as young as 3 months when vaccinated and none of the 86 dairy and beef heifers in the young age group were over 6 months old.[1,2] Of the 258 challenged heifers in the older age group, one was 8 months old when vaccinated, 64 were 10 to 12 months old, 117 were 10 to 16 months old, 67 were 12 to 14 months old, and 9 were 14 to 23 months old.[6,8-10,14] Serologic test results after test-eligible ages were reached were not available on the challenged heifers and certain others belonging to experimental dose groups. Program testing is often done on nontest-eligible heifers when age and vaccination histories are not available. Such testing is required for quarantine release and post-quarantine release tests. Therefore, it was considered appropriate to have a nontest-eligible category.

Statistical Analysis

The Chi-square procedure was used for the statistical analysis of the data.[15] Tables of the Chi-square distribution from Geigy were used for tests of significance since they are tabulated down to the 0.05% level.[16] The data from Table 16-1 were used in examining the significance of card test results. Table 16-2 contains all of the challenge data found for this review.

However, part of the data in Table 16-2 were not appropriate for statistical analysis and were excluded from the statistical analysis. One part of the eliminated data consisted of 30 heifers challenged with 9.4 x 10⁶ CFU of virulent *Brucella*. They were eliminated since only 2 of 11 heifers inoculated with the lower vaccine dose range were culture positive for the challenge strain while 7 of 10 heifers inoculated with the higher vaccine dose range were culture positive for the challenge strain.

Not only was the difference in isolation rate in a direction opposite of expectation but the difference was significant at the 2.5 percent level. Since there is no logical explanation for this significant reversal of outcome, these data were eliminated.

A decision was then made to eliminate 27 other heifers from the same experiment that were challenged with a higher level of 5.2 x 10⁷ CFU of virulent *Brucella*. This was done for purposes of consistency.

There were 21 other heifers challenged with a high level of 1 x 10⁸ CFU of

Table 16-1. Card Test Results Following Vaccination with *Brucella abortus* Strain 19

Age at vaccination	Card test results§	Nontest-eligible* (Dose)‡		Test-eligible† (Dose)‡	
		$9 \times 10^6 - 1 \times 10^9$	$3 \times 10^9 - 1 \times 10^{10}$	$9 \times 10^6 - 1 \times 10^9$	$3 \times 10^9 - 1 \times 10^{10}$
3-8 months	Positive	(a) 0	(c) 1**	(e) ...	(g) 1++
	Negative	79	88	...	64
9-23 months	Positive	(b) 5‡‡	(d) 5§§	(f) 8***	(h) 10+++
	Negative	378	108	137	26

* = female dairy cattle < 20 months of age; female beef cattle < 24 months of age.

† = female dairy cattle ≥ 20 months of age; female beef cattle ≥ 24 months of age.

‡ = colony forming units (CFU).

§ = 148 were rose bengal plate test (RBPT) results.

** = 4.5 x 10⁹ CFU at 3 - 6 months; RBPT positive at 13 - 16 months.

++ = 5 x 10⁹ CFU at 8 months; card test positive at 24 months.

‡‡ = 3 given 1 x 10⁹ CFU at 10 - 14 months; 2 given 5 x 10⁸ at 10 - 12 months.

§§ = 1 x 10¹⁰ CFU at 10 - 14 months.

*** = 3 x 10⁸ - 1 x 10⁹ CFU at 12 - 14 months; RBPT positive at 24 months.

+++ = 6 given 5 x 10⁹ CFU at months; 4 given 3 x 10⁹ at 10 - 12 months; card test positive at 24 - 27 months.

Table 16-2. Isolation Rate of Challenge Strains of *Brucella abortus* Following Exposure of Nonvaccinated and Strain 19 Vaccinated Heifers

Age at vaccination	Challenge Dose*	Nonvaccinated	Isolation rate by strain 19 dose* groups		
			9×10^6 - 1×10^9	3×10^9 - 1×10^{10}	Total†
3-6 months	1×10^7	23/30 (76.7%)	28/60 (46.7%)	5/26 (19.2%)	33/86 (38.4%)
8-23 months‡	6×10^6	11/20 (55.0%)	9/50 (18.0%)	1/17 (5.9%)	10/67 (14.9%)
	9.4×10^6	7/9 (77.8%)	2/11 (18.2%)	7/10 (70.0%)	9/21 (42.9%)
	1×10^7	77/92 (83.7%)	43/103‡ (41.7%)	6/39 (15.4%)	49/142 (34.5%)
	5.2×10^7	8/9 (88.9%)	8/10 (80.0%)	7/8 (87.5%)	15/18 (83.3%)
	1×10^8	10/11 (90.9%)	6/10 (60.0%)	...	6/10 (60.6%)
Totals§		113/141 (80.1%)	68/184 (37.0%)	21/74 (28.4%)	89/258 (34.5%)
Total**		136/171 (79.5%)	96/244 (39.3%)	26/100 (26.0%)	122/344 (35.5%)

* = colony forming units.

† = vaccinated groups only.

‡ = 1 heifer was 8 months old (no isolation); the rest were at least 10 months old.

§ = 8 - 23 months group.

** = both age groups.

virulent *Brucella* and they were also eliminated.

The additional 21 heifers were eliminated for two reasons. There were only 10 vaccinated heifers at that challenge level with all being inoculated at the lower vaccine dose range and none at the higher vaccine dose range. This left a totally inadequate number of heifers for drawing inferences about isolation rates at the higher challenge levels of 5.2×10^7 and 1×10^8 CFU of virulent *Brucella* with no inference being possible for isolation rates of the challenge strains due to vaccine dose differences.

Results

Serology

Card and RBPT results following vaccination are shown in Table 16-1. Of 233 heifers vaccinated at 3 to 8 months of age, two (0.86%) were positive. Both had been given the higher dose range of 3×10^9 to 1×10^{10} CFU Strain 19 (groups c and g). A dairy heifer in group c was one of 10 that were vaccinated with 4.5×10^9 CFU at an age range of 3 to 6 months. She was RBPT positive when the same 10 heifers were tested when 13 to 16 months old. A beef heifer in group g was one of 17 given 5×10^9 CFU Strain 19. She was estimated to be 8 months old when inoculated and was card test positive at 24 months of age.

Of 677 heifers vaccinated at 9 to 23 months of age, 28 (4.14%) were card or RBPT positive. Of the 383 in group b, 5 (1.31%) beef heifers were card test positive before they had become 24 months old. Three were given 1×10^9 CFU when 10 to 14 months of age and two were given 5×10^8 at 10 to 12 months. Of the 113 in group d, five (4.42%) beef heifers were card test positive before reaching 2 years of age. All five had been inoculated with 1×10^{10} CFU when 10 to 14 months of age. Of the 145 in group f, eight (5.52%) beef heifers were RBPT positive at 24 months of age. All 8 had been given a vaccine dose range of 3×10^8 to 1×10^9 CFU when 12 to 14 months old. Of the 36 in group h, 10 (27.78%) beef heifers were card test positive when 24 to 27 months old. Six were given 5×10^9 CFU at 9 months of age and four received 3×10^9 at 10 to 12 months.

Vaccination Dose and Age Affects on Surveillance

Table 16-3 shows the description of the Chi-square tests of significance as conducted on the card test data. The results of the statistical tests done on these data have important ramifications in considering the affects of vaccination dose and age on the effectiveness of the Market Cattle Identification (MCI) system. Tables 16-4 to 16-8 show the data that were ab-

Table 16-3. Description of Chi-square Tests Involving Card Test Data

Nontest-eligible - Low age vaccinates - Low vs High dose vaccinates
Nontest-eligbile - Old age vaccinates - Low vs High dose vaccinates
Nontest-eligible - Low dose vaccinates - Low age vs Old age vaccinates
Nontest-eligible - High dose vaccinate - Low age vs Old age vaccinates

Test-eligible - Old age vaccinates - Low vs High dose vaccinates
Test-eligible - High dose vaccinates - Low age vs Old age vaccinates

Low age - High dose vaccinates - Nontest-eligible vs Test eligible
Old age - Low dose vaccinates - Nontest-eligible vs Test eligible
Old age - High dose vaccinates - Nontest-eligible vs Test eligible

Nontest eligible - All 4 groups of age and dose vaccinates - 3 d.f.

Old age - All 4 groups of dose and eligibility vaccinates - 3 d.f.

stracted from Table 16-1 and tests of significance of the comparisons described in Table 3.

Dose and age affects on test-eligible heifers

Table 16-4 shows the results of the Chi-square tests of significance involving nontest-eligible heifers. Differences due to dose for the 3 to 8 month old (lower age) group are insignificant with a probability between 40 and 30%. In contrast, differences for the 9 to 23 month old (higher age) group are significant with a probability between 5 and 2.5% of occurring by chance alone. This indicates that the effects of high dose are of concern only for older age vaccinates.

Differences due to age are insignificant for both low-dose and high-dose vaccinates with probability levels of between 40 and 30% and between 20 and 10% respectively. While the difference between age groups for the high-dose vaccinates is not significant, perhaps due to inadequate sample size, there is an indication that age at vaccination for the high-dose vaccinates could be of concern in the MCI surveillance program.

An illustration of the effect of sample size is seen in the right hand side of Table 16-4 where the differences between low and high dose for the higher age groups and between low age and high age for the high-dose groups have the same order of magnitude. Yet only one of the comparisons is significant.

Table 16- 4. Chi-Square Tests of Card Test Data within Nontest-Eligible Vaccinates Comparing Dose andComparing Age.

Nontest-eligible vaccinates

Vaccine dose	3 to 8 months old				9 to 23 months old			
	Pos.	Neg.	Total	% +	Pos.	Neg.	Total	% +
Low dose	0	79	79	0.0	5	378	383	1.3
High dose	1	88	89	1.1	5	108	113	4.4
Total	1	167	168		10	486	496	

Chi-square value - 0.8930 - 4.2977
Probability Between 40% and 30% - Between 5% and 2.5%

Nontest-eligible vaccinates

Vaccination age	Low dose vaccinates				High dose vaccinates			
	Pos.	Neg.	Total	% +	Pos.	Neg.	Total	% +
3 to 8 mo. old	0	79	79	0.0	1	88	89	1.1
9 to 23 mo. old	5	378	383	1.3	5	108	113	4.4
Total	5	457	462		6	196	202	

Chi-square value - 1.0426 - 1.8826
Probability Between 40% and 30% - Between 20% and 10%

Table 16-5 shows the test of significance among all four dose and age groups shown in Table 16-4 for the nontest-eligible classification. This test represents 3 degrees of freedom (3 df) with the differences barely lacking significance with a probability between 10 and 5%. This is reflected in the fact that only one of the comparisons shown in Table 16-4 had significance at the 5% level.

Table 16-6 shows the results of the Chi-square tests of significance involving test-eligible heifers. Since there were no vaccinates for the low age, low dose combination, only two comparisons could be made for test-eligible vaccinates. The differences between the low and high dose groups

Table 16-5. Chi-Square Tests of CardTest Data within Nontest-Eligible Vaccinates Comparing Dose and Age Jointly

	Nontest-eligible Vaccinates			
	Pos.	Neg.	Total	% +
3 to 8 mo. old & Low Dose	0	79	79	0.0
3 to 8 mo. old & High Dose	1	88	89	1.1
9 to 23 mo. old & Low Dose	5	378	383	1.3
9 to 23 mo. old & High Dose	5	108	113	4.4
TOTAL	11	653	664	

Chi-square value - 7.0907 for 3 d.f.
Probability Between 10% and 5%

for high age vaccinates and between the low age and high age groups for the high dose vaccinates were both significant at the 0.05% level.

Eligibility effects in low and high dose and low and high age vaccinates

Table 16-7 shows the Chi-square tests of significance between nontest-eligible and test-eligible heifers in low and high dose and low and high age vaccinates. As noted above, there were no vaccinates for the low dose, low age test-eligible combination. The difference between nontest-eligible and test-eligible heifers for the low age and high dose comparison was insignificant with a probability of between 90 and 80%.

The differences between nontest-eligible and test-eligible heifers in both comparisons involving high age vaccinates were highly significant with a probability of between 1 and 0.5% in low dose vaccinates and less than 0.05% in high dose vaccinates.

This finding is worthy of discussion since the direction of the difference is in the opposite direction of what might be expected. One might expect the test-eligible heifers to have a lower serologic positive rate than the nontest-eligible heifers. There might be a number of explanations for this occurrence.

In the case of the low dose vaccinates, the seropositive heifers in the nontest-eligible group had been examined with the card test while the test-eligible positive heifers were examined with the RBPT. However, in the case of the high dose vaccinates, both groups of positive animals were tested with the card test.

Table 16-6. Chi-Square Tests of Card Test Data within Nontest-Eligible Vaccinates Comparing Dose and Comparing Age

Test-eligible vaccinates

Vaccine dose	3 to 8 months old				9 to 23 months old			
	Pos.	Neg.	Total	% +	Pos.	Neg.	Total	% +
Low dose	0	0	0	N.A.	8	137	145	5.5
High dose	1	64	65	1.5	10	26	36	27.8
TOTAL	1	64	65		18	163	181	

Chi-square Value - No low dose group 15.9573
Probability - Less Than 0.05%

Test-eligible vaccinates

Vaccination age	Low dose vaccinates				High dose vaccinates			
	Pos.	Neg.	Total	% +	Pos.	Neg.	Total	% +
3 to 8 mo.old	0	0	0	N.A.	1	64	65	1.5
9 to 23 mo. old	8	137	145	5.5	10	26	36	27.8
TOTAL	8	137	145		11	90	101	

Chi Square Value - No 3-8 Month group - 16.4364
Probability - Less Than 0.05%

Table 16-8 shows the significance test among all dose and eligibility groups from Table 16-7 for high age vaccinates. This test represents 3 df and has a significance level of less than 0.05% reflecting the high amount of significance between the nontest-eligible and test-eligible heifers for the high dose and high age vaccinates shown in Table 16-7.

Challenge Studies

The isolation rates of challenge strains of *B. abortus* following experimental exposure are shown in Table 16-2. Of 60 heifers vaccinated with 9×10^{8} to 1×10^{9} CFU (lower dose) Strain 19 at 3 to 6 months of age (lower age), 28 (46.7%) were culture positive for the challenge strain (1×10^{7} CFU dose; the median challenge dose). Of 26 lower age heifers inoculated with 3×10^{9} to 1×10^{10} CFU (higher dose) Strain 19, the challenge strain (median dose) was isolated from 5 (19.2%). Of 30 nonvaccinated controls (NVC) used in

Table 16-7. Chi-Square Tests of Card Test Data within Low, Dose, High Dose, Young Age, and Old Age Vaccinates Comparing Test Eligibility

Low dose vaccinates

Test-eligibility	3 to 8 months old				9 to 23 months old			
	Pos.	Neg.	Total	%+	Pos.	Neg.	Total	%+
Nontest-eligible	0	79	79	0.0	5	378	383	1.3
Test-eligible	0	0	0	N.A.	8	137	145	5.5
TOTAL	0	79	79		13	515	528	

Chi-square value - No 3-8 month group - 7.7692
Probability Between 1% and 0.5%

High dose vaccinates

Test-eligibility	3 to 8 months old				9 to 23 months old			
	Pos.	Neg.	Total	%+	Pos.	Neg.	Total	%+
Nontest-eligible	1	88	89	1.1	5	108	113	4.4
Test-eligible	1	64	65	1.5	10	26	36	27.8
TOTAL	2	152	154		15	134	149	

Chi-square value - 0.0504 - 16.4459
Probability Between 90% and 80% - Less than 0.05 %

---

these experiments, 23 (76.7%) were found infected following the same challenge dose.

Five different challenge doses were used on groups of heifers that had been vaccinated when 8 to 23 months old (higher age) (Table 16-2). Only one was 8 months old and the rest were at least 10 months old. Of 50 lower dose heifers, nine (18.0%) were found infected following a challenge strain dose of 6 x 10⁶ CFU (the low challenge dose). The challenge strain (same dose) was isolated from one (5.9%) of 17 higher dose heifers and 11 (55.0%) of 20 NVC. The next group received a challenge strain dose of 9.4 x 10⁶ CFU. The isolation rate was 18.2% (2 of 11) in the lower dose heifers, 70.0% (7 of 10) in the higher dose heifers, and 77.8% (7 of 9) in the NVC. Of 142 vaccinated heifers given a challenge strain dose of 1 x 10⁷ CFU (the median dose), the isolation rate was 41.7% (43 of 103) in the lower dose group, 15.4% (6 of 39) in the higher dose group, and 83.7% (77 of 92) in the NVC. Of 18

Table 16-8. Chi-Square Test of Card Test Data within 9 to 23 Month Old Vaccinates Comparing Test Eligibility and Dose Jointly

	9 to 23 months old vaccinates			
	Pos.	Neg.	Total	% +
Low dose and nontest-eligible	5	378	383	1.3
High dose and nontest-eligible	5	108	113	4.4
Low dose and test-eligible	8	137	145	5.5
High dose and test-eligible	10	26	36	27.8
TOTAL	28	649	677	

Chi-square value   59.2110 for 3 d.f.
Probability - Less than 0.05%

vaccinated heifers given a challenge strain dose of 5.2 x 10^7 CFU, the isolation rate was 80.0% (8 of 10) in the lower vaccine dose group, 87.5% (7 of 8) in the higher dose group, and 88.9% (8 of 9) in the NVC. Of 10 lower dose vaccinated heifers, the challenge strain (1 x 10^8 CFU dose) isolation rate was 60.0% (6 of 10), and 90.9% (10 of 11) in the NVC.

Effect of vaccination age and dose and challenge dose on isolation rate

In considering the amount of protection against virulent *Brucella* in relation to the effect of age at vaccination, vaccine dose, and challenge dose, it was noted above that not all of the data in Table 16-2 were appropriate for statistical analysis. The data actually analyzed are shown in Table 16-9. The description of the Chi-square tests of significance of isolation results are shown in Table 16-10. Tables 16-11 to 16-16 show the data that were abstracted from Table 16-9 and tests of significance of the comparisons described in Table 16-10.

Table 16-11 shows the results of tests of significance of the effect of dose of vaccine on lower age heifers versus NVC when challenged with a median dose of virulent *Brucella*. There were two vaccine dose groups and NVC. The differences among all three groups were significant at 0.05%.

The difference between the NVC and the low dose group had a significance level between 1 and 0.5% while the difference between the NVC and the high dose group had a significance level of less than 0.05%. There was a significant affect of increased dose of vaccine with the difference between the low dose group and the high dose group having a probability of between 2.5 and 1%.

Table 16-9. Isolation Rate of Challenge strains of *Brucella abortus* after Exposure of Nonvaccinated and Strain 19 Vaccinated Heifers. One Middle Challenge and Both High Challenge Experimental Groups Removed.

Vacc. age	Challenge*	No vaccine		Isolation rate by Strain 19 dose* groups					
				Low Dose		High Dose		Total†	
3-6mo.	1×10^7	23/30	(76.7)	28/60	(46.7)	5/26	19.2	33/36	(38.4)
8-23 mo.§	6×10^6	11/20	(55.0)	9/50	(18.0)	1/17	(5.9)	10/67	(14.9)
	1×10^7	77/92	(83.7)	43/103§	(41.7)	6/39	(15.4)	49/142	(34.5)
Total**		88/112	(78.6)	52/153	(34.0)	7/56	(12.5)	59/209	(28.2)
Total††		111/142	(78.2)	80/213	(37.6)	12/82	(14.6)	92/295	(31.2)

*colony forming units
†vaccinated groups only
§1 heifer was 8 months old (no isolation); the rest were at least 10 months old.
**8 - 23 months group.
††both age groups.

Table 16-10. Description of Chi-Square Tests Involving *Brucella* Challenge Data

Low age vaccinates	Low vs High dose vaccinates
Low age vaccinates	Low Dose vaccinates vs Non-vaccinates
Low age vaccinates	High Dose vaccinates vs Non-vaccinates
Low age vaccinates	All 3 groups of dose and non-vaccinates - 2 d.f.
Old age & Low challenge	Low vs High dose vaccinates
Old age & Low challenge	Low dose vaccinates vs Non-vaccinates
Old age & Low challenge	High dose vaccinates vs Non-vaccinates
Old age & Low challenge	All 3 groups of dose and Non-vaccinates - 2 d.f.
Old age & Median challenge	Low vs High dose vaccinates
Old age & Median challenge	Low Dose vaccinates vs Non-vaccinates
Old age & Median challenge	High dose vaccinates vs Non-vaccinates
Old age & Median challenge	All 3 groups of dose & Non-vaccinates - 2 d.f.
Median challenge	Low age controls vs Old age controls
Median challenge & Low dose vaccinates	Low age vs Old age vaccinates
Median challenge & High dose vaccinates	Low age vs Old age vaccinates
Median challenge	All 6 groups of Low vs Old age vaccinates - 5 d.f.
Old age non-vaccinated controls	Low vs Median challenge
Old age Low dose vaccinates	Low vs median challenge
Old age High dose vaccinates	Low vs median challenge
Old age Vaccinates	All 6 groups of vaccine & challenge doses - 5 d.f.

Table 16-11. Chi-Square Tests of *Brucella* Challenge Data for Comparisons within 3 to 6 Months Vaccination Age and Median Challenge Vaccine Trials.

3 to 6 months vaccination age & median challenge vaccine trials

	Pos.	Neg.	Total	% +
No vaccine controls	23	7	30	76.7
Low dose vaccine	28	32	60	46.7
High dose vaccine	5	21	26	19.2
TOTAL	56	60	116	

Chi-square value - 18.5303 for 2 d.f.
Probability - Less than 0.05%

No vaccine controls	23	7	30	76.7
Low dose vaccine	28	32	60	46.7
TOTAL	51	39	90	

Chi-square value - 7.3303
Probability - Between 1% and 0.5%

No vaccine controls	23	7	30	76.7
High dose vaccine	5	21	26	19.2
TOTAL	28	28	56	

Chi-square value - 18.3795
Probability - Less than 0.05%

Low dose vaccine	28	32	60	46.7
High dose vaccine	5	21	26	19.2
TOTAL	33	53	86	

Chi-square value - 5.7739
Probability - Between 2.5% and 1%

Vaccine Dose Effects in High Age Heifers
with Low Challenge

Table 16-12 shows the results of tests of significance of effect of vaccine dose on higher age heifers versus NVC when challenged with a low dose

Table 16-12. Chi-Square Tests of *Brucella* Challenge Data for Comparisons within 8 to 23 Months Vaccination Age and Low Challenge Vaccine Trials

8 to 23 months vaccination age & low challenge vaccine trials

	Pos.	Neg.	Total	% +
No vaccine controls	11	9	20	55.0
Low dose vaccine	9	41	50	18.0
High dose vaccine	1	16	17	5.9
TOTAL	21	66	87	

Chi-square value - 14.5256 for 2 d.f.
Probability - Between 0.1% and 0.05%

No vaccine controls	11	9	20	55.0
Low dose vaccine	9	41	50	18.0
TOTAL	20	50	70	

Chi-square value - 9.5830
Probability - Between 0.5% and 0.01%

No vaccine controls	11	9	20	55.0
High dose vaccine	1	16	17	5.9
TOTAL	12	25	37	

Chi-square value - 10.1166
Probability - Between 0.5% and 0.01%

Low vaccine controls	9	41	50	18.0
High dose vaccine	1	16	17	5.9
TOTAL	10	57	67	

Chi-square value - 1.4671
Probability - Between 30% and 20%

of virulent *Brucella*. As with the case above, there were two vaccine dose groups and the NVC. The differences among all three groups had a probability level between 0.1 and 0.05%.

The difference between the NVC and the low dose group had a significance level between 0.5 and 0.01% while the difference between the NVC and the high dose group also had a significance level between 0.5 and 0.01%. There was not a significant effect of increased dose of vaccine since

Table 16-13. Chi-Square Tests of *Brucella* Challenge Data for Comparisons within 8 to 23 Months Vaccination Age and Median Challenge Vaccine Trials

8 to 23 months vaccination age & median challenge vaccine trials

	Pos.	Neg.	Total	% +
No vaccine controls	77	15	92	83.7
Low dose vaccine	43	60	103	41.7
High dose vaccine	6	33	39	15.4
TOTAL	126	108	234	

Chi-square value - 62.2446 for 2 d.f.
Probability - Less than 0.05%

	Pos.	Neg.	Total	% +
No vaccine controls	77	15	92	83.7
Low dose vaccine	43	60	103	41.7
TOTAL	120	75	195	

Chi-square value - 36.1278
Probability - Less than 0.05%

	Pos.	Neg.	Total	% +
No vaccine controls	77	15	92	83.7
High dose vaccine	6	33	39	15.4
TOTAL	83	48	131	

Chi-square value - 55.0537
Probability - Less than 0.05%

	Pos.	Neg.	Total	% +
Low dose vaccine	43	60	103	41.7
High dose vaccine	6	33	39	15.4
TOTAL	49	93	142	

Chi-square value - 8.6996
Probability - Between 0.5% and 0.1%

the difference between the low dose group and the high dose group had a probability of between 30 and 20%. This contrasts with the level of significance due to increased vaccine dose in low age vaccinates challenged with a median dose of virulent *Brucella* and reflects to some degree the higher number of animals per group in the case of low age at vaccination and median challenge dose.

Table 16-14. Chi-Square Tests of *Brucella* Challenge Data for Comparison Between Vaccination for Each Vaccine Dose in Median Challenge Vaccine Trials

3-6 and 8-23 months vaccination age and median challenge vaccine trials

	Pos.	Neg.	Total	%+
3-6 month old no-vaccine controls	23	7	30	76.7
8-23 month old no-vaccine controls	77	15	92	83.7
TOTAL No-vaccine controls	100	22	122	

Chi-square value - 0.7562
Probability - Between 40% and 30%

	Pos.	Neg.	Total	%+
3-6 month old low dose vaccine	28	32	60	46.7
8-23 month old low dose vaccine	43	60	103	41.7
TOTAL Low dose vaccinates	71	92	163	

Chi-square value - 0.3732
Probability - Between 60% and 50%

	Pos.	Neg.	Total	%+
3-6 month old high dose vaccinates	5	21	26	19.2
8-23 month old high dose vaccinates	6	33	39	15.4
TOTAL High dose vaccinates	11	54	65	

Chi-square value - 0.1641
Probability - Between 70% and 60%

Vaccine Dose Effects in High Age Heifers with Median Challange

Table 16-13 shows the results of tests of significance of effect of vaccine dose on higher age heifers versus NVC when challenged with a median dose of virulent *Brucella*. As with the cases above, there were two vaccine dose groups and the NVC. The differences among all three groups had a probability level of less than 0.05%.

The difference between the NVC and the low dose group also had a significance level of less than 0.05% as did the difference between the NVC and the high dose group. In all three tests of significance, there were extremely high chi-square values. There was a highly significant affect of increased dose of vaccine, with the difference between the low dose group

Table 16-15. Chi-Square Tests of *Brucella* Challenge Data for Comparison Between Vaccination Age Among all Vaccine Dose by Age Groups for Median Challenge Vaccine Trials

	Pos.	Neg.	Total	%+
3-6 month old Low dose vaccinates	28	32	60	46.7
8-23 month old Low dose vaccinates	43	60	103	41.7
3-6 month old High dose vaccinates	5	21	26	19.2
8-23 month old High dose vaccinates	6	33	39	15.4
Total for two doses	82	146	228	

Chi-square value - 14.8132 for 3 d.f.
Probability - Between 0.5% and 0.1%

	Pos.	Neg.	Total	%+
3-6 month old No-vaccine controls	23	7	30	76.7
8-23 month old No-vaccine controls	77	15	92	83.7
3-6 month old Low dose vaccinates	28	32	60	46.7
8-23 month old Low dose vaccinates	43	60	103	41.7
3-6 month old High dose vaccinates	5	21	26	19.2
8-23 month old High dose vaccinates	6	33	39	15.4
TOTAL Controls and doses	182	168	350	

Chi-square value - 81.4973 for 5 d.f.
Probability - Less than 0.05%

and the high dose group having a probability of between 0.5 and 0.1%.

The percentage difference between the low dose and high dose isolation rates was about the same as was the case with the difference for increased vaccine dose for low age vaccinates challenged with a median dose of virulent *Brucella*. However, the level of significance in the lower age dose groups had a higher probability of between 2.5 and 1%. This reflects the much higher number of animals per group in the case of the high age at vaccination with median challenge as compared to the low age at vaccination and median challenge.

Effect of Age at Vaccination with Median Challenge for Each Dose

Table 16-14 shows comparisons between low age and high age vaccinates challenged with a median dose of virulent *Brucella;* each vaccine

Table 16-16. Chi-Square Tests of *Brucella* Challenge Data for Comparisons Between Low and Median Challenge Level for each Vaccine Dose and Among all Vaccine Dose by Level of Challenge Groups within 8 to 23 Month Vaccination Age.

8-23 month vaccination age low & median challenge vaccine trials

	Pos.	Neg.	Total	%+
8-23 mo. low challenge controls	11	9	20	55.0
8-23 mo. median challenge controls	77	15	92	83.7
Total 8-23 mo. controls	88	24	112	

Chi-square value - 8.0348
Probability - Between 0.5% and 0.1%

	Pos.	Neg.	Total	%+
8-23 mo. low dose & low challenge	9	41	50	18.0
8-23 mo. low dose & median challenge	43	60	103	41.7
Total 8-23 mo. low dose vacciantes	52	101	153	

Chi-square value - 8.4608
Probability - Between 0.5% and 0.1%

	Pos.	Neg.	Total	%+
8-23 mo. high dose & low challenge	1	16	17	5.9
8-23 mo. high dose & median challenge	6	33	39	15.4
Total high dose vaccinates	7	49	56	

Chi-square value - 0.9774
Probability - Between 40% and 30%

	Pos.	Neg.	Total	%+
8-23 mo. low challenge controls	11	9	20	55.0
8-23 mo. median challenge controls	77	15	92	83.7
8-23 mo. low dose & low challenge	9	41	50	18.0
8-23 mo. low dose & median challenge	43	60	103	41.7
8-23 mo. high dose & low challenge	1	16	17	5.9
8-23 mo. high dose & median challenge	6	33	39	15.4
Total 8-23 mo. low & median challenge	147	174	321	

Chi-square value - 95.6014 for 5 d.f.
Probability - Less than 0.05%

dose group or NVC. In the case of the NVC for the low age and high age heifers, there was no difference in isolation rates with the chi-square value having a probability of between 40 and 30%.

In the case of the low dose-low age and low dose-high age groups, there also was no difference in isolation rates with the chi-square value having a probability of between 60 and 50%. In the case of high dose-low age and the high dose-high age groups, there also was no difference in isolation rates with the chi-square value having a probability of between 70 and 60%.

Table 16-15 shows the results of a test of significance with 3 df among the four low and high dose groups shown in Table 16-14. This test gives a chi-square value which has a probabilty of occurring by chance between 0.5 and 0.1%. This table also shows the results of a test of significance with 5 df among all six groups shown in Table 16-14. This test gives a chi-square value which has an extremely low probability. The complete lack of significance reflected in the results of the three tests shown in Table 16-14 means that the high level of variation reflected in the two tests in Table 16-15 was due to the use of vaccine and the vaccine dosage level.

Vaccine and challenge dose effects in older age heifers

Table 16-16 shows the results of tests of significance between the low and median challenge doses for older age-low vaccine dose heifers, older age-high vaccine dose heifers, for NVC, and among all groups within the older age vaccinates.

The difference between the low and median challenge doses in the NVC was significant with a probability of between 0.5 and 0.1%. The difference between the low and median challenge doses in the low vaccine dose heifers also was highly significant with the same probability of between 0.5 and 0.1%.

However, the difference between the low and median challenge doses in the high vaccine dose heifers was not significant with a high probability of between 40 and 30%. This lack of significance in the high dose heifers is due partly to a smaller number of heifers in the two high dose groups as compared to the NVC and the low vaccine dose groups.

The Chi-square test among all six groups within the older age heifers has a probability of much less than 0.05%. This reflects an extreme amount of overall variation due to the effect of vaccine, vaccine dose, and the effect of challenge dose among the six older age groups.

Discussion

There is much disappointment that the current Strain 19 dose for calfhood vaccination has not brought about a reduction in post-vaccination serum-antibody titers. Positive sero test results cause marketing constraints to be placed on cattle until a diagnosis is made. Production capability is lost when sero-positive cattle are slaughtered. A significant level of Strain 19-induced titers increases the costs of brucellosis surveillance. This has resulted in serious consideration for changing to a vaccine dose lower than 3×10^9 CFU.

The data in this review indicate that heifers should be vaccinated before they reach 9 months of age. It would be preferable by many to state that they should be vaccinated before estrous cycles begin. The data also indicate that if heifers are inoculated with Strain 19 after they become 9 months old, a dose no higher than 1×10^9 CFU should be used, in order to significantly reduce retained antibody titers.

However, the primary purpose for Strain 19 vaccination is to raise the resistance of cattle to $B. abortus$ infection. The data in this review indicate that both younger and older age heifers given a Strain 19 dose of 9×10^6 to 1×10^9 CFU are not adequately protected against a virulent $Brucella$ exposure dose of 1×10^7 CFU. This finding supports a recent recommendation of a United States Animal Health Association Brucellosis Committee Subcommittee that the Strain 19 dose should not be lowered for calfhood vaccination.

Summary

Data were obtained from several sources and analyzed as to the effects of age at vaccination and dose of $Brucella abortus$ Strain 19 on post-vaccination card and rose bengal plate test results. Of 233 heifers vaccinated at 3 to 8 months of age, 79 were given a Strain 19 dose of 9×10^6 to 1 $\times 10^9$ colony forming units (CFU) and 154 were inoculated with 3×10^9 to 1 $\times 10^{10}$ CFU. Of 677 heifers vaccinated at 9 to 23 months of age, 528 received the above lower dose range and 149 were given the higher 3×10^9 to 1×10^{10} dose range.

Fewer sero-positive test results were found in younger heifers given the higher dose range compared to older heifers given the higher dose range. Sero-positive test results were less in older heifers given the lower dose range compared to older heifers given the higher dose range.

Of the 910 vaccinated heifers, 344 were challenged during their first pregnancy with virulent strains of $Brucella$. Challenge strain isolation rates were analyzed in 295 of the 344. Challenge strain infection was significantly less in both age groups that had been given the higher vaccine dose.

References

1.   Davies G, Cocks E, Hebert N. *Brucella abortus* (Strain 19) vaccine: (a) determina-

tion of the minimum protective dose in cattle; (b) the effect of vaccinating calves previously inoculated with anti-*Brucella abortus* serum. *J Biol Stand* 1980;8:165-175.

2. Deyoe BL, Dorsey TA, Meredith K, Garrett L. Reduced doses of *Brucella abortus* in cattle (abstract). *Proceedings*, 84th Annual Meeting of the USAHA 1980;163-164.

3. Hinshaw ER, Noon T. Unpublished data from University of Arizona herds; December 1985.

4. Oregon Department of Agriculture. Unpublished data obtained from one herd on November 25, 1985.

5. Confer AW, Buening GM, Espe BH, Smith RA. Antibody responses of heifers vaccinated with reduced doses of *Brucella abortus* Strain 19. The Bovine Practitioner 1983;18:174-178.

6. Deyoe BL, Dorsey TA, Meredith KB, Garrett L. Effect of reduced dosages of *Brucella abortus* Strain 19 in cattle vaccinated as yearlings. *Proceedings*, 83rd Annual Meeting of the USAHA 1979;92-104.

7. Herr S, Bosman PP, Ehret WJ, Te Brugge LA, Williamson CC, Pieterson PM. Brucellosis serology: reduced dose S19 vaccination of yearling heifers versus the use of the standard dose at 5-7 months of age in a clean herd. *J S Afr Vet Assoc* 1986;57:215-219.

8. Alton GG, Corner LA. Vaccination of heifers with a reduced dose of *Brucella abortus* Strain 19 vaccine before first mating. *Aust Vet J* 1981;57:548-550.

9. Adams LG, Crawford RP, Heck FC, Nielsen KH, Williams JD. Unpublished data from Texas A & M University; 1987. 40th Annual Brucellosis Research Conference, & USAHA, 1987.

10. Texas A & M University. Unpublished data from herd # 017. (USAHA,1987).

11. Texas A & M University. Unpublished data from herd # 018.

12. Texas A & M University. Unpublished data from Arizona group.

13. Texas A & M University. Unpublished data from Texas group.

14. Confer AW, Hall SM, Faulkner CB, Espe BH, Deyoe BL, Morton RJ, Smith RA. Effects of challenge dose on the clinical and immune responses of cattle vaccinated with reduced doses of *Brucella abortus* Strain 19. *Vet Microbiol* 1985;10:561-575.

15. Snedecor GW, Cochran WG. *Statistical Methods*. 6th edition. Iowa State University Press. Ames, Iowa 1967.

16. Lentner C. Geigy Scientific Tables. Vol. 2. *Introduction to statistics. Statistical tables. Mathematical formulae.* 8th edition, Ciba-Geigy Co. West Caldwell, New Jersey 1982.

Chapter Seventeen

Development of Live
Brucella Vaccines

L. *Garry Adams*

The ultimate mission of research on infectious diseases is their prevention. Protection of susceptible hosts by vaccination still remains one of the best methods to accomplish this mission. This approach was exemplified early in this century by Bang who reported in 1906 that infection of cattle with virulent *Brucella abortus* often leads to immunity.[1] He recommended that heifers be vaccinated with a heavy suspension of cultured *B. abortus* sometime before first breeding. The protection afforded by this method of vaccination was determined by reduction in the rate of abortion rather than by the rate of protection against infection. However using this approach, vaccination by Bang and other workers with uncontrolled quantities of cultured *B. abortus* of variable virulence frequently caused disease in many cattle rather than preventing it. Because of these problems, efforts were begun to find strains of reduced virulence which could be used as live vaccines to provide safe protective immunity in cattle.[2] It also became evident that killed vaccines could be a viable alternative approach to the problems associated with live vaccines; however, development of killed vaccines for cattle are addressed elsewhere in this volume.

Vaccination against most bacterial diseases, including brucellosis, has been largely unimproved during the last 100 years, many vaccines have been used continuously with little major improvements. Advances in immunology and bacterial genetics now provide new approaches for developing safer and more effective bacterial vaccines. These two fields of research facilitate the quest for 1) specific protective immunogens by inserting genetic information encoding protective immunogens into replicating sub-unit vector vaccines, and 2) development of genetically stable mutants, practically eliminating the problem of virulent revertants of attenuated vaccine strains. Both of these approaches can be used to address the observation that optimal protective immunity against some bacterial diseases, particularly against intracellular pathogens such as *B. abortus* can quite likely best be accomplished by vaccination with either attenuated live bacteria which imitate infection-induced immunity, or appropriate expression of specific sub-unit protective immunogens in attenuated replicating microbial vectors.

Historical Perspectives on Former and Current Live *Brucella* Vaccines

Because early killed *B. abortus* vaccine preparations were not effective in protecting cattle,[1] several investigators used various combinations of live field strain isolates, doses and inoculation routes in an attempt to protect cattle. Among the live strains evaluated as vaccines in cattle were *B. abortus* Strain 19,[3] *B. abortus* Strain 45/20,[4] mucoid variants of *Brucella suis*,[5] non-agglutinogenic *B. abortus* Strain B,[6] (e) *Brucella melitensis* Strain Rev. I,[7,8] and *Brucella suis* Strain 2.[9] Of these, only two, Strain 19 and Rev. I, have been used continuously as live vaccines in large and small ruminants respectively; however, a brief review of the origins and characteristics of each of these vaccines serve as a point of departure for discussing strategies for developing new live *Brucella* vaccines.

In 1923, John Buck, a U.S. Bureau of Animal Industry veterinary bacteriologist at the Beltsville Research Center, isolated a virulent strain of *B. abortus* from the milk of a registered Jersey cow named Victor's Lady Matilda, but when he left the organism at room temperature for a year, it became naturally attenuated and stabilized.[10] Buck called the isolate Strain 19 because it was his 19th stock culture in a series that he used in his vaccine research.

Over the next three decades Buck,[3] Cotton et al.,[11,12] and several other investigators[13-19] demonstrated that various doses and routes (subcutaneous, intradermal, conjunctival, and oral) of Strain 19 stimulated significant protection (usually between 65-75%) against abortion and often infection in sexually immature cattle against varying experimental doses, routes of challenge and virulent strains of *B. abortus*. Strain 19 was demonstrated not to revert to virulence *in vivo*[20] and to provide near life time immunity in sexually immature and adult cattle.[16,21,22] To provide whole herd immunity and to reduce persistent titers, the dosage of Strain 19 was reduced for sexually immature[21,23] and adult cattle without compromising protection[24-31] based on suggestions of previous workers.[15,32-37] Although reduction in dosage has alleviated some of the problems associated with Strain 19 vaccination, several disadvantages remain to be eliminated:

1. residual serum and milk antibody titers which complicate accurate serodiagnosis of field strain infection
2. persistent Strain 19 infection of vaccinates
3. the stigma of being identified as adult vaccinates from an infected herd
4. infectivity for man
5. narrow tolerance of the vaccination age and sex restrictions
6. difficulty in consistent low-dose delivery of viable organisms
7. occasional occurrence of arthritis and endotoxic shock

8. the constant necessity to carefully maintain vaccine seed stock having smooth antigenic and non-erythritol utilization characteristics.[25,30,38-42]

The chemical compound, erythritol, was discovered by Pearce et al.[43] to be a growth stimulant for most *Brucella* spp. and was proposed to be related to the host genitalia tissue tropism of brucellae. Strain 19 is CO_2 independent and inhibited by thionin, penicillin, and safranin.[39,44] Strain 19 is also uniquely inhibited by erythritol because it lacks a single enzyme-d-erythulose 1-phosphate dehydrogenase, which probably represents a recently acquired mutation[42] with a frequency of erythritol-utilizing revertants of 1:10$^{-5.44}$ to 1:9 x10^{-5}.[38] Numerous studies have attempted to demonstrate a correlation between the virulence of brucellae and their ability to metabolize erythritol; however, the inhibition of the growth of Strain 19 and its inability to oxidize erythritol was shown by Meyer[45] to be coincidental with, but unrelated to, its stabilized level of attenuation.

Similarly, in the early 1920s McEwen[4] isolated smooth *B. abortus* Strain 45 from cattle which was demonstrated to be relatively avirulent yet stimulated protective immunity in guinea pigs. While attempting to restore virulence to Strain 45 by serial passage through guinea pigs, McEwen[46] discovered that the 20th passage was rough but that by the 40th passage it had virulence comparable to field strains. He subsequently found that live cultures of the 20th guinea pig passage of *B. abortus* Strain 45, i.e. Strain 45/20, conferred protective immunity; however, when live Strain 45/20 was injected into pregnant cows, it reverted to a smooth pathogenic form that resulted in infection, abortion, and production of smooth agglutinins. Taylor[47] later compared intravenous injections of Strain 45/20 and Strain 19 in pregnant cows and observed that clinical disease was caused by smooth revertants of Strain 45/20 which required higher CO_2 for primary isolation. In contrast, Strain 19 retained its cultural and biological characteristics even after seven intravenous serial passages through pregnant cows. Although the infectivity of Strain 45/20[46,47] and stimulation of smooth agglutinins in cattle[48,49] made its use as a live vaccine impractical, the concept of using live rough mutants to induce protective immunity without stimulating cross reactive antibodies was originated.

In 1957, Elberg and Faunce[7] reported isolating a smooth attenuated *Brucella melitensis*, designated Strain Rev. I, from a streptomycin-dependent population growing in streptomycin deficient medium and demonstrated the strain induced significant protection without shedding against virulent experimental challenge in goats. Alton and co-workers[50-53] and others[54] subsequently reported no reversion to virulence and long term (2 to 3 years) protective immunity in goats and sheep although Rev. I frequently caused abortion in pregnant animals, was occasionally excreted in milk, and stimulated persisting agglutinins which interfered with diagnostic tests for extended periods of time. Rev. I was much more protective against virulent *B. melitensis* challenge in sheep and goats than was *B. abortus* Strain 19.[54,55] Rev. I was also documented to induce significant protection against virulent *B. abortus* challenge in cattle.[8,40]

Since 1971, millions of doses of *Brucella suis* Strain 2 have been reported to be used in China as an oral vaccine for effective prevention of brucellosis in sheep, goats, cattle, and swine.[9] *B. suis* Strain 2 is a laboratory-adapted strain attenuated by serial transfer on culture media for several years. *B. suis* Strain 2 is a smooth biotype 1 which is less virulent than Strain 19[9] and Rev. I[56] in mice and guinea pigs[57] although no studies of human susceptibility have been reported. Discriminatory antibiotic and enzyme marker assays fail to differentiate *B. suis* Strain 2 from divergent field strains.[58] *B. suis* Strain 2 was demonstrated to be remarkably stable by five serial passages each through guinea pigs, pregnant ewes, goats, and sows as monitored by spleen counts in guinea pigs.[9] Oral doses between 5 and 50 x 10[9] cfu are protective in sheep, goats, cattle and swine, stimulating serum agglutinins and complement fixing antibodies for up to nine months with a duration of immunity of 4-5 years in sheep. Interestingly, when *B. suis* Strain 2 is injected subcutaneously or intramuscularly (as opposed to oral administration of up to 5 x 10[11] cfu), it causes abortion in sheep, and goats.[9] Bosseray and Plommet[56] reported that *Brucella suis* Strain 2 induces immunity against *B. abortus* Strain 544 in mice equivalent to that produced by Strain 19 and Rev. I although immunity against *B. melitensis* waned somewhat with time which was thought to be related to the A-serotype specificity and/or its decreased ability to colonize lymph nodes. Mustafa[59] reported 71.2% and 53.6% protection (average = 55.3%) with oral dosages between 3.75 and 10 x 10[9] cfu in sheep and goats respectively following experimental challenge at 27 weeks post-vaccination with 5 x 10[6] cfu each of *B. melitensis* biotype 1 and 2 virulent field isolates. The *B. suis* Strain 2 vaccine was safe as none of the pregnant sheep or goats aborted following vaccination nor did they shed the vaccine strain in milk or vaginal discharges and only 2.25% had retained agglutinin titers after one year. Although the *B. suis* Strain 2 vaccine was considered to reasonably immunogenic, these levels of protection are significantly (χ^2= 70.1, p < 0.001) lower than the 82.7% reported by Xin.[9]

The molecular and genetic nature of the attenuating spontaneous mutations of these live *Brucella* vaccines has not been determined. Although the molecular basis for these spontaneous mutations could probably be painstakingly determined through site-specific mutagenesis and DNA sequencing, in all likelihood it will be more efficient to develop new live *Brucella* vaccines through modern molecular biology techniques. Approaches and rationale are developed in the following discussion.

Studies on cross-immunity with live virulent homologous and heterologous *Brucella* spp. and attenuated vaccines may also provide evidence to support approaches for developing improved live *Brucella* vaccines. In contrast to the results reported with the Chinese *B. suis* Strain 2 vaccine protecting cattle, Washko et al.[40] reported that cows fed *B. suis* failed to be protected against *B. abortus* challenge nor did Strain 19 protect against *B. suis* challenge in cattle[61] or swine.[62] *B. melitensis* Rev. I protected cattle against *B. abortus*[8] with no evidence of Rev. I shedding and goats were protected against *B. melitensis*[55] challenge, but *B. abortus* Strain 19 was much less protective against *B. melitensis* challenge in goats.[55] *Brucella neotomae* was demonstrated to protect goats and sheep against virulent *B. melitensis* challenge.[54]

These data demonstrate that homologous *Brucella* spp. are usually more protective than heterologous *Brucella* spp. within a given livestock species, but in some cases heterologous *Brucella* spp. may induce protective immunity equal to homologous *Brucella* spp. With the exception of swine, the general hierarchy of immunizing capacity of either vaccine or field strains of *Brucella* spp. for cattle, goats, and sheep is proposed to be *B. melitensis* (*B. neotomae* ?) ≥ *B. suis* > *B. abortus*. In swine, the immunogenic hierarchy apparently is *B. suis* ≥ *B. melitensis* > *B. abortus*. It should also be noted that smooth strains of *Brucella* spp. (e.g. *B. abortus* Strain 19, *B. melitensis* Rev. I, and *B. suis* Strain 2) are generally more protective in most livestock species than rough strains.

Such an overall hypothesis on the immunizing hierarchy of *Brucella* spp. may not be completely acceptable; however, with the possible exception of *Brucella ovis*, there is a very close genetic yet subtle unique relatedness among *Brucella* spp. and strains. The evidence to support this proposal has been documented by Verger et al. Hoyer and McCullough,[64] O'Hara et al.[65] Allardet-Servent *et al.*[66] and Muzny et al.[67] which in a general sense further supports a genetic basis for cross protection. Indeed, Bricker et al.[68] recently demonstrated by Western blotting that a 31-kilodalton protein extracted from *B. abortus* was conserved and expressed in the six recognized species of *Brucella* (except *B. ovis*) and eight biovars of *B. abortus*. Interestingly, and somewhat in parallel with proposed *Brucella* immunogenic hierarchy, *B. melitensis* had the strongest and most consistent Western blot reaction with the 31-kilodalton protein, as opposed to *B. abortus* from which it was originally derived. Thus, the documented cross-protection is medicated presumably through genetically encoded immunogenic epitopes shared between *Brucella* spp. and provides a fundamental basis to successfully produce live, safe, genetically engineered vaccines for several livestock species without stimulating persisting antibodies cross reactive in serodiagnostic tests for field strain infections.

Fundamental Biosafety and Efficacy Requirements for Live *Brucella* Vaccines

To provide the appropriate protection against brucellosis that will meet the needs of the livestock industry, national disease prevention programs and consumers alike, live *Brucella* vaccines[15,30,69-71] should:

1. not produce disease in vaccinated animals
2. prevent infection in both sexes at any age
3. prevent abortion and sterility
4. provide long term protection against infection and abortion with a single vaccination
5. not stimulate persistent antibodies interfering with accurate serodiagnosis of field strain infections
6. not be transmitted to other animals if the vaccine strain establishes a long-term latent infection
7. be biologically stable, practically excluding virulent revertants under *in vitro* and *in vivo* conditions
8. not be pathogenic for man
9. not contaminate meat and milk products
10. be readily grown in large-scale fermentation technology.

Obviously, each of the currently employed live *Brucella* vaccines has its own peculiar advantages and disadvantages within a given livestock species; however, clearly from the literature, *B. suis* Strain 2 has the greatest spectrum of livestock species cross-protection utility, followed by *B. melitensis* Rev. I and lastly *B. abortus* Strain 19. Each of these smooth strain-based vaccines produces long-term immunity with a single injection, but, depending upon the age at vaccination, stimulates some degree of residual agglutinating antibody titers which frequently confuse serodiagnosis of field strain infections. While *B. suis* Strain 2 apparently is not shed from the host, *B. melitensis* Rev. I and *B. abortus* Strain 19, which are biologically stable relative to reversion and lack of transmission to homologous or heterologous hosts, occasionally establish prolonged residual infections resulting in abortion and are shed at variable rates in biological fluids and excretions; hence, they pose a potential public health risk through contaminated meat and milk products. Strain 19 is restricted for use only in female cattle due to sterility problems in males. *B. melitensis* Rev. I[72] and *B. abortus* Strain 19[73-75] are both pathogenic for man. Because of these disadvantage of the current live *Brucella* vaccines and the continuing worldwide incidence of brucellosis in animals and man,[76,77] development of live, safe, and efficacious vaccines that do not possess have these drawbacks but do stimulate protective immunity against the major pathogens of the genus *Brucella* is highly desirable and justified.[40,53,78]

Rationale and Basic Requirements for Developing New Live *Brucella* Vaccines

Fundamental Requirements

Active immune prophylaxis should provide for elimination of the infection and prevention of subsequent reinfection. To improve the rate of progress of new vaccine development, several questions fundamental to the host-parasite interaction resulting in either acquired immunity or disease should be answered. Without a fundamental understanding of the pathogenesis of infection and the basic immunologic response during the infection and disease processes, vaccine development will be plagued with difficulties and adverse conditions, especially when a long-term immunity is desired. Certainly, of the early events in the infectious process, the interaction of the exposed bacterial cell surface with cellular receptors and other organelles is a critical event in determining bacterial survival in the host and often determines tissue/organ tropisms.[79] The bacterial surface is not static, but remarkably plastic, determined primarily by the microenvironment, which may indicate that, in the case of intracellular pathogens, virulence determinants must be expressed *in vivo* for live vaccines to be effective.[79,80] Knowledge of these events may provide an avenue for active immune intervention. Identification and understanding of virulence determinants and the role they play in pathogenic mechanisms is crucial in developing vaccines to inhibit the natural process of infection.

Specific Requirements

It has become increasingly evident that identification of immunizing B-cell and T-cell immunodominant epitopes is tantamount to significantly improving recombinant or synthetic vaccines against several diseases.[81,82] Presentation of the antigen to the immune system is a critical step in immunization. Macrophages, Langerhans cells, reticular cells, and B-cells can effectively present antigens. Additionally, recent evidence confirms that B-cells predominantly recognize conformational (or discontinuous) determinants directly, which allows them to process the antigen and express fragments on its cell surface in association with class II (Ia) MHC products so that the T-cell receptor can recognize the antigen in the context of the combined antigen-MHC complex.[81,83,84] This complex is in turn recognized by activated T-helper cells to form a trimolecular complex which results in secretion of the appropriate cytokines to act on B-cells to differentiate, proliferate, and secrete antibody. T-cells mainly recognize either unprocessed (primary sequence) monomeric antigen in association with class I MHC product complexes, generating suppress or cytotoxic T-cells or processed (unfolded or fragment) oligopeptide antigens of the molecule in association with class II MHC product complexes to generate helper/regulatory T-cells.

In general, immunodominance is determined by factors intrinsic and extrinsic to the structure of the antigenic site.[82] Extrinsic factors are determined by the way the antigen is processed by the host into fragments, but mostly by the strict correlation between the specific MHC molecule used to present the antigen and the dominant antigenic site. Apparently, some products of natural antigen processing also contain structures which may hinder binding to some MHC molecules or T-helper cells; hence, the possibility of actually improving the natural immune response exists.[85] Intrinsic structural features of dominant antigenic sites are determined by the presence of helices with hydrophobic residues on one side and hydrophilic residues on the other side of the molecule. Hence, the immunogenic antigens (matched B-cell and T-helper-cell epitopes) in new vaccines must be available or presented in the appropriate manner to be recognized and induce optimal long-term immunity.

State of Knowledge of Protective *Brucella* Immunogens and Virulence Factors

Protective Immunogens

Why are *B. abortus* Strain 19, *B. melitensis* Strain Rev. I, and apparently *B. suis* Strain 2 live vaccines as successful as they are? Bang[1] and others demonstrated that the natural infection usually gave life-long immunity. These stable attenuated strains emulate the natural infection-induced immunity by replicating with a transient persistence in the appropriate cells for a least a few weeks to provide an increasing immunogenic stimulus (persisting antigen effect) for specific and nonspecific responses resulting in long-lived immunity, probably due to memory cells. Notably, humoral and cellular immune responses are both stimulated by *B. abortus* Strain 19, *B. melitensis* Strain Rev. I, and apparently by *B. suis* Strain 2 vaccine strains[7,86-89] against a series of carbohydrate and protein antigens both common and distinct to *Brucella* spp.[90]

Given that cell envelopes of most gram-negative bacterial cells, including *Brucella*, are comprised of three major components- lipopolysaccharide, phospholipid, and proteins- and that methods to prepare cell envelopes and separate inner and outer membranes with or without peptidoglycans are available, unraveling the complexities of protective immunity still remains a formidable undertaking. Extensive periodic reviews of the immunity to *Brucella* infection in several hosts have been published providing a gradual understanding of the antigens involved.[40,69,88,90] Detailed reviews by Sowa, Winter, Canning, Smith, and Plommet (see Sowa and Hancock in this volume) with regard to outer membranes, lipopolysaccharides, killed vaccines preparations of *Brucella* as well as host B-cells, T-cells, and macrophages interactions have been presented. Winter and collaborators[91-96] have extensively characterized outer membrane proteins of *Brucella* and found them to be remarkably conserved in all *Brucella* strains and species, suggesting that these proteins could potentially induce cross-species protective immunity. Gomez-Miguel[97] identified a Braun-like lipoprotein bound to the peptidoglycan of *Brucella*.

Recently, Dubray[70] reviewed the status of protective *Brucella* antigens and concluded that with the exception of smooth lipopolysaccharide (S-LPS) induced active[98-101] and passive monoclonal antibody[102,103] immunity studies in mice no other protective antigens (much less protective epitopes) have been identified. Vendrell et al. reported in the poster session of this symposium (this volume abstract no. 27) that murine IgG2a and IgA monoclonal anti-membrane protein antibodies were protective. While SDS, phenol extracted, and cell envelope *Brucella* antigens containing S-LPS were protective,[70,104] *Brucella* porins and outer membrane preparations in other studies have failed to be protective in active[100] and monoclonal antibody passive[102] immunity studies in mice. Winter et al.[92,104] and Baldwin et al.[105] demonstrated specific cell mediated immune responses to outer membrane proteins in cattle.

We (Adams et al., unpublished data) have demonstrated that neither adjuvanted (MDP, TDM, and MPL in 1% squalane) *B. abortus* f5p S-LPS (11% protein) alone, native *B. abortus* outer membrane proteins 1, 2, and 3 plus 7 and 8 kilodalton proteins purified from "O"-polysaccharide-deficient (OPS⁻) *B. abortus* mutants alone, nor *E. coli*-cloned fusion products of *B. abortus* outer membrane proteins 1, 2, and 3 were protective in cattle. However, adjuvanted outer membrane protein-peptidoglycan complexes from OPS⁻ *B. abortus* mutants protected 47% of experimentally challenged cattle as compared ($p < 0.05$) to non-vaccinated controls. Brooks-Alder and Splitter[106] demonstrated that Strain 19-vaccinated cows had specific bovine blood mononuclear cell proliferative responses to SDS-PAGE-separated Western blot *Brucella* proteins in the molecular weight ranges of group 2 and 3 outer membrane proteins. We (Adams et al., unpublished data) have also demonstrated that Strain 19 vaccinated cows produce antibodies to these outer membrane proteins. However, the use of outer membrane proteins[107,108] as vaccines against enteric, but apparently not non-enteric, bacteria remains controversial,[109-112] because of 1) the difficulty of obtaining outer membrane proteins absolutely free of LPS contamination,[110,113] 2) unknown *in vivo* effects on cell envelope properties,[114] 3) shielding or inaccessibility of outer membrane proteins caused by OPS of lipopolysaccharides,[113,115] and 4) difficulty of purifying outer membrane proteins without destroying protective capacity.[110] This brief discussion of protective antigens serves to illustrate that molecular definition of *Brucella* immunogenic antigens is largely incomplete and in a state of confusion in the natural host.

Virulence Factors

The smooth lipopolysaccharide complex was identified early by Smith et al.[116,117] as being a major virulence factor in intracellular survivability. A correlation between the virulence and intracellular behavior of strains *B. abortus* and their susceptibility to H_2O_2 was demonstrated by Smith et al.[118] Frenchick[119] found that unidentified substances in water soluble extracts from virulent (Strain 2308) but not avirulent (Strain 19) strains of *Brucella abortus* inhibited phagolysomal fusion in murine macrophages. Canning and collaborators[120,121] recently demonstrated 5'-guanosine monophosphate and adenine to inhibit iodination function of bovine neutrophils. Beck et al. (this volume, abstract no. 23) reported the presence of superoxide dismutase in *Brucella* in the poster session. Glew, Ficht, Adams et al. (unpublished data) analyzed several *Brucella* spp. to find they contained unusually high concentrations of acid phosphatase similar to recent findings of Fields et al. [122] and Finlay et al.[123] They found that the genes encoding acid phosphatase (*phoP*) and its regulator (*phoN*) in *Salmonella* are inducible and linked to resistance to host defensins, thereby increasing their virulence and intracellular survivability. The fundamental nature of major *Brucella* virulence mechanisms certainly requires further elucidation.

In general, other than the smooth lipopolysaccharide complex and nucleotides, the factors for virulence of *Brucella* spp. are not understood. In summary, other than smooth lipopolysaccharide, specific immunogenic determinants have not been defined. The literature supports the concept that the host employs anti-OPS antibodies to promote clearance and phagocytosis of *Brucella* after initial infection thereby retarding but permitting "transient persistence" of bacterial proliferation so that development of longer term cell-mediated immunity can occur. Clearly, the status of knowledge of protective immunogens and virulence factors indicates that these two subjects are worthy of high research prioritization.

Strategies for Development of New Live
Brucella Vaccines

Assuming that for optimal immunity against brucellosis: 1) antibodies are required for immune clearance and 2) sensitized T-helper-cells and delayed hypersensitivity T-cells of the macrophage activating type are required for containment, killing, and elimination of *Brucella* spp., then it follows that identification of B-cell and T-cell epitopes and/or modified virulence factors for effective delivery to the host is the next logical step. Furthermore, because the predominant natural exposure in brucellosis is *per os*, oral delivery of the immunogen to the gut-associated lymphoid tissue (GALT) which stimulates generalized secretory,[124] humoral,[125] and cellular[126] immune responses may well be the optimal route for vaccination.

Identifying Virulence Factors

Availability of genetic and molecular data for the basis of pathogenicity and virulence will provide the foundation for achieving protection against diseases, such as brucellosis. Because microbial pathogenicity is a multigenic trait, dissection and identification of each factor and its genetic basis is in itself a formidable task. However, Falkow and collaborators[127-129] have succinctly and eloquently outlined a molecular strategy for the genetic analysis of bacterial pathogenesis. It is modeled after the Henle-Koch postulates and can be briefly stated as follows: 1) the phenotype or property should be associated with pathogenic strains or species of the genus, 2) specific inactivation or deletion of the gene(s) associated with the suspected virulence trait should reduce pathogenicity or virulence, and 3) reversion or allelic replacement of the mutated gene should restore pathogenicity.[127,128] Monospecific antibodies to a defined gene product that inhibits pathogenicity or virulence can be used as an acceptable alternative to the molecular Koch's postulates approach.

Recently Falkow and collaborators[129-133] used this strategy to compare homogenic bacteria differing from each other by a single determinant of pathogenicity, the ability to invade mammalian cells. They cloned the genes for pathogenic determinants using cosmid cloning vectors, thereby establishing the entire genetic library into a few hundred *E. coli* colonies. Next, the DNA fragments having the genetic segments retaining the invasive trait were identified and sequential subcloning by the use of appropriate restriction endonucleases was used to yield the smallest DNA fragment encoding the desired phenotype. Specific DNA-directed protein synthesis by the gene encoded by the smallest cloned genetic segment was then done through the minicell *in vitro* translation system. Finally they sequenced the nucleotides of the gene encoding the invasive trait to deduce the complete primary structure of the gene product.[129]

Since *Brucella* is more fastidious, this may not be as easily attained, because neither efficient bacteriophage mediated transfer systems nor plasmids have been identified. Smith and Heffron[134] used P1 bacteriophage and pDG4 plasmid; and Ficht et al. (unpublished data), who also used P1 bacteriophage were able to introduce one Tn5 insertion at a frequency of 10.[10-11] This makes reintroduction of genetic sequences into *Brucella* to fulfill the molecular Koch's postulates approach difficult but not impossible. As an adaptation of the molecular Koch's postulates approach, Finlay, Heffron, Falkow, and collaborators[122,123,135] in a series of elaborate experiments used Tn10 mutagenesis to inactivate genes encoding virulence factors detectable in an *in vitro* macrophage assay (MS or macrophage survival) to identify new inducible *Salmonella* virulence factors for adherence, invasion, and intracellular survival. While applying similar strategies to *Brucella* will not be without its difficulties, fundamental data on the genetic and molecular basis for virulence should be generated to allow development of better live *Brucella* vaccines.

Identifying B-cell and T-cell Epitopes

Neutralizing polyclonal or monoclonal antibodies are reacted with solubilized antigens from the pathogen in radioimmunoprecipitation, Western blotting, or other procedures to identify the intact native (conformational, folded, non-linear) immunogenic molecules for subsequent purification from the pathogen. Two basic approaches may then be used to identify the immunogenic B-cell epitopes. Frequently, direct amino acid sequence analysis of the native molecule may be attempted first to predict the structural antigenic determinants through computer-assisted hydropathicity analysis. These results form the basis for synthesizing a series of overlapping oligopeptides which when reacted with the neutralizing and antipeptide monoclonal antibodies in competitive inhibition assays are used to identify and map the 6 to 20 amino acid protective B-cell epitopes within the native molecule.[136,137] B-cell epitopes have also been identified by cloning the entire gene encoding the mature molecule identified from the pathogen and then subcloning and expressing overlapping segments of DNA as fusion products. The fusion products, which have the potential advantage of more natural conformational folding and glycosylation, are then reacted with the neutralizing monoclonal antibody to map the protective B-cell epitopes.[138]

For identification of T-helper-cell epitopes, peripheral blood monocytes from protected animals are stimulated in a proliferative assay with representative sections of Western blots of SDS-PAGE separated proteins of the pathogen[139] to identify intact native antigenic molecules. As in the identification of B-cell epitopes, subsequent to identifying, sequencing, computerized analysis for amphipathic helices, and synthesizing an overlapping series of oligopeptides from the identified native antigenic molecule, T-cells, preferably cloned T-helper-cells shown to be protective in adoptive transfer experiments, are stimulated with the series of oligopeptides to identify the protective T-helper-cell epitopes.[82] Because T-cells recognize fragments (or unfolded, processed forms) of the antigen molecule, only the primary sequence is usually important in defining T-cell epitopes, as contrasted with the B-cell epitopes which best recognize folded, topographic conformational determinants of the native form. Thus, it may be less difficult to analyze the T-cell epitope because all that is required is the amino acid sequence and the secondary structural features predictable by computer analysis.

Attenuation by Gene Deletion

This strategy involves the development of non-reverting avirulent *Brucella* strains having deletion mutations yet retaining virulence and colonization antigens which can colonize and persist in at least a single regional lymph node (e.g. cervical/prescapular with subcutaneous vaccination or GALT/mesenteric with oral vaccination) but with much less capacity than with field strain infection. Moreover, it will be necessary that the mutational defects be virtually impossible to be repaired under *in vivo* or *in vitro* conditions.

Several stable *Salmonella* non-virulent mutant vaccines have been developed by 1) the *Salmonella typhi galE⁻* (Ty 21a) mutant produced by Germanier and Furer[140] through nitrosoguanidine mutagenesis which was protective in man, 2) the *Salmonella typhimurium aroA* (SL1479) irreversible auxotrophic mutant produced by Hosieth and Stocker[141] through Tn10 transposon mutagenesis which was protective in mice,[141,142] sheep,[142] and cattle,[143-147] 3) the *S. typhimurium cya⁻ crp⁻* (SR-11) irreversible double deletion mutant produced by Curtiss and Kelly[148] through Tn10 transposon mutagenesis which was protective in mice, and 4) the *Shigella flexneri aroD⁻* auxotrophic mutant produced by Lindberg et al.[149] through Tn10 transposon mutagenesis which protected monkeys. The specter of reversion using attenuated living vaccines is always a matter of concern, but this possibility has been virtually eliminated by complete deletions of whole genes from the genome, particularly where double deletions of distant genes has been accomplished, thus addressing this concern (i.e. frequency of reversion <10⁻¹⁴). Clearly, these approaches to producing auxotrophic or other mutants of *Brucella* have application to live vaccine development.

Use of Attenuated Bacterial Vaccines for Antigen Delivery

The live avirulent mutant *Salmonella* vaccines mentioned above have been proven effective and safe in several species of animals, including man, sheep and cattle. A natural extension of these vaccines is to use them as delivery systems to carry foreign genes encoding protective determinants in a near-native state. This mode of delivery may be ideally suited, because B-cell epitopes, T-helper-cell epitopes, hydrophobic membrane anchoring sequences, cell growth and differentiation inducer cytokines can be incorporated into the recombinant vaccinal strain of bacteria. The major caveats to this strategy are that (a) the inserted B-cell epitopes and T-helper-cell epitopes are indeed protective, (b) adequate level of expression of the foreign protein occurs, (c) correct immunogenic form of protein is expressed, and (d) expression of the foreign gene occurs in the correct place, i.e. usually on the cell surface or secreted.

Successful examples fulfilling all or most of these criteria of this strategy include elicitation of immune responses or with protection against (a) cholera toxin as recombinant flagellin protein,[150] (b) β-galactosidase,[151] (c) malaria circumsporozoite protein,[152] (d) streptococcal colonization and virulence antigen,[142] and (e) heat labile *E. coli* enterotoxin(LT-B)[153] either administered orally or parenterally. Obviously, pending correct identification of protective *Brucella* B-cell epitopes and T-helper-cell epitopes, use of irreversible avirulent *Salmonella* (or other recombinant bacterial vectors, e.g. *E. coli* [154]) vaccine strains, as a delivery system becomes possible and offers the advantage of immunizing against brucellosis and salmonellosis simultaneously.

Use of Attenuated Viral Vectors for Antigen Delivery

Although adenoviruses, herpes simplex, varicella zoster virus, and baculovirus have been used as replicating sub-unit vectors, to date the vaccinia virus has proved to be the most successful viral vector, because of its 1) capacity to have large segments, i.e. several antigens, of DNA effectively inserted, 2) prior successful history of safe use in man, 3) broad host range, 4) utility to express a broad variety of functional antigens and cytokines in near-native form, 5) T7 bacteriophage RNA polyermase amplified foreign gene expression, and 6) successful use in animals.[155] Vaccinia however does have some disadvantages in that it may produce irritating lesions in primary recipients which in a very small percentage of vaccinates, particularly those immunocompromised, develop serious life threatening complications. Vaccinia virus recombinants for successfully protecting against viral diseases, e.g. rabies,[156] rinderpest[157] and vesicular stomatitis,[158] and bacterial diseases, e.g. diphtheria, [159] have been developed. Like the attenuated bacterial vaccine delivery system, the attenuated viral vector system for antigen delivery has the potential for developing replicating sub-unit *Brucella* vaccines. However, the same fundamental requirements are necessary, namely that 1) the inserted B-cell epitopes and T-helper-cell epitopes are indeed protective, 2) adequate level of expression of the foreign protein occurs, 3) correct immunogenic form of protein is expressed, and 4) expression of the foreign protein occurs in the correct place.

Present State of Development of New Live *Brucella* Vaccines

Attenuation by Gene Deletion

Smith and Heffron[134] through transposon mutagenesis have provided a system to define virulence factors and develop avirulent *Brucella*. Using Tn5 transposon mutagenesis and monoclonal anti-OPS side chain antibodies, we have produced a series of *B. abortus* mutants from Strain 2308 and Strain 19 selecting for OPS and non-virulent (survivability) strains in mice and *in vitro* macrophage survivability assays. Of these non-smooth mutant strains, some have been characterized to have residual splenic infection in BALB/c mice similar to Strain 19 but not to produce cross-reactive anti-OPS antibodies. Goats inoculated with two of these mutants (1 x 10⁹ cfu subcutaneously) did not produce cross-reactive anti-OPS antibodies and the mutants were not detected in urine, feces, saliva, blood, or tears weekly for 120 days or at necropsy in 40 tissues representative of the lymphoreticular and reproductive systems (Adams, L. G. and Ficht, T. A., unpublished data). Bovine macrophage survivability studies demonstrated that the two mutant strains survive intracellularly very similar to Strain 19. Long term *in vitro* passage has failed to demonstrate any reversion to virulence or smoothness and passage through mice has not revealed reversion to virulence. Pending final local, state, and federal approval, we propose to evaluate these transposon mutants as vaccines against virulent (Strain 2308) challenge in cattle under "outside-the-laboratory" quarantine confinement conditions.

Use of Attenuated Bacterial or Viral Vectors for Antigen Delivery

As previously stated, significant progress has been made on understanding the genetic relatedness of the species of *Brucella*[63-65,67,160] and the nucleotide sequence of the 16S rRNA from *B. abortus* Strain 1119 was reported to have a close relationship with *Agrobacterium tumefaciens* 16S rRNA;[161] however, this work needs to be extended to constructing a physical and genetic map of the *Brucella* genome which is prerequisite to exploiting immunogenic and virulence functions for purposes of vaccine development. Ficht et al.,[162,163] Sanborn et al.,[164] Mayfield et al.[165] Rossetti et al. (this volume, abstract no. 12), Wergifosse *et al.* (this volume abstract no. 16), Marquis et al. (this volume abstract no. 18), and Roop et al. (this volume, abstract no. 14) have isolated, by cloning, and often sequenced the nucleotide of all or portions of genes encoding several *Brucella* outer membrane proteins. Additionally Sanborn et al.[164] also have cloned a gene encoding a carbohydrate epitope of *B. abortus* LPS and demonstrated its antigenicity in mice.

Using an *E. coli* system, Ficht *et al.* expressed portions of *B. abortus* omps 1, 2, 3 and 8 kilodalton genes as fusion products which subsequently were demonstrated to be antigenic, but not protective when injected with an adjuvant into cattle (Adams et al., unpublished data). Ficht et al. (Ficht, in press) then determined the complete nucleotide sequence and flanking regions of *B. abortus* omp 2 and demonstrated that this gene or portions of it are repeated in a short sequence of *Brucella* DNA. Mayfield et al.[165] cloned and expressed with the native promoter, the complete gene for a soluble 31 kilodalton cell surface (i.e. at or near the surface) *B. abortus* membrane protein in *E. coli* which was shown to be immunogenic in mice by Bricker et al.[48] With this level of genetic and immunologic information available for several *Brucella* surface antigens, the next obvious step was to insert these genes into an attenuated bacterial or viral vaccine strain as a delivery system and evaluate the antigenicity and immunogenicity. Indeed, Stabel et al.[167] inserted the *Brucella* gene coding for the 31 kilodalton protein into the *Salmonella typhimurium cya-crp-* (4064) double deletion mutant and orally vaccinated mice and swine. Antibody specific for *Brucella* was detectable in serum and saliva of both species by day 21 and the recombinant organism persisted for over 21 days in mice and up to 14 days in swine, indicating that *Salmonella typhimurium cya- crp-* is an effective oral vaccine vector. From a mechanistic point of view for antigen delivery, these results are considered to be quite encouraging for the potential of producing new live *Brucella* vaccines. Likewise, this strategy implicitly requires that the correct immunizing epitope(s) be chosen to stimulate protective immunity, thus the continuing need to further characterize the immunizing *Brucella* molecules and their protective T-cell and B-cell epitopes.

As suggested by Mitchell[168] for cutaneous leishmaniasis, perhaps also new live vaccines for brucellosis, either recombinant or mutant in origin, should have several T-helper-cell and T-cell delayed hypersensitivity epitopes with fewer B-cell epitopes such that T-helper-cell and T-cell delayed hypersensitivity stimulation would primarily occur through macrophages and reticular cell presentation rather than B-cells, because T-cells of the macrophage-activating type are apparently required for immunity while antibodies reinforce the resistance.

Evaluation and Approval of Live *Brucella* Vaccines

InVitro Assays and *In Vivo* Assays in Laboratory Animals

It will be essential to evaluate as many aspects of potential live *Brucella* vaccines as possible under *in vitro* conditions using peripheral blood monocytes,[105,169] macrophages[122,123,135,170-172] and other tissue culture systems. Subsequent to encouraging *in vitro* results, candidate live vaccines should be evaluated in mice using a standardized procedure[99] under BL3 containment. Although a mouse model is not ideal, Plommet[99] regarded studies in mice useful as follows: 1) negative responses are correct indicators of reduced immunogenicity, 2) live vaccine immunogenicity is correctly assessed, but 3) for killed or subunit vaccines other animal models should be considered. Elberg[88] considered that "studies in which the mouse spleen is accepted as the index for the animal's response to infection and then only for very short periods postchallenge, suggest that the immunity referred to in much current research is ephemeral, in which only superinfection is being studied. Such work, while of great interest for itself, is of little guidance in translating to the natural infection in the natural host." Laboratory animal studies may be used for purposes of guidance in selecting vaccine candidates, but not for a direct indication of protective immunity in the natural host.

Primary Host Species

Ultimately evaluation of live mutant or recombinant *Brucella* vaccines in the natural host species using a standardized virulent challenge protocol will be required, which in the case of larger livestock species becomes problematic from the standpoint of long-term (i.e. up to 365 days for cattle) BL3 containment for adequate numbers of pregnant animals to allow valid statistical comparisons. Guidelines have been proposed for conducting such studies under "outside-the-laboratory" quarantine confinement conditions which, following an environmental assessment, await final local, state, and federal approval (Adams et al., USDA, Office of Agricultural Biotechnology, Agricultural Biotechnology Research Advisory Committee Hearing, Washington, D. C., Jan. 1989).

Conclusions

As a basis of departure in this review , I have strived to present a historical perspective of current live *Brucella* vaccines and their disadvantages as they relate to modern vaccine development strategies. Studies of cross-immunity and genetic relatedness imply the general hierarchy of immunizing capacity to be *B. melitensis* (*B. neotomae* ?) ≥ *B. suis* > *B. abortus*. This unifying and converging concept encourages the possibility of developing a live vaccine that will protect against all species of *Brucella* in their natural hosts. Certainly the safety and protective capacity requirements will be higher for new live *Brucella* vaccines and much better genetic definition of the vaccine strains will be necessary.

Before new approaches to vaccine development are undertaken, several questions fundamental to the host-parasite interaction resulting in either acquired immunity or disease should be answered. However, without a fundamental understanding of the pathogenesis of infection and the basic immunologic response during the infection and disease processes, vaccine development will be plagued with difficulties and adverse conditions, especially when a long-term immunity is desired. Identification and understanding of virulence determinants and the role they play in pathogenic mechanisms is crucial in developing vaccines to inhibit the natural process of infection. Identification of immunizing B-cell and T-helper-cell immunodominant epitopes is tantamount to significantly improving recombinant vaccines as well as the immunogenic antigens (matched B-cell and T-helper-cell epitopes) of new vaccines being presented appropriately to be properly recognized to induce optimal long-term immunity.

Molecular definition of *Brucella* immunogenic antigens is largely incomplete and in a state of confusion in the natural host. Other than the smooth lipopolysaccharide complex and nucleotides, the factors for virulence of *Brucella* spp. are not understood. Clearly, the status of knowledge of protective immunogens and virulence factors indicates that these two subjects are worthy of high research priority. Strategies for determining virulence factors and molecular characterization of B-cell and T-cell epitopes of immunogens are presented. Strategies for attenuation of *Brucella* by mutagenesis and construction of replicating sub-unit *Brucella* vaccines using existing bacterial or viral vaccine strains as an antigen delivery system are presented. Finally, in spite of the lack of fundamental knowledge of the genetic and molecular basis for virulence and immunogenicity, results from recent progress in the development and evaluation of new live *Brucella* vaccines demonstrate that the possibility of producing improved live vaccines has now become a probability.

References

1. Bang B. Infectious abortion in cattle. *J Comp Pathol* 1906;19:191-202.
2. Cunningham B. Brucellosis Symposium. Part III. Vaccines and brucellosis. *Ir Vet J* 1968;22:128-131.
3. Buck JM. Studies of vaccination during calfhood to prevent bovine infectious abortion. *J Agric Res* 1930;41:667-689.
4. McEwen AD, Roberts RS. Bovine contagious abortion. The use of guinea-pigs in immunisation studies. *J Comp Pathol Ther* 1936;49:97-117.
5. Huddleson IF, Bennett GR. The vaccinal immunizing value of a mucoid-growth phase of *Brucella suis* against brucellosis in cattle. *Mich St Coll Agric Exp Sta Bull* 1948;31:139-156.
6. Sieiro F, Rosenbusch C. Comparative immunity experiments in cattle using live vaccines prepared from nonagglutinogenic and agglutinogenic *Brucella abortus* strains. *Am J Vet Res* 1952;13:476-485.
7. Elberg SS, Faunce Jr K. Immunization against *Brucella* infection. VI. Immunity conferred on goats by a non-dependent mutant from a streptomycin-dependent mutant strain of *Brucella melitensis*. *J Bacteriol* 1957;73:211-217.
8. Van Drimmelen GC, Horwell FD. Preliminary findings with the use of *Brucella melitensis* Strain Rev. I as a vaccine against brucellosis in cattle. *Bull Off Int Epizoot* 1964;62:987-995.
9. Xin X. Orally administratable brucellosis vaccine: *Brucella suis* Strain 2 vaccine. In: eds. *Vaccine 86.* 1989;212-216.
10. Graves RR. Story of John M. Buck's and Matilda's contribution to the cattle industry. *J Am Vet Med Assoc* 1943;102:193-195.
11. Cotton WE, Buck JM, Smith HE. Efficacy and safety of abortion vaccines prepared from *Brucella abortus* strains of different degrees of virulence. *J Agric Res* 1933;46:291-314.
12. Cotton WE, Buck JM, Smith HE. Further studies of vaccination during calfhood to prevent Bang's disease. *J Am Vet Med Assoc* 1934;85:389-397.
13. Haring CM, Traum J. Observations of pathogenic and antigenic effects of *Brucella abortus*, United States Bureau of Animal Industry Strain 19. *J Agric Res* 1937;55:117-128.
14. Berman DT, Beach BA, Irwin MR. A comparison of the effects of subcutaneous and intracaudal vaccination of sexually mature cattle with *Brucella abortus* Strain 19. *Am J Vet Res* 1954;15:406-411.
15. Manthei CA. Evaluation of vaccinal methods and doses of *Brucella abortus* Strain 19. *Proc Annu Meet US Livestock Sanit Assoc* 1952;56:115-125.
16. Manthei CA, Mingle CK, Carter RW. Duration of immunity to brucellosis induced in cattle with Strain 19 vaccine. *Proc Annu Meet Am Vet Med Assoc* 1951;88:128-141.
17. Manthei CA, Mingle CK, Carter RW. Comparison of immunity and agglutinin response in cattle vaccinated with *Brucella abortus* Strain 19 by the intradermal and subcutaneous methods. *Proc Annu Meet US Livestock Sanit Assoc* 1952;56:100-114.
18. Crawford AB. Vaccination against bovine brucellosis. *J Am Vet Med Assoc* 1947;110:99-102.

19. Lawson JR. Strain 19 and the control of brucellosis. *Vet Rec* 1950;62:823-830.
20. Mingle CK, Manthei CA, Jasmin AM. The stability of reduced virulence exhibited by *Brucella abortus* strain 19. *J Am Vet Med Assoc* 1941;78:208-209.
21. Deyoe BL, Dorsey, TA. Immunogenicity of reduced dosages if *Brucella abortus* Strain 19 in cattle vaccinated as calves. Unpublished data.
22. McDiarmid A. The degree and duration of immunity in cattle resulting from vaccination with S19 *B. abortus* and its implication in the future control and eventual eradication of brucellosis. *Vet Rec* 1957;69:877-879.
23. Deyoe BL, Dorsey TA, Meredith K, et al. Reduced doses of *Brucella abortus* in cattle. USAHA 1980;163-163.
24. Alton GG, Corner LA, Plackett P. Vaccination of pregnant cows with low doses of *Brucella abortus* Strain 19 vaccine. Aust Vet J 1980;56:369-372.
25. Deyoe BL, Dorsey RH, Meredith KB, et al. Effect of reduced dosage of *Brucella abortus* Strain 19 in cattle vaccinated as yearlings. Proc Annu Meet US Animal Health Assoc 1979;83:92-104.
26. Nicoletti P. A preliminary report on the efficacy of adult cattle vaccination using Strain 19 in selected dairy herds in Florida. Proc Annu Meet US Animal Health Assoc 1976;80:91-106.
27. Nicoletti P, Jones LM, Berman DT. Adult vaccination with standard and reduced doses of *Brucella abortus* Strain 19 vaccine in a dairy herd infected with brucellosis. J Am Vet Med Assoc 1978;173:1445-1449.
28. Nicoletti P, Jones LM, Berman DT. Comparison of the subcutaneous and conjunctival route of vaccination with *Brucella abortus* Strain 19 vaccine in adult cattle. J Am Vet Med Assoc 1978;73:1450-1456.
29. Nicoletti P. The effects of adult cattle vaccination with Strain 19 on the incidence of brucellosis in dairy herds in Florida and Puerto Rico. Proc Annu Meet US Animal Health Assoc 1979;83:75-80.
30. Barton CE, Lomme JR. Reduced-dose whole herd vaccination against brucellosis: a review of recent experience. J Am Vet Med Assoc 1980;177:1218-1220.
31. Alton GG. Recent developments in vaccination against bovine brucellosis. Aust Vet J 1978;54:551-557.
32. Worthington RW, Mulders MSG, McFarlane IS, et al. A serological investigation on adult cattle vaccinated with *Brucella abortus* Strain 19. Onderstepoort J Vet Res 1973;40:7-12.
33. Haring CM, Traum JT. The effect of *Brucella abortus* Strain 19 on cattle of various ages and its bearing on adult cattle vaccination. Proc Annu Meet US Livestock Sanit Assoc 1943;47:42-46.
34. Hisatsune K, Kondo S, IguChi T, et al. Sugar composition of lipopolysaccharides of family Vibrionaceae. Absence of 2-keto-3-deoxyoctonate (KDO) except in *Vibrio parahaemolyticus* O6. Microbiol Immunol 1982;26:649-664.
35. Manthei C. Summary of controlled research with strain 19. Proc Annu Meet US Livestock Sanit Assoc 1959;63:91-97.
36. Davies G, Cocks E, Hebert N. *Brucella abortus* (Strain 19) vaccine: (a) determination of the minimum protective dose in cattle; (b) the effect of vaccinating calves previously inoculated with anti-*Brucella abortus* serum. J Biol Stand 1980;8:165-175.
37. Haring CM, Traum J, Maderious WE. Vaccination against brucellosis. J Am Vet Med Assoc 1947;110:103-107.
38. Corner LA, Alton GG. Persistence of *Brucella abortus* Strain 19 infection in adult cattle vaccinated with reduced doses. Res Vet Sci 1981;31:342-344.
39. Thomas EL, Bracewell CD, Corbel MJ. Characterization of *Brucella abortus* strain 19 cultures isolated from vaccinated cattle. Vet Res 1981;108:90-93.
40. Elberg SS, Fitzhugh HA, King, NB, et al. *Brucellosis Research: An Evaluation.* Washington, DC: National Academy of Sciences, 1977.

41. Crawford RP, Heck FC, Williams JD. Experiences with *Brucella abortus* strain 19 vaccine in adult Texas cattle. J Am Vet Med Assoc 1979;173:1457-1461.

42. Brown GM, Love EL, Pietz DE, et al. Characterization of *Brucella abortus* Strain 19. Am J Vet Res 1972;33:759-764.

43. Pearce JH, Williams AE, Harris-Smith PW, et al. The chemical basis of virulence of *Brucella abortus*. II. Erythritol, a constituent of bovine foetal fluids which stimulates the growth of *Brucella abortus* in bovine phagocytes. Br J Exp Pathol 1962;43:31-37.

44. Jones LM, Montgomery V, Wilson JB. Characteristics of carbon dioxide-independent cultures of *Brucella abortus* isolated from cattle vaccinated with Strain 19. J Infect Dis 1965;115:312-320.

45. Meyer ME. Metabolic characterization of the genus *Brucella* V. Relationship of strain oxidation rate of l-erythritol to strain virulence for guinea pigs. J Bacteriol 1966;92:584-588.

46. McEwen AD. The virulence of *B. abortus* for laboratory animals and pregnant cattle. Vet Rec 1940;52:97-106.

47. Taylor PW. Bactericidal and bacteriolytic activity of serum against gram-negative bacteria. Microbiol Rev 1983;47:46-83.

48. Diaz R, Jones LM. The immuno-diffusion method for the identification of cattle vaccinated with *Brucella abortus* Strain 45/20. Vet Rec 1973;93:300-302.

49. Corbel MJ. The immune response to *Brucella abortus* 45/20 adjuvant vaccine in terms of immunoglobulin class. Dev Biol Stand 1975;31:141-144.

50. Alton GG, Elberg SS, Crouch D. *Brucella melitensis* vaccine. The stability of the degree of attenuation. J Comp Pathol 1967;77:293-300.

51. Alton GG, Elberg SS. Rev. I. *Brucella melitensis* vaccine. A review of ten years of study. Vet Bull 1967;37:793-800.

52. Alton GG. Duration of the immunity produced by Rev. I. *Brucella melitensis* vaccine. J Comp Pathol 1966;76:241-253.

53. Alton GG. Control of *Brucella melitensis* infection in sheep and goats - a review. Trop Anim Health Prod 1987;19:65-74.

54. Jones LM, Entessar F, Ardalan A. Comparison of living vaccines in producing immunity against natural *Brucella melitensis* infection in sheep and goats. J Comp Pathol 1964;74:17-30.

55. Morgan WJB, Littlejohn AI, Mackinnon DJ, et al. The degree of protection given by living vaccines against experimental infection in goats. Bulletin/WHO 1966;34:33-40.

56. Bosseray N, Plommet M. Souche vaccinale *B. suis* 2. Virulence, immunogenicite, caracteres marqueurs. FAO/WHO Meeting on Oral/Conjunctival Brucellosis Vaccine 1988;2.

57. Garcia-Carrillo CB. *B. suis* Strain 2 vaccine. FAO/WHO Meeting on Oral/Conjunctival Brucellosis Vaccine 1988.

58. MacMillan AP, Gill KPW. Differentiation of *B. suis* Strain 2 from field strains. FAO/WHO Meeting on Oral/Conjunctival Brucellosis Vaccine 1988.

59. Mustafa AA. Field oriented trial of the Chinese *B. suis* Strain 2. vaccine in Libya. FAO/WHO Meeting on Oral/Conjunctival Brucellosis Vaccine 1988.

60. Washko FW, HutChings LM, Donham CR. Studies on the pathogenicity of *Brucella suis* for cattle. Am J Vet Res 1948;8:343-349.

61. Washko FW, HutChings LM. Susceptibility of cattle to *Brucella suis* following vaccination with *Brucella abortus* Strain 19. Am J Vet Res 1952;13:24-25.

62. Manthei CA. Research on swine brucellosis by the Bureau of Animal Industry. Am J Vet Res 1948;9:40-43.

63. Verger JM, Grimont F, Grimont PAD, et al. *Brucella*, a monospecific genus as shown by deoxyribonucleic acid hybridization. Int J System Bacteriol 1985;35:292-295.

64. Hoyer BH, McCullough NB. Polynucleotide homologies of *Brucella* deoxyribonucleic acids. *J Bacteriol* 1968;95:444-448.
65. O'Hara MJ, Collins DM, DeLisle GW. Restriction endonuclease analysis of *Brucella ovis* and other *Brucella* species. *Vet Microbiol* 1985;10:425-429.
66. Allardet-Servent A, Bourg G, Ramuz M, et al. DNA polymorphism in strains of the genus *Brucella*. *J Bacteriol* 1988;170:4603-4607.
67. Muzny DM, Ficht TA, Templeton JW, et al. DNA homology of *Brucella abortus* Strains 19 and 2308. *Am J Vet Res* 1989;50:
68. Bricker BJ, Tabatabai LB, Deyoe BL, et al. Conservation of antigenicity of a 31-kDa *Brucella* Protein. *Vet Microbiol* 1988;18:313-325.
69. Olitzki AL. Studies on the antigenic structure and virulent and non-virulent Brucellae with the aid of the agar gel precipitating technique. *Br J Exp Pathol* 1959;40:432-440.
70. Dubray G. Protective antigens in brucellosis. *Ann Inst Pasteur (Microbiol)* 1987;138:84-87.
71. Dougan G, Smith L, Heffron F. Live bacterial vaccines and their application as carriers for foreign antigens. In: Bittle JL, Murphy FA, eds. *Vaccine Biotechnology*. New York:Academic Press, 1989;271-273.
72. Spink WW, Hall JW, Finstad J, et al. Immunization with live *Brucella* organisms: results of safety test in humans. *Bull WHO* 1962;26:409-420.
73. Spink WW, Thompson H. Human brucellosis caused by *Brucella abortus*, Strain 19. *JAMA* 1953;153:1162-1165.
74. Human brucellosis due to Strain 19. *J Am Vet Med Assoc* 1974;165:989.
75. Plastridge WN. Bovine brucellosis: a review of the literature on diagnosis and control. *Proc Annu Meet US Livestock Sanit Assoc* 1954;58:135-179.
76. Matyas Z, Fujikura T. Brucellosis as a world problem. In: Valette L, Hennesen W, eds. *Developments in Biological Standardization*. Karger, Switzerland;1984:3-20.
77. Alton GG, Plommet M. Brucellosis summit in Geneva. *WHO Chron* 1986;40:19-21.
78. Kaplan MM. A summary of the present status of brucellosis. *WHO Chron* 1950;5:1-4.
79. Brown MR, Anwar H, Costerton JW. Surface antigens *in vivo*: a mirror for vaccine development. *Can J Microbiol* 1988;34:494-498.
80. Ellwood DC, Tempest DW. Effects of environment on bacterial cell wall contect and composition. *Adv Microb Physiol* 1972;7:83-117.
81. Ada GL. Antigen presentation and enhancement of immunity: An introduction. In: Brown H, Chanock RM, Lerner RA, eds. *Vaccines 86*. New York:Cold Spring Harbor Laboratory, 1986;105-108.
82. Berzofsky JA. Immunodominance of T-cell epitopes: Applications to vaccine design. In: Lerner RA, Ginsberg H, Chanock RM, et al, eds. *Vaccines 89*. New York:Cold Spring Harbor Laboratory, 1989;27-31.
83. Schwartz RH. The role of gene products of the major histocompatibility complex in T-cell activation and cellular events. In: Paul WE, ed. *Fundamental Immunology*. New York:Raven Press, 1984;379.
84. Nestorowicz AG, Laver G, Jackson DC. Antigenic determinants of influenza virus hemagglutinin. X. A comparison of the physical and antigenic properties of monomeric and trimeric forms. *J Gen Virol* 1985;65:1687-1693.
85. Murphy BR. Summary. In: Lerner RA, Ginsberg H, Chanock RM, et al, eds. *Vaccines 89*. New York:Cold Spring Harbor Laboratory, 1989;27-31.
86. Kaneene JM, Nicoletti P, Anderson RK, et al. Cell-mediated immune responses in cattle adult-vaccinated with *Brucella abortus* Strain 19 and in cattle infected with *Brucella abortus* field strain. *Am J Vet Res* 1979;40:1503-1509.
87. Mandecki W. Oligonucleotide-directed double-strand break repair in plasmids of *Escherichia coli:* a method for site-specific mutagenesis. *Proc Natl Acad Sci*

USA 1986;83:7177-7181.

88.   Elberg SS. Immunity to *Brucella* infection. *Medicine (Baltimore)* 1973;52:339-356.

89.   Wilkinson R, Cargill C, Lee K. Humoral and cell-mediated immune responses in non-pregnant heifers following infection and vaccination with *Brucella abortus.* *Vet Immunol Immunopathol* 1988;18:379-383.

90.   Corbel M. Recent advances in the study of *Brucella* antigens and their serological cross-reactions. *Vet Bull* 1985;55:927-942.

91.   Verstreate DR, Creasy MT, Caveney NT, et al. Outer membrane proteins of *Brucella abortus:* isolation and characterization. *Infect Immun* 1982;35:979-989.

92.   Winter AJ, Verstreate DR, Hall CE, et al. Immune response to porin in cattle immunized with whole cell, outer membrane, and outer membrane protein antigens of *Brucella abortus* combined with trehalose dimycolate and muramyl dipeptide adjuvants. *Infect Immun* 1983;42:1159-1167.

93.   Santos JM, Verstreate DR, Perera VY, et al. Outer membrane proteins from rough strains of four *Brucella* species. *Infect Immun* 1984;46:188-194.

94.   Verstreate DR, Winter AJ. Comparison of sodium dodecyl sulfate-polyacrylamide gel electrophoresis profiles and antigenic relatedness among outer membrane proteins of 49 *Brucella abortus* strains. *Infect Immun* 1984;46:182-187.

95.   Douglas JT, Rosenberg EY, Nikaido H, et al. Porins of *Brucella* species. *Infect Immun* 1984;44:16-21.

96.   Moriyon I, Gamazo C, Diaz R. Properties of the outer membrane of *Brucella*. *Ann Inst Pasteur (Microbiol)* 1987;138:89-91.

97.   Gomez-Miguel MJ, Moriyon I, Lopez J. *Brucella* outer membrane lipoprotein shares antigenic determinants with *Escherichia coli* Braun lipoprotein and is exposed on the cell surface. *Infect Immun* 1987;55:258-262.

98.   Plommet M. Brucellosis and immunity: humoral and cellular components in mice. *Ann Inst Pasteur (Microbiol)* 1987;138:105-110.

99.   Plommet M, Serre A, Fensterbank R. Vaccines, vaccination in brucellosis. *Ann Inst Pasteur (Microbiol)* 1987;138:117-121.

100.   Winter AJ, Rowe GE, Duncan JR, et al. Effectiveness of natural and synthetic complexes of porin and O polysaccharide as vaccines against *Brucella abortus* in mice. *Infect Immun* 1988;56:2808-2817.

101.   Montaraz JA, Winter AJ. Comparison of living and nonliving vaccines for *Brucella abortus* in BALB/c mice. *Infect Immun* 1986;53:245-251.

102.   Montaraz JA, Winter AJ, Hunter DM, et al. Protection against *Brucella abortus* in mice with O-polysaccharide- specific monoclonal antibodies. *Infect Immun* 1986;51:961-963.

103.   Limet J, Plommet A, Dubray G, et al. Immunity conferred upon mice by anti-LPS monoclonal antibodies in murine brucellosis. *Ann Inst Pasteur (Immunol)* 1987;138:417-424.

104.   Winter AJ, Rowe GE. Comparative immune responses to native cell envelope antigens and the hot sodium dodecyl sulfate insoluble fraction (PG) of *Brucella abortus* in cattle and mice. *Vet Immunol Immunopathol* 1988;18:149-163.

105.   Baldwin CL, Verstreate DR, Winter AJ. Immune response of cattle to *Brucella abortus* outer membrane proteins measured by lymphocyte blastogenesis. *Vet Immunol Immunopathol* 1985;9:383-396.

106.   Brooks-Alder B, Splitter GA. Determination of bovine lymphocyte responses to extracted proteins of *Brucella abortus* by using protein immunoblotting. *Infect Immun* 1988;56:2581-2586.

107.   Brass JM. The cell envelope of gram-negative bacteria: new aspects of its function in transport and chemotaxis. *Curr Top Microbiol Immunol* 1986;129:1-92.

108.   Benz R. Structure and function of porins from gram-negative bacteria. *Annu Rev Microbiol* 1988;42:359-393.

109.   Gilleland HE JR, Parker MG, Matthews JM, et al. Use of a purified outer

membrane protein F (porin) preparation of *Pseudomonas aeruginosa* as a protective vaccine in mice. *Infect Immun* 1984;44:49-54.

110. Teale AJ, Baldwin CL, Ellis JA, et al. Alloreactive bovine T lymphocyte clones: an analysis of function, phenotype, and specificity. *J Immunol* 1986;136:4392-4398.

111. Kuusi N, Nurminen M, Saxen H, et al. Immunization with major outer membrane proteins in experimental salmonellosis of mice. *Infect Immun* 1979;25:857-862.

112. Gilleland HE, Matthews-Greer JM. Perspectives on the potential for successful development of outer membrane protein vaccines. *Eur J Clin Microbiol* 1987;6:231-233.

113. Wilke-Greiser I, Moennig V, Thon D, et al. Characterization of monoclonal antibodies against *Brucella melitensis*. *Zentralbl Veterinarmed [B]* 1985;32:616-627.

114. Brown MRW, Williams P. The influence of environment on envelope properties affecting survival of bacteria in infections. *Annu Rev Microbiol* 1985;39:527-556.

115. Roy S, Scherer MT, Briner TJ, et al. Murine MHC polymorphism and T cell specificities. *Science* 1989;244:572-575.

116. Fitzgeorge RB, Solotorovsky M, Smith H. The behavior of *Brucella abortus* within macrophages separated from the blood of normal and immune cattle by adherence to glass. *Br J Exp Pathol* 1967;48:522-528.

117. Smith H, Fitzgeorge RB. The chemical basis of the virulence of *Brucella abortus* V. The basis of intracellular survival and growth in bovine phagocytes. *Br J Exp Pathol* 1964;45:174-186.

118. Smith H. Mechanisms of microbial pathogenicity. *Sci Basis Med Annu Rev* 1968;24:53-70.

119. Frenchick PJ, Markham RJF, Cochrane AH. Inhibition of phagosome-lysosome fusion in macrophages by soluble extracts of virulent *Brucella abortus*. *Am J Vet Res* 1985;46:332-335.

120. Canning PC, Roth JA, Deyoe BL. Release of 5'-guanosine monophosphate and adenine by *Brucella abortus* and their role in the intracellular survival of the bacteria. *J Infect Dis* 1986;154:464-470.

121. Bertram T, Canning P, Roth J. Preferential inhibition of primary granule release from bovine neutrophils by a *Brucella abortus* extract. *Infect Immun* 1986;52:285-292.

122. Fields PI, Groisman EA, Heffron F. A *Salmonella* locus that controls resistance to microbicidal proteins from phagocytic cells. *Science* 1989;243:1059-1062.

123. Finlay BB, Heffron F, Falkow S. Epithelial cell surfaces induce *Salmonella* proteins required for bacterial adherence and invasion. *Science* 1989;243:940-943.

124. Elson CO, Ealding W. Generalized systemic and mucosal immunity in mice after mucosal stimulation with cholera toxin. *J Immunol* 1984;132:2736-2741.

125. McCaughan G, Basten A. Immune system of the gastrointestinal tract. *Int Rev Physiol* 1983;28:131-157.

126. Brown A, Hormaeche CE, Demarco de Hormaeche R, et al. An attenuated aroA *Salmonella typhimurium* vaccine elicits humoral and cellular immunity to cloned beta-galactosidase in mice. *J Infect Dis* 1987;155:86-92.

127. Falkow S. Molecular Koch's postulates applied to microbial pathogenicity. *Rev Infect Dis* 1988;10:S274-S276.

128. Falkow S, Small P, Isberg R, et al. A molecular strategy for the study of bacterial invasion. *Rev Infect Dis* 1987;9:S450-S455.

129. Weiss AA, Falkow S. The use of molecular techniques to study microbial determinants of pathogenicity. *Philos Trans R Soc Lond [Biol]* 1983;219-225.

130. Isberg RR, Falkow S. A single genetic locus encoded by *Yersinia pseudotuberculosis* permits invasion of cultured animal cells by *Escherichia coli* K-12. *Nature* 1985;317:262-264.

131. Miller VL, Falkow S. Evidence for two genetic loci in *Yersinia enterocolitica* that

can promote invasion of epithelial cells. *Infect Immun* 1988;56:1242-1248.

132. Isberg RR, Voorhis DL, Falkow S. Identification of invasin: a protein that allows enteric bacteria to penetrate cultured mammalian cells. *Cell* 1987;50:769-778.

133. Small P, Isberg R, Falkow S. Comparison of the ability of enteroinvasive *Escherichia coli, Salmonella typhimurium, Yersinia pseudotuberculosis,* and *Yersinia enterocolitica* to enter and replicate within Hep-2 cells. *Infect Immun* 1987;55:1674-1679.

134. Smith LD, Heffron F. Transposon Tn5 mutagenesis of *Brucella abortus*. *Infect Immun* 1987;55:2774-2776.

135. Fields PI, Haidaris CG, Swanson RV, et al. Virulence determinants of *Salmonella* required for survival in macrophages. In: Brown F, Chanock RM, Lerner RA, eds. *Vaccines 86*. New York: Cold Spring Harbor Laboratory, 1986;205-211.

136. Houghten RA. Facile determination of exact amino acid involvement in peptide antigen-monoclonal antibody interactions. In: Chanock RM, Lerner RA, Brown F, et al, eds. *Vaccines 87*. New York:Cold Spring Harbor Laboratory, 1987;1-6.

137. Berzofsky JA. Intrinsic and extrinsic factors in antigenic structure. *Science* 1985;229:932-934.

138. Putney SD, Rusche JR, Javaherian K, et al. Mapping of the principal human immunodeficiency virus neutralizing epitope. In: Ginsberg HS, Brown F, Lerner RA, et al, eds. *Vaccines 88*. New York:Cold Harbor Springs Laboratory, 1988;253-258.

139. Young DB, Lamb JR. T lymphocytes respond to solid-phase antigen: A novel approach to the molecular analysis of cellular immunity. *Immunology* 1986;59:167-171.

140. Germanier R, Furer E. Isolation and characterization of Gal E Mutant TY 21a of *Salmonella typhi:* a candidate strain for a live, oral typhoid vaccine. *J Infect Dis* 1975;131:553-558.

141. Hoiseth SK, Stocker BAD. Aromatic-dependent *Salmonella typhimurium* are non-virulent and effective as live vaccines. *Nature* 1981;291:238-239.

142. Mukkur TK, McDowell GH, Stocker BAD, et al. Protection against experimental salmonellosis in mice and sheep by immunisation with aromatic-dependent *Salmonella typhimurium. Med Microbiol* 1987;24:11-19.

143. Smith BP, Reina-Guerra M, Hoiseth SK, et al. Aromatic-dependent *Salmonella typhimurium* as modified live vaccines for calves. *Am J Vet Res* 1984;45:59-66.

144. Smith BP, Reina-Guerra M, Stocker BAD, et al. Vaccination of calves against *Salmonella dublin* with aromatic-dependent *Salmonella typhimurium. Am J Vet Res* 1984;45:1858-1861.

145. Lindberg AA, Robertsson JA. *Salmonella typhimurium* infection in calves: cell-mediated and humoral immune reactions before and after challenge with live virulent bacteria in calves given live or inactivated vaccines. *Infect Immun* 1983;41:751-757.

146. Robertsson JA, Lindberg AA, Hoiseth S, et al. *Salmonella typhimurium* infection in calves: protection and survival of virulent challenge bacteria after immunization with live or inactivated vaccines. *Infect Immun* 1983;41:742-750.

147. Curtiss R, Goldschmidt RM, Fletchall NB, et al. Avirulent *Salmonella typhimurium* delta-*cya* oral vaccine strains expressing a streptococcal colonization and virulence antigen. In: Ginsberg H, Brown F, Lerner RA, et al, eds. *Vaccines 88*. Washington, DC: American Society for Microbiology, 1988;155-160.

148. Curtiss III R, Kelly SM. *Salmonella typhimurium* deletion mutants lacking adenylate cyclase and cyclic AMP receptor proteins are avirulent and immunogenic. *Infect Immun* 1987;55:3035-3042.

149. Lindberg AA, Karnell A, Stocker BAD, et al. Development of an auxotrophic oral live *Shigella flexneri* vaccine. In: Ginsberg H, Brown F, Lerner RA, et al, eds. *Vaccine 88*. Washington, DC: American Society for Microbiology, 1988;146-150.

150. Newton SMC, Jacob CO, Stocker BAD. Immune response to cholera toxin epitope inserted in *Salmonella flagellin. Science* 1989;244:70-72.

151. Dougan G, Hormaeche CE, Makell DJ. Live oral *Salmonella* vaccines: potential use of attenuated strains as carriers of heterologous antigens to the immune system. *Parasite Immunol* 1987;9:151-160.

152. Sadoff JC, Ballou WR, Baron LS, et al. Oral *Salmonella typhimurium* vaccine expressing circumsporozoite protein protects against malaria. *Science* 1988;240:336-338.

153. Clements JD. Use of mutants of *Salmonella* as vaccine vectors. In: Lerner RA, Ginsberg H, Chanock RM, et al, eds. *Vaccines 89*. New York:Cold Spring Harbor Laboratory, 1989;283-289.

154. Charbit A, Boulain JC, Ryter A, et al. Stable expression of a eukaryotic epitope at the surface of *Escherichia coli* and the construction of "exposition vectors." In: Chanock RM, Lerner RA, Brown F, et al, eds. *Vaccines 87*. New York:Cold Spring Harbor Laboratory, 1987;68-71.

155. Ginsberg HS. Summary. In: Chanock RM, Lerner RA, Brown F, et al, eds. *Vaccines 87*. New York:Cold Spring Harbor Laboratory, 1987;441-444.

156. Kieny MP, Lathe R, Drillien R, et al. Expression of rabies virus glycoprotein from a recombinant vaccinia virus. *Nature* 1984;312:163-166.

157. Yilma T, Hsu D, Jones L, et al. Expression of rinderpest genes in vaccinia virus recombinations: Protective immunization of cattle. In: Lerner RA, Ginsberg HS, Chanock RM, et al, eds. *Vaccines 89*. New York:Cold Spring Harbor Laboratory, 1989;383-386.

158. Mackett M, Yilma T, Rose JK, et al. Vaccinia virus recombinants: expression of VSV genes and protective immunization of mice and cattle. *Science* 1985;227:433-435.

159. Phalipon A, Kaczorek M. Presentation of viral epitopes on diphtheria toxin: A potential bivalent vaccine. In: Ginsberg HS, Chanock RM, Brown F, et al, eds. *Vaccine 89*. New York:Cold Spring Harbor Laboratory, 1989;463-471.

160. Allardet-Servent A, Bourg G, Ramuz M, et al. DNA polymorphisms in strains of the genus *Brucella. J Bacteriol* 1988;170:4603-4607.

161. Dorsch M, Moreno E, Stackebrandt E. Nucleotide sequence of 16S rRNA from *B. abortus. Nucleic Acids Res* 1989;17:1765-1765.

162. Sanborn, MR, Sherwood, JL, Keyser, GC, et al.: Cloning and expression of *Brucella abortus* outer membrane protein genes in *E. coli*. Abst D-50 Annual Mtg, ASM, pg 80, 1987.

163. Ficht TA, Bearden SW, Sowa BA, et al. A 36-kilodalton *Brucella abortus* cell-envelope protein is encoded by repeated sequences closely linked in the genomic DNA. *Infect Immun* 1988;56:2036-2046.

164. Sanborn, M.R., Sherwood, J. L., Keyser, G. C., et al. Cloning and expression of a carbohydrate epitope of *Brucella abortus* LPS, in *E. coli*, and its use as a subunit vaccine in mice. Abst. Annual Mtg. ASM, 1988.

165. Mayfield J, Bricker B, Godfrey H, et al. The cloning, expression, and nucleotide sequence of a gene coding for an immunogenic *Brucella abortus* protein. *Gene* 1988;63:1-9.

166. Sanborn MR, Sherwood JL, Keyser GC, et al. Cloning and expression of a carbohydrate epitope of *Brucella abortus* LPS, in *E. coli*, and its use as a subunit vaccine in mice. *ASM* p. 112, 1988.

167. Broes A, Fairbrother JM, Larivière S, et al. Virulence properties of enterotoxigenic *Escherichia coli* O8:KX105 strains isolated from diarrheic piglets. *Infect Immun* 1988;56:241-246.

168. Mitchell GF. Injection versus infection: the cellular immunology of parasitism. *Parasitol Today* 1987;3:106-111.

169. Stephan RN, Conrad PJ, Saizawa M, et al. Prostaglandin E2 depresses antigen-

presenting cell function of peritoneal macrophages. *J Surg Res* 1988;44:733-739.

170.	Harmon BG, Adams LG, Frey M. Survival of rough and smooth strains of *Brucella abortus* in bovine mammary gland macrophages. *Am J Vet Res* 1988;49:1092-1097.

171.	Harmon BG, Templeton JW, Crawford RP, et al. Macrophage function and immune response of *Brucella abortus* naturally resistant and susceptible cattle. In: Skamene E, ed. *Genetic Control of Host Resistance to Infection and Malignancy.* New York:Alan R. Liss, Inc., 1985;345-354.

172.	Harmon BG, Adams LG. Assessment of bovine mammary gland macrophage oxidative burst activity in a chemiluminescence assay. *Am J Vet Res* 1987;48:119-125.

Chapter Eighteen

Regulatory Policies for Field Testing Experimental Recombinant- Derived Veterinary Biological Products

David A. Espeseth and

George P. Shibley

Recent advances in molecular and cellular biotechnology have made possible the production of veterinary viral or bacterial vaccines by means of recombinant DNA (rDNA). The establishment of appropriate procedures for regulating the commercialization of these emerging rDNA products is a national and international issue which has been debated extensively in all countries where this technology is developing. This paper will discuss the current policy and processes that have been established for the regulation of these products within the United States Department of Agriculture (USDA) and more specifically within Biotechnology, Biologics, and Environmental Protection (BBEP) of the Animal and Plant Health Inspection Service (APHIS).

Regulation of rDNA-derived products is based on the principle that these products are not significantly different from similar products produced by conventional methods. Thus, existing statutes[1] provide a basic network of agency jurisdiction over both research activities and licensure of veterinary biological products. This existing network has been used to form the basis for the coordinated framework for regulating biotechnology products and research activities that fall under the jurisdiction of the USDA.

Current authorities and regulatory jurisdiction for biotechnology products were defined in two Federal Register publications.[2,3] A proposed coordinated framework for regulating biotechnology was published on December 31, 1984. This was followed by the June 26, 1986, publication describing the regulatory policies of individual Federal Departments and the policies for review of research conducted or supported within these Departments.

Biological Product Categories

For the purposes of licensing under the Virus-Serum-Toxin Act (VSTA), veterinary biological products derived by rDNA techniques or developed from hybridomas are classified into three broad categories, depending on the biological characteristics of the new products and on safety considerations.[4]

Category I comprises inactivated products prepared from recombinant DNA-derived vaccines, viruses, bacterins, bacterin-toxoids, viral subunits, or bacterial subunits (Table 18-1). These nonviable or killed products pose no risk to the environment and present no new or unusual safety concerns. Monoclonal antibody (hybridoma) products used prophylactically, therapeutically, or as components of diagnostic kits are also included in this category. (Tables 18-2 and 18-3 contain examples of some of these products.)

Category II comprises products containing live microorganisms that have been modified by adding or deleting one or more genes (Table 18-4). Deleted genes may code for virulence, oncogenicity, enzyme activity, or other biochemical function. Added genes may result in the expression of unique marker antigens or the production of novel biochemical byproducts. Precautions must be taken to ensure that this addition or deletion of specific genetic information does not impart increased virulence, pathogenicity, or survival advantages in these organisms compared with those found in wild-type forms. Genetic modification shall not confer on the microorganism any changes that result in the following: undesirable new or increased adhesive or invasive ability, undesirable colonization properties, or undesirable survival patterns, within the animal host. It is important that genes added or deleted do not compromise the safety characteristics of these organisms. In most cases the safety characteristics of the organisms are improved, so that they cannot pose any new threat to humans, other animal species, or the environment.

Category III consists of products using live vectors to carry recombinant-derived foreign genes that code for immunizing antigens and/or other immune stimulants. Live vectors may carry multiple recombinant-derived foreign genes and are capable of efficiently infecting and immunizing host animal species. Two classes of viral vectors are currently being used, the lytic viruses (such as polyoma and SV-40) and the so-called shuttle vectors based on retroviruses. Live vectors currently being evaluated include vaccinia virus, bovine papillomavirus, herpesviruses, adenoviruses, SV-40 virus, and yeasts. When used as live vectors of foreign genes, the new rDNA organisms must be fully characterized and compared with the parent virus. Concerns for safety to humans and animals, and concerns for impact on the environment must be addressed in an Environmental Assessment or Environmental Impact Statement before such products can be considered for experimental field trial or licensing.

Table 18-1. Licensed Biotech Products, Category IA: Bacterins

Product Code No.	Licensed	Establishment Firm	No.	Date Licensed
Escherichia Coli Bacterin (for swine)	26R8.44	Salsbury Labs.	195	12/23/82
Escherichia Coli Bacterin-Toxoid (for swine)	7850.00	Norden Labs.	189	3/15/83
Escherichia Coli Bacterin (for swine)	7900.R0	Salsbury Labs.	195	10/5/83
Escherichia Coli Bacterin-Toxoid (for swine)	2648.08	Norden Labs.	189	6/29/84
Escherichia Coli Bacterin (for swine)	26R8.56	Norden Labs.	189	7/16/84

Testing of Experimental Products

The provisions of Title 9, Code of Federal Regulations (CFR), Part 103.3 describe the type of information required to evaluate the shipment of unlicensed biological products for experimental purposes, such as for field safety or efficacy tests prior to licensing. Recently the VSTA was amended by the Food Security Act of 1985 to require persons shipping experimental veterinary biological products intrastate, as well as interstate and for export, to obtain authorization from the Deputy Administrator. According to 9 CFR 103.3, "No person shall ship or deliver for shipment any unlicensed biological product for experimental use in animals without approval from the Deputy Administrator (of BBEP)." These amended regulations now permit APHIS to supervise all experimental uses of veterinary biological products under outside containment conditions in the United States or for export.

As with veterinary biologics produced by conventional procedures, rDNA products must be shown to be pure, safe, potent, and efficacious,

Table 18-2. Licensed Biotech Products, Category I-B-I: Therapeutic or Prophylactic Use

Product	Code No.	Licensed Firm	Establishment No.	Date Licensed
Escherichia Coli Monoclonal Antibody (for newborn cattle)	3525.00	Molecular Genetics Inc.	284	11/8/87
Pseudorabies Virus Monoclonal Antibody	3800.00	Molecular Genetics Inc.	284	4/16/87

Table 18-3. Category I-B-2: Diagnostic Test Kits

Product	Licensed Firm	Establishment No.
Equine Infectious Anemia Antibody Test Kit	TechAmerica Group, Inc.	272
Avian Reovirus Antibody Test Kit	Kirkegaard & Perry Labs	350
Feline T-Lymphotropic Lentivirus Antibody Test Kit	AgriTech Systems, Inc.	313
Feline Leukemia Virus Antigen/ Feline T-Lymphotropic Lentivirus Antibody Test Kit	AgriTech Systems, Inc.	313
Pseudorabies Virus gp-X Antibody Test Kit	AgriTech Systems, Inc.	313

Table 18-4. Category II: Live Gene Deleted

Product	Firm	Establishment No.
Pseudorabies Vaccine, Modified Live Virus	Biologics Corporation	272
Pseudorabies Vaccine, Modified Live Virus	Agrion Corporation	213
Pseudorabies Vaccine, Modified Live Virus	Syntrovet Incorporated	314
Pseudorabies Vaccine, Modified Live Virus	Fermenta Animal Health	272

and not worthless, contaminated, dangerous, or harmful. Assurance of safety in all products has included the responsibility to ensure that products do not have any adverse effects upon the environment and do not harm animal and human health. To ensure that safety concerns are fully respected, regulations have also been amended to require a person wishing to import or ship a veterinary biological product anywhere in or from the United States to provide any additional information needed by the Deputy Administrator for proper assessment of the impact of the product on the environment. Such additional information will apply to live vaccines and may include (but is not necessarily limited to) demonstrating nonpathogenicity and nonreversion to virulence by means of a number of backpassages in the host animal. APHIS may require studies to determine the fate of the organism when injected into the host, and the ability of the organism to shed, transmit, and maintain itself in a livestock population. Persons may also be requested to define the stability and survival of the organism in the environment.

The authorization procedures required for shipment of biological products and the guidelines for review of applications to conduct field trials with live products from categories II and III will be considered on a case-by-case basis. The controlled movement of biological products from physical containment to field situations will be accomplished in three stages:

1. Movement from stringent containment conditions (containment level 4) to quarantined field conditions (containment level 3).

2. Restricted field tests (containment level 2).

3. Unrestricted geographical distribution after a license has been issued (level 1).

Certain experiments involving release into the environment of any organism containing rDNA (as described in Section III-A of National Institutes of Health (NIH) Guidelines) have required Recombinant DNA Advisory Committee (RAC) review and NIH and Institutional Biosafety Committee (IBC) approval before initiation. The Office of Recombinant DNA Activities (ORDA), however, has amended this review and approval procedure by permitting submission of such requests for approval to the Federal agency that has jurisdiction for review and approval of the experiment. Once approved by that Federal agency, the experiment may proceed without NIH review or approval. Thus, the shipment of rDNA veterinary biological products and their release from contained facilities will require APHIS authorization.

APHIS approval is required, for example, to move rDNA vaccines from stringent containment to quarantine trials, and again from quarantine trials (level 3) to restricted field trials (level 2). Each request to conduct field trials in accordance with the provisions of 9 CFR 103.3 must include the following information:

1. A letter of permission from the regulatory authority in each State

involved.

2. A description of the product, serial number of the lot of experimental product to be used, recommendations for use, and results of preliminary safety research conducted in containment, including:

    a. Biological characteristics of the modified organism compared to the parental organisms.

    b. All safety testing results.

    c. Molecular biology of the modified organism, including source and function of the DNA sequence used to modify the organism, vector description, and genetic stability.

    d. Some of the physical and chemical factors which can affect survival, reproduction, and dispersal.

3. A proposed general plan covering the methods and procedures for evaluating the product and for maintaining records of the quantity of experimental product prepared, shipped, and used. In the event of unanticipated adverse effects of the modified organism, proposed methods of biological or physical control and retrieval should be included in this plan.

4. A tentative list of the names and addresses of the proposed recipients and the quantity of experimental product to be shipped to each individual.

5. Copies of labels or label sketches with the statement "Notice! For Experimental Use Only - Not For Sale" or equivalent.

6. Any information the Deputy Administrator may require in order to assess the product's impact on the environment.

Quarantined Field Trials

Quarantined field trials will be conducted under conditions acceptable to the Deputy Administrator, BBEP, where there is adequate evidence of biological and/or physical control of the rDNA organisms. Note that each study in this category will be conducted only in quarantine facilities maintained as described in proposals approved by the Deputy Administrator. Facilities shall be maintained and operated in an appropriate way to prevent dissemination of any communicable disease. Test facilities will be inspected by a Veterinary Medical Officer from APHIS to determine if they comply with the guidelines discussed below.

Physical Requirements of the Facility

Generally the facility should be located and constructed so as to prevent test animals from having physical contact with animals outside the facility. The holding area should be of sufficient size to prevent overcrowding of animals in quarantine. The facilities should be constructed with materials which can withstand cleaning and disinfection. Doors, windows, and other openings should be provided with screens to prevent birds and insects from entering. A safe and effective program will be required to control insects, ectoparasites, and avian and mammalian pests. Facility specifications shall comply with applicable federal, state, and local laws, and with regulations relating to pollution control and the protection of the environment.

Sanitation and Security

The applicant shall arrange for a water supply adequate for use in cleaning and disinfecting the facility. All feed and bedding used in the approved quarantine facility shall originate from an area not under quarantine and shall be stored in the test facility in a vermin-proof storage area. Facilities must be adequately equipped to incinerate or effectively disinfect bedding and solid waste at the conclusion of the study.

Upon the death or destruction of test animals, the applicant shall arrange for the disposal of carcasses by procedures acceptable to the Deputy Administrator. Surviving animals can be slaughtered if there is evidence that organisms are no longer present or pose no risk to the environment.

Field Testing

To permit and encourage research with recombinant DNA-derived live vaccines, using restricted field trials outside quarantine, the Deputy Administrator of BBEP may authorize a person or firm to ship unlicensed biological products for the purpose of evaluation. The evaluation would involve treatment of a limited number of animals in different locations under open field conditions, level 2. Appropriate data must be submitted so that the agency can determine if the conditions of the proposed restricted field trials are adequate to prevent the spread of disease. Prior to authorizing use of the unlicensed product in limited field trials, the Deputy Administrator will require the applicant to provide information so that the agency can assess the product's impact on the environment, in compliance with the provisions of the National Environmental Policy Act (NEPA).

The information needed for this Environmental Assessment (EA) includes purpose and need, alternatives, affected environment, environmental consequences, and consultation with other agencies. The EA presents and discusses scientific data and other information relevant to the field tests and trials conducted out of containment. It is intended to provide the general public with documentation of the USDA's view of the environmental effects that may be associated with these limited field releases. The following format will be used to prepare the EA:

Section I, Purpose and Need - This section describes the proposed action and includes a concise statement of the problem and the agency program or action designed to deal with the problem.

Section II, Alternatives - All alternatives that were considered are discussed by identifying the impact of each alternative and the benefits and problems associated with each course of action.

Section III, Affected Environment - The effects of alternatives on each aspect of the environment are discussed.

Section IV, Environmental Consequences - Here the problems and benefits of the program action are discussed. When considering rDNA live vaccines, the benefits and problems of the experimental product are compared with conventional licensed products.

Section V, Consultation - This section lists all consultants or other contacts who have worked on the assessment, as well as all coordination activities with other agencies and organizations.

Section VI, Conclusion - This section gives the conclusion statement indicating that APHIS has reached a decision concerning whether or not the action will significantly affect the quality of the human environment. All cited references and personal communications are presented in Section VII. If it is concluded that restricted field studies would not have an adverse impact on the environment, the agency will publish its findings in the Federal Register and the field trial may be initiated 30 days following publication.

Four types of scientific information will be required by APHIS when considering the release of rDNA products from containment level 4 to conduct quarantine or restricted field trials under containment levels 3 and 2, respectively: human safety, ecological concerns, characterization of the vaccine virus, and animal safety (Tables 18-5 through 18-8, respectively).

In addition to providing this type of information for preparation of the Safety Factor Evaluation (see below) or the EA, the following data would be very appropriate in support of the testing of a live rDNA bacterial product—survival and reproduction of the engineered microorganism, interactions with other organisms in the environment, effects of the introduced organism on ecosystem function if applicable, scale and scope of the planned introduction and frequency of introduction. The biological characteristics of the engineered trait, the biology of the parental organism and the environment where the introduction is planned must all be a part of the ecological risk assessment. The organism's host range and ability to adapt to or affect other animal species may also need to be investigated.

Table 18-5. Limited Field Trial with Live Vectored Experimental Product: Human Safety Concerns

* Probability of human exposure
* Possible outcomes of human exposure
* Effect of gene manipulation on pathogenicity in man
* Risk associated with widespread use of the vaccine

Table 18-6. Limited Field Trial with Live Vectored Experimental Product: Ecological Concerns

* Extent of release into the environment
* Persistence of vector in the environment
* Extent of exposure to nontarget species
* Behavior of parent virus and vector in nontarget species
* Potential of vector to infect nonvertebrate organisms
* Physical and chemical factors that can affect survival, reproduction, and dispersal of vaccine

Table 18-7. Limited Field Trial with Live Vectored Experimental Product: Characterization of the Vaccine Virus

* Characteristics of parent virus
  -Identification, sources, and strains
  -Reproduction and capacity for genetic transfer
* Source, description, and function of foreign genetic material
* Method of accomplishing genetic modification
* Genetic stability, expression, and potential for recombination of the vaccine virus
* Advantages and disadvantages of the modified virus compared with conventional products
* Comparison of the modified organisms with the parents
* Route of administration

Table 18-8. Limited Field Trial with Live Vectored Experimental
Product: Animal Safety Concerns

- Fate of the vaccine in target and nontarget species
- Potential of shed and/or spread from vaccinate to contact target and
  nontarget animals
- Reversion to virulence resulting from back passage in animals
- Effect of overdose in target and potential nontarget species
- Relative safety when compared with conventional vaccines
- Extent of the host range and the degree of mobility of the vector
- Safety in pregnant animals and in offspring nursing vaccinated
  animals

Table 18-9 summarizes the containment levels and release categories
and describes the authorization required for approval at each level. Inevi-
tably, the review cycle includes review and approval of the test by an Institutional Biosafety Committee (IBC) as well as by state animal health
regulatory authorities. With live vectored biologics that raise public
health concerns, such as with vaccinia vectored experimental veterinary
biologics, state public health officials will also be involved in the review
and may need to approve the trial at the state level.

The quarantine trial, a test using a limited number of animals in
essentially quarantined conditions, requires APHIS to prepare a Safety
Factor Evaluation, which is a document that evaluates all parameters of the
trial including an inspection of test facilities. This quarantined experimental field test does not require the publication of an EA but does require
that documentation of the analysis that was conducted be prepared and
filed.

Although further refinements and adjustments may be necessary as
knowledge of rDNA products expands, procedures for review and approval of rDNA veterinary biological products that have been established
in the United States provide an appropriate balance of flexibility and control. As a result, new rDNA products should be marketed in a manner that
maintains the public confidence.

Table 18-9. Summary of Containment Levels and Release Categories

Category	Description	Authorization
Stringent containment (level 4)	Basic research conducted in filtered air voluntary compliance	If federally funded, IBC, NIH-RAC Guidelines, otherwise
Quarantine containment (level 3)	Host animal testing in non-filtered air	IBC, State, Federal (9 CFR 103), Safety Factor Evaluation
Restricted field trial (level 2)	Experimental products being evaluated under field conditions	IBC, State, Federal (9 CFR 103), EA and FONSI
Unrestricted geographic distribution (level 1)	USDA licensed product	EA and FONSI[*] USDA license

FONSI = Finding of No Significant Impact

References

1. 21 U.S.C, p. 151-158.
2. Federal Register, December 31, 1984 49:(252)50856-50907.
3. Federal Register, June 26, 1986 51:(123)23302-23350.
4. Federal Register, June 26, 1986 51:(123)23339.

PART SIX

DIAGNOSIS, EPIDEMIOLOGY, AND ECONOMICS OF BRUCELLOSIS

Chapter Nineteen

Leishmaniasis and Malaria: DNA Probes for Diagnosis and Epidemiological Analysis

Dyann F. Wirth

Parasitic diseases are still prevalent in many parts of the world, causing both human suffering and economic loss. Major efforts to control and even eradicate parasitic diseases have met with some success (for example, elimination of malaria from the southern United States and Cuba), but, in many developing tropical countries, parasitic diseases remain major health problems. Such diseases can pose a significant barrier to economic development, and their control is an important goal for improved world health. Intensive research is being devoted to the development of new control measures for many parasitic diseases. These control measures include development of vaccines and new chemotherapeutic agents as well as improved vector control strategies. Previous experience has demonstrated the need for extensive baseline information before the introduction of any control program and the need for continued monitoring of the control program to assess its effectiveness. These diseases have complex life cycles involving vectors of transmission and intermediate hosts, both of which have an impact on transmission of the disease and can affect the outcome of any control measure.

Recent developments in biotechnology, including the use of monoclonal antibodies and recombinant DNA, have provided new tools for the collection of information on these diseases and have the potential for providing more extensive and detailed information on the parasite in the infected human and in insect vectors. This article discusses on the potential impact of these new methodologies on epidemiological studies of two parasitic diseases, leishmaniasis and malaria, for which new methods of detection, both in man and insect vectors, have been developed. These diseases are caused by parasitic protozoa of the genera, *Leishmania* and *Plasmodium*. Each of these genera has a unique life cycle. Each poses a separate set of problems for epidemiological studies and for eventual control.

Leishmaniasis

Human leishmaniasis is caused by at least 14 different species and subspecies of the genus *Leishmania*. The clinical manifestations of the disease depend in part on the infecting *Leishmania* organism. The disease falls into three general categories: simple cutaneous disease, which is often self-limiting; mucocutaneous disease, which involves the destruction of nasal tissue; and visceral disease, a systemic infection that is often fatal if untreated. In fact, the diseases share relatively few properties except that they are caused by organisms of the same genus and, in humans, the parasite grows in the phagolysosomal vesicles of macrophages. Epidemiological studies over the last 25 years have shown that, in general, leishmaniasis is a zoonotic disease; the parasite is transmitted to man from a reservoir mammalian host by a phlebotomus sandfly vector during a blood meal. Of the numerous *Leishmania* species infective for mammals, only a subset can infect and cause disease in humans. Presumably, this selectivity is a combination of factors including the intrinsic susceptibility of humans and the feeding habits of the sandfly vector. Enormous effort has been devoted to the isolation and characterization of *Leishmania* organisms that infect man and to the identification of the principal mammalian reservoirs and species of phlebotomus vector.[1] The result of many such studies has been the correlation of particular clinical manifestations with certain species or subspecies of the parasite (See Table 19-1 for summary).

The identification of *Leishmania* species is based on a variety of ecological, biological, biochemical, and immunological criteria.[2] Each cultured isolate of the parasite has been analyzed by the use of one or more of these criteria and categorized as to species and subspecies. Certain controversies remain as to whether organisms isolated in distant geographic locations but sharing certain common properties belong to the same or distinct subspecies of *Leishmania*. For example, *L. mexicana garnhami*[3] isolated in Venezuela is very similar to *L. mexicana amazonensis* isolated in Brazil as determined by isoenzyme profiles and monoclonal antibodies,[4] but there are conflicting results as to its growth characteristics in sandfly vectors.[7] Whether these organisms represent strains of the same subspecies or distinct subspecies cannot be resolved because there is no single generally accepted method for species identification in the genus *Leishmania*. This uncertainty complicates comparison of the disease epidemiology in distinct geographic locations and represents a potential limitation on the transfer of control measures from one geographic location to another. The World Health Organization has addressed this problem by establishing a set of reference strains for the various species and subspecies to be used for comparison and classification of new isolates.

Table 19-1. Major Leishmania Species Causing Human Disease

Disease	SpeciesPrimary*	Geographic Location
Cutaneous leishmaniasis	*L. mexicana mexicana*	Mexico, Central America
	L. mexicana amazonensis	Brazil Amazon region
	L. mexicana pifoni	Venezuela
	L. major	Southern USSR, Middle East
	L. tropica	Asia, southern Europe, northern and western Africa
	L. braziliensis guyanensis	Northern, southern America
	L. braziliensis panamensis	Central America
	L. braziliensis peruviana	Peru
Diffuse cutaneous disease	*L. mexicana amazonensis*	Brazil, Amazon region
	L. aethiopica	Ethiopia and Kenya
Mucocutaneous disease	*L. braziliensis braziliensis*	Western and northern South America
Visceral disease	*L. donovani*	India
	L. donovani infantum	Mediterranean area
	L. chagasi	Northern South America

*Based on Marinkelle, C.J., *The Control of Leishmaniasis.*[9]

The diverse nature of leishmaniasis clearly requires a diverse control program with specific targets for each focus of the disease. This will require more extensive collection of baseline data with regard to the infecting *Leishmania* species in humans, the relevant sandfly vector, and the principal mammalian reservoir of the particular species or subspecies. These data must be collected at each focus for proper implementation of any control program directed at either the sandfly vector or the mammalian reservoir. For control measures that involve identification and treatment of patients, accurate, rapid diagnosis of leishmaniasis must be achieved before treatment with relatively toxic chemotherapeutic agents is begun.[9]

One of the major problems in further analysis of the ecology and epidemiology of the disease is the extremely laborious task of identifying the parasite. All of the work documenting the species and subspecies of *Leishmania* is dependent on the isolation of the organism either directly in culture or after passage through a susceptible laboratory animal, most commonly the hamster. This has several limitations, namely the number of samples that can be handled at any one time, the time it takes to grow the parasites and subsequently type them, and perhaps more important, the selection from an otherwise mixed population of parasites of those species that grow either *in vitro* or in experimental animals. A method of direct identification of *Leishmania* parasites from lesions, sandfly vectors, and intermediate mammalian reservoirs is necessary if broader epidemiological studies involving large numbers of samples are to be initiated.

Current diagnosis of leishmaniasis is achieved either by direct examination of a tissue biopsy or by means of a delayed type hypersensitivity test referred to as the Montenegro test.[9] Neither of these methods is able to distinguish *Leishmania* species or subspecies, and the Montenegro test cannot distinguish current from previous infections. For certain forms of leishmaniasis, the most effective control measures may be the direct treatment of infected patients[10] and will require specific diagnosis of *Leishmania* species or subspecies from lesion material in order to design treatment regimens that minimize morbidity and mortality [for review see (11)]. For example, cutaneous infection with *L. braziliensis* is often associated with subsequent mucocutaneous disease, and early diagnosis could facilitate treatment and perhaps reduce the frequency of mucocutaneous disease.

DNA Probes in the diagnosis of leishmaniasis

A new methodology based on DNA probes specific for the various *Leishmania* species was developed. To provide a direct diagnosis of patients with leishmaniasis and to eliminate the need for culturing parasites before species identification.[12] This methodology allows direct diagnosis from lesion material without requiring of isolation of the parasite. Such direct diagnosis of *Leishmania* species, which had not been possible with any of the existing methodologies, provides the basis for the clinical management of this disease. In the initial studies, the DNA probes, which were based on total kinetoplast DNA (kDNA), could differentiate the major species complexes in the New World, *L. mexicana* and *L. braziliensis*. Subsequent experiments in which recombinant DNA methodologies were used resulted in the development of DNA probes that can differentiate species, subspecies and even distinct isolates of the parasite [12-17]

The basis for the DNA probes is the minicircle, which is a highly repeated small circular DNA molecule found within the mitochondria of the parasite. It has no apparent function and has an apparent high rate of DNA sequence divergence as measured by restriction site polymorphism and DNA hybridization studies.[18-22] In the New World *Leishmania*, the kDNA minicircles isolated from *L. mexicana* do not share any sequence homology with those isolated from *L. braziliensis*.[12-13] These differences in DNA sequence have provided the basis for a DNA probe that can distinguish the two *Leishmania* species directly when material obtained from a lesion is applied to nitrocellulose.

These DNA probes have been used to diagnose leishmaniasis in patients from the Institut du Tropical de Medicine de Manaus[23] (Table 19-2). In each case, the results of the DNA probe were compared to standard diagnostic tests, including the Montenegro test (see above), histopathology, and culturing and subsequent characterization of the parasite. As can be seen in Table 19-2, the DNA probe detected the disease in 32 of the 43 patients who had positive results in the Montenegro test. This observation may mean that in some patients, the parasite density was below the detection limit of the assay, which, based on laboratory experiments, is as few as 50 organisms in a single spot on nitrocellulose. There are cases in which organisms were cultured from lesions that were originally negative. Another possibility is that the delayed-type hypersensitivity test detected either a previous infection or a cross-reacting antigen from another type of infection.[24] A third possibility is that the parasite in the lesion is of a type not recognized by the kDNA probe; however, every parasite that has been isolated from a lesion has reacted with either the *L. braziliensis* or *L. mexicana* kDNA probes.

The DNA probe clearly detects infections in more patients than either histopathology or culturing. Although this probably results from the greater sensitivity of the DNA probe than these other methods, it may also represent false positives in the DNA probe method. Because there is no single standard for the detection of parasites, the exact determination of false positives is not possible. However, in 10 cases in which histopathology failed to detect parasites and the result of the DNA probe was positive, the culturing of the parasites clearly demonstrated their presence. The question of the false positive reaction with DNA probes has been tested experimentally. These kDNA probes did not hybridize with touch preparations of uninfected tissue from several animals and from a limited number of human lesions that subsequently proved not to be due to leishmaniasis. In addition, these DNA probes did not react with *Trypanosoma cruzi*, malaria, or *Escherichia coli*. Further evidence that the number of false positives with the kDNA probes is relatively low was obtained by testing duplicate touch preparations of each lesion with kDNA from both *L. mexicana* and *L. braziliensis*. In every case in which there was a reaction with the kDNA probe, it was specific for either *L. mexicana* or *L. braziliensis*, and the duplicate lesion showed no reaction above background. When parasites were isolated from these lesions and subsequently tested by kDNA hybridization, the original identification was confirmed. An alternative method of limiting the number of false positive reactions due to nonspecific binding of labeled DNA to tissue or blood is to perform *in situ* hybridization and examine each preparation under the microscope as

Table 19-2. Comparison of Diagnostic Tests for Leishmaniasis

Diagnostic Test	No. of patients
Montenegro positive	43
Hybridization positive	32
L. mexicana DNA probe	2
L. braziliensis DNA probe	30
Culture positive	27
Histopathology	17

suggested by Barker and co-workers.[15] This is a very time-consuming and expert process not easily adapted to large numbers of samples.

One of the limitations of the kDNA minicircle as a hybridization probe is that, although it can distinguish the major species complexes of New World cutaneous leishmaniasis, the kDNA minicircle from each complex is homologous to all the subspecies and it is therefore impossible to distinguish subspecies.[12,13] This identification of subspecies is important clinically because certain manifestations of the disease are specific to the parasite subspecies; it is also important in the description of any intermediate host or insect vector carrying a particular subspecies. In addition, our work and the work of others has indicated that, in the Old World *Leishmania* species causing cutaneous and visceral disease, kDNA sequence homology occurs among different species.[12,16,17,24,25-27] For example, kDNA isolated from *L. major* hybridizes with both of the other cutaneous species, *L. tropica* and *L. aethiopica*, and with the visceral strain *L. donovani*.[17]

Therefore a new approach is required for the development of DNA probes that can distinguish subspecies in New World cutaneous leishmaniasis and differentiate the species complexes of the Old World isolates. Several groups have used recombinant DNA methods to develop such DNA probes with these narrower specificities, see Table 19-3.[14-17,26,28-30] The method has been to clone restriction fragments of a kDNA minicircle and to use these cloned subfragments as more specific probes for species, subspecies, and even isolates. The general observation from this body of work is that, within the minicircle population, there are DNA sequences that have undergone rapid sequence divergence and can thus serve to differentiate even closely related organisms.[28] In addition, we have shown that this sequence divergence can occur within a single minicircle. A nested set of deletions of a single cloned minicircle fragment from *L. mexicana amazonensis* was generated and then tested for hybridization specificity. The full-length minicircle had a similar specificity to total

Table 19-3. Hybridization Specificities of Cloned Kinetoplast DNA Fragments

Source	Specificities	Reference
L. donovani	species	28
L. infantum	species	28
L. donovani	visceral complex	16
L. chagasi	non-Indian visceral	16
L. major	isolate	17
L. mexicana	species	30
amazonensis	subspecies	30
	isolate	30
L. major	isolate	14
L. tropica	isolate	14
L. aethiopica	isolate	14

and two deletions demonstrated species- and isolate-specific hybridization patterns.[30]

The next step for the utilization of DNA probes will be in the detection of infected insect vectors and intermediate hosts. Preliminary laboratory experiments show that parasites can be detected in infected sandflies that have been squashed directly on nitrocellulose.[31] This approach must now be tested in the field. Similarly, laboratory-based experiments have demonstrated that parasite infections can be detected in tissue touch preparations from animals experimentally infected;[12] however, both the intensity of infection and the target tissue in natural hosts will be different and thus the DNA probes must be tested directly in field-extracted material. These will be compared with alternate methods developed for antigen detection in insect vectors and infected animals.[32-34]

The DNA probe methodology should be readily adaptable to field situations. Once the tissue biopsy or sandfly vector is obtained, it is applied directly to nitrocellulose or other solid supports and is stable in this form indefinitely. Thus samples could be collected from distant sites and returned for processing. The major disadvantage of this methodology is the requirement for a radioisotope. Alternative methods of labeling DNA, which are being developed and tested for such biological specimens, should be useful in field situations.

Malaria

Human malaria is caused by the four major *Plasmodium* species, *P. falciparum, P. vivax, P. malaria,* and *P. ovale.* In most parts of the world, the prevailing parasite species is *P. falciparum,* which causes the most severe form of the acute disease and is often fatal in children.[37] *Plasmodium vivax,* the next most prevalent disease is characterized by relapses caused by parasites that remain in the liver in a latent form. The parasite is transmitted by various species of the anopheline mosquito to the human host. The sporozoite, the infectious form of the parasite released from mosquito salivary glands, initiates the exoerythrocytic cycle in the liver. Subsequently developed merozoites invade erythrocytes, and the asexual cycle continues through the course of the infection. A subset of the infected erythrocytes develop into gametocytes, the form can develop in mosquitoes, and results in disease transmission. There is no significant animal reservoir for this disease.

Malaria is among one of the major infectious diseases in the world, with acute clinical malaria affecting some 90 million to 100 million people per year according to the World Health Organization estimates.[38]

Elimination of malaria worldwide has proved to be a difficult goal, and thus current efforts are devoted to the control of malaria.[39] During the eradication program, several problems arose that will have an impact on any control program. Among these problems is the widespread resistance of anopheline vectors to insecticides,[40] the emergence of *P. falciparum* strains resistant to chloroquine, the primary chemotherapeutic agent, and the subsequent development of multidrug resistant parasite strains.[41] New approaches to control measures include improved conventional methods of vector controlling and chemotherapy and the development of innovative measures including vaccines for the malaria parasite and biological control of anopheline vectors.

The parameters of malaria transmission and disease prevalence have been studied for the last 40 years in many parts of the world. Mathematical models of disease transmission have been developed based both on entomological factors and human factors such as immunity.[42-46] In addition, epidemiological studies have demonstrated an association of malaria prevalence with certain variants in erythrocytes, sickle cell trait,[47-49] glucose-6-phosphate dehydrogenase deficiency,[50,51] Duffy blood-group antigens[52,53] and recently, alpha-thalassemia.[54] These studies have shown that malaria is a complex and dynamic disease that is varied throughout the world. Thus any control program must take into consideration the multiple factors that can affect malaria transmission and must measure these factors in each situation. For this to be achieved, it is imperative that new and efficient means of measuring both entomological and human factors on a large scale be implemented.

DNA Probes in the Detection of Malaria Infection

Both vaccine and future drug trials will require a sensitive and rapid method for detecting parasites. Currently, malaria infection is determined by the use of a thick smear stained with Giemsa. This method is both specific and sensitive for the diagnosis of malaria but has severe limitations when large numbers of samples must be handled in a timely fashion, as will be the case for the collection of baseline data for many of the vaccine trials and chemotherapy studies. A trained microscopist is required for each determination, and this is time-consuming, tiring, and potentially subject to reader bias, especially when large numbers of slides must be read in a short time period. Thus alternative methods for handling large numbers of samples are necessary.

DNA probes specific for human malaria have been developed by several groups,[55,56] and recent work by Barker et al.[57] has demonstrated that the DNA probe specific for *P. falciparum* can be used to detect malaria infection directly in finger-stick blood samples from infected patients. The DNA probes specific for *P. falciparum* are dispersed, highly repeated DNA sequences isolated from the *P. falciparum* genome using recombinant DNA technology. In laboratory and field testing, the pPF14 probe[57] is specific for *P. falciparum* and does not react with *P. vivax*, the other major human malaria. The DNA methodology is as sensitive as routine microscopy, detecting parasite densities as low as 40 parasites per microliter of blood. As can be seen in Table 19-4, the DNA probe method detects *falciparum* infection in 129 of 632 patients compared with the 121 detected by routine examination of Giemsa-stained thick smears. Subsequent examination of duplicate slides by expert microscopists confirmed the DNA probe diagnosis in those patients missed by routine microscopy.

The DNA probe method offers the advantage of a standardized procedure that can be used in a batchwise fashion on large numbers of samples. An important feature of this methodology is that it is reproducible over a large number of samples and should be less subject to reader bias. In addition, in our recent work, we have been able to correlate the intensity of DNA hybridization with parasite density and thus the DNA probes may also provide information on the intensity of infection. One limitation of the correlation of hybridization intensity with parasite density is the potential for variation in the number of repeated target sequences in different *P. falciparum* strains. The DNA probe methodology now must be tested in an epidemiological study to assess its general usefulness.

TABLE 19-4. Comparison of DNA Probes Specific for *P. falciparum*

Diagnostic Test	No. of patients*
Clinic microscope positive	121
DNA positive	129
Clinic negative	511
DNA negative	503

*Patient population consists of 632 patients examined at malaria clinics of the Malaria Division of the Thailand Ministry of Public Health in either Bangnamron or Chantiburi, Thailand in July 1985. Blood was collected by digital puncture into a heparinized capillary and treated as a previously described.[47] Malaria thick smears were prepared in the routine manner for diagnosis at the clinic. A separate set of slides, both thin and thick smears, was prepared and subsequently analyzed by malaria experts.[57]

Development of the Polymerase Chain Reaction to Amplify DNA Signals

The recent development of a method to amplify target DNA sequences has greatly enhanced the sensitivity of our DNA probes and will now allow the use of non-radioactive methods to detect target sequences. We have tested the polymerase chain reaction (PCR) developed by Cetus Corporation and have been able to demonstrate a million-fold amplification of target DNA sequences in both the *Leishmania* spp. kDNA system and for *P. falciparum*- and *P. vivax*-specific DNA probes. In each case, the cloned target DNA has been sequenced and oligonucleotide primers based on this sequence have been used in the PCR reaction. Target DNA has been successfully amplified from purified DNA, tissue samples, and blood samples and from formalin-fixed, paraffin embedded tissue sections. In addition, we have been able to amplify sequences directly from infected insect vectors. This methodology is successful in the laboratory and should be readily adaptable to field use.

Conclusion

The application of new methods of biotechnology to the epidemiology of leishmaniasis and malaria is in its initial phases. The new tools offer distinct advantages with regard to specificity, sensitivity, and ease of use for large numbers of samples when compared to existing methodologies. These new tools have enormous potential for their contribution to new knowledge on the transmission and prevalence of these diseases. Before these methods are generally accepted for use, they must be extensively tested under field situations and modified to provide the relevant information important for epidemiological analysis.

The work reported here was supported by support from the UNDP, World Bank, World Health Organization Special Programme for Research and Training Tropical Diseases, NIH (AI 21365, AI 19392), and The John D. and Catherine T. MacArthur Foundation.

References

1. Lainson R. *Trans R Soc Trop Med Hyg* 1983;77:569; Lainson R, Shaw JJ, *Nature* (London) 1973;273:595 (1978).
2. Chance ML, Walton BC, eds. *Biochemical Characterization of Leishmania,* Geneva: UNDP/World Bank/WHO, 1982.
3. Scorza JU et al. *Trans R Soc Trop Med Hyg* 1979;73:293.
4. Momen H, Grimaldi G. *Trans R Soc Trop Med Hyg* 1984;78:701.
5. Miles MA et al. *Trans R Soc Trop Med Hyg* 1980;74:243.
6. Lainson R. *Proceedings of the 3rd Venezuelan Congress of Microbiology and Symposium on Leishmaniasis,* Bouquisimeto, Venezuela,1983.
7. Lainson R, Shaw J. In *Biology of Kinetoplasitdae 2,* W.H.R. Lunden, Evans, eds. London: Academic Press, 1979;1-116.
8. Peters W, et al. *J Roy Soc of Med* 1983;76: 540.
9. Montenegro, *An Fac Med Univ Sao Paulo* 1926;1:323.
10. Marinkelle CJ. *Bull World Health Organization* 1980;58:807.
11. Deane LM, Grimaldi G. *Leishmaniasis.* Chang, Bray, eds. Amsterdam: Elsevier, 1985.
12. Wirth DF. D McMahon-Pratt. *Proc Natl Acad Sci* USA 1982;79:6999.
13. Barker DC, Butcher J. *Trans R Soc Trop Med Hyg* 1983;77:285.
14. Kennedy, WPK. *Mol Biochem Parasitol* 1984;12:313.
15. Barker DC, et al. *Parasitology* 1985;91:S139.
16. Lopes UG, Wirth. DF. *Mol Biochem Parasitol.* (in press)
17. Wirth DF, Rogers WO. *Rapid Detection and Identification of Infectious Agents.* D Kingsbury, S Falkow, eds. New York: Academic Press, 1985.
18. Englund PT. *J Biol Chem* 1979;254:4895.
19. Kidane GZ, Hughes D, Simpson L. *Gene* 1984;27:265).
20. Jackson PR et al. *Am J Trop Med Hyg* 1984; 33:808.
21. Steinert M, Van Assel S. *Plasmid* 1980;3:7.
22. Lopes UG, et al. *Parasitology* 1984;70: 8.
23. Roger et al. (In preparation.)
24. Aston DC, Thornley AP. *Trans R Soc Trop Med Hyg* 1970;75:537.
25. Arnot, DF, Barker DC. *Mol Biochem Parasitol* 1981;3:47.
26. Barker DC, Arnot DF. *Eur J Cell Biol* 1980;22:124.
27. Spithill TW, et al. *J Cell Biochem.* 1984;24:103.
28. Lawrie JM, et al. *Am J Trop Med Hyg* 1985;34:257.
29. Frasch ACC, et al. *Mol Biochem Parasitol* 1985;4:163.

30. Togers WO, Wirth DF. In preparation.
31. Perkins P, Wirth DF. Unpublished observations.
32. McMahon-Pratt David DJ. *Nature.* London 1981;291:581.
33. CC Jaffe *et al., J Immunol* 1984;133:440(1984)
34. McMahon-Pratt et al. *J Immunol* 1985;134:1935.
35. Frankenberg, et al. *Am J Trop Med Hyg* 1985;34:266.
36. McMahon-Pratt D, et al. *Am J Trop Med Hyg* 1983;32:1268.
37. Cohen S, Lambert PH. In: *Immunology of Parasitic Infections.* S Cohen and KS Warren, eds. Blackwell, Oxford, England, 1982, p. 422.
38. *World Health Statistical Quarterly,* 1984;37:130-161.
39. *World Health Organization Technical Report Series,* No. 640 (1979).
40. *World Health Organization Technical Report Series,* No. 655 (1980).
41. *World Health Organization Technical Report Series,* No. 711 (1984).
42. McDonald G. *Tropical Diseases Bulletin,* 1952;49:81.
43. G. Mcdonald, *Proc Roy Soc Trop Med* 1955;48:295.
44. Bruce-Chwatt JA. *Tropical and Geographic Medicine* 1976;28:1-8.
45. J.A. Najera, *Bulletin of the World Health Organization* 1974;50:449-457.
46. Molineaux L, Gramiccia G. *The Garki Project* Geneva: World Health Organization, 1980;109-115.
47. Haldane, JBS. *8th International Congress Genet* 1949;35:267-273 (Hereditas Luppl.)
48. JH Walker, LJ Bruce-Chwatt, *Trans R Soc Trop Med Hyg* 1956;50:511
49. A.F. Fleming, *Ann Tro Me Parasitol* 1979;73:161.
50. Luzzato L., et al. *Bulletin of the World Health Organization* 1974;50:195.
51. L. Luzzato, Blood 1979;54:961.
52. Miller LH, et al. *N Engl J Med* 295, 302 (1976).
53. L. H. Miller et al. *Am J Trop Med Hyg* 1978;27:1069.
54. Flint JL, et al. *Nature* London1986; 321, 744-750.
55. Y. Pollack et al. *Am J Trop Med Hyg* 34, 663.
56. E. McLaughlin et al. *Am J Trop Med Hyg* 1985;34:837.
57. Barker RB, et al. *Science* 1986;231:1434.

Chapter Twenty

Current and Future
Serological Methods

Peter F. Wright snd
Klaus H. Nielsen

Introduction

"Although a number of tests are employed in the serological diagnosis of bovine brucellosis, we are still looking for the perfect test, a simple rapid test which will detect an infected animal early in the incubation period as well as at all subsequent stages of the disease. Furthermore, this test should not react with serum from vaccinated cattle as it is now evident that vaccination of cattle will have to continue and increase in certain heavily infected areas. Until such an ideal test is devised, we will have to make the best possible use of those presently available." These are the introductory remarks of the late Dr. Lois M. Jones[1] (1924-1986) in a paper which she had delivered here at this conference in 1976. Over a decade has elapsed and a number of new serological techniques have been applied to brucellosis serology, but are we now any closer to that "ideal test?"

The application of new serological techniques to the diagnosis of bovine brucellosis will not necessarily result in a markedly improved test from a diagnostic standpoint. It is necessary to consider new techniques not only in view of what we have recently learned from research developments but also in view of what we have already learned from conventional serology. In this review, we shall attempt to focus on the diagnostic perspective with respect to antigens and antibodies and their relevance in current and new serological techniques.

Classical Serology

It is quite clear that the agglutination tests have historically played a very prominent role in brucellosis serology and it is safe to say that for the most part it is still true today. The agglutination tests, as simple as they may seem, have been intensively studied with respect to their serological and diagnostic performance and a number of modifications have been intro duced, driven by the need for greater diagnostic specificity. For future consideration, it is important to understand these modifications from an immunological view point.

Table 20-1 compares the reactivity of the four major bovine isotypes in the conventional assays most widely used in brucellosis serology.[2] The standard or serum agglutination test (SAT) performed at a neutral pH demonstrates a high analytical sensitivity in the detection of all the bovine isotypes with the important exception of IgG$_1$. As pointed out by Dr. Alton[3] at this meeting 13 years ago, the SAT has been repeatedly shown to have poor diagnostic sensitivity when compared to other conventional tests. This, however, does not imply that the SAT will demonstrate a high diagnostic specificity. In fact, its diagnostic specificity is also very poor, especially when the test is interpreted at 30 IU.[4]

The buffered plate antigen test (BPAT) and the card or Rose Bengal test (RBT) are referred to as the buffered agglutination tests. Although the antigens differ with respect to bacterial staining and cell concentrations, they are both buffered[5] to a pH of 3.65. These tests were developed based on the observation that bovine IgG$_1$ agglutinates very poorly except at an acid pH[1]. As can be seen in Table 20-1, both the BPAT and Card tests are comparable and demonstrate a greater analytical sensitivity in the detection of IgG$_1$ when compared to IgG$_2$. Notably, IgM and IgA are not reactive in this study, although it has been previously reported that IgM is reactive in the card test.[1] The BPAT and the card tests may differ somewhat in diagnostic performance but it is generally agreed that they exhibit greater diagnostic sensitivity and specificity than the SAT.[6,7]

In an effort to enhance diagnostic specificity, sera have been treated to minimize or eliminate IgM reactivity in the SAT. Most commonly, the agglutinating activity of IgM has been removed by precipitation from the test sample with Rivanol or destroyed by cleavage with 2-mercaptoethanol (2ME).[1] Like the buffered agglutination tests, the Rivanol and 2ME agglutination tests (Table 20-1) detect only IgG$_1$ and IgG$_2$ isotypes; however, the analytical bias in favor of the detection of IgG$_1$ over IgG$_2$ is not nearly as great as in the buffered tests. It is interesting to note that treatment with Rivanol or 2ME promotes the reactivity of IgG$_1$ as this isotype is not normally reactive at a neutral pH but on the other hand, the reactivity of IgG$_2$ is reduced. Given that the diagnostic specificity may be enhanced by the elimination of IgM reactivity, the diagnostic sensitivity may also be enhanced by the promotion of IgG$_1$ reactivity.

The complement fixation test (CFT) demonstrates (Table 20-1) the highest degree of analytical sensitivity in the detection of IgG$_1$ among the classical tests. Furthermore, IgG$_1$ appears to be the only isotype detectable in this test. The reactivity of IgM in the CFT is subject to differences of opinion[1,3,8] but the diagnostic performance of the CFT would support that IgM is not reactive under standard test conditions. The diagnostic sensitivity of the CFT is slightly lower than that of the buffered agglutination tests but its diagnostic specificity is the highest of any of the classical

Table 20-1. Analytical Sensitivity of Classical Assays in the Detection of Affinity Purified Anti-*B. abortus* Antibody Isotypes[2]

Assay	IgM	IgG_1	IgG_2	IgA
SAT*	20	—[+]	125	650
BPAT[s]	—	550	5500	—
CARD[s]	—	600	7500	—
RIV**	—	1550	2750	—
2ME**	—	1500	2600	—
CFT[++]	—	210	—	—

*Standard agglutination test, ng of isotype required to agglutinate 75% of cells under standard test conditions.
[+]No reaction in any assay at isotype concentrations as great as 20,000 ng/ml.
[s]Buffered plate agglutination test and card test, ng of isotype required to agglutinate cells under standard test conditions.
**Rivanol and 2 mercaptoethanol agglutination tests, ng of isotype required to agglutinate 75% of cells under standard test conditions.
[++]Complement fixation test, ng of isotype required to fix 1.5 $^{CH}50$ units of guinea pig complement under standard test conditions.

tests.[4,7] This is likely due to its high analytical sensitivity in the detection of IgG_1 only.

The differences in the diagnostic performances of these classical tests are primarily based on their biases in the detection of the major antibody isotypes. Diagnostic specificity is certainly increased when IgM reactivity is abrogated either generally or by selective means such as ethylene diamine tetrauretic acid (EDTA) treatment.[9] Although IgA is produced in the response to infection, its diagnostic importance appears to be minimal, probably owing to its very low concentration in bovine serum.[10] Diagnostic specificity may be further increased by the additional elimination of IgG_2 as in the CFT. As the detection of both of IgM and IgG_2 is reduced or eliminated, there is a decrease in diagnostic sensitivity but this decrease is less than what might be expected. It may very well be that the enhanced analytical sensitivity of the CFT in the detection of IgG_1 compensates for its isotype restriction.

It has been pointed out[1] that there may be an inherent danger in dismissing the diagnostic importance of IgM at very early stages of infection. Although IgM may be the first isotype produced in response to infection, the switch to IgG occurs very rapidly in our experience. In addition, it has been our experience that the IgG_1 response is predominant and that the IgG$_2$ response is much more variable. We would therefore suggest that an immunoassay of high analytical sensitivity for IgG$_1$ alone may offer a better combination of diagnostic sensitivity and diagnostic specificity than the classical assays in current use.

In the preceding discussion, no mention has been made of the problems in brucellosis serology which are attributable to the response to Strain 19 vaccination or the response to other bacteria exhibiting cross-reacting antigens. While diagnostic specificity has been improved through the restriction of the isotypes detected in the classical tests, the problems stated above are not resolved. All of the tests thus far described make use of the same antigen, the whole cell of *B. abortus*. As will be discussed later, specific antigenic epitopes may be the key to differentiating these reactors from infected cattle.

Conventional Serology

Given the shortcomings of the classical serological tests using whole cell antigens, a great deal of research has been directed toward the identification of the diagnostically relevant antigens of *Brucella*.[11,12] Some antigenic extracts were then applied to conventional serological techniques other than the classical assays.

It has been well established that the immunodominant antigen involved in the response to infection is the smooth lipopolysaccharide (SLPS). It is responsible for the reactivity observed in the classical tests which is easily demonstrated by the lack of reactivity of the rough strains in these assays. The SLPS has been used in two hemolytic assays: the indirect hemolysis test (IHLT)[13] and the hemolysis-in-gel test (HIGT).[14] In both cases,[4,15] the diagnostic sensitivity of these tests was higher than that of the CFT; however, the diagnostic specificity was considerably lower. Combined with the fact that the problem of differentiating different types of reactors had not been resolved with the use of SLPS, neither of these tests have found wide acceptance.

A polysaccharide antigen, originally designated as poly B, showed promise in the differentiation of infected from vaccinated reactors[16] in a radial immunodiffusion (RID) test. As will be discussed later, this antigen is actually the polysaccharide component of the "O" chain of the SLPS. Differentiation was in fact possible with the immunodiffusion technique but the diagnostic sensitivity was very low compared to assays using whole cells or SLPS.[17,18] As a consequence, this test was not diagnostically acceptable.

Primary Binding Assays

Over the course of the last decade or so, there has been a tremendous amount of effort expended on the development of primary binding assays for the diagnosis of brucellosis. We have summarized these efforts (about 60) in a publication which is currently in press.[19] For this review, we will make only general comments on these developments.

Radioimmunoassay (RIA) procedures which have been applied to brucellosis serology vary considerably. Indirect, competitive and even antigen capture systems have been developed. Antigens have ranged from whole cells to soluble antigens to extracts. In some systems, specific isotypes were targeted using isotype specific antisera or protein A, while in others broad specificity antiglobulins were used. Amplified detection systems were also applied in some cases. In general, the analytical sensitivity of the RIA is very high which would impart a high diagnostic sensitivity. However, the diagnostic specificity of any given RIA would be influenced by its isotype specificity. The predominant antigen in all of these assays is the SLPS whether on the whole cell or prepared otherwise. None of these assays are capable of differentiating infected from vaccinal reactors. Given the inherent problems associated with the use of radioisotopes, RIA techniques have not found wide acceptance.

Fluoroimmunoassay (FIA) techniques have also been applied to a limited extent. Again, both indirect and competitive systems have been developed. Most recently, a particle concentration FIA has been developed by a commercial diagnostic firm in the United States. As in the RIA techniques, the antigen preparation used has been variable but SLPS has remained the immunodominant antigen. More recent techniques have made use of fluorometers for a more objective assessment of antibody binding. FIA techniques demonstrate a high diagnostic sensitivity and again, the diagnostic specificity would be influenced by its isotype specificity. At present, none of the FIA techniques are capable of distinguishing between different types of reactors.

Enzyme immunoassay (EIA or ELISA) techniques have been extensively applied to brucellosis serology, far more so than RIA or FIA techniques. Over half of the publications in the literature on primary binding techniques pertain to the indirect ELISA alone, not to mention variations on the technique. We have extensively reviewed the various aspects of ELISA techniques in recent publications.[19,20,21]

A wide variety of antigen preparations have been used in the ELISA technique. While SLPS has been the immunodominant antigen in the majority of preparations, carbohydrate and protein antigens have been applied in some laboratories. Various enzyme systems have been used, the most common being horseradish peroxidase. Both monoclonal and polyclonal antibody reagents have been employed. Antiglobulin specificities have covered all combinations of isotypes. In general, the same comments made with respect to the RIA and FIA techniques are applicable to the ELISA techniques in terms of diagnostic sensitivity and specificity. However, indirect ELISA techniques are gaining in acceptance in the diagnostic laboratory and are routinely being used in several countries including Australia, Canada, and the United States. Also, there have been recent developments which show promise in the differentiation of infected cattle from vaccinates and cross-reactors.

Indirect ELISA

At our federal laboratory, we have extensively studied the indirect ELISA technique in terms of diagnostic performance. Details of our current protocol and its application are described elsewhere.[19] In this review, we will describe briefly some of the factors which we have found to contribute to assay performance in terms of diagnostic sensitivity and specificity.

For the indirect ELISA, a semi-purified preparation of SLPS is used as the antigen.[22] In comparing SLPS preparations from S 413, S 1119-3, and S 19, we have not found any appreciable differences in diagnostic performance. If the SLPS is further purified by nuclease and protease digestion and column chromatography, the SLPS does not adsorb to polystyrene microplates as uniformly as the semi-purified preparations. We suspect that the purified SLPS tends to form spontaneous micelles in aqueous solution which do not adsorb efficiently. The net result of using a highly purified preparation is an increase in non-specific background activity in the assay, due to its poor adsorption characteristics, with a concomitant loss of diagnostic specificity and sensitivity.

The type of polystyrene microplate will also have an effect. When high binding efficiency plates are used, non-specific background levels are also increased, resulting in the same effect as stated above. This is likely due to the enhanced protein adsorption characteristics of these plates. Low to medium binding efficiency plates will actually adsorb more SLPS and offer lower non-specific backgrounds in the assay.

Even the choice of enzyme substrate system will affect diagnostic performance. It has been our experience that the more analytically sensitive the substrate system, the more prone it is to non-specific interactions. This serves to lower diagnostic specificity and to a lesser extent diagnostic, sensitivity.

The isotype specificity of detection reagent will greatly effect diagnostic performance. The analytical sensitivities of three anti-bovine conjugates are compared in Table 20-2. A commercial polyclonal (prepared in rabbit) anti-bovine IgG (H+L) demonstrated a high analytical sensitivity in the detection of isotypes IgG_1 and, in progressively lesser degrees, IgG_2, IgM, and IgA. A monoclonal anti-bovine light (L) chain, specific for a common determinant on both lamda and kappa chains, demonstrated a very high and near equal sensitivity in the detection of all isotypes. A monoclonal anti-bovine IgG_1 demonstrated a very high analytical sensitivity in the detection of its specific isotype alone.

All of the above reagents have been diagnostically assessed in our indirect ELISA. In comparison to the BPAT, all of the ELISA detection reagents met or surpassed this screening test in terms of diagnostic sensitivity. The diagnostic specificities of these reagents decreased in the order of anti-IgG_1 then anti-IgG (H+L) with anti-L chain demonstrating the lowest specificity. The anti-IgG (H+L) conjugate equalled the BPAT in terms of diagnostic specificity. In comparison to the CFT, all of the ELISA detection reagents surpassed this confirmatory assay in terms of diagnostic sensitivity with the anti-IgG_1 having the highest sensitivity. The diagnostic specificities decreased as above and all specificities were lower than that of the CFT.

These results are not unlike what has been discussed in the comparison of the classical serological techniques. As the isotypes detected are narrowed to the point where IgG_1 alone is detected, the diagnostic specificity of the ELISA is increased. The diagnostic sensitivity of the ELISA was not compromised by the use of the monoclonal anti-IgG_1 reagent and in fact it increased. This would support our earlier suggestion that a high analytical sensitivity in the detection of IgG_1 alone may result in a better combination of diagnostic sensitivity and specificity. In this study, the diagnostic specificity using the anti-IgG_1 reagent was slightly lower (by less than 0.5%) than that of the CFT. However, over a great many years, CFT reactors have been culled from Canadian herds and this may have introduced a bias in favor of CFT specificity.

The indirect ELISA using SLPS and anti-IgG_1 does not circumvent the problems associated with S 19 vaccinates and cross-reactors. In fact, its higher analytical sensitivity in the detection of IgG_1 increases its sensitivity in the detection of calfhood vaccinates, more so than the other detection reagents studied in this ELISA. This would suggest that IgG_1 is the prevalent isotype remaining after vaccinal titres decline. This is perhaps not surprising since this isotype is predominant in the response to SLPS.

Competitive ELISA

The potential for using highly specific monoclonal antibodies in competitive ELISA techniques for improved diagnosis has been subject to discussion for a number of years. Monoclonal antibodies have been produced to a number of antigenic determinants on the surface of *Brucella*[23,24]

Table 20-2. Analytical Sensitivity of Indirect and Competitive ELISAs in the Detection of Affinity Purified anti-B. abortus Antibody Isotypes[2]

Assay	IgM	IgG_1	IgG_2	IgA
I Pc H/L*	660	310	440	890
I Mc L#	45	100	120	110
I Mc G_1§	—'	105	—	—
C Mc 'O'**	<10	<10	<10	<10

'Indirect ELISA, polyclonal anti-IgG (H+L) conjugate, minimum ng/ml of isotype resulting in an optical density of 1.0 under standard test conditions.
#Indirect ELISA, monoclonal anti-Light chain conjugate, minimum ng/ml as above.
§Indirect ELISA, monoclonal anti-IgG_1 conjugate, minimum ng/ml as above.
**Competitive ELISA, monoclonal anti-"O" polysaccharide conjugate, minimum ng/ml of isotype resulting in complete inhibition of conjugate binding.
'No reactivity at isotype concentrations as great as 20,000 ng/ml.

and applied in competitive assays with limited success.[25,26] A competitive ELISA has recently been developed in Dr. Nielsen's laboratory which shows promise in the differentiation of the response of field-infected cattle from the response to vaccination or exposure to cross-reacting organisms.[27] To understand the proposed mechanism for this differentiation, it is necessary to understand the nature of the antigen and monoclonal antibodies raised to its epitopes.

The SLPS of Brucella consists of a lipid A component which is linked to the "O" chain polysaccharide by a short carbohydrate core. The "O" chain polysaccharide of Brucella abortus is a linear, homopolymer of 4,6-dideoxy-formamido-alpha-D-mannopyranosyl residues exhibiting 1,2 glycosidic linkages throughout its length. The "O" chain polysaccharide of B. melitensis is exactly the same except for the substitution of a 1,3 glycosidic linkage between each series of four 1, 2 linkages.[28] Furthermore, it is now recognized that the poly B antigen is actually the free "O" chain polysaccharide with only a small remnant of the core still attached and that this antigen may be purified from either B. abortus or melitensis.[18]

The substituted linkage appears to be responsible for the occurrence of the classical A and M antigens based on monoclonal antibody studies.[28] Further studies by this research group have suggested that there are both unique and common epitopes on the respective "O" chains. In addition, some of these epitopes are univalent while others are multivalent. It is believed that the multivalent epitopes reside along the length of the polymer, whereas the univalent epitopes are located at the terminal portion of the chain.[29] One monoclonal in particular (designated Ys-T9-2), which was raised against *Yersinia enterocolitica* 0:9, is capable of precipitating free "O" chain from *Y. enterocolitica, B. abortus* and *B. melitensis*. It is thought that this monoclonal has specificity for a common, multivalent epitope defined by the short series of 1,2 linkages described for *B. melitensis*.

Cross-reactions between *B. abortus* and *Y. enterocolitica* 0:9 are understandable in that their "O" chain polysaccharides are identical.[29] The crossreactions observed between *Brucella* and other Gram negative bacteria are related to N-acyl derivatives of 4-amino-4,6-dideoxy-D-manno-pyranose units found in the "O" chain polysaccharides of these other bacteria.[28] The monoclonal antibody described above does not bind to these cross-reacting antigens.

As previously stated, the SLPS is immunodominant in the response to both field strains and S 19; however, this common, multivalent epitope appears to be only weakly immunogenic. It is hypothesized that antibody to this epitope is only produced in significant amounts after prolonged or chronic exposure of a dosage such as that offered by field infection.[27] Vaccinated (S 19) cattle appear to produce only a transient response to this epitope except under circumstances where a persistent infection with the vaccine strain may be established. Based on the reactivity of the "O" chain polysaccharide in the RID test, it may be further hypothesized that the immunodominant epitopes may be univalent, possibly occurring at the terminal portion of the chain and are incapable of participating in a precipitin reaction.

The competitive ELISA is based on the reagents described above and the method is detailed elsewhere.[19,27] The purity and the presentation of the polysaccharide antigen on the surface of the polystyrene microplate are critical points. The antigen must be free of SLPS as this contaminant will preferentially adsorb to the plate. Only low to medium binding microplates allow the optimal presentation of this linear epitope. In studies using this polysaccharide antigen in an indirect ELISA format, the immunodominant epitopes were reactive when adsorbed to high-binding-capacity but not lower-binding-capacity microplates. Although some degree of discrimination is possible in the indirect ELISA, a greater degree is achieved in the competitive ELISA.

The analytical sensitivity of the competitive ELISA is shown in Table 20-2. All bovine isotypes compete effectively against the monoclonal antibody for binding to this particular epitope. The analytical sensitivity of this assay is far greater than that of any of the indirect ELISAs developed in our laboratory.

The data for the indirect ELISA shown in Figure 20-1 highlights the problem associated with vaccinates in this assay. These sera were specifically selected based on reactor and infection status. They represent those seropositive reactors that were vaccinated as calves with S19 and, were greater than 18 months of age at the time of testing. This group also includes some cattle that became infected with the vaccine strain as proven by bacteriological culture. At a diagnostic threshold of 0.300 OD units, all 100 vaccinates are considered to be seropositive. Of these, 34 cattle are persistently infected with S19 and as can be seen, are not serologically distinguishable from those non-infected cattle which demonstrate elevated post-vaccinal titers. Sera from 132 healthy cattle which have not been vaccinated have been included for comparison and represent what may be expected of routine diagnostic submissions. Although not illustrated in this figure, the majority of S19 calfhood vaccinates (>95%) tested after 18 months of age would appear as a sub-population of OD values within the upper limits of the negative OD range (ie., in the 0.200-0.300 range). The sera from 132 field strain-infected cattle, confirmed by bacteriological culture, have also been included for comparison. The age old dilemma still exists in that, based on reactivity in the indirect ELISA, infected (field or vaccine strain) reactors cannot be differentiated from those non-infected vaccinates which have been described above.

The data in Figure 20-2 demonstrates the enhancements to diagnostic differentiation afforded by the competitive ELISA. This figure represents an expanded group of sera tested more recently in the competitive ELISA and the sera in the preceding figure are included in the total. All of the 34 cattle persistently infected with S19 demonstrate inhibition activities of 70% or greater. By comparison, 275 field strain-infected cattle demonstrate similar inhibition activities. All of the 123 non-infected vaccinates demonstrate inhibition activities of 40% or less with the majority of sera showing inhibition activities of 20% or less. By comparison, 273 healthy cattle demonstrate inhibition activities of 20% or less. Based on these data, it would appear that infected (field or vaccine strain) cattle may be differentiated from vaccinated cattle based on reactivity in the competitive ELISA. It would also appear that there is no loss of diagnostic sensitivity or compromise of diagnostic specificity with this assay.

The competitive ELISA in its present format is not without some limitations. Approximately 20% of these cattle (data not shown) vaccinated with S 19 may demonstrate a transient immune response of sufficient magnitude to be detectable for a period of about two months post-vaccination. However, this is still an improvement over conventional serology and the indirect ELISA. Data from experimental infection studies[27] would suggest that the onset of an immune response detectable in the competitive ELISA may be slower than that of the response detectable by the indirect ELISA. This may be due to the weak immunogenicity of this particular epitope in comparison to other immunodominant epitopes of the SLPS which are reactive in the indirect ELISA. To clarify whether or not this will

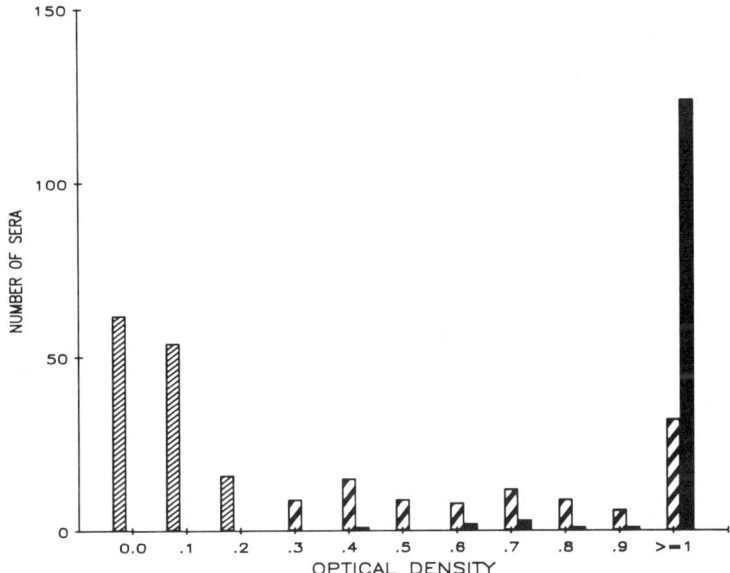

Figure 20-1. Comparison in the Indirect ELISA of Groups of Selected Sera from Negative (Light Bar), S 19-Vaccinated and Vaccine Strain-Infected (Medium Bar) and Field Strain-Infected (Dark Bar) Cattle. Data are expressed as OD_{414nm} and grouped in class intervals of 0.1 units with the lower class limit indicated on the axis.

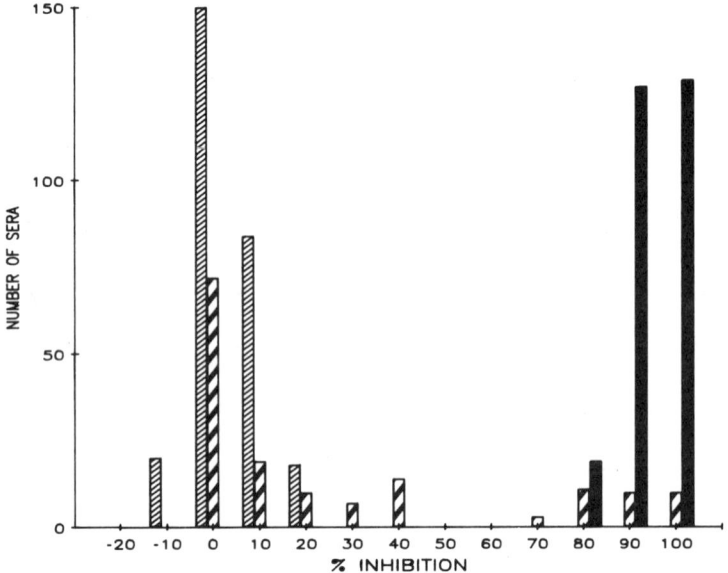

Figure 20-2. Comparison in the Competitive ELISA of Groups of Selected Sera from Negative (Light Bar), S 19-Vaccinated and Vaccine Strain-Infected (Medium Bar) and Field Strain-Infected (Dark Bar) Cattle. Data are expressed as percent inhibition relative to the monoclonal reagent in buffer alone and are grouped in class intervals of 10% with the upper class limit indicated on the axis.

have an effect on diagnostic sensitivity, both the indirect and competitive ELISAs will have to be compared with respect to relative sensitivity over a period of time in a herd where natural infection is present.

Summary

From the analysis of classical serology, it is apparent that diagnostic specificity is enhanced by restricting the antibody isotypes detected. Although all isotypes may be detected, the predominant isotype associated with infection appears to be IgG_1 and it is detectable very early in the immune response. Both the buffered agglutination tests (BPAT and card) and the CFT demonstrate an analytical bias in favor of the detection of this isotype. The high diagnostic sensitivities of the buffered agglutination tests combined with their simplicity have made these assays highly successful as screening tests. The high diagnostic specificity of the CFT has made it the most reliable confirmatory test.

The problem of serologically differentiating infected cattle from those that have been vaccinated or exposed to cross-reacting organisms has not been resolved through the use of the SLPS in either hemolytic or primary binding assays. It is apparent that the SLPS is the immunodominant antigen in response to infection and vaccination. As well, the antigenic epitopes responsible for cross-reactivity also reside on the SLPS. Although these assays offer enhanced diagnostic sensitivity, diagnostic specificity in general has not been improved.

Of the primary binding assays, the indirect ELISA has been the most extensively studied. Using SLPS as the antigen, the diagnostic specificity and sensitivity of this assay may be modulated by altering the isotype specificities of the antiglobulin reagent. We are currently modifying our indirect ELISA using a monoclonal anti-IgG_1 for use as a high-volume screening assay. Given our brucellosis-free status in Canada, it is important to use a screening test of high diagnostic sensitivity for surveillance purposes. In addition, for any country involved in the export of cattle, it would be wise to identify any reactor (vaccinate or otherwise) that could be interpreted as infected by classical serology.

Characterization of the "O" chain polysaccharide of the SLPS has resulted in the development of a competitive assay based on a monoclonal specific for a common and repeating epitope on the polysaccharide. At present, this assay would appear to differentiate infected from S 19-vaccinated cattle. In the near future, we will be conducting a large field trial using the indirect ELISA as a screening test and the competitive ELISA as a confirmatory test and comparing their performances to the BPAT and

CFT respectively.

Given the current progress in the development of ELISA techniques, we now stand at the threshold of what could very well be the future brucellosis serology. We have the tools and the understanding but now there is a need to develop them into a diagnostic system which is internationally acceptable. The use of monoclonal detection reagents offers a degree of standardization that has never before been achieved. In addition, we now have the potential for developing analytical anti-*Brucella* antibody standards through monoclonal technology. Dr. Nielsen has recently produced a monoclonal bovine IgG₁ antibody which is reactive with an immunodominant epitope of the SLPS. Characterization of the SLPS and its "O" chain polysaccharide will allow a much higher degree of standardization of antigen production in the future. We are currently collaborating with Dr. Dubray and Dr. Zygnunt at INRA in France on methods of antigen standardization. Through genetic engineering, it may be possible to clone the relevant antigens into bacteria that are safer to handle and easier to grow. Dr. Rigby's group at our Institute has had some success in the expression of *Brucella* "O" chain antigens by *E. coli*. The potential for developing very simple and rapid field tests may exist if the proper epitopes could be presented in an assay such as the latex agglutination test.

In summary, are we any closer to the "ideal test" of which Dr. Jones spoke? In our opinion, the answer is yes but the true measure of success will be the development and application of an internationally accepted diagnostic system for brucellosis.

References

1. Jones M. *Brucella* Antigens and Serologic Test Results. *Bovine Brucellosis: An International Symposium*, Crawford RP, Hidalgo RJ eds. College Station: Texas A&M University Press, 1977;40-48.

2. Nielsen K, Heck FC, Wagner GG, Stiller J, Rosenbaum B, Pugh R, Flores E. Comparative assessment of antibody isotypes to *Brucella abortus* by primary and secondary binding assays. *Prev Vet Med* 1984;2:197-204.

3. Alton G. Development and Evaluation of Serological Tests. *Bovine Brucellosis: An International Symposium*, Crawford RP, Hidalgo RJ eds. College Station: Texas A&M University Press, 1977;61-71.

4. Dohoo IR, Wright PF, Ruckerbauer GM, Samagh BS, Forbes LB. A comparison of five serological assays for bovine brucellosis. *Can J Vet Res* 1986;50:485-493.

5. Alton GG, Jones LM, Angus RD, Verger JM. *Techniques for the Brucellosis Laboratory*. Institut Nacional de la Recherche Agronomique, Paris, FR 1988; pp 71-77.

6. Pietz D. *Brucella* Antigens and Serologic Test Results. *Bovine Brucellosis: An International Symposium*, Crawford RP, Hidalgo RJ eds. College Station: Texas A&M University Press, 1977; 49-60.

7. Morgan WJB. The Diagnosis of Brucellosis in Britain. *Bovine Brucellosis: An International Symposium*, Crawford RP, Hidalgo RJ eds. College Station: Texas

A&M University Press, 1977; 21-39.

8. Nielsen K, Duncan JR. Bovine IgM: does it fix guinea pig complement in the absence of bovine complement components? *Vet Immunol Immunopathol* 1987;14:335-343.

9. Nielsen K, Stilwell K, Stemshorn B, Duncan R. Ethylene diaminetetraacetic acid (disodium salt)-labile bovine immunoglobulin M Fc binding to *Brucella abortus*: a cause of nonspecific agglutination. *J Clin Microbiol* 1981;14:32-38.

10. Nielsen K, Duncan JR, Stemshorn B, Ruckerbauer G. Relationship of humoral factors (antibody and complement) to immune responsiveness, resistance and diagnostic serology. *The Ruminant Immune System*, Butler JE ed. New York: Plenum Press, 1981; 367-389.

11. Raybould TJG. Antigens of diagnostic significance in *Brucella abortus*. *Can J Microbiol* 1982;28:557-566.

12. Stemshorn BW. Recent progress in the diagnosis of brucellosis. *Devel biol Standard* 1984;56:325-340.

13. Plackett P, Cottew GS, Best SJ. An indirect haemolysis test (IHLT) for bovine brucellosis. *Aust Vet J* 1976; 52:136-140.

14. Ruckerbauer GM, Stemshorn BW, Nielsen KH. An hemolysis-in-gel test for anti-*Brucella* antibody in cattle serum. *The Ruminant Immune System*. Butler JE ed. New York: Plenum Press, 1981; 782-783.

15. Nicoletti P, Carlsen WB. Indirect hemolysis test in the serodiagnosis of bovine brucellosis. *Am J Vet Res* 1981; 42:1494-1497.

16. Diaz R, Garatea P, Jones LM, Moriyon I. Radial immunodiffusion test with *Brucella* polysaccharide B for differentiating infected from vaccinated cattle. *J Clin Microbiol* 1979;10:37-41.

17. Jones LM, Berman DT, Moreno E, Deyoe BL, Gilsdorf MJ, Huber JD, Nicoletti P. Evaluation of a radial immunodiffusion test with polysaccharide B antigen for the diagnosis of bovine brucellosis. *J Clin Microbiol* 1980; 12:753-760.

18. Cherwonogrodzky JW, Nielsen KH. *Brucella abortus* 1119-3 O-chain polysaccharide to differentiate sera from *B. abortus* S-19 vaccinated and field-strain-infected cattle by agar gel immunodiffusion. *J Clin Microbiol* 1988;26:1120-1123.

19. Wright PF, Nielsen KH, Kelly WA. Primary binding assay techniques for the serogiagnosis of bovine brucellosis: enzyme immunoassay. *Animal Brucellosis*, Nielsen KH, Duncan JR eds. Boca Raton: CRC Press, 1989; in press.

20. Nielsen KH, Wright PF, Kelly WA, Cherwonogrodzky JW. A review of enzyme immunoassay for detection of antibody to *Brucella abortus* in cattle. *Vet Immunol Immunopathol* 1988;18:331-347.

21. Wright PF, Nielsen KH. Application of enzyme immunoassay in veterinary medicine: serodiagnosis of bovine brucellosis. *Nonisotopic Immunoassay*, Ngo TT ed. New York: Plenum Press, 1988;129-146.

22. Nielsen K, Wright PF. Enzyme immunoassay and its application to the detection of bovine antibody to *Brucella abortus*. Agriculture Canada, Animal Diseases Research Institute, Nepean, ON 1984;1-121.

23. Holman PJ, Adams LG, Hunter DM, Heck FC, Nielsen KH, Wagner GG. Derivation of monoclonal antibodies against *Brucella abortus* antigens. *Vet Immunol Immunopathol* 1983;4:603-614.

24. Bundesen PG, Wyatt DM, Cottis LE, Blake AE, Massingham WA, Fletcher G, Street G, Welch JS, Rylatt DB. Monoclonal antibodies directed against *Brucella abortus* cell surface antigens. *Vet Immunol Immunopathol* 1985;8:245-260.

25. Schurig GG, Hammerberg C, Finkler BS. Monoclonal antibodies to *Brucella* surface antigens associated with the smooth lipopolysaccharide complex. *Am J Vet Res* 1984; 45:967-971.

26. Rylatt DB, Wyatt DM, Bundesen PG. A competitive enzyme immunoassay for the detection of bovine antibodies to *Brucella abortus* using monoclonal antibodies.

Vet Immunol Immunopathol 1985;8:261-271.

27. Nielsen K, Cherwonogrodzky JW, Duncan JR, Bundle DR. Enzyme-linked immunosorbent assay for differentiation of the antibody response of cattle naturally infected with *Brucella abortus* or vaccinated with Strain 19. *Am J Vet Res* 1989;50:5-9.

28. Bundle JR, Cherwonogrodzky JW, Caroff M, Perry MB. The lipopolysaccharides of *Brucella abortus* and *B. melitensis*. *Ann Inst Pasteur/Microbiol* 1987;138:92-98.

29. Bundle DR, Gidney MAJ, Perry MB, Duncan JR, Cherwonogrodzky JW. Serological confirmation of *Brucella abortus* and *Yersinia enterocolitica* 0:9 O-antigens by monoclonal antibodies. *Infect Immunity* 1984;46:389-393.

Chapter Twenty-one

Challenges to the Epidemiology of Infectious Diseases in the Next Decade

Alfred S. Evans

I am not a veterinarian, and certainly not an expert on brucellosis. However, I can make a small claim to having worked on some zoonotic diseases, such as Newcastle disease of chickens,[1-9] rabies,[10] leptospirosis,[11] California encephalitis virus, in conjunction with Wayne Thompson at the University of Wisconsin,[12] and Teschen virus of pigs in conjunction with Dorothy Horstman while with the Army in Germany.[13] This talk is directed primarily at challenges to the epidemiology of human infectious diseases in the next decade but I will also try to emphasize the important role that diseases arising from animals and birds will play in those developments and the need for close collaboration with infectious disease specialists in veterinary medicine and public health. I can not do this without acknowledgment of my long-term friendships with Jim Steele, formerly at the Centers of Disease Control, and with the late Bob Hanson from the University of Wisconsin, for both of whom I have the highest respect and regard.

My presentation is based in part on past publications on the theme of infectious disease epidemiology,[14-17] but more particularly on papers given within the past month in Beijing, China[17] and at the National Institute of Health in this country, the latter in co-authorship with Robert Shope.[18] I will emphasize both specific infectious diseases and the methodology used to study them. I will be largely concerned with viral rather than bacterial infection, although it has been my pleasure to edit epidemiology books concerned with both.[19-20] Persons interested in methodology in epidemiology studies are referred to a recent book on the subject.[21]

My priority list of the major challenges in human infectious disease epidemiology for now and in the next decade is presented in Table 21-1. I wish to discuss several issues in more detail, but not necessarily in the order listed.

Retroviruses

In my view, control of the retrovirus infections of humans, HIV-1 and 2 and HTLV-1, is and will remain our major challenge now and in the decade or so to come.

Five years ago I presented some thoughts on the past, present, and future of infectious disease epidemiology at a meeting of the International Epidemiological Association.[14] At the time of that presentation, the infectious diseases occupying the most space in two of our most prominent journals, the *New England Journal of Medicine* and the *Lancet*, were AIDS, leading the list, followed by viral hepatitis, herpes infections, and malaria. Four years later, the 1988 indexes of these journals show the same pattern, as portrayed in Table 21-2, and now include many papers dealing with the virus itself, the human immunodeficiency virus (HIV-1) which destroys the immune system and leads to the syndrome we call AIDS.

While doubts on the necessary and sufficient role of this virus in the causation of AIDS have been raised by a prominent virologist, Dr. Duesberg,[22,23] there is no question in my mind that public health policy must be based on control of HIV transmission, if we are to reduce the impact of this dreadful epidemic. A related virus, designated as HIV-2, also can lead to AIDS and is the predominant infection in certain parts of Africa.

Given the current and projected number of persons with AIDS and HIV infection, as shown in the Table 21-3, I can predict that these topics will dominate our journals, our medical hospital practice, our health insurance, our national costs for health care, as well as many other aspects of our society over the next decade or longer. For example, in 1992 alone it is predicted that 80,000 new cases of AIDS will occur in the United States, compared with the cumulative total of almost 100,000 since the syndrome was first recognized in 1981. Even if all transmission were to cease today, there are well over one million persons in the United States already infected with HIV most of whom will fall ill over the next decade. I predict that, while there will be a declining incidence in homosexuals, the rate of incidence in I.V. drug users, heterosexual contacts of current cases, and infants of infected mothers will continue to rise and produce wide and profound effects on our health care system and on the very fabric of our society in endemic areas.

The worldwide picture is equally alarming, with over 375,000 cases reported currently and some 500 million infected on a global basis. It is imperative that countries where HIV has not spread, or is just emerging, mount extensive educational programs on how the virus is transmitted and ways to prevent it. Asia is a high priority in my view. The pernicious circle of drug addiction (especially cocaine and crack), poverty, crime, and prostitution of both males and females must not be allowed to establish itself there, as it has in urban centers of the United States and some other centers of the developed world. HIV is also invading our college populations, and vigorous educational efforts must be carried out now, led by the students themselves, to try to halt its spread in this setting. I also suggest that our national programs not be directed at HIV alone, but on the wider

Table 21-1. Priorities for the Epidemiology of Infectious Diseases in the Next Decade

---

1. Control retroviruses (HIV-1, HIV-2, HTLV-1).

2. Control other high-incidence infections.

3. Expand and improve immunization programs.

4. Recognize and control new infectious agents.

5. Increase early diagnosis and detection of epidemic diseases.

6. Improve surveillance in developed and developing countries including surveillance of animal and avian diseases.

7. Apply molecular techniques to epidemiology and control of infectious diseases and to their pathogenesis.

8. Train more epidemiologists, especially for developing countries, and train more in epidemiology, molecular biology and genetics in developed countries to meet future challenges.

9. Expand the concept of the hospital epidemiologist to outpatient departments and clinics.

10. Seek to understand the pathogenesis of disease in both the community and in the individual as a basis for prevention.

---

and more acceptable aim of control of all sexual and blood-borne diseases.[24,25] These now include HIV, HTLV-1, hepatitis B, hepatitis A, syphilis, and cytomegalovirus. I wish to emphasize the growing threat of of HTLV-1 in I.V. drug users, which can lead to adult T cell leukemia, tropical spastic paresis, and perhaps other diseases. HTLV-1 may amplify the growth of HIV, since it infects the same cells. Such widened programs would also benefit the efforts against other venereal infections and tuberculosis, whose incidence and clinical severity are increasing in HIV-infected persons. Effective behavioral control of just hepatitis type B (HBV) would also greatly reduce the transmission of the other infections which are spread by the same routes, including HIV, since HBV is said to be some ten times more infectious than HIV.

Table 21-2. Number of Papers Devoted to Infectious Disease Subjects in the *New England Journal of Medicine* and the *Lancet* in 1989

New England Journal of Medicine (Jan.-Dec., 1988)			*Lancet* (Jan.-July, 1988)	
1. AIDS and ARC	62	1.	HIV	76
2. HIV	54	2.	AIDS	44
3. Herpes viruses	8	3.	Herpes V.	29
EBV	4		EBV	1
CMV	3		CMV	17
HSV	1		HSV	9
			HHV-6	12
4. Jap. B and vaccine	5	4.	Hepatitis	23
5. HTLV-1	4	5.	Malaria	14
6. Malaria	4	6.	Legionaires	10
7. Tuberculosis	4	7.	Salmonella	7
8. Hepatitis	4	8.	HTLV-1	5
9. Meningococcal Dis.	3	9.	Listerosis	5
10. Legionella	3	10.	Measles	3

I challenge you veterinarians to increase your efforts to understand the pathogenesis and spread of simian retroviruses that induce AIDS-like syndromes in monkeys and to seek other animal models of HIV infection, perhaps a species such as the genetically susceptible transfected mouse under study at the National Institutes of Health. These models are desperately needed to judge the effectiveness of new therapies and new approaches to prevention such as CD4 receptor blocking agents, interferon, and other immunological modalities.

Other Infectious Agents

In addition to the retroviruses, it can be predicted that other viruses demanding our attention over the next decade will include hepatitis B virus (HBV), despite the encouraging results with the new vaccines, Delta hepatitis and the non-A, non-B hepatitis viruses, and herpes infections, including the newly discovered herpes virus type 6 (HHV-6), (recognized as responsible for exanthem subitum and some cases of mono-like illnesses) provide new challenges. Papilloma virus will be of increasing long-term goals for control, respectively. The slow virus infections will be

Table 21-3. AIDS Update, February 1989

United States	1988*	1992**
New cases***	28,000	80,000
Cumulative cases	70,000	365,000
Cumulative deaths	35,000	263,000
HIV infected	1-1.5 million	
I.V. Drug users		
New York and New Jersey	15-20%	
Los Angeles and Seattle	5%	

Worldwide 1988*

Total cumulative cases	377,000
Africa (mostly heterosexuals)	200,000
N. America	110,000
Latin America	40,000
Europe	25,000
Australia, New Zealand, and Pacific	1,500
Asia	500

Total HIV infected - about 5 million

From: Center for Disease Control, World Health Organization, and the *New York Times*, Feb. 5, 1989.

*approximate number
**estimated
***Pattern - Changing from homosexual to greater percent I.V. drug users, their sexual partners, and their children (1000 now with 84% in Blacks and Hispanics).

increasing through organ transplants and in HIV-infected persons. Certainly, malaria and schistosomiases will be with us for a long time.

Immunization Programs

Hopefully, those childhood infections against which the World Health Expanded Program in Immunization (EPI) is directed, namely diphtheria, pertussis, tetanus, poliomyelitis, measles, and tuberculosis, will be under control by the end of this century. The greater thrust now provided through the participation of other organizations such as UNICEF, the Rockefeller Foundation, the Child Survival program, and others offers hope that realistic goals will be met, albeit not the original WHO goal of immunization of all children by the year 1990.

The major deterrents to success in developing countries are the general problems of getting the mothers to bring the children back for the 3 or 4 shots required, the problems of transport of materials and vaccine in difficult terrain, especially in the rainy season, and the maintenance of the cold chain. Specific problems are the difficulty of getting a good antibody response to measles vaccine in the presence of maternal antibody, poor immune response to oral polio vaccine in certain African and other countries, and the need for a better pertussis vaccine. A priority list for improved or needed vaccines for both developing and developed countries was recently prepared by the National Institute of Allergy and Infectious Disease and the Institute of Medicine, National Academy of Sciences (USA)[26] and is shown in Table 21-4. Progress has already been made on an improved HBV vaccine based on HBV DNA insertion into a yeast carrier. A much more potent and standardized inactivated poliomyelitis vaccine has been developed and tested and is equal in potency to oral poliomyelitis vaccine (OPV); it is immunogenic in geographic areas where OPV has failed. A more potent Edmundson-Zagreb Measles vaccine that overcomes much of the maternal antibody problem has been produced in Yugoslavia and had successful field trials, but has not yet been adopted by the World Health Organization. Several new, sometimes conjugated *Haemophitus influenzae* vaccines have been tested in Finland and the United States and been found effective in children over 18 months of age; under that age where much disease still occurs, the vaccine has not been sufficiently immunogenic. Encouraging results with killed and live cholera typhoid vaccines are being reported, and several attenuated pertussis vaccines are in development. The possibility that new types of time-release adjuvants can periodically release their antigens at defined intervals over a long period of time, thus eliminating the need for repeated injections, is on the far horizon and has been successfully used for certain animal vaccines. As mentioned earlier, several trials of bovine and monkey derived rotavirus vaccines are underway, as are both live and killed vaccines against hepatitis A virus (HAV) infections. However, HIV, RSV gonococcal, chlamydia, syphilis, and malaria vaccines seem to be in the more distant future.

Our main practical problem today is getting the effective vaccines that we now have into those that need them, and within the window of time after the disappearance of maternal antibody and before the onset of natural exposure occurs as in measles infection. It is not only children that present vaccine problems but also the elderly, whose use of tetanus, influenza, pneumococcal, and perhaps HBV vaccines is far below what we can and should attain In this older group antibody levels are dropping

Table 21-4. Vaccine Priorities

United States		Developing Countries	
1.	Hepatitis B	1.	*Strep. pneumoniae*
2.	Respiratory syncytial virus	2.	*Plasmodium* spp.
3.	*H. influenzae* Type B	3.	Rotaviruses - 3 types
4.	Influenza	4.	*Salmonella typhi*
5.	Varicella - Zoster	5.	*Shigella* spp.

If technical developments permit, strep Group B and *N. gonorrhoea* would be placed on the list above (from reference 26).

from childhood vaccines or from natural infections to which they were exposed to earlier in life, so that childhood infections and reactivated viral and bacterial infections are of increasing importance as our senior citizens grow in number and in their life-span. This problem will be confounded by the close and often unsanitary environment in many of our homes for the elderly, much like our day care nurseries are today. I would put influenza, *H. influenzae*, hepatitis viruses, respiratory syncytial virus, and recurrent herpes viruses on the high risk group of infections for this group. Care of the elderly and of AIDS patients will compete for our health budget in a difficult ethical dilemma, since neither group can be expected to be financially contributing members of society, even after our best medical care is rendered.

Emergence of New Viruses and New Infections

What new agents can we expect in the future? Several levels in the emergence of new viruses and their subsequent involvement of humans are shown in Table 21-5. I wish to explore some of these levels with you in more detail, as derived from a presentation given earlier this month by Robert Shope and myself at an NIH conference on "Emerging Viruses and Viral Infections."[18] The evolution of agents in nature usually involves one or more changes in viruses as they pass through human, animal, or avian hosts. These are depicted in Table 21-6 and include mutation; recombination of animal/avian strains with human strains as in influenza; and the emergence of genotypic variants as they multiply in human or animal hosts, as found with poliovirus, Epstein-Barr virus, and other herpes viruses.

Certain general concepts involved in the geographic and transport factors of newly emerged agents are depicted in Table 21-7. The umbrella concept of malaria hiding many other diseases, as promoted by my associate, Dr. Wilbur Downs at Yale, is an important one to remember. In an endemic area, malaria parasites are commonly present in the blood of both healthy and diseased persons so that persons with a febrile illness are often passed off with a diagnosis of malaria when many other infections may be the real cause of the illness. Perhaps there are similar ubiquitous agents in animals, such as various common parasitic infections, that may mislead the veterinarian, and discourage further investigation into the real cause of the illness. "Challenge the diagnosis," says Dr. Downs, and it is good advice for practitioners of both human and veterinary medicine.

Several factors that result in human exposure to new or pre-existing agents are depicted in Table 21-8. All involve movement of some type: 1) The human host moves to new sites where the agent is present, 2) The infectious agent is moved by human, animal, avian, insect carriers, or even tissues or cells from these hosts, to a susceptible population, and 3) Agents are introduced into portals of entry in humans that were not previously involved with that agent. New invasive diagnostic procedures, organ transplants, or unusual sexual practices are examples of this. Is there an equivalent of homosexual transmission in the animal kingdom?

In addition to emergence in nature, new viruses or our immunosuppressive drugs may lead to reactivation of old and new agents. In addition, our improving technology and curiosity are discovering new agents in old syndromes (*Legionella pneumophila* and the new TWAR chlamydial agents as causes of pneumonia), or old agents are producing new syndromes (parvo virus as cause of erythema infectiosa). Some examples of new or recrudescent viral infections are given in Table 21-9. It should be noted among this audience how many of these diseases are zoonotic infections. Could more intensive surveillance systems and newer diagnostic and seroepidemiological methods have predicted these infections earlier and prevented epidemic spread to other animals and to humans? Such predictive surveillance is one of the great challenges to infectious disease specialists in both human and veterinary medicine.

New syndromes of bacterial or of unknown cause are shown in Table 21-10. Kawasaki disease is an exanthem that peels, has mucous membrane involvement, and later involves other organs, especially the heart, with some 15-20% developing coronary artery disease, of which aneurysms are the most common. The disease occurs mostly under age two and is most frequent in Japan, where it was first recognized in 1967. Over 100,000 cases have since been reported. It also occurs in this country and other developing countries. Its etiology is a mystery and a great challenge for pediatric infectious disease workers in the next decade.

Finally, new environments for the interaction of the agent and of the host may result in new associations or the spread of old infections as shown in Table 21-11.

Table 21-5. Levels in the Emergence of Viruses and of Host-Virus Interactions

LEVEL

I. Agent evolving in nature.

II. Agent has evolved but effective human contact has not yet occurred.

III. Effective exposure, infection, and a new disease occur. (New agent, new disease).

IV. Previously latent or non-pathogenic agent produces disease in compromised host (old agent, new disease).

V. Known viruses in search of diseases or known diseases in search of viruses or the accidental tourist. Unknown viruses in search of unknown diseases.

Early Diagnosis and Detection

Given the existence of new agents and the possibility of their involvement in human population, how shall we set up systems for their early detection? Some suggestions are offered in Table 21-12. Similar early detection and sentinel systems are important in recognizing new or emerging infectious agents in animals. Veterinarians must work closely with those detecting human infections. Indeed, I favor combined units because most of the new human infections are likely to emerge from animals or birds or to have counterpart infections in those species.

Other Challenges in Infectious Disease Epidemiology

I have spent most of this lecture dealing with the emergence of new agents and new agent-host interactions, but there are also other important challenges facing us in infectious disease epidemiology to which I referred in Table 21-1. Of very high priority is the need for improved systems of surveillance in both developed and developing countries, utilizing the

Table 21-6. Factors Bearing on Viral Evolution.

Viral mutation	From human passage of virus or in animals by zoonotic agent
Viral recombination	Recombinants involving human, ani-mal, and avian viruses
Genotypic variation	Arising from passage in normal or immunocompromised hosts
Emergence of New Viral Properties	Genetic alterations affecting viru lence, transmission, tissue, tropisms, etc.
New animal viruses	Retroviral infection of non-human primates may lead to emergence of latent viruses capable of infecting humans
Interspecies infection	Viruses non-pathogenic for one species may be pathogenic for another species

tremendous power that the computer and improved methods of national and international communication bring to this task. Similar challenges must exist in veterinary medicine. In addition, there is an acute need for the training of more epidemiologists, especially for the developing world. I have had many veterinarians take my course in infectious disease epidemiology in the Summer Graduate Program in Epidemiology, started in 1965 at the University of Wisconsin, moved from there to the University of Minnesota from 1967 to 1987, and now at the University of Michigan. I have welcomed such students, but it is important for veterinarians to develop their own courses that focus entirely on animal and avian diseases, especially the zoonotic infections important to humans.

The relationship between viruses and malignant and chronic diseases deserves more emphasis. We have the fine studies of Marek's lymphoproliferative disease of chickens, of renal cancer in leopard frogs, of hepatitis viruses and liver cancer in woodchucks and in the Peking duck, and of feline leukemia virus in cats as examples. These are also important prototypes of human cancer and their pathogenesis.

Time does not permit discussion of other priorities on the list, but I do wish to emphasize the importance of seroepidemiological methods in both human and veterinary medicine, since so many infections are not clinically expressed. Laboratory methods using serologic tests and new molecular techniques represent important tools in prospective serological studies, such as those now being conducted in the homosexual populations at high risk to HIV infections. Prospective seroepidemiological studies have also been of enormous importance in recognizing the possible causative role of Epstein-Barr virus in infectious mononucleosis,[22-29] in African Burkitt's lymphoma[30] and more recently in Hodgkin's disease.[31] The prospective cohort studies of Beasley et al.[32] on the relationship of hepatitis B (HBV) to hepato-cellular cancer in Taiwan have led to the current trials of HBV vaccination of newborns in highly endemic areas for prevention of this malignancy by eliminating infection with its main causal factor, HBV. If successful, it will be the first human cancer preventable by a vaccine. In this effort, we follow in your footsteps in developing herpes vaccine to prevent Marek's lympho-proliferative disease in chickens. We have much to learn from one another and many exciting challenges to face together in the future. I hope this discussion will put another strand in the bond of that relationship.

Summary

This presentation has attempted to delineate some of the challenges facing human infectious disease epidemiology in the next decade. I have tried to relate some of these to similar challenges in veterinary medicine and to stress the overlap between the two. In human diseases, HIV infection, AIDS, and other associated retroviral diseases constitute now, and for the foreseeable future, the biggest challenge in infectious disease epidemiology that we face. Indeed, I regard AIDS as one of the major problems of our society, which will affect almost all avenues of human endeavor. Other retroviruses, such as HTLV-1, are also important, and various hepatitis viruses, herpes viruses, Lyme disease, and tuberculosis are also important challenges for the next decade. The effective use of current vaccines in our children, especially in developing countries, is one area in which we are making important progress, but I do not predict that any of these infections will be eradicated in the next decade as was smallpox. But enormous decreases in measles and poliomyelitis should occur, with their possible elimination in some developing countries. New agents will emerge, and we must be prepared to recognize them early and institute early control measures. A good surveillance system in both human and veterinarian medicine is critical to these ends. The future will bring important new tools such as molecular biology, monoclonal antibody and rapid diagnostic techniques to bear on problems of transmission, pathogenesis, and vaccine development. It will be an exciting time, and we should be training young scientists in epidemiology, genetics and microbiology so that they are capable of meeting these challenges.

Table 21-7. Geographic and Transport Factors: General Concepts

1. Viruses may evolve in situ in isolated and focal geographic areas and betransported to human communities by human migration, arthropod vectors, animals, and birds.

2. Viruses evolving in indigenous hosts often cause inapparent infection.

3. When viruses are transported to new ecosystems, new geographic areas, or new hosts, they often emerge as "new diseases."

4. In order to emerge, viruses need receptive soil, appropriate transport mechanisms, and a non-immune host .

5. Remember "The umbrella of Malaria" - many new diseases and viruses may hide beneath it.

6. Seek new diseases within old clinical syndromes.

Table 21-8. Factors Favoring Effective Contact Between Humans and New or Pre-existing Viral Agent

FACTOR	EXAMPLES
1. Travel and exploration	Tropics, ocean depths, space archeological diggings
2. Human movement	Migration from remote rural to urban settings
3. Animal movement	Migration or transport into new ecosystems and into new susceptibles
4. Arthropod or other vector carriage	Either alone or via birds, airplanes, food, humans
5. Organ movement	1. Human or animal organs for human transplantation 2. Animal organs for tissue culture
6. New portals of entry	New or old agents introduced by new route due to behavioral changes or invasive medical procedures.

Table 21-9. Examples of New or Recrudescent Viral Diseases

DISEASE	AREA (YEAR)	RISK FACTORS
AIDS	USA (1981 on)	Introduction of HIV homosexual & IV spread
Arg. Hem. fever	Argentina ('73)	Rodent exposure maize harvesting
Bol. Hem. fever	Bolivia ('64, '71)	Rodent exposure in houses
Ebola fever	Zaire and Sudan	Patient contact (1976) needle spread
Epid. Poly-arthritis	Pacific Area	Mosquito borne
Lassa fever	Nigeria ('69,'89) Liberia, Sierra Leone ('70-'74)	Hospital exposure Rodent exposure
Marburg disease	Germany, Yugoslavia ('67), South Africa ('75)	Exposure to monkey culture
Rift Valley fever	Egypt ('77)	Local outbreak, wind, mosquitos, camels
Yellow fever	Nigeria ('79-'80)	Sylvan outbreak, viremic tourists, home water storage

Table 21-10. Recent NewBacterial Diseases of Unknown Cause

DISEASE	ETIOLOGY FACTORS	POSSIBLE RISK
1. Chronic fatigue syndrome		Unknown Stress, depression, ?EBV
2. Kawasaki disease	Unknown	Rug shampoo, swamps
3. Legionaire's disease	*L. Pneumophilia*	cooling towers, smoking
4. Lyme disease	*B. burgdorferi*	Exposure to infected ticks
5. Toxic shock	Staphlococci	Highly absorbant tampons

Table 21-11. Special Environmental Hazards

EXPLORATION

1. Arctic and Antarctic
2. Bottom of the ocean
3. Space flight
4. Under the earth
5. Remote tropical settings

SOCIAL

1. Day care centers
2. Nurseries
3. Homes for the elderly
4. Prisons
5. Recruit camps
6. Polaris submarines
7. Massive sit-ins

IATRAGENIC

1. Needle puncture
2. Biopsies
3. Invasive procedures
4. Organ transplants
5. Artificial insemination
6. Vicarious pregnancy

Table 21-12. Early Detection of New Viruses and New Diseases

---

1.   Establish sentinel surveillance and serological units in high-risk areas for emerging viruses supported, if possible, by a high-level laboratory or at least a rapid transport system to one. Monitor and collect blood and other secretions from febrile illnesses.

2.   Prepare a mobile team and laboratory under the CDC or WHO, staffed by highly trained microbiologist, epidemiologists, entomologists, etc. , that is prepared to leave on a moment's notice to investigate an outbreak of disease anywhere in the world.

3.   Set up a "red alert" reporting system for hospital, especially in high-risk areas to report unusual cases or epidemics.

References

1. Evans AS, Curnen EC. Serological studies on infectious mononucleosis and other conditions with human erythrocytes modified by Newcastle disease virus. *J Immunol* 1948;58:323-335.
2. Evans AS. Serological studies on infectious mononucleosis, viral hepatitis, and other conditions with human erythrocytes modified by Newcastle virus: a comparison of the virus strain employed. *J Immun* 1959;64:411-420.
3. Evans AS, Melnick JL. Attempts to produce lymphopenia in rabbits following the intravenous inoculation of certain viruses. *J Inf Dis* 1950;86:223-25.
4. Evans AS. The occurrence of Newcastle disease antihemagglutinin in human sera and its relationship to mumps virus. *J Immun* 1951;67:529-538.
5. Evans AS. Newcastle disease neutralizing antibody in human serum and its relationship to mumps. *Am J Hyg* 1954;60:204.
6. Evans AS. Pathogenicity and immunology of Newcastle disease virus (NDV) in man. *Am J Pub Health* 1955;45:742-745.
7. Evans AS. The interaction of serum with erythrocytes modified by Newcastle disease virus. *J Immun* 1955;74:391-396.
8. Evans AS. The laboratory diagnosis of Newcastle disease in man. *Am J Clin Path* 1956;26:163.
9. Evans AS. Newcastle disease, the virus and its relation to human illness. *Health* 1960;14:12-14.
10. Evans AS. Rabies in Wisconsin. *Wisconsin Med J* 1963;62:329-333.
11. Allen V, Sueltman S, Evans AS. Leptospirosis in Wisconsin. *Am J Public Health* 1965;55:1936-1944.
12. Thompson WH, Evans AS. California virus studies in Wisconsin. *Am J Epid* 1965;81:230-234.
13. Evans AS, Horstman DM. Unpublished studies of Teschen virus of pigs and it relationship to poliovirus carried out in the U.S. Army 98th General Hospital, Munich, Germany, 1950-1952.
14. Evans AS. Ruminations on infectious disease epidemiology: retrospective, curspective, and prospective. *Intl J Epid* 1985; 14:205-211.

15. Evans AS, Brachman PS. Emerging issues in infectious disease epidemiology. *J Chr Dis* 1986;39:1105-1124.
16. Evans AS. Subclinical epidemiology. The first Harry A. Feldman Memorial Lecture. *Am J Epid* 1987;125:545-555.
17. Evans AS. Thoughts on the future of infectious disease epidemiology. Presented at the International Scientific Conference on Epidemiology, April 24-26, 1989, Beijing, China.
18. Evans AS, Shope RS. Assessing geographic and transport factors. Presented at Conference on Emerging Viruses and Virus Infections, National Institute of Allergy and Infectious Diseases, National Institutes of Health, Bethesda, Maryland, May 2-3, 1989.
19. Evans AS ed. Viral Infections of Humans. *Epidemiology and Control.* 3rd ed., New York: Plenum Press, 1989.
20. Evans AS, Feldman HA. *Bacterial Infections of Humans. Epidemiology and Control.* Plenum Press, NYC, 1982.
21. Kelsey J, Thompson D, Evans AS. *Methods in Observational Epidemiology.* Oxford Press, NY 1982.
22. Duesberg P. Retroviruses as carcinogens and pathogens. Expectations and reality. *Cancer Res* 1987;47:1199-1226.
23. Duesberg P. HIV is not the cause of AIDS. *Science* 1988; 241:524-516.
24. Evans AS. Does HIV cause AIDS? An historical perspective. *JAIDS* 1989;2:107-113.
25. Evans AS. The multiple benefits of an AIDS control program. *JAIDS* 1988;1:415.
26. National Institute of Allergy and Infectious Diseases. Program for accelerated development of new vaccines. 1985 progress Report, NIH, Bethesda, 1985.
27. Evans AS, Neiderman JC, McCollum. Seroepidemiological studies of infectious mononucleosis with EB virus. *New Eng J Med* 1968;279:1121-1127.
28. Sawyer RN, Evans AS, Niederman JC, McCollum RW. Prospective studies of a group of Yale University freshmen. I. Occurrence of infectious mononucleosis. *Yale J Biol Med* 1971;123:263-269.
29. Hallee TJ, Evans AS, Jiederman JC, Brooks CM, Voegtly JC. Infectious mononucleosis at the U.S. Military Academy: A prospective study of a single class over four years. *Yale J Biol Med* 1974;47:182-195.
30. de Thé G, Geser, A, Day NE, Tuber PM, Williams EH, Beir DP, Smith PG, Dean A, Bornkamm GW, Feorino P, Henle W. Epidemiological evidence for causal relationship between Epstein-Barr virus and Burkitt's Lymphoma from Ugandan prospective study. *Nature* 1978;274:756-761.
31. Mueller N, Evans AS, Harris NL and members of the EBV-HD collaboration. Hodgkin's disease and EBV. Evidence of elevated antibody prior to diagnosis. *New Eng J Med* 1989;320:696-701.
32. Beasley RP, Hwang L-V, Lin C-C, Chien C-S. Hepatocellular carcinoma and hepatitis B virus: a prospective study of 22,707 men in Taiwan. *Lancet* 1981;2:1129-1133.

Chapter Twenty-two

Regulatory Program Decision Making Through Brucellosis Epidemiologic and Econometric Simulation Modeling

Stephen H. Amosson

and Raymond A. Dietrich

Introduction

As governments faced rising costs in the early 1970s, concern spread over government involvement in animal health programs and the efficiency with which regional and national programs were conducted. Government officials, producer groups, and others involved in brucellosis control began to have questions that were difficult to answer: Should the government be involved? Can eradication of the disease be achieved? Is a control or eradication policy the most cost effective? What combinations of program components are the most effective?

These questions led to the development of bio-economic simulators. These simulators provided a mechanism for projecting the future effects of current and proposed programs on disease prevalence, changes in benefits and/or losses from the disease, and program costs. Legislators, government officials, and producer groups can use such data and information in determining the effectiveness or ineffectiveness of current and proposed animal health programs.

The purpose of this paper is to examine the development, use, and empirical implications of bio-economic simulators in modeling bovine brucellosis. We will trace the evolution of bio-economic simulators employed to model bovine brucellosis; examine the development process of the last bio-economic simulator, BRUSIM; discuss the empirical implications derived from the two studies in which BRUSIM has been employed; and discuss the potential uses, limitations, and improvements that can be made in BRUSIM.

Review of Literature

In 1975, bio-economic simulation of the brucellosis eradication program in England and Wales was conducted by Hugh-Jones, Ellis and Felton.[1] This study was based on a stochastic computer simulation of a 100-herd model representing dairy and beef herds of England and Wales. Disease spread was simulated using a Monte Carlo random number technique with probability ranges discerned epidemiologically relevant. Varying herd management assumptions were used to be representative of the population; the model assessed and monitored within-herd infection spread, the amount of time to clean up the herd and the physical losses of beef and milk. The model, which generalized the simulation results to all the herds in England and Wales, yielded benefit/cost ratios 1.1 to 2.2 for the British Compulsory Eradication scheme, depending on the inclusion of losses.

A second Monte Carlo-based study was conducted by Roe and Morris[2] to evaluate the Australian brucellosis program. The model was designed to simulate range conditions, herd structure and population characteristics for any designated region. A 10% sample of the animals in the geographic area was simulated with each animal being represented on an individual animal basis. A Monte Carlo simulation determines the epidemiological sequence of events that can occur to the animals given the characteristics of the cattle population. Results indicated a 5.03 benefit/cost ratio for a test-and-slaughter eradication program, compared to a 2.96 benefit/cost ratio for a continued-vaccination program, when compared to a no-program option.

The previously mentioned Monte Carlo studies have an appealing characteristic, the ability to demonstrate the range of potential outcomes that can occur within an affected herd. This type of analysis allows for the evaluation of the timing of testing given varying sets of herd characteristics and environmental factors such as herd size, density, and frequency of testing.

The Monte Carlo approach leaves some major unanswered questions in evaluating national animal health programs. Brucellosis is a disease that is predominantly spread by infected animals coming in contact with clean animals. Therefore, the basic mode of disease spread is the purchase of infected replacements. In the Hugh-Jones et al. study,[1] the spread between herds was not modeled. Failure to account for the spread of infection diminishes the validity of macro program testing comparisons and the benefit-cost analysis.

The Roe and Morris Monte Carlo study[2] allowed for the spread from affected herds to non-affected herds. The probability of the spread of infection within the specified district (county) is proportional to the prevalence of infected breeding cattle within that district. The probability of a herd being infected from outside the district but within the region (state) is proportional to the prevalence of infected breeding cattle within that region. The spread to a district from the remainder of the country is assumed to be proportional to the percentage of infected breeding cattle in the matrix as a whole. The probability of purchasing breeding cattle from within a district is the same for all districts as is the probability of any district purchasing outside the district but within the region or from outside the region.

The Roe and Morris analysis also leaves unanswered some epidemiologic and operational considerations. First, the study used the assumption of homogeneous purchase of breeding cattle by all districts. In the U.S., the amount and location of breeding replacement purchases vary considerably by state. Second, no differentiation was made on the probability of purchasing replacements by herd size. Logically, a rancher owning a herd of 1,000 cows purchases more animals from different sources than a rancher owning a herd of 10 cows during any given year.

Third, it is questionable that the spread of brucellosis to clean herds is proportionate to the percentage of infected breeding cattle in the population under consideration. The present U.S. herd prevalence is at least three times the current animal prevalence rate. The spread to clean herds is dependent on such factors as number and frequency of purchases, number of breeding animals purchased, vaccination status, and producer and/or government monitoring of these purchased replacements.

A primary problem with Monte Carlo simulation modeling of macrobiological systems is the cost involved. Simulating the potential events for every breeding animal in a large population or a small representative sample involves the use of large amounts of computer. Further, simulating the probability of an event with a flat normal distribution, as was conducted in the Monte Carlo studies, yields nothing more than that probability times its outcome if the population is large enough. For example, if the probability of an infected animal aborting is 0.6 and 1,000 infected animals are simulated the expected number of abortions is 600.

In 1975, Carpenter[3] developed a linear programming model for evaluating California's brucellosis program. Using a partial budgeting approach for projecting benefits and costs over a 15-year planning horizon, it yielded benefit/cost ratios of 5.07 for a program featuring heavy vaccination and 3.82 for an eradication program

In 1979, Carpenter and Howitt[4] expanded on the use of linear regression and linear programming as a tool for brucellosis policy evaluation in California. The authors formulated an ordinary least squares regression equation that describes prevalence in period t (number of infected cows divided by total number of cows in California) as a function of prevalence in period t-1, percentage level of vaccination, level of surveillance and the level of animal health personnel in the program.

The solution to the linear programming problem (L.P.) yields the economically optimal levels of vaccination, market cattle idendication, (MCI) surveillance, and animal health personnel necessary to achieve eradication with a 15-year planning horizon. The major benefit of linear programming is the ability to perform ex-post sensitivity analysis at a relatively low cost. This analysis allows for the evaluation of changes in the planning horizon of eradication, cost of program components, effectiveness of program components, and physical constraints.

While Carpenter and Howitt point out some interesting possibilities for the use of linear programming, operational shortcomings arise from this approach. First, the MCI program consists of testing cull cows at the slaughter level and tracing infected cows (reactors) back to the herd of origin. The MCI effectiveness is a function of the total marketing of cull cows which tends to follow eight-year cycles. Therefore, there is no guarantee that there will be sufficient cull cows available to test as indicated by the L.P. solution. During years of heavy culling, the physical constraints of the MCI testing system may be overloaded, which could cause the MCI effectiveness to decrease. The effect of cattle cycles is a major determinant of the effectiveness of the MCI system and is not accounted for in the study.

Second, as vaccination increases, the number of infected animals in an affected herd decreases. Thus, the number of infected animals culled from affected herds decrease. Since detection of affected herds under the MCI system is dependent on the number of infected cows culled, the level of vaccination has an inverse affect on the effectiveness of the MCI system.[5,6] This relationship may yield multicollinearity problems, biasing the estimates of the effectiveness of both components in the regression equation.

Third, research by Amosson et al.[7] and Roe[8] indicates that the relationship between the MCI and/or vaccination programs and the prevalence rate takes the shape of a hyperbolic curve that stabilizes at a positive rate of infection. The linear extrapolation of the hyperbolic curve inherent in linear programming may yield an optimal eradication solution where it is totally unfeasible, thus, misleading policy makers about the effectiveness of the MCI and vaccination components.

Fourth, the effect of introduction of the disease by purchase of infected replacements from outside of California is not considered. This factor dampens the probability of achieving full eradication.

The use of linear programming as a tool for evaluating more animal health programs is questionable. The flexibility of L.P. to analyze potential program elements is intuitively appealing. Some of the problems with cattle cycles, model misspecification, and introduction of infection from other states can be handled within an L.P. framework. However, the overriding problems of row linear relationships between prevalence and program components, in conjunction with the bias created by multicollinearity between program components, severely limit the effectiveness of L.P. in evaluating brucellosis programs.

In 1977, Beal and Kryder[a] developed the first systems simulation model for evaluating proposed U.S. national brucellosis programs. This model divided the U.S. into five regions based on geographic location, surveillance program effectiveness, producer characteristics, and infection levels. Beef and dairy sectors were analyzed separately. Physical losses were estimated on a per-infected-animal basis and then aggregated on a regional and national basis. Physical losses were valued at 1975 prices over the 35-year simulation period with cow numbers and herd size structure being held constant.

Beal and Kryder were the first to use binomial methodology with brucellosis in simulating the probability of purchasing an infected replacement. Binomial methodology takes into account herd size, the number of purchases, the source of the purchases, inter-regional movement, and prevalence levels in determining the probability of a clean herd becoming infected.[a] They also introduced the use of sampling from hypergeometric distributions for estimating detection probabilities of infected herds under the MCI.

Results indicated declining but favorable benefit/cost ratios for the following: 1) an all out eradication program over the 1975-76 program, 2) a reduced present program, and 3) a voluntary vaccination program with no other surveillance, when compared to a no-program option. Econometric analysis of the Beal and Kryder[10,11] results yielded higher benefit/cost ratios but left the ranking of the alternative programs unchanged.

A subsequent effort by Amosson, Dietrich and Hopkin, the National Brucellosis Technical Commission (NBTC) bio-economic simulation model, used both an epidemiological model and a sector equilibrium econometric model. The NBTC system's simulation epidemiological model expanded on the Beal and Kryder model by 1) further delineating the U.S. into eight regions; 2) allowing for affected herds to move into a "quarantined status" (infected and detected), or an undetected infected status (This has a major impact on infection rates, disease spread and clean-up rates in the model); 3) allowing the disease to spread between beef and dairy herds while simulating them simultaneously; and 4) allowing for "early quarantine release" i.e., quarantined herds to be released from quarantine while still infected. Cow numbers and herd size structure were held constant over the model's 20-year planning horizon.

The NBTC sector equilibrium econometric model generated changes in consumer surplus, producer surplus, and total welfare for each alternative

---

[a] For elaboration on use of double binomial, triple binomial, and hypergeometric approximation in animal disease problems see Beal, V.C. Jr. *Regulatory Statistics*, Vols 1, 2-A, and 2-B. Veterinary Services, APHIS, USDA, Hyattesville, Maryland, May, 1988.

control program compared to a baseline projection which estimated the effects of the 1975-76 brucellosis program. Results revealed benefit/cost ratios ranging from 24.02 for whole herd vaccination (vaccinating calves and cows) to -12.48 for the no-program option. In general, adult vaccination programs of high prevalence regions yielded the highest benefit/cost ratios, followed by calfhood vaccination programs and the proposed eradication programs. All increased government funding programs yielded benefit/cost ratios greater than one.

Development of BRUSIM

An economic and epidemiologic analysis of a national and/or regional disease control program requires two types of models: an epidemiologic model and a welfare model. The epidemiologic model is necessary to simulate industry characteristics; incidence and spread of infection; the effects of various prevention, control, and/or eradication program components on the level of infection; and physical losses and associated producer, state, and federal expenditures (See Figure 22-1).

An economic welfare model is necessary to interpret the economic effects of the change in physical losses to consumers, producers and related industries. "TECHSIM," a general equilibrium econometric model, was developed to simulate the equity impacts.[12] TECHSIM consists of systems of equations describing the inter-relationships of industries involved in the crop and livestock sectors of the United States. The equations in TECHSIM were formulated using ordinary least squares and generalized least squares estimating techniques on historical data. Portions of TECHSIM have been published in various sources, therefore, this paper will primarily focus on the development of the epidemiologic simulation model, BRUSIM.

The NBTC epidemiologic systems simulation model served as the prototype in developing BRUSIM. The eight regions of the NBTC simulation model have been replaced with 16 regions in BRUSIM (See Figure 22-2). Six regions of BRUSIM (Northeast-Lake, Atlantic, Florida, Northern Plains, West, and California) are identical to NBTC regions. The other two NBTC simulation regions were further subdivided into ten regions in BRUSIM (Alabama, Kentucky, Mississippi, Tennessee, Arkansas, Louisiana, Oklahoma, West Texas and East Texas). Texas was divided into East and West regions to reflect differences in management practices, prevalence levels and Uniform Method and Rules (UM&R) classifications.

The 10 new regions represent areas that have or may undergo in the future, high levels of program activity due to high brucellosis prevalence levels. Program records indicate varying types and levels of program components have existed in these states since 1976. Delineation of these

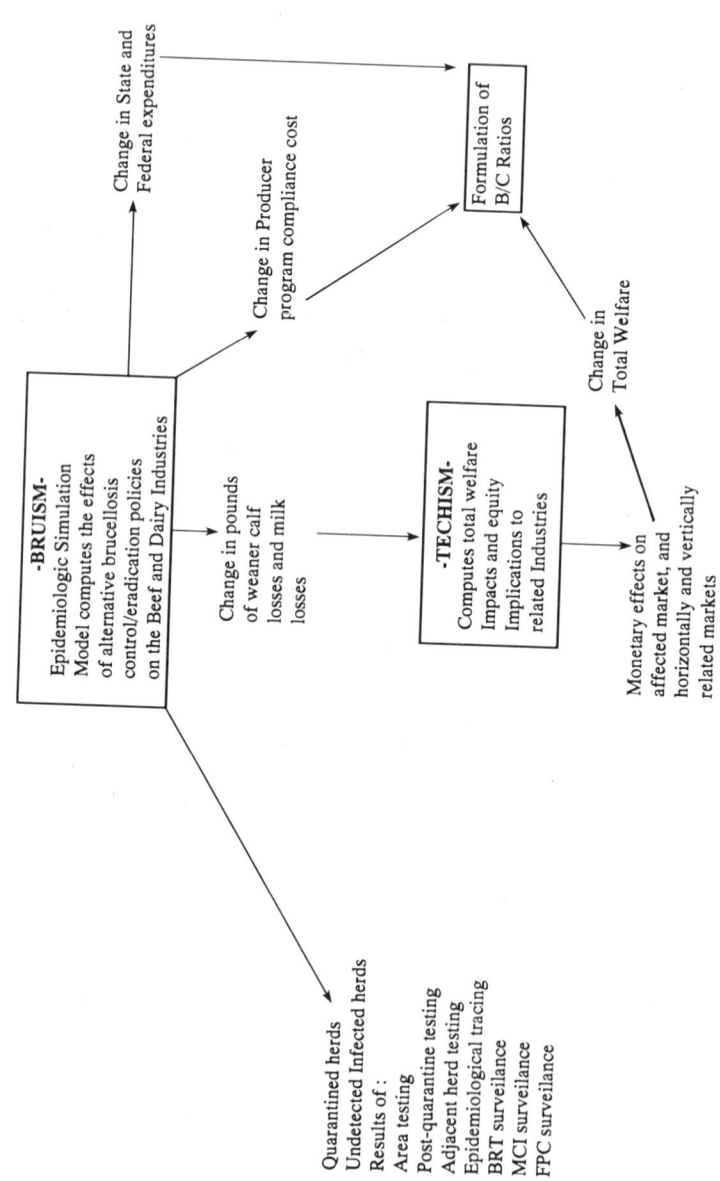

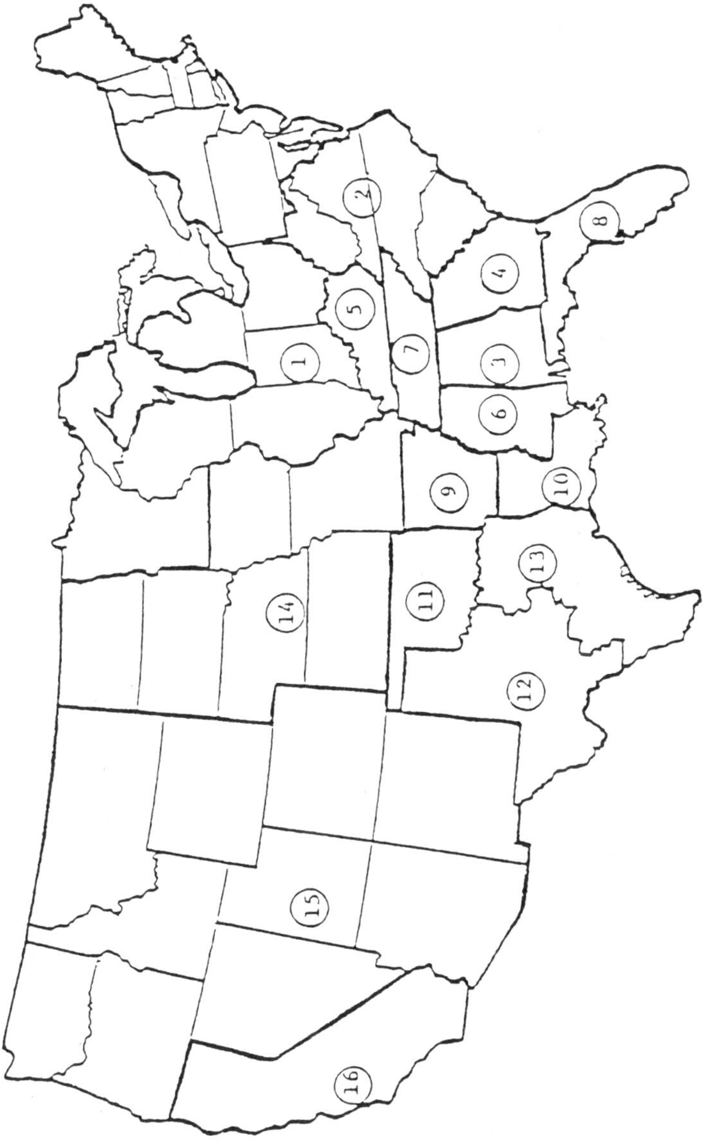

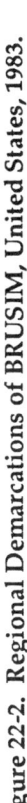

Figure 22-2. Regional Demarcations of BRUSIM, United States, 1983.

regions allows for a more accurate portrayal of program activities occurring in these regions.

A second major modification of the NBTC model in BRUSIM is separation of the effects of major program components. A series of equations representing MCI, first point of concentration (FPC) testing, adjacent herd testing, secondary epidemiologic tracing, post-quarantine testing, and area testing are contained in BRUSIM. The previous studies by Beal and Kryder[9] and Amosson et al.[7] accounted for changes in these program components through the efficiency of the MCI and BRT systems, and if applicable, modification in the rate of disease spread.

Linear and non-linear equations representing the effects of program components were estimated using ordinary least squares, theoretical distributions, and epidemiological judgement. Delineation of program components allows BRUSIM to be used determine the epidemiologic and economic efficiency of individual program components and/or combinations of program components.

Data for BRUSIM were obtained from both primary and secondary sources. Some of the basic information and epidemiologic data were obtained from the 1978 NBTC study. The NBTC data were supplemented and updated by information from the U.S. Department of Agriculture and U.S. Department of Commerce. Additional epidemiological data were obtained from a national survey of owners of quarantined herds and a survey of Texas producers with quarantined and non-quarantine herds. Data sources also included the expert judgement of NBTC personnel, brucellosis epidemiologists, and state and federal program officials. Specific parameters relating to herd characteristics, herd management, epidemiology, and physical losses used in BRUSIM for the beef and dairy sectors are shown in Table 22-1.

The annual results from BRUSIM are printed in five output sections for the beef and dairy sectors on a regional and national basis. The output sections printed are an epidemiological summary, a program component test summary, an epidemiological tracing component summary, state and federal expenditures, and producer expenditures (See Table 22-2).

Economic Analysis

Benefit-cost analysis was the primary criteria used in determining the economic acceptability and ranking of alternative programs. This criterion has been used widely in determining the economic efficiency of animal health programs.[1,7,9,10,11,13,14] Net benefits were defined as the change in the value of physical losses of meat and milk associated with alternative programs compared to the base program. Net costs were defined as the change in total cost from the base program to specified program alterna-

Table 22-1. Brusim Input Factors as Related to Region, Herd Size, Year of Infection and Quarantine, and Beef and Dairy Sector, 1984.

Input Matrix Description	Dimension of Matrix				Sector	
	Reg	HZ	Inf Year	Quar Year	Beef	Dairy
Total number of cows	X				X	X
Proportion of replacement purchased	X				X	X
Source ratio of replacements purchased		X			X	X
Total number of herds	X	X			X	X
Number of undetected affected herds	X	X	X		X	X
Quarantined herds	X	X	X	X	X	X
Average number of cows per herd	X	X			X	X
Undetected within herd infection rates	X	X	X		X	X
Undetected infected clean-up rates	X	X	X		X	X
Regional sales probability	X				X	X
BRT Rate	X					X
Cull Rate*					X	X
Replacement Rate*					X	X
MCI Rate	X				X	X
FPC Rate	X				X	X
FPC testing percentage	X				X	X
Quality control factor	X				X	X
Neighborhood spread factor	X	X			X	X
Weight loss for undetected infected			X		X	X
Weight loss for detected infected			X		X	
Milk loss for undetected infected	X		X			X
Milk loss for detected infected	X		X			X
Producer test per cow	X	X			X	X
Quarantine herd tests	X	X	X	X	X	X
Clean-up rate for quarantine herd tests	X	X	X	X	X	X
Residual infection rates	X	X			X	X
Weighted population proportions	X	X			X	X
Weighted infection rates	X	X			X	X
Area testing coefficients	X				X	X
Contact herd year keys*	X				X	X
Number of contact herds	X				X	X
Percent contact herds tested	X				X	X
Herdsize management parameter	X				X	
Owner testing percentage	X				X	X
Secondary Epidemiologic testing percentage	X				X	X
Post-quarantine testing percentage	X	X			X	X

*Dimensioned by model year

Table 22-2. Variable Included by Output Section of BRUSIM, United States 1983.

Output Section	Variables Included
Epidemiologic Summary	Year, Undetected Affected Herds, Quarantined Herds, Quarantined Infected Cows, Undetected Infected Cows, Total Infected Cows, Pounds of Calf Loss, Pounds of Milk Loss, Producer Costs and Cumulative Producer Costs Discounted
Program Component Test Summary	Year, FPC Cows Tested, MCI Cows Tested, MCI Herds Quarantined, MCI Reactor Rate, Herds Area Tested, Quarantined Area Test Herds, Epidemiologic Traced Herds Quarantined, Heifers Vaccinated and On Farm Tests
Epidemiological Tracing	Year, Adjacent Herds Tested, Adjacent Component Summary Herds Quarantined, Post-Quarantined Herds Tested, Post-Quarantined Herds Quarantined, Secondary Epidemiologic Herds Tested, Secondary Epidemiologic Herds Quarantined, Total Epidemiologic Herds Tested, and Total Epidemiologic Herds Quarantined
State and Federal Expenditures	Year, MCI, FPC, Area Test, Herd Depopulation, Epidemiologic Tracing, Vaccination, Quarantine Herd Testing, Fixed Cost and Total Cost Producer Expenditures Year, FPC, Area test, Post-Quarantine Testing, Private Testing, Secondary Epidemiologic Trace Testing, Adjacent Herd Testing, Vaccination, Quarantine Herd Testing and Total Cost

Contained only in printout of dairy sector.

tives.

Changes in benefits and costs were measured from a base model that held infection in a relatively "steady state" over the simulation horizon. The fundamental program components of the base program were the same as those employed in the NBTC study[7] and similar to the U.S. brucellosis control program existing during 1976. Gramlich refers to this type of benefit-cost analysis as the decision of the direction to take within the "black box,"[15] ie, the decision to eradicate or reduce the level of infection has been made and the question of how to improve the program to reach the goal is being considered.

This analysis does not include the monetary losses which accrue to humans from the contraction of brucellosis in the form of undulant fever. Placing a dollar value on the potential loss of life and health resulting from undulant fever was considered out of the scope of the study. It is anticipated that cases of undulant fever would decrease from current levels with the subsequent reduction in infection projected in the alternative programs considered.

A decrease in the prevalence of brucellosis yields a lower average cost to cattle producers through reduction in physical losses and abatement of preventive costs. The resultant increase in the supply of beef and milk due to decreases in physical losses can have varying effects. For example, the price of beef to consumers may fall, while grain producers may face increased demand; competing products such as pork, chicken and fish may also face reduced demand because of the relatively lower price of beef. Given these possible varying effects, it becomes imperative to assess the equity implications of bovine brucellosis control and/or eradication programs. Total net benefits from a general equilibrium supply and demand model represents the net effect of a change in infection not only to producers but also to consumers and related industries.

Economic theory provides a basis for the delineation of total net benefits into its components through measurements from general equilibrium solutions of the affected markets.[16] Thus, the impacts of changes in prevalence can be measured with respect to society, livestock producers, grain producers and other related industries on a national basis.

TECHSIM was utilized to evaluate the equity implications of the change in calf pound losses from the base model. TECHSIM does not include equations describing milk supply and demand relationships. Changes in milk supplies were evaluated at the U.S. average blend price received by producers for milk in 1982.[17]

Programs Evaluated By BRUSIM - TECHSIM

The BRUSIM - TECHSIM bio-economic simulator was used to analyze alternative U.S. Brucellosis programs in two recent studies. Eleven alternative programs were examined between the two studies.[14,18] The eleven programs simulated from 1976 to 2005 included the following:

1.   Base Program - Defined as the FY 1976 through FY 1984 brucellosis program with changes in program procedures that would result in the disease remaining at a relatively constant level from 1985 to 2005 the base program would serve as the basis from which changes in program efficiency could be measured for alternative bovine brucellosis programs. The market cattle identification system (MCI), first-point-of-concentration testing, and brucellosis ring testing were assumed to be the backbone of the surveillance system.

2.   Current (1976-84) Program - Defined as the existing 1976-84 bovine brucellosis program in the contiguous 48 states. This program was simulated to reflect a continuation of progress which has been made between FY 1976 and FY 1984 through FY-2005.

3.   Rapid Eradication - This scenario was modeled under (a) theoretical and (b) realistic modes.

a.   Theoretical mode - Assumed that obstacles relating to manpower and industry cooperation were nonexistent and that there would be strict adherence to the requirements of the Uniform Methods and Rules (UM&R).

b.   Realistic mode - Assumed that manpower and industry cooperation obstacles will continue to exist but that there would be strict adherence to the requirements of the UM&R by program authorities.

4.   Base Program with a 25% Increase in Program Efficiency in Class C Regions - This scenario assumed that 1984 base program assumptions would apply to all regions from 1985 to 2005. It further assumed that there would be a 25% increase in program efficiency in terms of adherence to the UM&R after 1984 in Class C regions.

5.   Base Program with a 25 % Decrease in Program Efficiency in Class C Regions - This scenario assumed that 1984 base program assumptions would apply to all regions from 1985 to 2005. It further assumed that there would be a 25 percent decrease in program efficiency in terms of adherence to the UM&R after 1984 in Class C regions.

6.   No State-Federal Program with No Vaccination - This   scenario assumed that a milk ordinance enforced would be for dairy cattle.

7.   No State-Federal Program with Calfhood Vaccination Supported by Industry - Two scenarios were modeled. Both scenarios assumed that annual federal funding will be limited to $6 million. Both also assumed that there would be a milk ordinance-enforced brucellosis program in cattle. One scenario assumed that vaccination would result in a 45% vaccination level of female calves entering the herd and the other assumed a 75% vaccination level of female calves entering the herd.

8.   Base Model Plus Adjacent Herd Testing - Two models were utilized to analyze the effectiveness of using adjacent herd testing. One model used the program component assumptions of the base model but imposed 100% adjacent herd testing of MCI-identified affected herds in all regions. The other model followed the same procedure as the first but assumed that adjacent herd testing was half as effective in identifying affected herds.

9.   Vaccination Programs - Three vaccination models were simulated to identify the benefits and costs of vaccination given current levels of infection. One model assumed a 40% vaccination level and a second model had a 75% vaccination level in all regions in the breeding cow herds within three and five years, respectively. Another scenario assumed that 75% of the cows were vaccinated within five years in the high-incidence states only. Levels and efficiencies of other program components remain unchanged from the base model for all vaccination scenarios.

10.   Combined Vaccination and Adjacent Herd Testing - This scenario analyzed the combined effects of vaccination and adjacent herd testing in high-incidence regions. This model assumed that 75% of the cows were vaccinated within five years in high-incidence regions and 100% adjacent herd testing was performed in these regions. The remaining program components remain unchanged from the base model.

Results and Discussion

A number of major conclusions and/or implications were reached in these studies from analyzing the results of the alternative program analyzed.

1.   All alternative programs evaluated which reduced the prevalence of brucellosis yielded positive economic results with respect to benefit-cost ratios and net benefits.

2.   The realistic eradication program appears to be the most effective program of the alternative programs analyzed since it ranked above other alternative programs, except the theoretical eradication program, in total benefits, net benefits, and benefit cost ratios. The theoretical eradication program demonstrated that the present "state of the art" within the U.S. bovine brucellosis program is capable of detecting sufficient number of infected herds for achieving eradication. Application and or utilization of current program components at higher efficiency levels through stricter adherence to the requirements of the UM&R and continuation of producer incentives via indemnity payments, along with the incorporation of a depopulation program, would likely result in an annual increase in program costs for a short interim period over the program costs currently incurred. However, simulation results of this study, as well as the recent experience of the Canadian Department of Agriculture, suggest that such

an approach would be cost effective while leading toward the goal of eradication.

3.   Vaccination will continue to play a "Jekyll and Hyde" role in control/eradication programs. Vaccination contributes substantially to the reduction within-herd spread and accelerates clean-up once affected herds have been identified, which may save the individual producer from economic ruin. However, this same reduction in within-herd spread causes a "masking" of detection under current disease surveillance systems, thus impeding the eradication process. It should be noted, in the event of decreases in program efficiency, vaccination may be essential for disease control. High regional vaccination levels reduce the relative spread between herds, preventing endemic outbreaks of infection.

4.   Vaccination is a cost-effective program practice in high-incidence regions. Results of the analysis indicate that the cost of vaccination may be partially or totally offset in high-incidence regions through the reduction in infection and the lower affected herd clean-up time required, resulting in a reduction in testing costs. Vaccination in low-incidence regions did not prove to be economically effective if program activity remained at adequate levels to maintain low-incidence status.

5.   Results revealed that adjacent herd testing could be a highly effective tool in bovine brucellosis control/eradication programs. A model employing 100% adjacent herd testing of all MCI-traced affected herds projected substantial reductions in prevalence and, in addition, total cost decrease over the simulation time horizon, compared to the base model. When the effectiveness of the estimated adjacent herd testing behavioral equation was reduced 50%, adjacent herd testing still resulted in major reductions in prevalence and total costs remained below the base model.

6.   A reduction in the prevalence will result in livestock producers losing economic rents (returns to fixed factors of production such as land and management). This is the result of an inelastic demand for red meat and these losses are partially shared by the competing red meat producers of pork and lamb. Symmetrically, consumers of livestock products will be the big winners. This suggests that the cost of a control/eradication program should at least be shared by the government.

Potential Uses of BRUSIM

In the past, the BRUSIM-TECHSIM bio-economic simulator has primarily been used to evaluate potential national programs in the U.S. These programs were the concern of legislators, producers groups U.S. Department of Agriculture taxpayers, and (USDA/APHIS) personnel. This represents only one of the major potential uses of BRUSIM. The following is a partial list of other potential uses of BRUSIM.

1. Tailoring Regional Programs - BRUSIM is divided into regions based on prevalence and industry characteristics. Central eradication programs could be designed and evaluated in BRUSIM that fit the particular prevalence and industry characteristics of that region.

2. Monitoring Function - BRUSIM could be used to monitor the results of program components used in a region by comparing projected results to actual numbers. This could identify certain program component implementation breakdowns or the ineffectiveness of a certain program component in a region.

3. Evaluation of Individual Program Components - While all current program components are presently simulated in BRUSIM, virtually nothing has been done to evaluate the cost effectiveness of the individual program components.

4. Risk Analysis - Vaccination slows disease spread and lowers within-herd infection but impedes detection through the primary surveillance systems. BRUSIM has the potential to evaluate such tradeoffs while considering the potential risk of future elimination of federal funding.

5. Optimal Allocation of Economic Resources - BRUSIM could be used to strategically plan where financial resources could most effectively be utilized between regions and program components in the case of reduced funding.

6. Program Component Interaction and Timing - BRUSIM could be used to investigate the interactions between program components. Also, it could be used to investigate the optimal timing and levels of program component implementation under limited manpower leading to an eradication goal.

7. Evaluation of Vaccine Development or New Program Components- With slight modifications, BRUSIM could evaluate the cost and epidemiologic effectiveness of new vaccines or new program components.

8. Evaluation of Related Diseases - The framework of BRUSIM could easily be adapted to evaluate other diseases that spread in a similar manner and/or could be identified in a similar manner to BRUSIM.

9. Adoption to Other Countries - By respecification of regions, industry characteristics, and program component efficiency level, the BRUSIM framework could be used in any country for evaluation of brucellosis or similar diseases.

BRUSIM Limitations and Potential Improvements

The major limitation of BRUSIM is the extensive amount of data required for the simulator, Table 22-1. This extensive data requirement may inhibit the adoption of BRUSIM for use in evaluating diseases in the species and potential use in other countries. The remaining limitations can be remedied through further development of the model, such as the following improvements:

1. Microcomputer Version - The current version of BRUSIM is a fortran-based program that runs on a main frame computer. Recent technological improvements in microcomputers make it possible for BRUSIM to be adapted for use on micros. The improvement would greatly increase the accessibility of BRUSIM for use by scientists and government officials.

2. Improved User Friendliness - The sophistication of BRUSIM now requires the user to be intimately familiar with the computer program to utilize it.

3. Improved Input Data and Behavioral Equations -The latest data used to estimate behavioral equations for BRUSIM was 1982. Data being developed by the National Animal Health Monitoring System and other sources could be used to improve and/or validate behavioral equations as well as improve the input data in BRUSIM.

In summary, the evolution of bio-economic simulation of bovine brucellosis was traced. Advantages and disadvantages of simulation models utilizing Monte Carlo, Linear Programming and binomial techniques were examined. The development of the last bio-economic simulator BRUSIM - TECHISM was examined in detail.

BRUSIM, a disease simulation model, was developed to measure the impact of various program components upon selected epidemiologic parameters and to determine costs and physical losses associated with brucellosis control/eradication programs given epidemiologic coefficients and economic criteria from 1976 through 2005. The U.S. was divided into 16 regions based on such factors as brucellosis prevalence, producer characteristics, and cattle population.

TECHISM, an econometric model, was used for determining the net benefits accruing to society, consumers, producers, and related industries as a result of decreases in beef and milk losses from alternative programs compared to a base program. The discounted values and associated program costs were used for determining benefit/cost ratios and related economic decision criteria.

This bio-economic simulator has been used in two studies to evaluate alternative U.S. bovine brucellosis programs. The major implications derived from these studies were as follows: 1) All control/eradication programs evaluated lead to reductions in yielded positive economic results, 2) A realistic eradication program appeared to be the most economically and epidemiologically effective, 3) Vaccination exhibits a "Jekyll and Hyde" effect, it substantially reduces within herd spread and accelerates affected-herd clean-up but causes a "masking" of detection under current disease surveillance systems, 4) Vaccination is a cost-effective program practice in high prevalence areas, 5) Adjacent herd testing appeared to be a highly epidemiologically and economically efficient program component, and 6) Consumers are the big winners from reductions in prevalence, suggesting the cost of a control/eradication program should be at least shared by the government.

The primary use of BRUSIM has been to analyze the epidemiologic and economic efficiency of alternative U.S. bovine brucellosis programs. Many other potential uses of the analytical capabilities of BRUSIM exist. BRUSIM could be utilized to tailor make regional programs, monitor program progress, evaluate individual program components, analyze risk, evaluate optimal allocation of resources under limited funding, analyze program component interaction and timing, and analyze the cost effectiveness of vaccines or new program components. In addition, the BRUSIM framework could be adopted for use in evaluating other diseases and for use in other countries with similar problems.

The extensive data requirements of BRUSIM may limit extension of its use in other countries and for evaluating diseases in other species. The use and results of BRUSIM can be enhanced by developing a micro-computer version of the program, improving the user friendliness, and updating the data bases from which input data and behavioral equations are derived.

References

1. Hugh-Jones ME, Ellis PR, Felton MR. An Assessment of the Eradication of Bovine Brucellosis in England and Wales. Study No. 19, University of Reading, England, 1975.
2. Row RT, Morris RS. The Integration of Epidemiological and Economic Analysis in The Planning of The Australian Brucellosis Eradication Program, in *New Techniques in Veterinary Epidemiology and Economics*, Proceedings of the Symposium, University of Reading, England, July 15, 1976.
3. Carpenter TE. A Report of the Bovine Brucellosis Eradication Program in California. California Dept. of Food and Agriculture. Sacramento, California, 1975.
4. Carpenter TE, Howitt R. A Linear Programming Model used in Animal Disease Control. In: WA Geering, RT Roe, LA Chapman eds. *Veterinary Epidemiology and Economics*, Brisbane, Australia: Watson Ferguson and Co., 1980;483-489.
5. Beal VC Jr. *Regulatory Statistics*, 5th edition. Veterinary Services, APHIS/USDA, Hyattesville, Maryland, 1975.
6. Amosson SH, Dietrich RA. Theoretical Basis and Empirical Implications of the Bovine Brucellosis Market Slaughter Testing Program in the United States. *Preventive Veterinary Medicine* 3(1984/5) 53-64, 1984.
7. Amosson SH, Dietrich RA, Hopkin JA. Report-National Brucellosis Technical Commission, Appendix B, Benefit-Cost Analysis. Prepared for APHIS, USDA, 1978.
8. Roe RT. The Application of Computer Simulation to the Planning of Public Investment in the Control of Animal Disease. Ph.D. Dissertation, University of

Melbourne, 1977.

9. Beal VC Jr and Kryder HA Jr. Brucellosis Program Analysis, APHIS, USDA, Hyattesville, Maryland, 1977.

10. Liu CI. An Economic Impact Evaluation of Government Programs: The Case of Brucellosis Control in The United Stated. *Southern Journal of Agricultural Economics*, July 1979: 163-168.

11. Teigen LD, Carman LM. The 10-Year Brucellosis Eradication Program: A Short-Term Analysis. CED/Forecast Support Group, USDA Working Paper, 1978.

12. Collins GS. An Econometric Simulation Model For Evaluating Aggregate Economic Impacts of Technological Change on Major U.S. Field Crops. Ph.D. Dissertation, Texas A&M University, 1980b.

13. McCauley EH, Nasser AA, New JC Jr, Sundquist WB, Miller WM. A Study of The Potential Economic Impact of Foot-And-Mouth Disease in The United States. TB-1597, Univ. of Minnesota, May, 1979.

14. Dietrich RA, Amosson SH, Crawford RP. Economic and Epidemiologic Analysis of U.S. Bovine Brucellosis Programs, Texas Agricultural Experiment Station Bulletin, B-1534, April, 1986.

15. Gramlich, EM. *Benefit-Cost Analysis of Government Programs*. Prentice-Hall, Inc. Englewood Cliffs, New Jersey, 1981.

16. Chavas, JP and Collins GS. Welfare Measures From Technological Distortions in General Equilibrium. *Southern Economics Journal* 48(1982):745-753.

17. U.S. Department of Agriculture, Crop Reporting Service. *Agricultural Prices - Annual Summary 1982*, Washington, D.C., June, 1983.

18. Amosson SH. Economic and Epidemiologic Implications of National Bovine Brucellosis Programs—A Case Study. Ph.D. Dissertation, Texas A&M University, 1983.

Chapter Twenty-three

Economic Losses Attributable
to Brucellosis

Richard P. Crawford, L. Garry Adams,
*J.ohn D. Williams, and R.aymond A. Dietri*ch

Most research on bovine brucellosis and programs recommending its eradication are justified by citing the effects of pathogenic field strains of *Brucella abortus* on livestock production. The most commonly mentioned signs of brucellosis are abortion, dead or weak calves, reduced milk yield, lower weaning weight, extended calving interval, and lower fertility.

Economic modeling and disease simulation using computers are recent additions to the research armament. Production coefficients for cattle with brucellosis are necessary to model brucellosis eradication programs and determine benefit/cost ratios. The 1978 report of the National Brucellosis Technical Commission (NBTC) stated that physical loss coefficients are a limiting factor in a simulation model of a complex disease such as brucellosis.[1] Most available data, especially the long-term effects of brucellosis on livestock production, are over 30 years old and some recent data are contradictory.[2]

Drs. Berman and Anderson of the NBTC reviewed the literature for data to support physical loss coefficients for brucellosis in cattle. In addition they analyzed program data from states and interviewed epidemiologists, state program supervisors, and experienced ranchers to arrive at the following physical loss coefficients for beef cattle that were used in the NBTC report. Sixty percent of the infected cows and bred heifers were expected to either abort or have calves that will die within seven days of birth during the first year of infection. An additional 22% were expected to have weak calves of which 10% will die and the weaning weight of the remaining will be decreased by 20%. During year two of infection the calf mortality due to abortion will decrease to 5% and the percentage with weak calves and reduced weaning weights will decrease to 17%. However in 15% of the cattle, sterility or a three month delay in conception can be expected. During year three of infection the calf mortality due to abortion is expected to decline further to 0.1%. The 13% with weak calves will result in an additional calf mortality of 1.3% (10%) before weaning and the weaning weights of the survivors will decrease by 20%. The slow breeders (three months) or sterile cows will decrease to 10%. Drs. Berman and Anderson also utilized a factor of 0.899 for Strain 19 (S19) vaccinated cattle with brucellosis which represented a 10.1% effectiveness of vaccination in reducing such physical losses as abortion, weak calves, etc. They stated that, although a high level of vaccination has been found to substantially reduce the likelihood of infection, it has only limited effectiveness in reducing physical losses should infection occur. The following research was designed and initiated to validate or determine physical loss coefficients for beef cattle with brucellosis.

Objectives

The objectives of this research were: 1) to measure the effect of S19 vaccination on calf mortality and natural recovery from B. abortus S2308 infection and 2) to quantitate reductions in reproductive functionality and calf weight attributable to persistent B. abortus S2308 infection in cattle.

Materials and Methods

Calf Mortality

This was determined following parturition of both non-vaccinated and Strain 19 (S19) vaccinated cattle which were challenged by inoculating 1 x 10^7 colony forming units (cfu) of B. abortus S2308 onto the conjunctiva of the eyes of primi-gravid cattle.[34] Non-pregnant heifers had been inoculated subcutaneously with doses of S19 that ranged from 1.0 x 10^8 to 1.0 x 10^{10} cfu approximately 9 months prior to challenge.[4] Calf mortality included abortions, term-calves that were dead including dystocias, and weak calves that died in the first month after birth.

Disease Classification

Isolation of B. abortus S2308 at parturition following challenge was considered evidence of infection and brucellosis; recovery from infection and brucellosis was failure to isolate B. abortus from later samples collected at subsequent parturitions and slaughter of cows that initially had brucellosis; and non-infected were cows from which B. abortus was never isolated including slaughter tissues.

Year Two and Three

Cross-bred (*Bos taurus* x *Bos indicus*) cattle with brucellosis were selected from those that were culture positive at parturition following challenge (year one). Controls include 15 non-vaccinated and 15 cattle vaccinated with 1×10^8 cfu of S19. Fifteen S19 vaccinated but non-challenged cattle that were randomly selected from the same foundation herd of the same age and breed phenotype. Two fertile bulls were added and the herd was maintained on a 120-acre pasture for two more gestations.

At Parturition

Milk and uterine samples were cultured for Brucella.[3,4] Calves were weighed and permanently tattooed.

Calf Weight

At approximately monthly intervals each calf was weighed. These weights were plotted to determine a growth curve for each calf.

Fertility

Days to conception was determined by the number of days from addition of the bulls (Day 0) to parturition of calf two minus 285 days; and the calving interval was the days between calf two and calf three.

Milk Production

Weight gain of each calf in the first 60 days was determined from the growth curve minus birth weight.

Beef Production

A 205-day weaning weight was determined for each calf by the method of the Beef Improvement Federation.[5]

Losses Attributable to Brucellosis

Losses attributable to brucellosis are those losses from cows with brucellosis in excess of non-infected controls.

Results

Calf mortality in 116 non-vaccinated heifers challenged with S2308 in five experiments is depicted in Table 23-1. The calf mortality in heifers with brucellosis ranged from 58% to 94% and the calf mortality in heifers that were not infected ranged from 0 to 50%. The calf mortality attributed to brucellosis, i.e. calf mortality in heifers with brucellosis minus calf mortality in non-infected heifers, ranged from 38% to 94%. The total of the five experiments was a calf mortality of 86% for heifers with brucellosis and 30% for non-infected heifers or 56% calf mortality attributed to brucellosis in non-vaccinated heifers. These data show a high calf mortality (30%) in non-infected heifers that was attributed to causes other than brucellosis. Four were abortions, two were dead-term calves, two were weak and died, and one died of dystocia.

Calf mortality in 156 S19-vaccinated heifers challenged with S2308 is depicted in Table 23-2. Calf mortality in heifers with brucellosis ranged from 33% to 100% and the calf mortality in heifers that were not infected ranged from 18% to 47%. The calf mortality attributed to brucellosis ranged from 15% to 53%. The total of the five experiments was a calf mortality of 86% for 51 heifers with brucellosis and 40% for 105 non-infected heifers or 46% calf mortality attributed to brucellosis in S19-vaccinated cattle. These data also show a high calf mortality (40%) in S19-vaccinated non-infected cattle that was attributed to causes other than brucellosis. Twelve were abortions, seven were dead-term calves, seven were weak calves that died, and 16 (38%) were dystocias that required intervention to deliver the calf which was either already dead or died. If these 16 dystocias in non-infected cows and the one that was in cows with brucellosis were omitted as sire related, the calf mortality in S19-vaccinated cattle attributed to brucellosis would be 84% minus 25% or 59%.

Table 23-3 is a summary of the mortality for year one in the two previous tables. A chi-square of less than 0.01 and 0.99 suggests that the live-dead ratio of calves from heifers with brucellosis and heifers without brucellosis, respectively, was not significantly affected by S19 vaccination prior to infection. Also the chi-square of 1.47 supports the conclusion that the distribution of calf mortality attributed to brucellosis and calf mortality attributed to causes other than brucellosis was not significantly affected by S19 vaccination. As expected, calf mortality was more likely to occur in heifers with brucellosis (86%) compared to heifers that did not have brucellosis (38%) and this is supported by the chi-square of 28.93; (P<0.005) which is highly significant.

Table 23-4 presents data that extends the calf mortality observed in cows with brucellosis to include years two and three. One S19-vaccinated cow aborted during year two and one non-vaccinated cow aborted during year three. All control cows had live calves. The calf mortality attributed

Table 23-1. Calf Mortality in Heifers Challenged with 1 x 10⁷ CFU *Brucella abortus* Strain 2308

| | | Brucellosis at Parturition | | | Mortality |
| | | Yes | | No | Attributed to |
Experiment No.	N*	Mortality	N*	Mortality	Brucellosis
		Cattle on Dirt			
003	31	94%	2	0	94%
004	24	88%	14	50%	38%
010	5	80%	0	0	80%
		Cattle on Concrete			
017	12	58%	1	0	58%
012	14	93%	13	15%	78%
TOTAL	86	86%	30	30%	56%

*N = number of observationscalves.

to brucellosis was significantly reduced in both year two and year three to 3% and again S19 vaccination was not a factor. This significant reduction in years two and three is supported by a chi-square of 35.88 and with two degrees of freedom the P is less than 0.005. One S19-vaccinated cow was never diagnosed pregnant and this cow had declining antibody titers and *B. abortus* was never isolated after year one. Therefore 97% of the cows with brucellosis that conceived had live calves in years two and three.

Table 23-5 depicts the fate of the 30 cattle with brucellosis that were monitored during years two and three. Nine non-vaccinated and eight S19 vaccinated cattle excreted *B. abortus* at the second and third parturition. Six non-vaccinated and seven S19-vaccinated cattle were culture negative at parturition of calf three and also at slaughter which followed the weaning of the calf. Therefore recovery or persistence of infection was not affected by S19 vaccination prior to infection.

In view of the fact that 13 (43%) of the cows infected with *B. abortus* recovered, the production coefficients for years two and three will be presented for cows with brucellosis (persistent infection), cows that recovered, and control cows that did not have brucellosis but which were in the same herd as the others. One of the 15 control cows was diagnosed pregnant but was found dead in the pasture before calving in year two and therefore n=14 for data from control cows.

Table 23-2. Calf Mortality in Strain 19 Vaccinated Heifers Challenged with 1 x 10⁷ CFU *Brucella abortus* Strain 2308

| | | Brucellosis at Parturition | | | Mortality |
| | | Yes | | No | Attributed to |
Strain 19 CFU	N*	Mortality	N*	Mortality	Brucellosis
		Cattle on Dirt			
1.0×10^8	23	100%	17	47%	53%
1.0×10^9	9	78%	30	40%	38%
1.0×10^{10}	6	100%	34	47%	53%
		Cattle on Concrete			
5.0×10^8	3	33%	11	18%	15%
2.5×10^8	10	70%	13	31%	39%
TOTAL	51	86%	105	40%	46%

*N = number of observations

Fertility was measured by the days to conception in year two (Table 23-6). The means of 21, 12, and 25 and medians of 17, 12, and 14 days to conception for brucellosis, recovered, and control cows, respectively, suggest good fertility for all groups with the majority becoming pregnant following first estrus. Fertility was also measured by the calving interval between calf two and calf three (Table 23-7). The means of 401, 361, and 457 and medians of 347, 343, and 448 days between parturitions for brucellosis, recovered, and control cows, respectively, suggest that control cows had more difficulty breeding back following calf two than the cows with brucellosis. Duncan's multiple range and chi-square of 6.74 (P< 0.05) both support a longer calving interval for controls. This statistical significance is probably the result of a drought that occurred in the summer and fall of year two. Body condition scores (BCS) of all cows were determined during the fall when calves were weaned. Minimum BCS is one (thin) and maximum is nine (fat).⁶ A mean BCS of 4.59, 4.90, and 4.39 occurred in brucellosis, recovered and control groups, respectively. A BCS of five or more is recommended to maintain a 12-month calving interval and 44%, 73%, and 21% of the brucellosis, recovered, and controls cows, respectively, had a BCS of five or more. Therefore the assumption was made that the control cows as a group suffered more from the drought than the other groups and this was reflected in the longer calving interval.

Table 23-3. Summary of Calf Mortality in Heifers Challenged with 1×10^7 CFU *Brucella abortus* Strain 2308 - Year 1

Strain 19	N*	Brucellosis at Parturition Yes Mortality	N	No Mortality	Mortality Attributed to Brucellosis
No	86	86%	30	30%	56%
Yes	51	86%	105	40%	46%
	$\chi^2 = <0.01$		$\chi^2 = 0.99$		$\chi^2 = 1.47$
TOTAL	137	86%	135	38%	48%

$$\chi^2 = 28.903; P < 0.005$$

*N = number of observations

There was one heifer with brucellosis that failed to conceive, i.e. was sterile, during year two and three. This was a S19-vaccinated cow that was negative to culture at the end of the experiment and therefore considered to have recovered from brucellosis.

Milk production of dams was estimated by the weight gain of calves in the first 60 days (Table 23-8). A growth curve was determined for each calf and the weight at 60 days after calving minus the birth weight was assumed to be the direct result of the milk production of the dam. The means of 107, 112, and 109 pounds, and medians of 103, 115, and 110 pounds for brucellosis, recovered, and control cows, respectively, suggest no significant reduction in milk production attributable to brucellosis during years two and three.

Beef production was determined by calculating a 205-day weaning weight for each calf that was adjusted for the age of the dam. The means of 363, 368, and 399 pounds for the brucellosis, recovered, and control cows, respectively, suggest that cows with brucellosis may wean lighter calves although the analysis of variance suggested non-significance. The medians of 358, 379, and 364 pounds for the brucellosis, recovered, and control cows, respectively, and chi-square also suggested no significant difference. (See Table 23-9)

The brucellosis cows weaned 13 male and 20 female calves with one abortion and the recovered cows weaned seven male and 16 female calves with one abortion during years two and three. The control cows weaned 16 male and 11 female calves with one male abandoned by the dam after a

Table 23-4. Summary of Calf Mortality Attributed to Brucellosis

Strain 19	Year 1		Year 2		Year 3	
	N*	Mortality	N*	Mortality	N*	Mortality
No	86	56%	15	0	15	7%
Yes	51	46%	14**	7%	14**	0%
TOTAL	137	48%	29	3%	29	3%

$$\chi^2 = 35.88; 2df, ; P < 0.005$$

*N = number of cattle with brucellosis
**1 cow never diagnosed pregnant during year 2 and year 3 - therefore N= 14

dystocia during years two and three. The 205-day weaning weight was adjusted to a male equivalent by adding 10% to the weight of the female calves and the combined weaning weights were also adjusted to reflect the average beef produced during each 365-day period.[7] These average pounds of beef take into consideration that no beef was produced by the cows that aborted, failed to conceive, or abandoned their calf. The means of 388, 393, and 382 pounds of beef and medians of 411, 441, and 404 pounds of beef for brucellosis, recovered, and control cows, respectively, suggest no difference between groups (See Table 23-10).

Due to the drought in year two and the extended calving interval for some cows, the calves in year three were weaned in two groups rather than one. The brucellosis cows weaned 11 calves in the fall and five calves in the spring of year three, and the control cows weaned seven and seven. A computer composite of the growth curves of calves from control cows weaned during the study is depicted in Figure 23-1.[8] During drought year two the composite growth curve suggests a daily weight gain of approximately one pound and during normal year 3 A a daily weight gain of 1.59 pounds per day. During year 3B which was in the winter and early spring, the calves and their dams were grazing highly fertilized and lush rye grass and the daily weight gain was 2.16 pounds per day. Figure 23-2 shows the computer composite growth curves of calves from persistently infected cows. During drought year two the composite growth curve suggests a daily weight gain of 0.91 pounds per day and during normal year 3A a daily weight gain of 1.54 pounds per day for calves from persistently infected cows. During year 3B the daily weight gain was 1.88 pounds for the five calves from infected cows grazing lush rye grass. These data suggest comparable weight gains in calves from infected and control cows on the same nutrition plane and are consistent with the positive correlation of

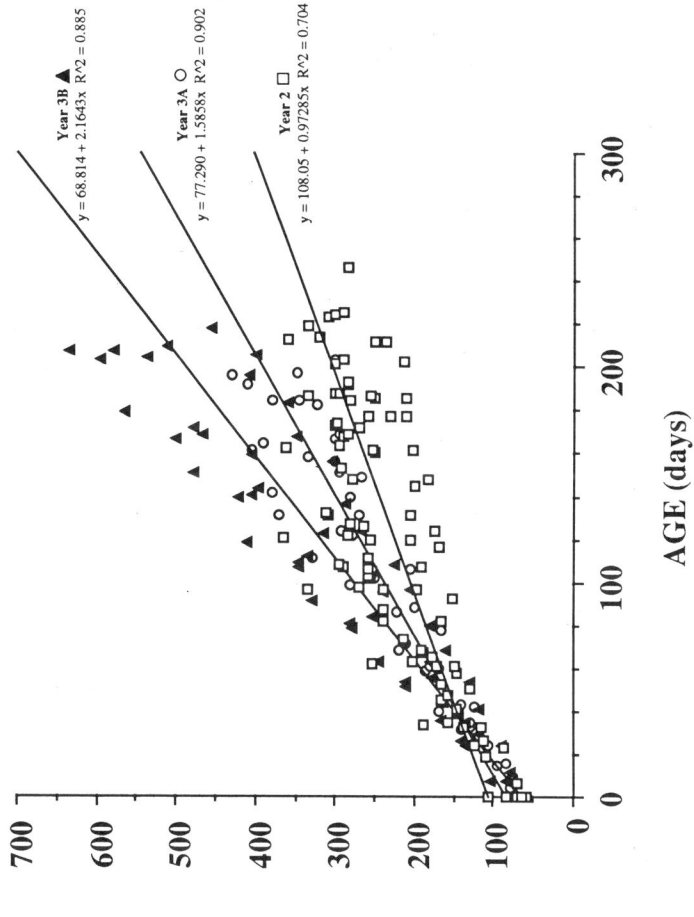

Figure 23-1. Growth Curves of Calves–Control Cows

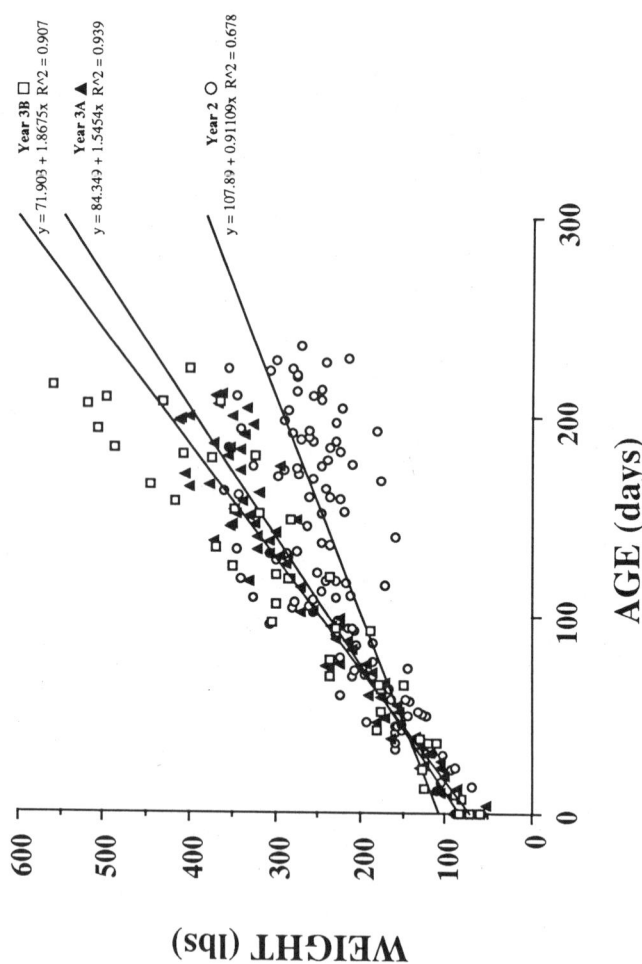

Figure 23-2. Growth Curves of Calves-Infected Cows

Table 23-5. Fate of 30 Cattle with Brucellosis

	Condition at end of third gestation	
Strain 19	Infected	Recovered*
No	9	6
Yes	8	7
Total	17	13
	$\chi^2 = 0.14$, not significant	

*Culture negative - both parturition and slaughter tissues

nutrition and beef production.

Discussion

The data in Table 23-3 suggest that 48% of the beef cows with brucellosis have a dead calf attributed to brucellosis during year one of infection. The remaining 38% mortality observed in these experiments was attributed to something other than brucellosis and was most probably influenced by the environment and/or experimental design of collection of samples from the dam and calf immediately following parturition plus weekly samples from the dams. Note that generally (Tables 23-1 and 23-2) the calf mortality in cows that did not have brucellosis was higher in groups on dirt than the groups on concrete. These heifers were tested serologically negative for brucellosis, leptospirosis, vibriosis, infectious bovine rhinotracheitis (IBR), and bovine virus diarrhea (BVD). Heifers that were culture-negative for *Brucella* at parturition were slaughtered for additional tissues for bacteriology. No attempt was made to measure milk production or calf growth in year one under these conditions of experimental design to test vaccine protection.

The calf mortality attributed to brucellosis was 56% for the 86 non-vaccinated heifers and 46% for the 51 S19-vaccinated heifers with brucellosis (Table 23-3). There were 17 calf deaths in S19-vaccinated heifers that were associated with a dystocia in a heifer with brucellosis and 16 in non-infected heifers. If these calf deaths were excluded as sire related, the calf mortality attributed to brucellosis would be 59% for S19-vaccinated heifers-84% minus 25%. Chi-square would be 0.32 and remain not significant. During years two and three, one abortion occurred in both S19-vaccinated and non-vaccinated cows. Therefore the data in this study support the hypothesis that S19-vaccination does not affect calf mortality in cows with

Table 23-6. Fertility in Beef Cattle

| | Days to conception* | | |
	Brucellosis	Recovered	Controls
Mean	21	12	25
Median	17	12	14
Range	0-78	0-41	2-84
N**	17	11	14

Analysis of variance and $\chi^2 - P > 0.05$; not significant

*Conception was calculated as calving date minus 285 days after bulls were released (Day 0)
**N = number of observations

brucellosis. The association of lower calf mortality in S19 vaccinated populations is probably due to the fact that vaccinated cattle contract brucellosis at a lower rate than non-vaccinated cattle. In these studies, if cows had brucellosis, the calf mortality was the same (not statistically different) for both S19-vaccinated and non-vaccinated cattle. Therefore the effect of S19 vaccination appears to be protection against infection and not protection against calf mortality if infection occurs.

The calf mortality of 48% attributed to brucellosis in the 137 vaccinated and non-vaccinated heifers in year one following infection is lower than the 62% calf mortality used by the NBTC-60% abortion plus 10% of the 22% with weak calves. The high calf mortality of 38% in heifers without brucellosis was subtracted from the 86% calf mortality observed in heifers with brucellosis to yield the calf mortality attributed to brucellosis. Mortality in non-infected cattle is normally low and was not considered in the 62% calf mortality used by the NBTC. The calf mortality in non-infected heifers in this study may have been affected more by the environmental stress than the calf mortality in heifers with brucellosis which resulted in a low estimate of calf mortality attributed to brucellosis. Both the NBTC and the results of this study agree that calf mortality is significantly reduced after year one.

This study did not attempt to measure weight loss in calves due to decreased milk production during year one. For years two and three the fertility, milk production, and calf weights from cows with brucellosis were not reduced when compared to either cows that recovered or non-infected control cows in the herd. Therefore the data from this study do not agree with the physical loss and infertility coefficients used by the NBTC.

Table 23-7. Fertility in Beef Cattle - Calving Interval - Days Between
Parturitions

	Brucellosis	Recovered	Controls
Mean	401	361	457**
Median	347	343	448**
Range	310-572	324-550	317-598
N*	16	11	14

*N = number of observations
**Probability <0.05 Duncan's Multiple Range
χ^2 = 6.74; significantly longer

The results of this study also do not agree with the 10.1% effectiveness of
S19 in reducing physical loss and infertility coefficients. Both this study
and the NBTC coefficients support the thesis that the majority of the losses
in cows with brucellosis occur in year one following exposure and infection.

The variation in the level of nutrition between year two and three and
within year three was unexpected and unfortunate. It is possible that
minor losses due to brucellosis could have been demonstrated if the
numbers had been larger and nutrition had been optimal. However all
cows with brucellosis, cows that recovered, and non-infected control cows
had equal access to what nutrients were available and the statistics support
no significant losses attributable to brucellosis in years two and three
following infection.

SUMMARY

In summary, losses attributable to brucellosis were those from cows
with brucellosis in excess of non-infected controls. Primi-gravid cross-
bred (*Bos taurus* x *Bos indicus*) heifer cattle were challenged conjunctivally
with 10^7 colony forming units (cfu) of pathogenic *B. abortus* S2308. Calf
mortality of 86% in 137 heifers with brucellosis and 38% in 135 heifers
without brucellosis was recorded. Therefore a calf mortality of 48%
attributed to brucellosis occurred in year one following challenge. Vacci-

Table 23-8. Fertility in Beef cattle - Weight Gain of Calves in 60 days* ci

	Brucellosis	Recovered	Controls
Mean	107	112	109
Median	103	115	110
Range	72-135	49-162	55-147
N**	33	23	27
Analysis of variance and χ^2 - P > 0.05; not significant			

*Growth curve at 60 days minus birth weight
**N = number of observation

Table 23-9. Beef Production - 205-Day Weaning Weights*

	Brucellosis	Recovered	Controls
Mean	363	368	399
Median	358	379	364
Range	222-552	227-565	256-648
N**	33	23	27
Analysis of variance and χ^2 - P > 0.05; not significant			

*Adjusted for age of dam
**N = number of observations

nation of heifers 9 months prior to challenge using doses from 10^8 to 10^{10} cfu of B. abortus S19 did not significantly reduce the calf mortality attributed to brucellosis in 51 culture-positive heifers in year one or the natural recovery from S2308 infection in the 15 that had been vaccinated with 10^9 cfu of S19 and monitored in years two and three following challenge. Calf mortality decreased significantly to only one additional abortion in 17 cows that were persistently culture-positive for S2308 during years two and three. No reduction in fertility, milk production, or calf weights attributed to brucellosis could be demonstrated in years two and three.

Table 23-10. Average Beef Production - Pounds Per Unit Per Year*

	Brucellosis	Recovered	Controls
Mean	388	393	382
Median	411	441	404
Range	196-495	0-554	207-476
N*	16	11	14
Analysis of variance and χ^2 - P > 0.05; not significant			

*Average 205-day weaning weight adjusted to male equivalent and 365-day calving interval.
**N = number of observations

Acknowledgments

This paper is dedicated to Dr. O.D. Butler of College Station, Texas. At the time the research was initiated Dr. Butler was Associate Deputy Chancellor for Agriculture for The Texas A&M University System. He has since retired and is currently a Professor Emeritus. When we started our search for a place to do the research we had no success, i.e. nobody wanted a herd of cattle with brucellosis. Dr. Butler knew the research needed to be done. He volunteered a pasture that he had leased and arranged for the Texas Agricultural Experiment Station to become the leasee. To further show his commitment, his registered Charlois cattle occupied pastures that were adjacent to the one that contained the diseased cattle during the entire time of the project.

References

1. National Brucellosis Technical Commission. Report to Animal and Plant Health Inspection Service, U.S. Department of Agriculture and U.S. Animal Health Association, August, 1978. Appendix B. Benefit-Cost Analysis, Stephen H. Amosson, Raymond A. Dietrich, and John A. Hopkin.
2. Crawford RP, Williams JD, Childers AB, et al. The effects of *Brucella abortus* on serology, bacteriology, and production in three Texas cattle herds. *Proc Annu Meet US Anim Health Assoc* 1978;82:89-105.
3. Crawford RP, Adams LG, Williams JD. Relationship of fetal age at conjunctival exposure of pregnant heifers and *Brucella abortus* isolation. *Am J Vet Res* 1987; 48:755-757.

4. Crawford RP, Adams LG, Williams JD. Relationship of days in gestation at exposure and development of brucellosis in Strain 19 vaccinated heifers. *Am J Vet Res* 1988;49:1037-1039.
5. Guidelines For Uniform Beef Improvement Programs. United States Department of Agriculture, Extension Service, Program Aid 1020, September 1981.
6. Herd DB, Sprott LR. Body condition, nutrition and reproduction of beef cows. Texas Agricultural Extension Service, Bulletin B-1526, College Station, TX.
7. Hammack SP. Personal communication, May 1989. Texas Agricultural Extension Service, Stephenville, TX.
8. Cricket Graph, Cricket Software, Malvern, PA. June 1986.

Chapter Twenty-four

Role of Wildlife in
Transmitting Brucellosis
Donald S. Davis

The general consensus of the scientific community has been and continues to be that the primary hosts of most species of *Brucella* are domestic animals and livestock. This opinion has been supported by the known epidemiology and the published literature. At the last International Symposium on Bovine Brucellosis in 1976, there was quite a bit of discussion about non-bovine (wildlife) hosts of brucellosis. The majority of the speakers though that wildlife in general was not a threat or major obstacle to the Federal Eradication Program at that time.

Well, several things have happened in the last 13 years to make us modify that belief somewhat. In some of those states where brucellosis has been successfully eliminated in domestic livestock, the primary source of the disease has become infected wildlife species. Human cases of brucellosis have been attributed to contact with infected wildlife, and wildlife have been identified as the source of infections in domestic livestock in several states.

Although the most common source of *Brucella* for livestock in the United States continues to be infected domestic livestock, the situation in some areas is changing. This is, in part based on numbers. The number of *Brucella*-infected elk and bison in the United States is estimated to be 20,000, and the number of infected feral swine exceeds 100,000. The number of *Brucella*-infected cattle is presently less than 10,000. Thus solely on a numerical basis, wildlife should be recognized as the largest potential source of *Brucella*. Other parameters such as the probability of interspecific contact and other behavioral differences generally result in spatial and temporal separation of wildlife and domestic livestock.

However, as the number of *Brucella*-infected domestic livestock is decreased (toward zero) within the United States, the relative importance and likelihood of transmission from a wildlife reservoir concomitantly increases. For instance, the probability of a wildlife source of infection for a cattle herd in Texas is miniscule when compared to the probability of a cattle to cattle transmission. In a brucellosis-free state such as Wyoming, however, the reverse is true. There are thousands of *Brucella*-infected elk and bison in western Wyoming, and the chances of a wildlife-to-cattle transmission are much greater than a cattle-to-cattle transmission. In those western states in the United States where brucellosis in domestic livestock is negligible, wildlife is viewed as the primary threat and is a continuing obstacle to the National Brucellosis Eradication Program.

Dr. Margaret Meyer quite correctly stated during the previous Brucellosis Symposium that, to say you have a wildlife "reservoir of infection, you have to not only find the organism, you have to show that it is transmitted from animal to animal in the reservoir and transmitted from the reservoir to domestic animals." This will be the main theme of this presentation. I will review what has become known concerning brucellosis and wildlife particularly since 1976 with emphasis on transmission.

Bison *(Bison bison)*

American bison *(Bison bison)* was the first wildlife species in the world to be identified as being infected with *Brucella*. Serologic evidence of the presence of brucellosis was first reported by Mohler[1] in 1917 from three bison cows from Yellowstone National Park, and the *B. abortus* bacterium was isolated in 1930 by Creech[2] from the testes of a bison bull killed on the National Bison Range, Moiese, Montana. Subsequent and more extensive serologic testing by Rush[3] in 1930 and by Tunnicliff and Marsh[4] in 1935 of bison sera from Yellowstone and Moiese indicated a *Brucella* reactor rate of 53% (58/110) and 60% (305/484) respectively. Six of six bison from Utah in 1965 were found to possess serum antibodies which reacted with *B. abortus* tube agglutination antigens at titers of 20 or greater.[5] From 1917 to 1985, 2,211 sera from Yellowstone Park bison have been tested for brucellosis; 817 (37%) have reacted positively and 181 (8.2%) were classified as suspects. During the period from 1962-1985, tissues from 87 Yellowstone bison were collected and cultured for *Brucella*. *Brucella abortus* biovar 1 was isolated from seven of these bison.[6]

Brucellosis in bison has also been a problem in Canada for some time. Moore[7] tested 37 sera collected from bison in Elk Island National Park, Alberta in the winter of 1946-1947, and 16.2% were found to be positive and 13.5% questionable. Corner and Connell[8] tested 343 bison sera from the same park in 1956, and 42.3% reacted to an agglutination test. Choquette et al.[9] (1978) reported that sera collected from 2,365 free-ranging bison on and near Wood Buffalo National Park, Alberta, and the Northwest Territories from 1959-1974 were tested for brucellosis and 31.7% reacted positively to the tube agglutination test. *Brucella abortus* was also cultured from bison with orchitis and arthritis.

All this background is to emphasize that the problem of brucellosis in bison is historically well established and that it is of considerable importance in some areas. On the basis of these data alone, we can say that two of the three criteria stated by Meyer for a wildlife reservoir have been met

by the bison. There have been many instances in the last 60 years in which
B. abortus has been isolated from bison, and this wildlife species obviously can maintain the infection by passing the organism from animal to
animal. Bison in both the United States and Canada have been shown to
be able to maintain *Brucella* infections in herds for many years without
contact with any infected livestock. The last criteria, that of transmission
to domestic livestock, is always the most difficult to document, but the case
has been made in several instances.

In two replications under controlled conditions, *B. abortus* stain 2308
was transmitted from experimentally infected bison to susceptible cattle.
The infected bison-to-susceptible cattle transmission was compared to an
infected cattle-to-susceptible cattle transmission under parallel and identical experimental conditions. There were no statistical differences between the two, meaning that bison-to-cattle transmission was as likely as
cattle-to-cattle transmission under those conditions.[10]

The first documented case of naturally occurring transmission of brucellosis from bison to cattle was reported in 1983 in North Dakota in a herd
of beef cattle on the same premises as a herd of bison. The cattle herd had
been tested and found to be free of *Brucella* reactors the previous year. In
July 1983, five adult female bison and one bull were sent to slaughter and
all six were found to be card, standard plate test, and Rivanol positive. The
remaining 21 bison were tested and 18 were found to be reactors. Upon
testing the 77 cattle in the herd, one cow reacted at 200 on the standard plate
test, was card positive, and rivanol 200. All the bison and the reactor cow
were slaughtered, blood and tissues collected, and submitted for laboratory examination. *Brucella abortus* biovar 1 was isolated from 13 of the
bison and the one reactor cow. The cattle herd was depopulated in
September 1983.[11]

Another instance of bison-to-cattle transmission is reported to have
occurred in 1987 in South Dakota in one cow in a herd of 1,100 beef cattle
that were pastured adjacent to a *Brucella*-infected bison herd. The cow had
been seen across the fence with the infected bison and subsequently
became card positive and Rivanol 100. *Brucella abortus* biovar 1 was
isolated from the tissues of this reactor cow after slaughter. None of the
other cattle in the herd were found to be *Brucella* reactive (Holland, 1989
personal communication).

The state of Wyoming (classified as brucellosis-free since 1985) has
now had four incidences in which the occurrence of brucellosis in domestic
cattle has been attributed to contact with infected bison (and or elk) after
extensive epidemiologic investigations (Swanson, 1989 personal communication).

These facts and the inability of the National Park Service to address the
issue have led to the current policy in the states of Wyoming and Montana
of killing all bison that leave the environs of Yellowstone Park. This last
winter more than 550 bison were killed by hunters under the control of the

Montana Department of Fish, Wildlife and Parks as the bison left the northern boundary of Yellowstone Park. This was done to prevent the possible spread of brucellosis into Montana cattle populations. Sera were collected from 465 of the bison and 53% (246) were found by a battery of serologic tests to be positive (reactive) for brucellosis. *Brucella abortus* biovar 1 was isolated from one of the Montana-hunter-killed bison (Ferlicka, 1989 personal communication).

In another situation, 16 bison from the herd that winters at the National Elk Refuge, Jackson, Wyoming, were killed as part of a herd reduction management plan and tissue samples were collected. Eleven of the bison were classified as *Brucella* reactors and *B. abortus* biovar 1 was isolated from three of the bison (Swanson, 1989 personal communication).

Of the remainder of public herds and privately owned bison in the United States, most are free of brucellosis. Through the use of tried and true brucellosis eradication and control methods (test, slaughter, and vaccination) the vast majority of bison herds in the United States are not presently infected with brucellosis. There is one exception in South Dakota where the largest privately owned bison herd of over 5,000 animals is presently under a quarantine for brucellosis. The problem of brucellosis in the Canadian bison herds is further complicated by the presence of tuberculosis and anthrax. Also the Canadians are facing the possibility of losing the last genetically pure and geographically isolated pool of the Wood bison subspecies (*B. b. athabascae*).

In summary, the bison/brucellosis issue continues to heat up particularly in the West where livestock producers are quick to point out that they were forced to go to the expense and considerable effort to eliminate brucellosis from their herds, and now the Federal Government is avoiding the issue with regard to the last significant foci of brucellosis in that area the free-ranging, publicly owned bison (and elk). Unfortunately, the issue is not that clear. The same bison are at times under the jurisdiction of the National Park Service (whose policies vary from Yellowstone to Grand Teton), the U.S. Fish and Wildlife Service, the National Forest Service, Wyoming Game and Fish, Montana Fish, Wildlife, and Parks, or the state veterinarians of Wyoming or Montana. Control of a herd depends on the herds location, which changes continually throughout the year.

Coordination at the highest levels of the U.S. Department of Agriculture and the U.S. Department of the Interior (and perhaps the Congress) will be necessary to effectively address this problem. One thing is certain, if the greater Yellowstone area continues to have less than normal precipitation, the park will not recover from the last three years of drought and the ravages of the fires of last winter. The intense overgrazing within the park will continue and so will the variable number of winter migrations out of the park. This, of course, will increase the chances of bison-to-cattle transmission and further inflame the livestock producers.

Elk (Wapiti) (*Cervus elaphus*)

Rush[3] in 1932 found the first serologic evidence of *Brucella* infections in elk when 13 of 67 serum samples from Yellowstone National Park were positive or suspicious on the plate agglutination test. Further serologic evidence of brucellosis in elk was documented in 1935 by Tunnicliff and Marsh[4] when they classified 6 of 32 elk from Yellowstone National Park as reactors to the agglutination test. They speculated that the elk population had become infected with brucellosis from an association with infected bison in Yellowstone National Park.

Honess and Winter[12] (1956) agreed with this theory and further stated that brucellosis had spread from domestic cattle to bison, and then from the infected bison to the elk. They based this belief solely on the fact that while bison were infected at a greater than 50% rate, elk on the same range were found to be infected with brucellosis at about a 10% rate. In Canada, Corner and Connell[8] in 1958 reported that of 221 elk sera collected from 1956 to 1957 in Elk Island National Park, four were suspicious and 25 were positive to the brucellosis agglutination test. In a serologic survey of wild ruminants in Colorado by Adrian and Keiss,[13] sera collected from 1967 to 1976 from 3,833 elk were tested by the rapid screening agglutination test for brucellosis. Ten were positive at a 1/25 dilution and one was positive at a 1/50 dilution. Vaughn et al.[14] in 1973 found none of 54 elk from Idaho to have detectable levels of *Brucella* antibodies. Three of 113 elk from Utah in 1978 tested by the slide agglutination test were found to be positive.[15]

The results of the most comprehensive serologic and bacteriologic survey of brucellosis in elk were reported by Thorne et al.[5] in 1978. They found brucellosis in 31% of 1,165 elk from Wyoming examined over a 5-year period by testing serum samples by the standard plate agglutination, buffered *Brucella* antigen, Rivanol, and complement fixation techniques. *Brucella abortus* biovar 1 was isolated from 17 of 45 elk. The results of this investigation indicated that "no single serologic test should be relied upon to diagnosis brucellosis in elk." In a separate report, Thorne et al.[16] discussed the clinical effects of experimental infections of elk with *B. abortus* Strain 2308 and the methods of transmission from experimentally infected to susceptible elk. In 1985, McCorquadale and DiGiacomo[17] reported a summary of serologic surveys for *B. abortus* in populations of elk in North America. Out of a total of 7,267 elk tested, 446 (6.1%) were classified as reactors.

Elk have been shown to be able to transmit brucellosis to non-infected elk and cattle in the same enclosure under experimental conditions.[16] A human case of brucellosis from an elk source was documented in 1988 in a Montana hunter that handled a fetus from a elk cow that he had shot (Ferlicka, personal communication). In Wyoming, there have been four separate instances where elk (and/or bison) have been determined, by epidemiologic evidence, as the source of *Brucella* infections in cattle herds. *B. abortus* biovar 1 isolates have been made from elk tissues in Wyoming and Montana on many occasions, and recent serologic surveys of the elk in the Jackson herd (the 8,000 to 11,000 on the National Elk Refuge) have shown the rector rate to vary from 30 to 50%.

Elk (from some areas) would also seem to satisfy the three criteria as defined by Meyer for a wildlife reservoir of brucellosis. Elk have some similarities with bison as wildlife reservoirs but they also have some obvious and important behavioral and ecological differences. There are three to four times more infected elk in the western United States than there are infected bison. The elk are much more widely distributed and migrate over a much larger area than the bison. So, in that sense, *Brucella*-infected elk may represent a larger threat to the surrounding livestock industries. Elk, however, are extremely synchronous in their breeding behavior, and therefore will probably abort over a shorter period than do bison. Many of the elk in that part of the country are feedground elk, meaning that they are fed on federal and state feeding grounds during the winter. This becomes a double-edged sword in terms of the transmission of brucellosis. The elk will most likely abort while they are on the feedgrounds surrounded by scores, if not hundreds, of other elk (and in some cases bison). This of course increases the chance of transmission to susceptible elk and therefore maintains the disease in elk populations. If the elk on the feed grounds are separated from cattle during the period when they are aborting, the probability of transmission from infected elk to susceptible cattle would be reduced. It is probably not a coincidence that virtually all elk herds heavily infected with brucellosis are "feeding grounds" elk.

Some investigators of the elk/brucellosis problem believe that in the absence of the winter feeding grounds, the disease would not persist in elk at the present levels. Elk are not as gregarious as bison or cattle and when elk cows have calves in the natural environment (not like the feeding grounds situation), the elk cow generally separates from other animals and seeks seclusion to have her calf. The elk calf is left out by itself for a period of days and is visited three or four times a day by its dam. Bison, by comparison, prefer to calve (or abort) near other animals (preferably other bison but a cattle herd will do). In this regard, infected female bison may represent a greater risk to sympatric cattle herds than an infected female elk. Nevertheless, elk, like the bison in certain regions of the western United States, have become important reservoirs of *B. abortus* and, as such, pose difficult problems for the states involved as well as the Federal Brucellosis Eradication Program.

Reindeer and Caribou *(Rangifer* spp.)

Serologic evidence of brucellosis in Alaskan Eskimo natives has been recorded since 1939. The infective agent was originally thought to be *B. abortus* and human cases were attributed to contact with domestic cattle or swine. In 1958-1959, *Brucella* spp. organisms were isolated from blood and bone marrow from two Eskimos in Alaska. The organisms resembled but were not identical to a strain of *B. suis*.[18] Epidemiologic evidence based on the occurrence of this non-typical strain of *Brucella* suggested that caribou or wild reindeer *(Rangifer tarandus)* were the animal reservoirs and the source of the human infections in Alaska.[19] Huntley et al.[20] in 1963 first isolated the *Brucella* organism from the Arctic caribou herd; they stated that this organism was pathogenic to humans and brucellosis was prevalent among the Alaskan native populations that were dependent upon caribou for food.

There has been some speculation that brucellosis may have been endemic in the prehistoric caribou of North America, while others believe that the disease was introduced into Alaska at the turn of the century by the reindeer brought from Russia. While there is some evidence to support each of these views, it is interesting to note that all of the isolates from North American reindeer and caribou are indistinguishable from those of Siberia from one another and are now classified as *B. suis* biovar 4.[21] More recently, serologic surveys in Alaska, Canada, and Siberia have documented the presence and distribution of brucellosis in caribou populations in North America and Russia.[22-27] Tessaro and Forbes[28] in 1986 reported a *B. suis* biovar 4 isolated from a barren ground caribou *(R.t. groenlandicus)* and presented an excellent review of the distribution of human and animal cases of brucellosis in Northern Canada. Attempts to vaccinate semi-domesticated herds of reindeer in Alaska with killed *B. abortus* Strain 45/20 have met with mixed results,[29] as have attempts to utilize Strain 19 vaccine in Russian reindeer.[30] In any case, *B. suis* biovar 4 is now recognized as a circumpolar etiologic agent of brucellosis with caribou and reindeer as its primary host but capable of infecting humans, dogs, and a variety of carnivorous hosts.[31] The documented presence of *B. suis* biovar 4 in a widespread and migratory wildlife reservoir species such as caribou of Alaska, Canada, and Siberia puts severe strains on the imagination when the realistic chances of the total success of governmental brucellosis eradication programs in the future are considered.

Feral Swine *(Sus scofa)*

Although not an indigenous wild species in North America, populations of feral swine (domesticated pigs that have returned to the wild state) are of sufficient number, ecological impact, and distribution to consider them wildlife in many areas, particularly in the southeastern United States. Brucellosis in feral swine in the continental United States was first reported by Wood et al.[32] in 1976 in South Carolina. Eighteen percent of 255 of the feral hogs tested were reactors as determined by the card, complement fixation, and the rivanol tests. *Brucella suis* biovar 1 was isolated from the lymph nodes of one boar. Twenty-four percent (10/42) of feral swine in Hawaii had been previously found to have low agglutination titers to *Brucella* antigens by Nichols[33] in 1962. Becker et al.[34] in 1978 tested 95 serums from feral swine trapped in Florida by the card, standard tube, complement fixation, and Rivanol precipitation test and found 50 (53%) to be positive to at least one test. Tissues were collected from nine swine and *B. suis* biovar 1 was isolated from the lymph nodes of all nine. The standard tube test was the only serologic technique utilized that detected *Brucella* antibodies in all culture-positive swine.

While investigating epidemiologic trends of brucellosis in Florida in 1977, Bigler et al.[35] reported that 22% of the (6/27) human cases of brucellosis during 1974 and 1975 were attributable to hunter contact with swine. Lawhorn[36] in 1984 reported that 8 out of 76 (11%) feral swine from southeast Texas were positive for brucellosis. The National Veterinary Services Laboratory, in Ames, Iowa, has isolated *B. suis* from over a dozen cattle in Florida over the last year (personal communications, Darla Ewalt, NVSL), and *B. suis* was also isolated from a cow in Texas (personnel communications, Jim Alexander, Texas Animal Health Commission). A report of transmission from a feral swine to a hunter has also been recently reported from California (Jessup, personal communication). The wide geographic distribution of feral swine and the fact that they are known to be capable of transmission of brucellosis to humans and domestic livestock should be of some particular concern to government agencies responsible for the control and/or eradication of this disease.

Other Wildlife Reservoirs of Brucellosis

The only other wildlife species that meets (at least partially) the criteria for a wildlife reservoir for brucellosis is the coyote (*Canis latrans*). Positive serologic reactions were first detected in two coyotes from Texas during a serologic survey in the United States conducted on seven species of wild carnivores from five states. Randhawa[37] et al. in 1977 reported agglutinin prevalence rates (which they attributed to *B. canis*) in 198 coyotes from Texas as 7.1, 8.9, and 6.7% as determined by the card test, the rapid slide agglutination test, and the salt 2-mercaptoethanol tube test respectively. Hoq[38] in 1978 reported *Brucella* agglutinins in 9 of 148 coyotes tested by the rapid plate agglutination technique. Davis[39] et al. in 1979 found 18% of 51 coyotes from eastern Texas to be serologically positive for brucellosis by several methods and *B. abortus* biovar 1 was isolated from 7 of 43 of the same coyotes.

Congenital transmission was also documented in the Texas coyotes. Davis[40] et al. in 1988 reported experimental infection of coyotes by feeding them mascerated bovine tissue that had been infused with 1 x 10⁸ CFU of *B. abortus* Strain 2308 per gram of tissue. These infected coyotes were capable of secondarily transmitting the *B. abortus* organism to susceptible cattle in the same isolation paddock and subsequent *B. abortus*-induced abortions in those cattle were observed under the confined experimental conditions. No cases of naturally occurring brucellosis transmission from coyotes to either domestic livestock or humans have been reported.

The prevailing theory on brucellosis in wild canids is that they generally become exposed by scavenging on placental membranes or the fetus from an aborting ruminant, and that, while they may (or may not) become infected, the wild canids do not under most circumstances play a preeminent role in the distribution of *Brucella* spp. in nature. These same canids are, however, excellent sentinel animals for the presence of brucellosis within an area and probably could be utilized more effectively as such.

Other wild and feral bovids may prove to be wildlife reservoirs in certain areas of the world. In the last 20 years, there have been several studies in relation to brucellosis and the African buffalo (*Syncerus caffer*). The earliest reported testing of African buffalo was in 1966 by Sachs and Staak[41] during their investigation of brucellosis in antelopes of the Serengeti when they tested four buffalo and found them to be negative. Roth[42] reported a positive agglutination titer in one buffalo from Rhodesia and a suspicious reaction in another from a total of 43 tested. Sachs et al.[43] reported that four of 23 African buffalo from northern Tanzania reacted to *Brucella* antigens. DeVos and Van Niekerk[44] in 1969 found 36 of 253 buffalo from Kruger National Park, South Africa, to be serologically reactive. Serologic evidence of brucellosis in 15 of 102 buffalo tested in Rhodesia was reported in 1972 by Condy and Vickers.[45] Kaliner and Staak[46] first isolated *B. abortus* biovar 3 from a buffalo in 1973 with orchitis from Tanzania. Gradwell et al.[47] in 1977 isolated *B. abortus* biovar 1 from four of 68 buffalo from Kruger National Park. Further serologic evidence of brucellosis in free-ranging African buffalo was reported in Rhodesia by Condy and Vickers[48] in 1976 and in South Africa by Herr and Marshall[49] in 1981. The latest report of brucellosis in African buffalo was by Waghela and Karstad.[50] They reported that 30% of the buffalo tested from the Masai Mara area of Kenya had detectable *Brucella* antibody levels. Waghela and Karstad[50] also stated that an increase in shared grazing and watering areas between wildlife and domestic cattle "makes the presence of infections by *Brucella* spp. in wildlife an important consideration in any program for control of brucellosis."

Brucellosis is also a problem in some populations of Asian buffalo (*Bubalis bubalis*). Zaki,[51] for instance, reported that, of 200 Asian buffalo tested in Egypt, 75 were found to be reactive. Recently *Brucella suis* biovar 4 (previously thought to be limited to reindeer and caribou and those animals which feed upon them) was for the first time reported in a muskox (*Ovibos moschatus moschatus*).[52]

Brucella spp. antibodies have been found in a myriad of other wildlife including several species of wild deer, African antelope, gazelles, wild carnivores, and even medium-sized omnivores. Even more disturbing is the fact that isolations of *Brucella* spp. have been made from the tissues of animals ranging in type and location from the capybara (*Hydrochaeris hydrochaeris*) in Venezuela[53-56] to a Rhodesian waterbuck (*Kobus ellipsiprymnus*),[57] to the muskox in the Arctic. The epidemiologic significance of this wealth of information is still uncertain other than the fact that brucellosis is indeed world-wide in its distribution.

Summary and Conclusions

McCorquodale and DiGiacomo[17] in 1985 in their review of brucellosis in wild ungulates and cattle stated that there "have been no published reports of wild ungulates hindering eradication of bovine brucellosis in any part of the world." While at face value that statement may be true, one must ask, in what country or area has brucellosis been successfully and truly eradicated where large numbers of free-ranging infected ungulates or wildlife are present?

A synonym for eradication is extermination and both literally mean to completely wipe out or destroy. The overwhelming existing evidence is that no species of *Brucella* is in any imminent danger whatsoever of extinction in spite of governmental pronouncements that areas or entire countries are "free of brucellosis." Rangiferine brucellosis in reindeer and caribou is circumpolar in distribution, well established in large populations of animals that migrate thousands of miles each year, and the source of disease in humans, domestic animals, and other wildlife species in the holarctic regions of the United States, Canada, Europe, and Russia.

Bovine brucellosis is being effectively combated in livestock in North America, but infected populations of bison and elk in Canada and the United States are of sufficient size and geographic distribution to create a real and serious threat to the livestock producers in certain areas of both countries. In the southeastern portion of the United States, feral swine have shown their ability to transmit brucellosis to cattle and humans. The exact distribution and prevalence of *Brucella*-infected feral swine in the United States are not known. The large number of African ungulates with brucellosis such as the African buffalo, the eland, the hippopotamus, impala, wildebeest, zebra, and kudu concerns those familiar with wildlife disease and the ease of exchange of disease between grazing wildlife and domestic livestock in Africa.[51] Mixed infections of brucellosis in capybara in South America may present problems for humans in those areas who utilize the capybara as a food source or for domestic livestock producers that are trying to eliminate brucellosis from their herds.

One should not overstate the issue of wildlife brucellosis. The majority of known *Brucella* infections are still in domestic livestock. However, in industrialized countries that picture is changing as brucellosis in domestic animals is being brought under some control, while wildlife brucellosis in these same countries is either fairly constant or increasing. The picture is not completely bleak. With the powerful modern tools of molecular genetics and biotechnology, new vaccines are being developed and improved diagnostic techniques are being presently evaluated. If and when these new methods of detecting and brucellosis are successfully developed and become available, then they must be combined with innovative strategies and delivery systems for use in free-ranging wildlife species. For it is in the prevention of brucellosis in wildlife populations (as well as in domestic animals) that any realistic hope for the control or eradication of the disease lies. The only other alternative, which is the elimination of wildlife reservoirs of brucellosis, is economically, ecologically, and aesthetically unacceptable.

References

1. Mohler JF. Annual Report of the United States Bureau of Animal Industry. 1917;106.
2. Creech GT. *Brucella abortus* infection in a male bison. *North Am Vet* 1930;11:35.
3. Rush WM. Bang's disease in the Yellowstone National Park buffalo and elk herds. *J Mammal* 1932;13:371.
4. Tunnicliff EA, Marsh H. Bang's disease in bison and elk in the Yellowstone National Park and the National Bison Range. *J Am Vet Med Assoc* 1935;86:745.
5. Thorpe BD, Sidwell RW, Bushman JB, Smart KL, Noyes R. Brucellosis in wildlife and livestock in west central Utah. *J Am Vet Med Assoc* 1965;146:225.
6. Clarke WW, Kopec JD. Report to the Brucellosis Committee. Movement of Yellowstone Park Brucellosis Infected and Exposed Bison. Proceedings of the 89th Annual Meeting, U.S. Animal Health Association, Milwaukee, WI, 1985:176.
7. Moore TA. A survey of buffalo and elk herds to determine the extent of *Brucella* infection. *Can J Comp Med* 1947;11:131.
8. Corner AH, Connell R. Brucellosis in bison, elk and moose in Elk Island National Park, Alberta, Canada. *Can J Comp Med* 1958;22:9.
9. Choquette LPE, Broughton E, Cousineau JG, Novakowski NS. Parasites and diseases of bison in Canada, IV. Serological survey for brucellosis in northern Canada. *J Wildl Dis* 1978;14:329.
10. Davis DS, Templeton JW, Williams JD, Kopec JD, Adams LG. *Brucella abortus* in Captive Bison I. Serology, Bacteriology, Pathogenesis, and Interspecific Transmission to Susceptible *Bos taurus* heifers. Submitted to the *J Wildl Dis* Feb 1989.
11. Flagg DE. A case history of a brucellosis outbreak in a brucellosis free state which

originated in bison. Proceedings of U.S. Animals Health Assoc 1983;87:171-172.

12. Honess RF, Winter KB. Diseases of wildlife in Wyoming. *Bul 9, Wyoming Game and Fish Commission,* Cheyenne 1956:279

13. Adrian WJ, Keiss RE. Survey of Colorado's wild ruminants for serologic titers to brucellosis and leptospirosis. *J Wildl Dis* 1977;13:429.

14. Vaughn HW, Knight RR, Frank RW. A study of reproduction, disease and physiological blood and serum levels in Idaho elk. *J Wildl Dis* 1973;9:296.

15. Thorne ET, Morton JK, Thomas GM. Brucellosis in elk. I. Serologic and bacteriologic survey in Wyoming. *J Wildl Dis.* 1978;14:74.

16. Thorne ET, Morton JK, Blunt FM, et al. Brucellosis in elk. II. Clinical effects and means of transmission as determined through artificial infection. *J Wildl Dis,* 1978;14:280.

17. McCorquadale SM, DiGiacomo RF. The role of wild North American ungulates in the epidemiology of bovine burcellosis: A review. *J Wildl Dis* 1985;21(4):251.

18. Meyer M.E. Species identity and epidemiology of *Brucella* strains isolated from Alaskan Eskimos. *J Infect Dis* 1964;114:169.

19. Toshach SR. *Brucella melitensis* in the Northwest Territories. *Can J Public Health* 1955;46:155.

20. Huntley BE, Philip ERN, Maynard JE. Survey of brucellosis in Alaska *J Infect Dis* 1963;112:100.

21. Meyer ME. Identification and virulence studies of *Brucella* strains isolated from Eskimos and reindeer in Alaska, Canada, and Russia. *Am J Vet Res* 1966;27:253.

22. Broughton E, Choquette LPE, Cousineau JG, Miller FL. Brucellosis in reindeer, *Rangifer tarandus* (L.), and the migratory barren ground caribou, *Rangifer tarandus groenlandicus* (L.), in Canada. *Can J of Zoolog* 1970;4:1023.

23. Davidov NN. On the epizootiology of brucellosis in domestic reindeer in Yakutia. *Proceedings of the Fifth All-Union Symposium on Biological Problems in the North* 1972. Magadan, 1974;229.

24. Gorban LV. Natural foci of brucellosis in the far north. *Microbial Epidermiol Immunobiol* 1977;8.

25. Zarnke R, Yuill TM. Serologic survey for selected microbial agents in mammals from Alberta. *J Wildl Dis* 1981;17:453.

26. Dieterich RA. Bacterial diseases: *In, Alaskan Wildlife Diseases.* RA Dieterich, ed. Fairbanks: University of Alaska Press, 1981;45.

27. Zarnke RL. Serologic Survey for selected microbial pathogens in Alaskan wildlife. *J Wildl Dis* 1983;114:169.

28. Tessaro SV, Forbes L B. *Brucella suis* biotype 4: A case of granulomatous nephritis in a barren ground caribou (*Rangifer tarandus groenlandicus* L.) with a review of the distribution of rangerifine brucellosis in Canada. *J Wildl Dis* 1986;22: 479.

29. Dieterich RA, Deyoe BL , Morton JK. Effects of killed *Brucella abortus* Strain 45/20 vaccine on reindeer later challenge-exposed with *B. suis* type 4. *Am J Vet Res* 1981;42:131, 1981.

30. Orloff E.S. Brucellosis in reindeer. *Proc. 17th World Vet Congr* Hanover 1963;1:585.

31. Neiland RA, King JA, Huntley BE, et al. The diseases and parasites of Alaskan wildlife populations, Part I. *Bull Wildl Dis Assoc* 1968;4:27.

32. Wood GW, Hendricks JB, Goodman DE. Brucellosis in feral swine. *J Wildl Dis* 1976;12:5796.

33. Nichols L Jr. Ecology of the wild pig. Hawaii Division of Fish and Games, PR Project W5-R-13, 1962:20.

34. Becker HN, Belden RC, Breault T et al. Brucellosis in Feral swine in Florida. *J Am Vet Med Assoc* 1978;173:1181.

35. Bigler WJ, Hoff GL, Hemmert WH, Tomas JA, Janowski HT. Trends of brucellosis

in Florida an epidemiologic review. *Am J Epidemiol* 1977;05(3):24.

36. Lawhorn B. Pseudorabies and brucellosis in East Texas piney wood rooter hogs. Park Producers, July-August, 1984:4.

37. Randhawa AS, Dieterich WH, Hunter CC, Kelly VP, Johnson TC, et al. Prevalence of seropositive reactions to *Brucella canis* in a limited survey of domestic cats. *J Am Vet Med Assoc* 1977; 171(3):267.

38. Hoq MA. A serologic survey of Brucella agglutinins in wildlife and sheep. *California Veterinarian* 1978;32:15-17.

39. Davis DS, Boeer WJ, Mims JP, Heck FC, Adams LG. *Brucella abortus* in coyotes. I. A serological and bacteriologic survey in eastern Texas. 1979;15(3):367.

40. Davis DS, Heck FC, Williams JD, Simpson TR, Adams LG. Interspecific transmission of *Brucella abortus* from experimentally infected coyotes (Canis latrans) to parturient cattle. *J Wildl Dis* 1988;24(3):533-537.

41. Sachs R, Staak, C. Evidence of brucellosis in antelopes of the Serengeti. *Vet Rec* 1966;79:857.

42. Roth HH. A survey of Brucellosis in game animals in Rhodesia. *Bull Epizoot Dis Afr* 1967;15:133.

43. Sachs R, Staak C. Serological investigation of brucellosis in game animals in Tanzania. Bull Epizoot Dis Afr 11968;6:91.

44. DeVos V, Van Niekerk CAWJ. Brucellosis in the Kruger National Park. *J S Afr Vet Med Assoc* 1969;40:331.

45. Condy JB, Vickers DB. Brucellosis in Rhodesian wildlife. *J S Afr Vet Med Assoc* 1972;43:175.

46. Kaliner G, Staak C. A case of architis caused by *Brucella abortus* in the African buffalo. *J Wildl Dis* 1973;9:251.

47. Gradwell DV, Schuttee AP, Van Niekerk CAWJ, et al. The isolation of *Brucella abortus* biotype 1 from African buffalo in the Kruger National Park. *J S Afr Vet Med Assoc* 1977;48:41.

48. Condy JB, Vickers DB. Brucellosis in buffalo (*Syncerus caffer*) in Wankie National Park. *Rhodesian Vet J* 1976;7:58.

49. Herr S, Marshall C. Brucellosis in free-living African buffalo (Syncerus caffer): A serological Survey, Onderstepoort. *J Vet Res* 1981;48:133.

50. Wagela S, Karstad L. Antibodies to *Brucella* spp. among blue wildebeest and African buffalo in Kenya. *J Wildl Dis* 1986;22:189.

51. Zaki R. *Brucella abortus* infection among buffaloes in Egypt. *Comp. Pathol* 1948;58:73.

52. Gates CC, Wobeser G, Forbes LB. Rangiferine brucellosis in a muskox, *Ovibos moshatus moschatus* (Zimmermann). *J Wild Dis* 1984;20(3):177.

53. Lord VR, Flores RC. *Brucella* spp. from capybara (*Hydrochoerus hydrochaeris*) in Venezuela: Serologic studies and metabolic charaterization of isolates. *J Wildl Dis* 1983;19:308.

54. Bello A, Mogollon P, Villegas M, et al. La brucelosis en los animales salvages: 1. El chigüire (*hydrochoerus hydrochaeris*). *Vet Trop* 1976;1:117.

55. Bello A, Mogollon P, Ramirez M, Rodriquez V, Laserna RD, Perez M, Moreno J, Lord RD. Brucelosis en chiguires del Estado Apure (*Hydrochoerus hydrochaeris.* Acta Cient Vene 1978;29-Supp 1:178.

56. Bello A, Lord VD, Mogollon P, Laserna RD, De Salmeron C, Ramirez M, Moreno J, Toro M, Ramos J. Estudio epidemiológico de la brucelosis en chiguires(*Hydrochoerus hydrochaeris*) del Estado Apure. *Acta Cient Venez* 1979; 30(1):31.

57. Condy JB, Vickers DB. The isolation of *Brucella abortus* from a waterbuck.

Chapter Twenty-five

Eradication of Brucellosis at the Herd Population Level: Part 1. A Producer's Perspective

John B. Armstrong

I am pleased to be included as a speaker in this Second International Symposium on Brucellosis. This symposium has provided an excellent overview of the recent knowledge that has been gained from sophisticated research on brucellosis during the last 10 years. The present session on diagnosis, epidemiology, and economics of brucellosis says much of what needs to be said about these subjects. My charge is to round out this session by providing a "bottom-line" assessment of the disease and the regulatory program from the perspective of the producer.

I want to give you some background on my involvement with brucellosis so you will better understand the perspective from which I will make my comments. I have been involved with brucellosis as a cattle producer for more than 40 years. I have dealt with the disease in my own herds and in the herds at the King Ranch, where we had to think about the disease from the standpoint of a worldwide corporation.

I became involved with the brucellosis issue in state and national level organizations of cattlemen many years ago and have continued that involvement. I was among those who seriously questioned the old regulatory program in the mid-1970s and who called for the studies that formed the basis of our new efforts.

I am also past Chairman of the Texas Animal Health Commission. During my tenure there, the new programs were defined for Texas and put into place. I am presently Chairman of the Brucellosis Committee of the U.S. Animal Health Association and Chairman of the National Cattlemen's Association Committee on Animal Health.

During the past 15 years, I have observed the major transition in the cattle industry caused by this disease. We have come from a situation in which Texas producers, threatened by a state embargo, were in near rebellion about a program they regarded as unworkable, to the present situation, in which most cattlemen feel positive about the progress that has been made and the possibility of actually achieving the ultimate goal of eradication. I assure you that this represents a dramatic turnaround in the industry. I will try to address key events that have caused this turnaround.

As I begin my remarks, I cannot help but recall the First International Symposium on Brucellosis held by Texas A&M and the Texas Agricultural Experiment Station in 1976. That symposium came at the peak of the concern about the old regulatory program. It probed key questions about what we needed to know and what was missing. It set the stage for an active program of research that has continued over the years. Texas A&M University has emerged as one of the key centers of excellence in research on brucellosis. The body of knowledge reflected in the presentations we have heard at this second symposium has expanded by at least a factor of two or more over the last few years.

In the next few minutes, I will express my own views and what I believe to be the views of my counterparts in the cattle business on several matters that are relevant to brucellosis in the industry:

1. Evolution of the program from the producer's viewpoint.
2. Major factors that allowed progress to occur.
3. Key research contributions impacting producers.
4. Evolving industry attitudes.
5. Plan for rapid completion of the brucellosis eradication program.

Evolution of the Program

You have already heard excellent presentations on key epidemiologic factors that have shaped the regulatory program in the 1980s and you will hear about future plans for the program in the next session. My comments are intended to briefly trace how the program has evolved in this critical decade from the industry's perspective.

I have mentioned the confrontation between Texas producers and regulatory officials in the mid-1970s. We believed that the old program was unworkable and unaffordable, and challenged the USDA to conduct a thorough scientific study of the program. We agreed in advance to live with the recommendations that evolved from such a credible study. We were fortunate to have excellent and dedicated people who conducted the "Blue Ribbon" study (The National Brucellosis Technical Commission) and recommended the elements of the new program. The National Academy of Science's report, completed in the same time period, provided a clear assessment of current knowledge on the disease. About that time, the first Texas A&M symposium was also held. The two studies and the symposium reflect a very high level of expert agreement on the major issues as is summarized in the (National Brucellosis Technical Commission Report, August 1978, Section 4,4-1):

all available evidence supports the conclusion that present biologic knowledge is adequate to achieve local eradication with continuing surveillance, if one is willing to accept the commission's definition for local eradication, as generally accepted for foot-and-mouth disease of cattle, vesicular exanthema of swine, and viscerotropic velogenic Newcastle disease of chicken and turkeys.

These studies, and the ensuing negotiations in the U.S. Animal Health Association, resulted in the development of a new regulatory program for brucellosis. The program began in the early 1980s and has continued to evolve through the rest of this decade. Progress has been good, the program has matured with experience, and producer attitudes are greatly improved.

The results of research conducted during this period have removed much concern about ambiguity and uncertainty on key points of disease management in the minds of producers and have given us important new tools. I will say more about this later on.

Texas and other Gulf Coast states have been and remain the largest source of new infection in the U.S. As the new program has progressed, and other states with fewer initial infections have made great progress, another factor has come into play that affects producer attitudes. The clean states have become increasingly concerned about importing animals from states with high levels of infection. Regulatory restrictions of states in clean areas, and the price differential for known clean animals, have created further producer incentives to clean up this disease in states like Texas.

Figure 24-1 (provided by USDA/APHIS) summarizes the status of the states across the U.S. with respect to level of infection. In September, 1988, there were 27 free states, 16 states with Class A status, 6 Class B states, and 1 state with B/C status This represents remarkable progress in this decade. Figure 24-2 shows the remarkable reduction in the number of reactors identified per year during the '80s. We are clearly on the move with excellent progress. Figure 24-3 shows the same kind of information as Figure 24-2, but for Texas, an example of a state with high prevalence. Progress is being made here too. Figure 24-4 shows a reduction in the number of quarantined herds in Texas at the end of each fiscal year. And Figure 24-5 shows a similar reduction in the number of newly detected infected herds over time.

As we sit together in this symposium in mid-1989, producer attitudes are generally very positive. Clear evidence shows that we are making progress. The program is much less laborious than it was in the last decade, and we can begin to see some real light at the end of the tunnel. I will return to this point later in the presentation to discuss a plan for rapid completion of the brucellosis program that could only be successful with the today's positive industry attitude.

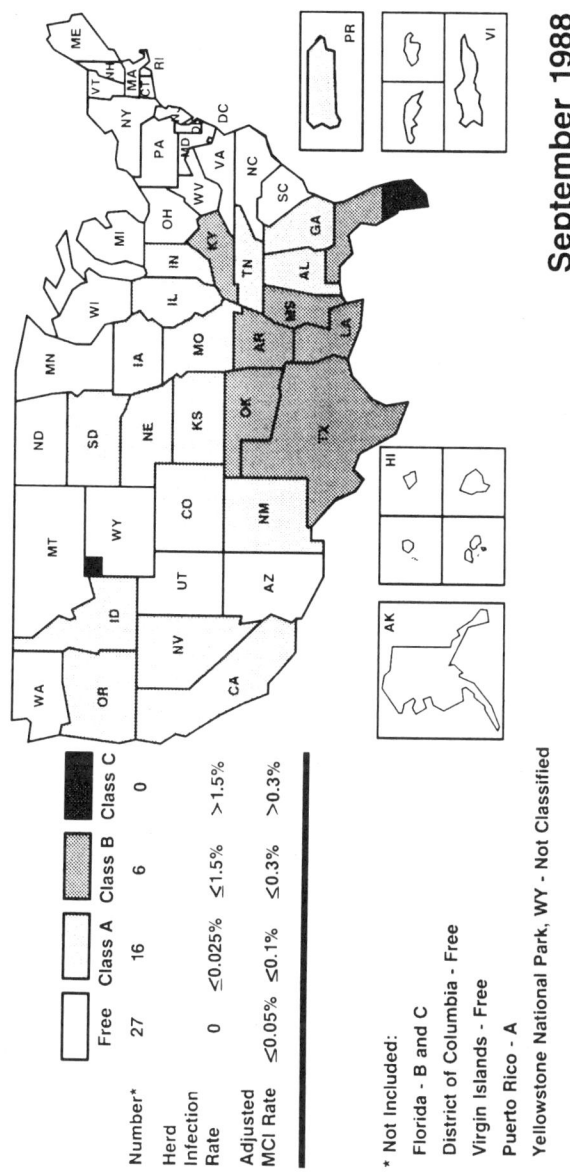

Figure 25-1. Cattle Brucellosis State Classification

Brucellosis Eradication
Blood Testing: Cattle

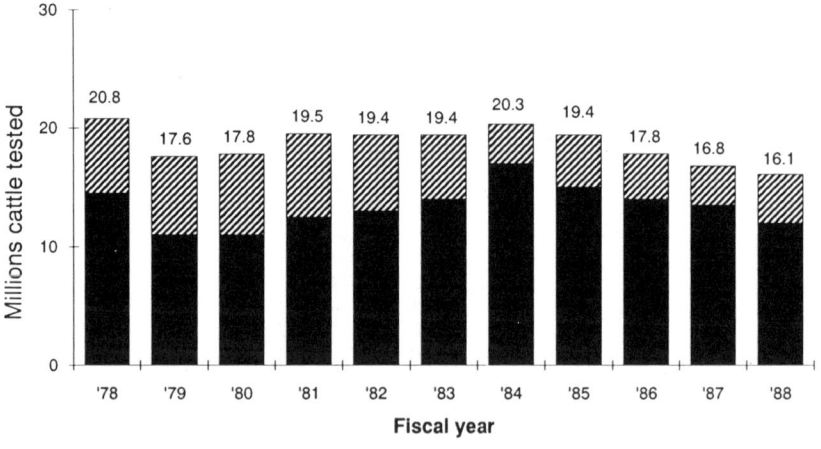

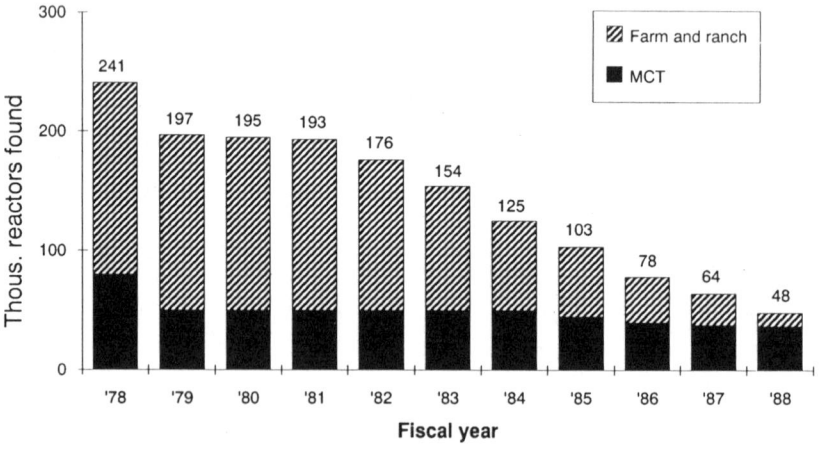

*Estimate

Figure 25-2. Brucellosis Eradication - Blood Testing: Cattle

BLOOD TESTING:
TEXAS CATTLE

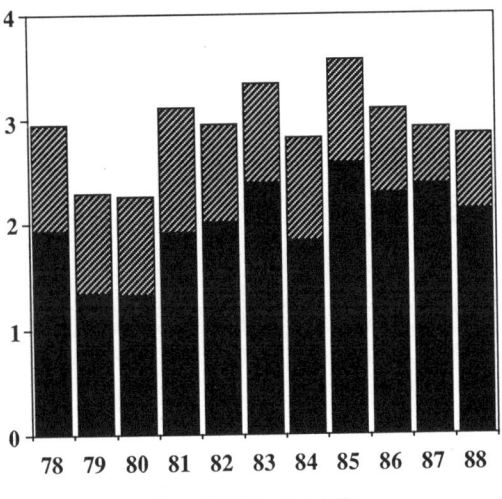

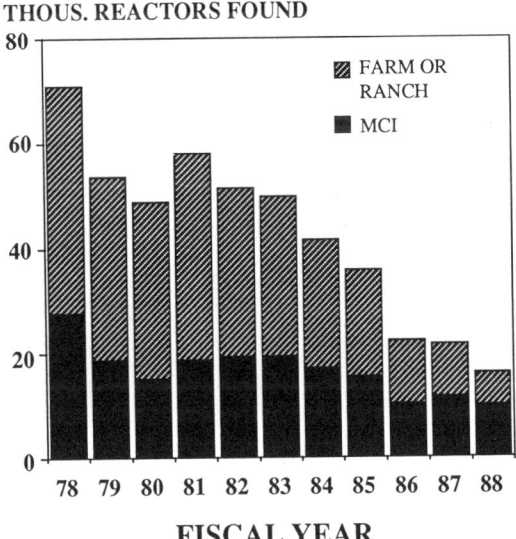

Figure 25-3. Blood Testing: Texas Cattle

Brucellosis Eradication in Texas
Number of Cattle Herds Quarantined*

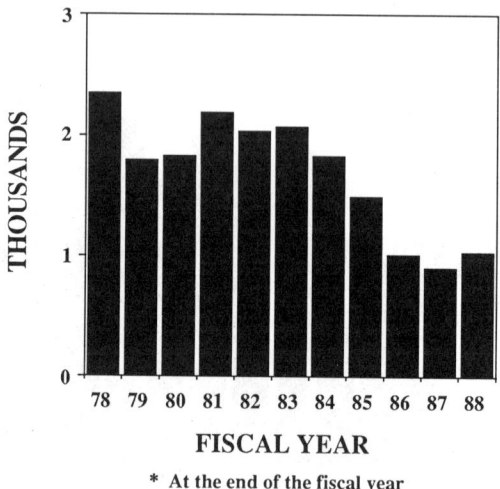

* At the end of the fiscal year

Brucellosis Eradication in Texas
Number of Newly Infected Herds

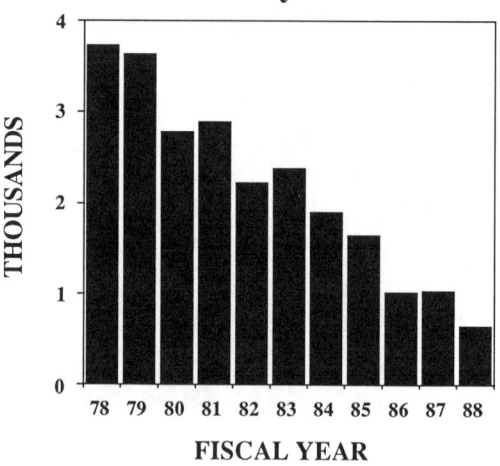

Figure 25-4. Brucellosis Eradication in Texas: Number of Cattle Herds Quarantined

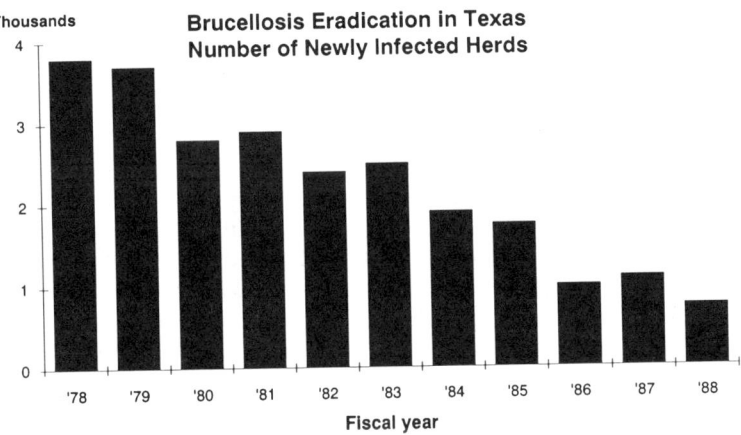

Figure 25-5. Brucellosis Eradication in Texas: Number of Newly Infected Herds

Major Factors that Permitted Progress

Beginning with the findings of the Blue Ribbon Committee (NBTC) and the National Academy report, and extending through the evolution of the new regulatory program in the '80s, one general theme has contributed to industry support for the new regulatory program. Although the theme sounds obvious and simple today, it was not always so. The theme is simply that, for the brucellosis program to be successful, it must be based on scientifically sound epidemiologic principles and it must be economically affordable to the industry. The new program has taken us a long way toward success using these principles.

Individual herd plans, involving more efficient use of epidemiologists and private veterinarians, have replaced the blind test-and-slaughter methods of the '70s. Adult vaccination in problem herds has significantly reduced the spread of infection and the cost of clean-up. Development of new diagnostics that do a much better job of separating the infected animal from the vaccinate have decreased costs, enhanced the maintenance of open market channels, and vastly reduced the frustration associated with false-positive reactions and unnecessary imposition of quarantine. The intensified testing and clean-up programs in high prevalence areas have been successful in several states, including Texas.

Key Research Contributions

In 1975, when the major concerns about brucellosis came to a head, there were very few laboratories either in the government arena or in universities that were conducting meaningful research on the disease. I know that the program at Texas A&M, which began in the summer of 1975, had less than $30,000 appropriated to it at start-up. Through increased state funding and acquisition of competitive grants from the federal government, as well as contributions from industry, this program is now funded at between $600,000 and $700,000 per year and involves a team of more than a dozen scientists. There are other laboratories in other states that have had a similar increase in effort.

While brucellosis is not a new disease, you have heard at this symposium how much new information has been learned about it in very recent years, and by implication, how little we knew before 1975. The opportunity to use new methods in modern biology have accelerated progress and given us some exciting new tools to use on this old problem.

Modern research has placed in proper perspective many of the common beliefs about the spread of the disease and its alternate hosts or disease reservoirs. We now have a better understanding of the possible role of coyotes or other carnivores in spreading the disease; as well as the possible role of deer, buffalo, or other wild ruminants. We also have an important new understanding of heifers from infected herds initially test negative and later reveals a latent infection when calving.

The revalidation of the use of adult vaccination with Strain 19 vaccine and the quantitative studies validating dosages and measuring residual titers, which were at Texas A&M, gave us a critically important tool for reducing the spread of infection and cost of herd clean-up.

New methods in biology have given us diagnostic tools with greatly enhanced sensitivity and precision, thus allowing regulatory officials to make a much more precise distinction between the infected animal and the vaccinate. As progress continues, we are obtaining the ability to use these more precise tests in the marketplace, rather than in referral laboratories, thus facilitating the flow of animals to markets and reducing unnecessary expense for the producers.

You have heard exciting reports at this symposium about the new vaccines that are being developed for brucellosis. The killed product and the new live recombinant vaccine being developed at Texas A&M, along with companion diagnostics, should bring us new tools at a critical time in the accelerated brucellosis eradication program.

Evolving Industry Attitudes

As I mentioned earlier, it is clear that producer attitudes about brucellosis and the regulatory programs have changed considerably in the last 10 years. There has always been a wide diversity of opinion in the industry about the disease and what should be done about it. Throughout the '50s, '60s, and '70s, prudent cattle and dairy producers effectively dealt with the disease by using good management and the available biological tools. Regulatory strategies, in retrospect, were not always optimal, and frustration, distrust, and animosity emerged as a result.

It has taken time to build the industry's confidence in the new program; in fact, some still believe that eradication is not an achievable goal and that the only problem with brucellosis is a regulatory one. However, it is my belief that the balance of industry thinking has clearly shifted from negative to positive and that producers generally support the program. Voluntary support is clearly the most vital ingredient of a successful program. Without the voluntary support of the industry, no level of regulatory resource can force compliance.

I am reminded of a statement made during the days of the old program that described an unscrupulous trader who stated that he had a pickup truck, gooseneck trailer, pair of cowboy boots, and a steel-trap mind, and that with these tools, he could overcome any regulations that could be written. I believe we have drastically reduced the number of people with this attitude.

As I have stated, the concern of our customers in other states about the risk of importing brucellosis, as well as the legal implications for the producer or his agent, has put pressure on the industry to make the program work.

The program has always been viewed differently by different parts of the livestock industry. Dairymen are interested in keeping a clean herd because they are under the constant scrutiny of the milk test. Registered breeders are clearly motivated to keep clean herds as a necessary condition for keeping their market channels open, especially overseas. Commercial cow-calf operators of substantial size have the resources and interests to deal with the disease and the regulatory program in an informed way. However, small part-time or hobby operators are sometimes less interested in eradication and have fewer facilities and other resources to manage the prevention program. This group represents a continuing challenge in terms of communication and compliance.

Communication continues to be a vital element in the campaign to clean up brucellosis. The Extension Service, especially here in Texas, has been an important part of the educational process. The Texas Animal Health Commission has also had an active role in public awareness and producer education. The state and national livestock organizations continue to play a critical role in maintaining awareness and communication. The U.S. Animal Health Association is a forum for hammering out agreements between the industry, the regulatory agencies, and the scientific community. We all need to continue to improve our effectiveness in dealing with state and federal governments in the law- and rule-making arena, and to speak out effectively on the matter of ensuring that adequate resources are available to make programs successful.

Looking Ahead: A Plan for Rapid Completion of the Brucellosis Eradication Program

I hope I have conveyed to you a sense that the beef cattle industry is generally positive about the present program and the progress that has been made. Nevertheless, I would also mention that we believe it is always a good idea to evaluate the situation and ask about ways to improve even a good effort. We can learn much from previous efforts to eradicate other diseases.

At some stage of clean-up in other disease eradication efforts, there came a point where a more intensive and often more expensive effort was needed to more effectively locate the last pockets of infection and to intensively engage in clean-up activities to remove these last traces of disease. This included the use of drastic techniques, such as herd depopulation, to reach the final goal.

The National Cattlemen Association's Animal Health Committee instructed me to ask APHIS to give this some thought and to present an alternative plan for the remaining effort to eradicate brucellosis. Dr. Jim Glosser has responded with a bold proposal (not stated as USDA policy at this point) that deserves consideration and support. As I mentioned, it builds on the experience involved in previous efforts to eradicate other diseases.

The National Cattlemen, along with representatives from the National Milk Producer's Federation, American Farm Bureau Federation, Livestock Marketing Association, Livestock Conservation Institute, U.S. Animal Health Association, and several state veterinarians and health commissions have reviewed the proposal and provided feedback to APHIS.

If this option is implemented, we believe that, within five years, all states will either be free or be in the qualifying process to acquire free status. This objective will only be attainable with adequate funding, producer cooperation, and aggressive administration at the local, state, and national level.

In the short-run, such a program would cost more money than is currently allocated. However, this is a case of spending more money now, and realizing significant savings in the long term. We are exploring ways to fund such a program. One way is for the Secretary of Agriculture to declare an emergency funding need which could be funded from the Commodity Credit Corporation. This approach was taken 10 years ago in the final phase of the hog cholera eradication program.

In conclusion, let me congratulate the organizers of this symposium here at Texas A&M for the success of this meeting and for the work they have accomplished during the last 10 years in research and education on this challenging disease. Producers feel positive about what has been done and where we are going. We all obviously need to continue to work together so that we in the United States can soon speak of this disease in the past tense.

Chapter Twenty-six

Eradication of Brucellosis
at the Herd Population Level:
Part II. A Producer's Perspective

Paul C. Genho

My presentation is essentially my viewpoint on the brucellosis eradication program. Of necessity then, it will follow a different format than the other presentations in this symposium. But, while I'm unable to follow the scientific format normally used in these kinds of presentations, it doesn't lessen my concern with what is happening here. Since I come from a "C" area of Florida, the brucellosis eradication program may have more impact on me than anyone here.

My training is as a production-oriented reproductive physiologist. My profession is as a manager. I raise cattle for a living. As a reproductive physiologist I'm concerned about brucellosis because I recognize brucellosis can be a devastating reproductive disease. As a manager, I'm concerned because I realize that the lowered reproductive performance in infected cows and the regulatory restrictions on moving quarantined animals means significantly reduced profits. I'm dedicated to the eradication of this disease.

I think it's important and, if I might brag a little, I want to announce to the entire world that our entire cow herd has, as of this past fall, reached the status of being certified free. For those of you who aren't aware of the process of becoming certified free, it requires two clean tests after the animals are all quarantined, 10 to 14 months apart, and an annual test thereafter. It sounds simpler than it really is. We do it because it allows us free movement of heifers to any area of the nation. The final paper work was recently completed. Our entire herd is certified free. My intent in this presentation is to outline some of the things I think assisted us in reaching this status and then to outline some of my feelings about the program and what I think the future direction of it should be.

Previous to 1980, the Ranch had not been supportive of the brucellosis eradication program. There were probably a number of reasons for this attitude. One of them was the federal government's on again, off again approach to calfhood vaccination. Another was questions about the effectiveness of calfhood vaccination, as well as the eradication program in general. No doubt the manager at that time felt he had more important items to deal with. And, to be candid, at that time there was probably the feeling held by many in Florida that even if there was a little brucellosis in our herds, it probably was not hurting us too much. In 1980, all replacement heifers were vaccinated for the first time. This was done with the old standard dose when the animals were approximately 12 months old. You can imagine the titer problems we had with those animals for a number of years.

In 1981, I was employed by the Ranch and assumed management of the herd health program. One of the early decisions I made was to "clean up" our herd as far as brucellosis was concerned. While this decision represented a commitment to eradication of the disease, it was not a priority item in my mind. It could not be. There were too many other items of greater economic importance that demanded my attention.

We did start calfhood vaccinating all heifers at 4 to 6 months of age. We also intensified collection of blood samples using fee basis veterinarians. In addition, we adult vaccinated one mature herd of around 2,000 head and totally depopulated another herd of approximately 2,000 cows we had just acquired. When we first bled this recently acquired herd, we found a fairly high incidence of the disease, and thus decided to depopulate rather than try to cleanup by bleeding. We stopped bringing outside females into our herd, thus eliminating the chance of reinfection. We instigated a limited breeding season (which incidentally, I feel is as vital a tool in eradication as calfhood vaccination or bleeding). The limited number of non-pregnant cows we kept were isolated in separate herds. Our reasoning was that this might reduce the chance of them infecting other animals if their reproductive failure was due to brucellosis. In other words, we did those things that one would generally prescribe to cleanup.

I might say that the incidence of the disease was never very high in any of our herds, except the one already mentioned which we disposed of shortly after acquiring it. As a result, we should have cleaned up quickly. Unfortunately, we made little if any progress for three or four years. Those herds that were clean to start with we got certified free right away. In those that were not, we continued to have low levels of infection.

After about four years of following this program, I was asked to attend a meeting of federal and state regulators, epidemiologists, and the veterinarians who were doing our work, as well as several of our people. The purpose of this meeting was to review our accomplishments and to modify our herd plan, if needed.

About midway through the meeting, I suddenly realized that the reason we were not making more progress in eradicating brucellosis was that no one was in charge of the program. Now do not misunderstand me. Everyone there was doing his job well. I am not in the least critical of what they were doing, but both the needed coordination of efforts and my attention to the program was missing. I'm a manager and what I was doing was to depend on others to manage an important program for me with only perfunctorial attention on my part. I decided right then and there that I was going to take charge of the program. In other words, I was going to see to it that we got cleaned up.

Because my knowledge of the disease and the program was limited, I recognized that I needed the best help I could get to accomplish this. As a result, in my view the regulators became tools to help me accomplish my goal of cleaning up instead of thorns in my side. The poor epidemiologist no doubt got tired of my very frequent phone calls trying to understand what was going on. My job was to apply judgment and the needed coordination. The herd plan became my plan, and I began to have major input into it. I made a few changes. Some were big changes, some were subtle. They weren't all my ideas, but they were all endorsed by me and the plan became what I wanted done.

For example, I began to insist on complete gathering at bleeding. That should seem obvious, but when you gather cattle from a large pasture with brush or woods in it, you frequently leave a cow or two. I instructed our men that we had to bring in every cow. I became a fanatic on the subject and we improved markedly in this area. In addition, every bleeding chart went across my desk and I personally reviewed each one. In fact, I called the state lab and had copies sent directly to me. I wanted no waiting in getting the results. Previously the charts went to the veterinarians who, at year end, gave them to our secretary for filing. He tried to coordinate pulling reactors and suspects directly with our foremen who didn't understand or weren't committed to the program. I didn't know how many reactors we were having.

Under the modified program I personally made sure reactors were pulled out promptly. We designated a highly isolated pasture to be a holding pasture for reactors and suspects awaiting slaughter. You can't always get a cow slaughtered the day you pull her out of the herd, so we designated an escape-proof pasture to be used only for reactors and suspects awaiting slaughter. This eliminated the occasional escape we were experiencing. It also allowed me to know for sure that the cow was actually removed from the herd. I insisted on a monthly inventory by tag number of the animals in the pasture. None ever again escaped.

We started transporting the blood samples at our expense to the state lab to allow us to have the rivanol result within 24 hours. This allowed us to remove the card test negative-rivanol positive animals that were being missed when we used only the card test to identify potential problem animals. You should understand that once cattle are turned out into the pastures, it's difficult to find one individual animal, regardless of what the test results say. We created what we called suspect herds within units. All titered cattle were added to this herd until their status could be determined. This sometimes meant we kept these suspect herds intact for 12 to 18 months, collecting blood samples from them frequently to assure ourselves that they were clean.

We had always separated our replacement heifers at weaning and managed them as a separate unit until after their first calf. Now, in addition, we started collecting samples from them at 18 months of age for information only. High titered animals were isolated from the balance of our replacement heifers until we could accurately determine their status. And finally, upon sound scientific recommendation, we adult vaccinated the two units of cattle of about 2,000 head each that we were having the most trouble cleaning up. I have no reluctance in recommending whole herd vaccination where persistent levels of the disease exist. The net result of this more intensive program was that we moved rapidly to cleaning up. Several additional management units of around 3,000 head were certified each year, until, as I mentioned, we have now achieved our goal of every unit being certified free.

This evolutionary process of going from resisting the program, to merely complying, to personal involvement in the process, to cleaning up is not limited to me. I believe the vast majority of the Florida producers I know today are at least complying and most are determined to clean up their herds. This is very different from the mood of eight or ten years ago, when resistance by many herd owners was common. This evolutionary attitude is due in part to efforts by both the National and Florida Cattleman's Associations and their Animal Health Committees' constant efforts to sell the program. Members of the Brucellosis Committee of the United States Animal Health Association were heavily involved in encouraging producers to begin eliminating brucellosis. John Armstrong, who shares a spot on this program with me, has been greatly involved.

In Florida, a special tribute needs to be paid to J. O. Pearce and Dan Childs, who have worked for years to get fellow producers' support. Florida Agriculture Commissioner Doyle Connor, Florida State Veterinarian Clarence Campbell, Dr. Paul Bectin, and a number of federal employees have contributed heavily to our progress in Florida. A special tribute should also be paid to the late Dr. Joe Hendrix, who in his outspoken way helped gain producers' support, as has the educational program recently sponsored by the Kerr Foundation. Pressure to clean up brucellosis caused by the recently enacted regulatory limitation on movement of heifers from "B" and "C" areas has no doubt helped focus producers' attention on the seriousness of the problem, but to totally ascribe the change in attitude to these rules and regulations would be inaccurate.

Because of this change in producers' attitude, major progress is being made. It is anticipated that within the very near future, Florida will reach the "B" status. This will be a major step in the eradication program, as the south half of Florida is the last "C" area in the nation.

I think there are two great lessons here. First, the disease can be eliminated; and second, the program *will work*. Eradication of brucellosis is more than elimination of the *Brucella abortus* organism. It will never be accomplished if the program is "owned" and directed by only the veterinarians, epidemiologists, and regulators. Cowboys, cattle, economics, physical terrain, and managers are all part of the necessary solution.

The information I have indicates that nationally there are only around 2,400 identified infected herds remaining. We've made major progress in just the last two or three years and the possibility of totally eradicating the disease seems a distinct reality today. Unfortunately, at this point federal funding to continue many of the key elements needed to eliminate these last pockets of infection is scheduled to be phased out. As I understand it, the present intent is for the USDA to have only a "residual" program. Funding for this residual program will be limited to that necessary to cover the cost of disease surveillance and enforcement of interstate regulations. If this is allowed to occur, progress in eradication brucellosis will suffer and in fact the possibility of losing some of what we've accomplished during the past several years is a distinct possibility.

It should seem obvious to even the most casual observer that, given the major progress we've made, at this point we should intensify rather than reduce our efforts to eradicate the disease completely. To back off in our efforts invites a loss of what we've gained. I strongly advocate continued and perhaps even increased funding for those programs that have resulted in the progress we have made. Among the programs needing continued funding are calfhood vaccination, adult vaccination, and possibly depopulation. I have never been a supporter of the indemnity program. I feel it is counterproductive to, on a continuous basis, pay producers a premium above market to have the disease. However, where residual pockets of the disease persist, I can see the merits of assisting producers by alleviating some of their financial loss if complete depopulation becomes necessary.

Now, if I may change the thrust of my presentation somewhat, I'd like to talk about the kind of problem we often have after eliminating brucellosis, with calfhood vaccination-induced, titered animals. They create major problems for the producers and will for the regulators. I have heard a number of scientists and regulators state that the reason we have high titers in calfhood vaccinated animals is because we vaccinate them when they are older than the recommended age. If you have made this statement, you've been wrong.

Everyone knows that vaccinating older animals will result in an increase in titered animals, but I also know from the many animals we vaccinate each year that a small percent of heifers vaccinated at the age of four to five months, later have titer levels that could result in them being classified as either suspects or reactors. I can make this statement because at Deseret we simply don't vaccinate any animals after six and one-half months of age that are kept as replacement heifers, and yet we continue to have a small number of titers show in these animals when they become test eligible. This is usually a greater problem at the time of first calving.

I heard one highly respected scientist say, a year or so ago, that only 1 in about 800 animals (if I recall the numbers he gave) would have elevated titers if vaccination was done at the right age. My experience would indicate that the number of titered animals would be a lot higher than 1 in 800 actual field vaccinations, but even if this is correct, the economic result to the producer of 1 in 800 animals potentially being falsely classified as a reactor is considerable.

One thing I hope we remember is that we do not quarantine animals, we quarantine herds, and if the herd of origin is 200 or 300 head, you're going to have that many animals quarantined. At our ranch, we consider each 3,000 cow unit as a herd, and thus one false reactor in 800 or even 1,000 or 2,000 cows would result in the loss of our ability to ship the heifers from that unit, given the present interstate regulation for movement of females. If you are not aware, present regulations require that heifers from "C" areas either be from certified herds, spayed, or "S" branded and sent to a quarantine lot, in order to move interstate. Loss of our certification then, would result in considerable economic loss.

A topic of discussion at the USAHA Brucellosis Committee meetings in Little Rock last October was the effect of the number of organisms in a dose of vaccine on such non-infected calfhood vaccination-induced residual titers. It has been postulated that a lower dosage vaccination would provide immunity similar to the present dose and at the same time reduce these false titers. Dr. Jan Huber's presentation tends to support this; however, the protection in lower dose vaccines was somewhat reduced. Concerns about maintaining sufficient numbers of organisms in the commercially available vaccines to provide an adequate immune response prevented the committee from recommending a reduction in the number of organisms.

However, the problem calfhood vaccination-induced titers in non-infected animals needs to be recognized as a serious economic problem by regulators as well as producers, and demands attention. We should recognize that if producers reach certified-free status and then begin to have problems with titers limiting to movement of their animals, their support for the program will wane. This problem will no doubt intensify for regulators as the number of infected herds continues to decrease, and the percent of heifers being vaccinated increases.

A somewhat similar problem exists with the recent increase in the number of *Brucella suis* cases found in cattle. On our ranch, we've identified one case per year for the last three years. Some of you may not be aware that a sizable feral swine population is present in many of the Southeastern states. Exposure of cattle to such feral swine no doubt is the source of the *B. suis* infection in these cattle. Eradication of the feral swine population is not a possibility, either physically or politically.

Unfortunately, as I understand it, the presently utilized serological test fails to differentiate between *B. abortus* and *B. suis*. Differentiation is only accomplished by milk or tissue culture. My experience is that successful isolation of *Brucella* strains from tissue samples, while high is far less than 100%. An animal may be infected with Strain 19 or *B. suis* and yet isolation may not be accomplished. Hence, if the epidemiologist, lacking adequate information, classifies an animal as a reactor, the whole herd origin would be quarantined for brucellosis when in reality they were non-infected for that particular disease. I do not have an answer for this problem, but have personally had to deal with the potential of this kind of an economic threat to our operation.

Finally, I'm personally gratified by the interest and progress being made in the research to improve the vaccines. I believe if one can be developed and released that it will greatly expedite our progress. Particularly, I see new vaccines as a possible solution to the calfhood vaccination-induced titer problem. I also feel that it will have wide acceptance by the producers. I'm a strong advocate of this and other related research. We need continued efforts in basic research such as is being reviewed during this symposium, but we also need continued field research to test applications and demonstrate the efficiency of our eradication program. Hopefully, adequate funding will be allocated to allow us to do those things that are necessary to complete the eradication of brucellosis from the cattle population.

PART SEVEN

NATIONAL PROGRAM POLICIES

Chapter Twenty-seven

Protection of Brucellosis-Free Areas from Reinfection

M. Davidson, A. Shimshony,
H. Adler, M. Banai, and A. Cohen

In many countries, brucellosis is still a serious economic problem, with regard to livestock, and a major public health hazard for human beings. Among 176 countries that responded to questionnaires distributed by the Food and Agricultural Organization (FAO), World Health Organization, and Office International des Epizooties (OIE) concerning disease occurrence and control in 1987,[1] two countries had never encountered brucellosis, 15 countries had completely eradicated the disease, 19 countries did not encounter the disease in 1987, and 140 countries were still infected.

Based on information submitted by 48 member countries of the OIE, Fensterbank[2] reported that 13 countries have eradicated brucellosis, 17 are in the process of advanced eradication, 8 have initiated a vaccination program primarily as a control strategy, and 10 have not yet defined applicable measures. Three basic modes of control are generally applied:
1. eradication by a "test and slaughter" system
2. vaccination scheme
3. a combination of the two methods.

The parameters to be considered in choosing the method of control include prevalence of the disease; type of husbandry and management; size of herds; movement and trade of animals; and technical and financial resources available.

Finally, the control scheme is completed by measures aimed at preventing reinfection.

History of the Disease in Israel

Gur[3] reviewed the history of the brucellosis disease in Israel. Until 1920 there were no reports regarding the incidence of brucellosis in Israel. Cases of the disease among cattle were first reported in 1923, after bulls were imported from Europe and Egypt.

In 1927, Smith[4] reported that 80% of the dairy cattle herds were infected by the disease at the prevalence rate of 15 to 20%. During that same year, an eradication program was initiated that applied the "test and eliminate" ("test and isolate") method of eradication on herds infected by *Brucella abortus*. The program was voluntary, requiring the herd owners' agreement. In herds with a low morbidity rate, positive cows were slaughtered or sold. In herds with a high morbidity rate, the infected cows were isolated in groups on the farm. As no control system was established on the regional or national level, infected cows were traded freely and continued to serve as a source of infection.

Every year the number of inspected dairy herds increased; in response to the diagnosis of the agglutination test and the isolation of the positive cows, the number of herds free of brucellosis rose significantly. Table 27-1 summarizes the operation of the "test and eliminate" eradication program in dairy herds from 1931 to 1947.

All of the isolates of the disease were that of *B. abortus*. In 1939, however, *B. melitensis* was first identified in a dairy cow, and in 1945 *B. melitensis* was again isolated from 19 dairy cows in two herds that had come into contact with infected sheep.

In 1947, the first vaccination attempt was made using Strain 19 vaccine, produced by the Central Veterinary Laboratory at Weybridge, U.K.

The history of the disease up to 1970 was summarized as follows.[5-8]

At the time of the declaration of the State of Israel (1948), the dairy cattle population consisted of about 20,000 head in agricultural settlements and about 6,000 in urban herds located near the big cities. Virtually all rural herds were free of brucellosis. The urban herds were heavily infected; 43% of these herds and 25% of the cattle had positive reactions to the agglutination test. Over 14,000 dairy cows and heifers were imported from the U.S.A. and Europe and were distributed to new and old settlements. Some of the imported cattle were found to be infected by *B. abortus* and reintroduced the infection into many free herds. A wave of abortions among dairy cattle caused heavy losses. All the dairy cattle, calves and adults in both rural and urban herds, had been vaccinated with S19. The incidence of abortion decreased from year to year.

Beef cattle imported from Turkey (1956) introduced the infection into many beef herds, and a second wave of abortions took place. Vaccination of beef herds with S19 suppressed the clinical disease. By order of the Minister of Agriculture (1960), all urban cattle were slaughtered and the owners were compensated. The main source of infection in Israel was thereby eliminated.

The epizootology and control of brucellosis practiced in Israel differ according to the type of cattle reared:

1. Dairy cattle of the Israeli Friesian breed are kept in closed and isolated confinement.

Table 27-1. Bovine Brucellosis Control 1931-1946 "Test and Isolate" Scheme - Dairy Cattle

Year	No. Settlements control	No. Cows control	No. Tests	No. Infected settlements	No. Positive tests	No. Settlements infected unit
1931	35	2,883	29,724	11	682	—
1933	54	3,302	19,991	20	422	—
1934	64	4,817	20,461	22	160	—
1935	89	6,426	26,362	12	142	—
1936	109	8,116	28,705	17	216	—
1937	125	8,295	34,000	21	195	—
1938	137	8,546	29,200	28	127	—
1939	135	8,828	40,168	11	120	10
1940	143	10,390	46,460	13	159	10
1941	150	12,357	48,535	7	49	8
1942	165	13,647	49,268	13	72	5
1943	173	15,436	49,836	14	104	5
1944	193	16,309	39,602	11	110	3
1945	201	16,984	44,116	18	53	4
1946	209	19,276	47,051	13	73	2

2. Beef cattle of different European breeds are kept on natural pasture with supplementary food when necessary.

3. Baladi cattle, originally an indigenous breed, are kept on natural pasture under semi-nomadic conditions.

In 1961, an "eradication scheme" was set up, based on the "test and slaughter" policy. Adult vaccination was discontinued. Vaccination with S19 was limited to 2 to 6 month old dairy and beef calves. Rules concerning the eradication of bovine brucellosis by virtue of the Animal Disease Ordinance of 1945 were issued by the Minister of Agriculture. The ordinance called for notification of the disease, detection, isolation and slaughter of infected animals, the declaration of an infected farm or settlement, the issue of compensation, vaccination, and disinfection.

The "test and slaughter" program among dairy cattle is based on the milk ring test run routinely on tank milk 2 to 4 times per year. In the case of a positive reaction, the test is repeated on the bulk milk of groups of cows. Cows in the positive groups are serologically tested using the serum agglutination test, the Rose Bengal test, and the complement fixation test. A bacteriological examination of the milk and organs of slaughtered animals is performed for epidemiological purposes.

Much effort was put into testing the blood of entire herds of beef and Baladi cattle. An average of 13,150 sera were tested annually during 15 years of an intensive eradication program (1970-1988), with an annual average of 85 slaughtered cattle compensated by the government.

Serious problems were encountered regarding the indigenous Baladi breed which lived under semi-nomadic conditions. A disease incidence rate exceeding 30% resulted in the slaughter of entire herds with full compensation to the owners.

The first confirmed outbreak of brucellosis in small ruminants occurred in 1953 in a flock of sheep imported from Turkey.[3] It is assumed that a few foci of the disease had existed prior to the import from Turkey. Extensive types of sheep and goats, particularly the migratory flocks, were involved. In 1957, 38.5% of the flocks had varying proportions of reactors.

In 1969, the Veterinary Services vaccinated young and adult ewes with Rev. 1 vaccine. Since 1980, due to several cases of abortions in vaccinated ewes, only females up to the age of 6 months have been vaccinated.

Eradication of the brucellosis disease in sheep by employing the "test and slaughter" policy has not been possible for economic reasons. Given the risk of reinfection from nomadic Baladi cattle and sheep flocks, the Veterinary Services continues to vaccinate heifer calves with S19.

The campaign against bovine brucellosis in Israel during the past 19 years (1970-1988) is summarized in Table 27-2. During the years 1970 to 1972, the number of infected settlements decreased. Brucellosis was virtually eradicated from all dairy herds. An increase in prevalence was again recorded from 1973 to 1980, especially among beef and Baladi cattle. During the years 1983 to 1987, all dairy herds were free of brucellosis. In

Table 27-2. Bovine Brucellosis Eradication 1970-1988

Year	Infected settlements				Isolates				Serol. diagnosis	Slaughtered	Vaccinated	Blood tests	Milk ring test
	Total	Dairy cattle	Beef cattle	Local cattle	Abortus Settl.	Abortus Isol.	Melitensis Settl.	Melitensis Isol.					
1970	3	1	–	2	1	3	2	4	–	35	31,478	9,972	–
1971	6	2	–	4	6	7	–	–	–	25	31,704	10,949	15,900
1972	8	1	3	4	8	22	–	–	–	22	39,312	12,076	15,800
1973	26	2	3	21	1	7	2	13	23	165	43,765	10,570	11,300
1974	26	4	3	19	4	15	2	13	20	152	47,063	13,358	13,600
1975	29	3	7	19	10	18	3	5	–	–	52,107	15,873	12,300
1976	40	14	8	18	14	18	8	13	18	258	47,568	19,868	14,001
1977	23		2	20	4	6	4	9	15	82	49,638	18,468	18,492
1978	23	6	4	13	8	8	3	3	12	95	49,612	14,316	18,594
1979	20	5	4	11	1	1	4	11	15	91	47,244	12,475	10,764
1980	20	1	9	10	4	5	5	6	11	103	48,896	12,498	7,356
1981	10	2	2	6	4	11	–	–	6	64	48,699	10,443	3,966
1982	12	2	6	4	1	1	2	2	9	20	48,331	12,752	3,865
1983	18		11	7	3	4	3	3	12	50	51,933	11,802	4,124
1984	5		1	4	1	1	–	1	4	24	56,146	10,782	3,411
1985	4			4	–	–	1	1	3	27	55,200	5,479	3,256
1986	1			1	–	–	1	1	1	13	52,219	4,531	3,413
1987	1			1	–	–	2	2	2	11	55,488	2,478	2,214
1988	1	1		–	–	–	1	9	–	21	58,962	4,111	2,511

Table 27-3. Annual Prevalence Rate of Brucellosis-Infected Herds 1970-1988

Years	Total	Dairy	Beef	Baladi
1970-1972	0.20%	0.08%	0.5%	0.4%
1973-1980	1.00%	0.30%	3.0%	2.4%
1981-1982	0.40%	0.10%	2.0%	0.6%
1983-1987	0.20%	0.00	1.2%	0.4%
1988	0.04%	0.06%	0.0%	0.0%

1988, one dairy herd was found infected by *B. melitensis*. Since 1985, no case of brucellosis among beef cattle was recorded. In the last three years, only two foci were found in Baladi herds, all caused by *B. melitensis*.

Table 27-3 summarizes the annual prevalence rate of brucellosis-infected herds among the different cattle breeds.

During the years 1970 to 1988, 205 cultures of *Brucella* spp were isolated from cattle at the Kimron Veterinary Institute. These cultures are listed in Table 27-4.

Protection of Bovine Brucellosis-Free Areas

In order to protect brucellosis-free herds and areas from reinfection, the potential sources of infection must be taken into consideration. Sources of reinfection may include the following:

1. Serologically negative, latent carriers of *Brucella* in herds free of the disease and under permanent inspection, which may become carriers at a later stage and excrete the organisms[10]

2. Heifer calves born to serologically positive dams or infected by contaminated milk who carry the latent disease until its appearance during puberty. This was reported to occur among 2.52% of such calves[11]

3. *B. abortus* in other animals, particularly in wild animals such as bison, elk, deer, coyotes, wild opossums, raccoons, and moose[12]

4. *B. abortus* in other farm animals such as sheep,[13] goat, pigs, camels, buffalo, dogs,[14] and horses

5. Other types of *Brucella* such as *B. melitensis* in sheep[15,16] and goats and *B. suis* in pigs

6. Strain 19 *Brucella* from a vaccinal source

7. Incidence of the disease among animals in neighboring countries;

8. Import of infected animals

9. Use of contaminated animal by-products for feedstuffs, particularly milk products

Table 27-4. *Brucella* spp. Cultures 1970-1988, Kimron Veterinary
Institute

	Isolates	*B. abortus*	*B. melitensis*
Dairy cattle	54	11 (20%)	43 (80%)
Beef cattle	27	22 (82%)	5 (18%)
Baladi cattle	124	88 (71%)	36 (29%)
TOTAL	205	121 (59%)	84 (41%)

To prevent reinfection of free areas, an effective monitoring system
must be set up and maintained, providing control over all the animals in
the country or region, with specific attention to nomadic cattle herds and
sheep flocks. Such a system was established in Israel to direct those vital
operations necessary for the control, diagnosis, prevention, and eradication of infectious diseases. It is based upon specific rules and orders
promulgated by the Minister of Agriculture.

Registering and Marking of Cattle

The "Registration, Ear-tagging and Transportation of Cattle" Rule
requires that every bovine from age 6 months must be officially ear-tagged
and registered. A state identity card for each bovine assigns a computerized number which matches the ear tag number. Listed on the card is all
vital information regarding the animal's identity, details and health status,
S19 vaccination, and other obligatory vaccinations. A non-obligatory
freeze-brand may also be applied to dairy cows; this marking consists of a
four-digit number, usually corresponding with the last four digits on the
state ear tag. If a herd or animal is placed under quarantine, the identity
card(s) is withdrawn and kept in the District Veterinary Office until the
termination of the quarantine period. The identity card is returned to the
Veterinary Services after the death or slaughter of the animal. The
registration and marking system enables individual monitoring of every
bovine in all of the nation's herds.

Movement Control

Any movement of the animals, either for breeding or slaughter purposes, and any change of ownership, must be approved by a veterinary
officer. This permit is entered on the identity card which must accompany
the animal throughout its life. A surveillance system is set up on the roads
to check identity cards and permits of transported animals.

Regulatory Procedures against Infectious Diseases

The Veterinary Services authorities must carry out all measures for diagnosing, preventing, and eradicating all notifiable diseases as required by the Animal Disease Ordinance; likewise, the animal owners are required to carry out the instructions issued. All operations required by law are carried out by the State Veterinary Services, including veterinarians and stock inspectors under the authority of regional veterinary offices across the country. Every operation is recorded and reported periodically to the managing board of the Veterinary Services. Israel's clinical Veterinary Service is run by the "Hahaklait" Cooperative Farmers Society for Livestock Insurance and Clinical Veterinary Service. Medical aid is offered through regular weekly visits and emergency calls to care for sick animals. Clinical veterinarians are required to report to the Veterinary Services all notifiable diseases. A central laboratory, Kimron Veterinary Institute (K.V.I.), is maintained by the Department of Agriculture to carry out all tests for notifiable and other diseases. The department for brucellosis also serves as a national reference laboratory for the Ministry of Health and for hospitals.

Regular Surveillance System for Brucellosis
Dairy cattle

The testing of pooled fresh milk four times a year using the milk ring test procedures allows for effective supervision and early detection of infection among the herd. In the case of a positive reaction in the tank milk, the bulk milk of groups of 10 cows is tested. In a group found positive, each individual cow must be tested serologically using the three accepted methods: the Rose Bengal test, the agglutination test, and the complement fixation test.

The limitation of this method is that the infected milk is diluted in large amounts of milk pooled from large dairy herds. A satisfactory solution has been found by adding milk fat to the tested milk and by determining the amount of tested milk according to the number of cows in the herd. During 1982, one positive cow which had excreted *B. melitensis* organisms in her milk was found from among the 300 milking cows in the herd. The milk ring test is effective in cattle in diagnosing every species of *Brucella*. It is important to note that this method is not sufficiently satisfactory for the individual diagnosis of an infected cow. A cow at the stage of secreting *Brucella* organisms in her milk will certainly be a positive reactor, as opposed to an infected cow who does not secrete those organisms at that stage. During an outbreak of *B. melitensis* in a large dairy herd in 1988, positive cows were found in a serological test after the diagnosis of the milk ring test had shown negative. In smaller family milk herds, two samples are tested annually.

Beef Cattle

Serological tests are run on herds once every five years. Herds that have had recently been declared disease-free are tested more frequently, particularly local Baladi breed beef cattle, both nomadic and semi-nomadic. For this purpose, the Veterinary Services have set up regional cattle pens in pasture areas. Blood samples of beef cattle drawn in slaughter houses are sent to the laboratory for serological testing. Fetuses, placenta, and sera from cows that have aborted are also taken for laboratory testing, particularly during waves of abortion. In artificial insemination centers, bull calves are tested serologically at an isolation station, and twice a year as adult bulls at the station itself.

Special attention is paid to single cows that test positive in the serological tests. These cows may be experiencing a cross-reaction with occasional microorganisms or other bacteria such as *Yersinia* spp., *Vibrio* spp., *Salmonella* spp., or E. coli, as in the case of mastitis,[17] or they may be experiencing a positive reaction to the S19 vaccine (particularly up until one year after the vaccination). A unique phenomenon among dairy heifers is the reaction to S19 which may localize in the joints causing arthritis, giving a positive serological reading. At the K.V.I., *Brucella* S19 was isolated from the synovial fluids taken in a case of gonitis. Among all the methods for differential diagnosis developed recently, the most effective is still the complement fixation test.[18] Isolation of reactors and repeated testing within 2 to 4 weeks offer the most reliable information. Singleton and other persistent reactors must be slaughtered, and their organs must be tested bacteriologically after slaughter.

Sheep

One of the most difficult problems relating to the policies for protecting cattle in free zones from brucellosis, is the presence of *B. melitensis* among sheep. Cattle are sensitive to *B. melitensis*; from 1970 to 1988, 205 *Brucella* spp. were isolated in Israel, of which 41% were *B. melitensis* and 59% were *B. abortus*. Sheep were diagnosed following abortions, screening tests, and incidence of the disease in man using serological and bacteriological methods that identified the biotypes of bacteria for epidemiological follow-up. To prevent direct contamination, the infected sheep flocks were quarantined and iron-branded, and cattle that came into contact with them were tested.

Vaccination

According to the International Zoo-Sanitary Code, when the brucellosis infection rate in a country or region is reduced to under 0.2% of all cattle and to under 1% of all herds, the country or region respectively, is designated as a brucellosis-free zone. At this stage, vaccination of calves with S19 is discontinued to prevent post-vaccinal serological reactions; the region may then be certified with the "officially bovine brucellosis-free" status. The success of the eradication program among cattle in Israel should have permitted, in fact, the cessation of vaccination. However, given the presence of B. melitensis among small ruminants, it was decided to continue the vaccination policy for all cattle, including dairy cattle, and not exclusively for cattle that come into contact with sheep. Approximately 65 to 75% of all vaccinated cattle are generally resistant to exposure, while the remaining 25 to 35% may become infected[19] but generally do not abort,[20] thus reducing the danger of infection. Following experimental challenge of vaccinated cattle, 25% of the cows became infected. Yet, vaccinated animals continually exposed to reinfection may, in time, became infected and act as carriers of the germ, without actually showing clinical evidence of the disease. Under conditions of field exposure, vaccination offers immunity against abortion for five or more subsequent lactations.

When breakdowns occur, they are primarily due to excessive exposure to Brucella, usually at an advanced age, and not to the enhanced virulence of the organism.[21] There is insufficient evidence regarding cross-immunity between the various spp. of Brucella. There is information regarding the vaccination of sheep in the U.S.S.R. with S19 vaccine against B. melitensis, as well as the vaccination of lambs with Rev. 1 vaccine against B. ovis.[22] The accepted assumptions and experience with field outbreaks of B. melitensis prove that the B. abortus S19 vaccine may render adequate protection against B. melitensis as well. During the first stage of a recent outbreak of the disease in a dairy herd, more non-vaccinated cows (24.1%) became infected than did vaccinated cows (8.3%); at a later stage of the outbreak, more adult cows (20%) became infected than did younger cows (7%) (see Tables 27-6 and 27-7). Today, all calves are vaccinated at 2 to 6 months with S19 in all bovines including the Baladi herds; this program will continue until the brucellosis eradication program among sheep is completed. At the same time, an intensive vaccination program of 2-to 7-month-old female lambs and kids with Rev. 1 vaccine is being carried out, in order to decrease the number of aborting ewes, thus preventing the source of direct contamination of cattle. Every vaccinated animal is marked by the piercing of its ear, and it may thus be identified for a number of years.

Preventing Contamination from Other Sources

Purchase of Animals for Breeding Purposes
Transport permits issued by the Veterinary Officer, based on information regarding the animals' health status at their farm of origin, prevent reintroduction of the disease into free herds. The purchase of sheep is also conditional on a screening test of the flock (10%) and evidence that the sheep have been vaccinated (a pierced ear). It is understood that as long as the sheep are diseased, the transmission of the disease by sheep can not be effectively controlled.

Other Domestic Animals
In farms that tested positive or were suspected to be positive during the eradication program and the surveillance follow-up, the domestic animals were tested as well. Surveys indicated that dogs, horses, animals in zoological gardens, camels, pigs and others (excluding cattle, sheep and goats) tested negative for both *B. abortus* and *B. melitensis*.

Wild Animals
There is a law in Israel which protects wild animals; the law forbids hunting protected wild animals and determines which animals may be hunted, in which areas and during which seasons. The most prevalent wild ruminants in Israel are the gazelle and the ibex. It is feasible that infected animals which abort may contaminate the pasture or grass harvested for feed. In 1982 *B. melitensis* was diagnosed in one cow in a large dairy farm; it was suspected that the alfalfa supplied to the housed dairy cows had been infected by a gazelle. That same year, 98 gazelles underwent serological screening; three reacted positively to the Rose Bengal test, one was suspected-positive in the agglutination test and all responded negatively to the CFT. Surveys such as these continue among animals tested after hunting.

Imported Animals
All imports of sheep and cattle are liable to certification by local state authorities that they have come from brucellosis-free farms and that they have been negatively tested. Upon arrival in Israel, the animals are quarantined and serologically tested again. It is important to consider that many countries do not vaccinate calves against brucellosis. The importing of non-vaccinated bovines may expose them to infection by *B. melitensis* in Israel.

Infected Animals in Neighboring Countries
Neighboring countries in the Middle East have reported the presence

of brucellosis among sheep, goats and cattle in their area, and these may serve as a source of infection and renewed outbreak of the disease among sheep, goats and cattle in Israel. Israel's borders are protected by a security fence which prevents direct contact with animals in the neighboring countries. The movement of animals from the controlled territories into Israel proper is forbidden.

Nutritional Management as a Source of Reinfection by *Brucella*

With the reduced profitability of the agricultural farm, many efforts have been made to make use of industrial by-products for animal feedstuffs so as to lower production costs. One of the most common feedstuffs products for dairy cattle is whey processed in industrial dairies. These plants generally make use of sophisticated equipment with excellent modern pasteurization systems. The major danger may be found in the smaller, non-supervised plants and in occasional breakdowns in the larger plants. As long as brucellosis exists in dairy sheep, the potential danger of contamination exists as well. The greatest danger is that of *per os* contamination, by consumption of food which contains large numbers of bacteria.

Many animals could be infected simultaneously despite the fact that the cattle were vaccinated with S19. The outbreaks of *B. melitensis* among cattle in Israel were mostly sporadic, with a low incidence of disease; they occurred following contact with infected sheep. In 1976 an outbreak of *B. melitensis* was reported in a 300-cow dairy herd which had received whey from a nearby dairy plant. Thirty-seven dairy cows were ordered slaughtered and were compensated by the state. Six dairy farmers who drank unpasteurized milk from the milk tank became ill.[23] In 1988 there was a serious outbreak of *B. melitensis* at another dairy farm with 300 milking cows.

Given the importance of this subject in the context of protecting free zones from brucellosis, the following description of the last mentioned outbreak of brucellosis in a dairy herd is presented.

An Outbreak of *Brucella melitensis* in a Dairy Cattle Herd

The B.H. farm in northern Israel had a dairy herd consisting of 300 cows, 132 heifers, 197 heifer calves and 80 bull calves for a total of 709 head in the herd. The average yearly milk yield was 9000 kilogram per dairy cow in 1987 and 1988 . Heifer calves were vaccinated at the age of 2 to 6 months with S19 vaccine. All vaccinations were recorded on the calves' identity cards.

In December 1987, 75 beef cows were purchased from Germany; these imports were non-vaccinated Simmental cows born in 1985. The cows were retained in a closed group close to the dairy farm. These cows had been serologically tested for brucellosis twice in Germany prior to their export, and again in December 1987 at the quarantine station in Israel. All tests were negative.

The milk ring test was routinely run on tank milk three times a year. In 1988, the milk was tested on January 5 and on May 24. All tests were negative. On November 2, 1988, the third test of the tank milk was run and was found positive. Following this positive test, a group milk test was taken. All the cows in the positive groups were tested serologically in the laboratory using three methods - the RBT, the SAT, and the CF. Following three consecutive weekly MRT, 124 cows were serologically tested, 16 of which were found positive and immediately slaughtered.

At the same time, 285 dry cows and calves were tested serologically. Two calves born in 1987, one of which had not been vaccinated, were found positive and slaughtered. The 75 Simmental cows were tested serologically as well, and one was found positive. An EDTA seroagglutination test[24] was carried out in the laboratory to verify the specificity of the test, and the final diagnosis of brucellosis was confirmed. Milk samples were tested bacteriologically; large numbers of the *B. melitensis* biotype 3 organism were isolated. In a number of the tested and slaughtered cows, *Brucella* was isolated in the retropharyngal lymph nodes, the udders and the mammary glands. The subsequent surveillance for detection of infected cows included the following tests: a weekly MRT test of all milk cows in the herd, a monthly serological test using the three testing methods on all cattle head in the herd, and starting from January a weekly serological test of the high risk groups of cows around parturition. Table 27-5 summarizes the incidence of the disease in the herd.

Epidemiology

Period of Infection

Contamination occurred during 1988, following the serological test of the beef cattle (December 1987), and following the last negative milk test (24.5.88). Antibodies appeared in the blood 1 to 3 months after infection in accordance with the pregnancy status of the cow. The estimated time of infection was some 3-5 months before the disease was discovered. The high level of titer, 1:640 - 1:2560, found in 9 of the 11 cows first diagnosed by SAT (Table 27-8) as well as the particularly high level of bacteria isolated in the milk support this assumption.

Table 27-5. *Brucella melitensis* on the B.H. Farm

	No. head	Not vaccinated	Slaughtered		Aborted	
			No. head	Not-vaccinated	No. head	Serolog. positive
Cows	300	8	36	5	17	6
Pregnant heifers	71	2	3	-	-	-
Inseminated heifers	61	2	2	1	-	-
Vaccinated calves	104	-	-	-	-	-
Non-vaccin. calves	93	93	-	-	-	-
Bull calves	80	80	-	-	-	-
Simmental	75	75	30	30	-	2
Total	784					

Source of Infection

The following possibilities were tested:
The Farm's Purchase of Animals - Dairy heifer calves, the Simmental cows and 2 beef bulls were acquired during 1987 and 1988. They were all tested as was the farm of origin, and were found negative.

Contact with Sheep and Goats in Neighboring Pastures - The dairy herd is a closed unit that remains in contained yards and does not graze.

Infection by Contaminated Feed - The feed ration in a dairy herd includes 4 major components: silage, concentrates, hay, and whey. Silage and hay are made of corn, legume, and cereals. The possibility was tested that the grass was contaminated by infected sheep and goats in pasture. The ambiental conditions (summer temperature), germ resistance, the technology involved in preparing the silage, and the epidemiology of the infection do not support this theory. The food concentrates are composed primarily of grains and protein from an external source common to many farms. The quantity of whey consumed daily at the farm is 25,000 liters. An adult cow drinks 30 to 40 liter daily. Whey is produced primarily from the cheese of dairy cattle, but also from the cheese of dairy sheep and goats. A pipeline system carries the whey to drinking basins in each of the yards. Every animal receives whey in its ration. The simultaneous and massive outbreak of the disease, 23 cows in two months, in a flock which is generally vaccinated, necessarily indicates the presence of a high bacterial level. It is plausible that the source of this contamination was in sheep and goat whey, a particular shipment of which was not properly pasteurized, due to some technical failure. A bacteriological examination of the whey in the tank and in the pipeline after discovery of the disease was negative. Six additional dairy herds in the region which received whey from the same source, were tested a number of times after the outbreak and were found negative.

The Vaccination Situation

The farm's calves are vaccinated with S19 4 times a year at the age of 2 to 6 months. Nevertheless, it was found that due to technical difficulties, eight dairy cows had not been vaccinated during the period prior to the outbreak. Of the first 18 cows to be infected, five (27.7%) were found to be non-vaccinated. Together with the Simmental cows and heifers, there were 87 non-vaccinated cows in the herd at the onset of the outbreak. Of the non-vaccinated cows, 41.4% were found serologically positive, while only 8.3% of the vaccinated cows were positive (Table 27-6). It is accepted that 65 to 75% of the vaccinated animals are resistant to infection.[19] The remaining 25 to 35% of vaccinated animals may become infected but

Table 27-6. Incidence of Slaughter and Abortions among Vaccinated and Non-Vaccinated Cows - B.H.

	No. cows	Infected No.	Slaughtered %	Infected aborted No.	Infected aborted %	% out of infected
Non-vaccinated (includ. 75 Simmental)	87	36	41.4	4 2 (Sim.)	4.6	19
Vaccinated	419	35	8.3	4	0.9	11.4
TOTAL	506	71	11.5	8	1.6	22.2

usually do not abort, and the risk of horizontal infection is low.[20] Under field conditions, vaccination with S19 offers immunity and prevents abortion for a period of 4 to 5 lactations.[21]

The incidence rate among adult cows (5 to 8 years old) was 20%, as compared with 7% among the younger cows (Table 27-7).

Abortions

During 1988 17 cows in the herd (5.6%) aborted. The average abortion rate in the region's herds is 4.4%. Eight of the cows (of which two were Simmental) that aborted were found to be serologically positive.

From Table 27-6 it is evident that the percentage of positive aborting animals among those not vaccinated was 4.6%, as compared to 0.9% among those vaccinated. *B. melitensis* was isolated from the aborted fetuses and lymph nodes of three cows, two of which were non-vaccinated Simmental and one of which was a 5-year-old vaccinated Israeli dairy cow. *B. abortus* in exposed cattle causes a high abortion rate, followed by massive horizontal infection and high infection rate. In contrast, it is acceptable to believe that *B. melitensis* does not cause a high rate of abortions among cattle, and therefore the spread of the disease and the morbidity rate in the herd are low. As stated previously, vaccination of calves lowers the risk of abortion.

Course of the Disease

The initial source of infection in the flock was particularly massive. Sensitive cows, primarily those not vaccinated that had been exposed to a high level of bacteria, were infected by the disease. It is plausible that infection was spread *per os* by very contaminated sheep whey - in a one-time occurrence. During the first stage of the outbreak, 82% of the infected cows were concentrated in two adjacent groups: C and E (see Table 27-9). The explanation for this may lie in the large quantity of whey that these groups received as they were situated close to the whey tank (gravitational flow) and the large quantity of whey that these cows tend to drink in general - 40 liters per day.

The serological reaction in cows 4 to 6 months pregnant may appear four weeks after infection, as opposed to 10 weeks later in non-pregnant cows or cows in the early stages of pregnancy (up to 2 months). From these factors it may be assumed that all cows slaughtered in November and December, and some of those slaughtered in January, were infected from the initial source of infection by food.

It may be suspected that the organism remained in the whey pipeline in a caseous precipitate with the proper pH. The system was washed and disinfected with a chlorine solution following the outbreak.

Table 27-7. Infected Dairy Cows According to Age Groups - B.H.

Year of birth	No. of cows	% of herd	Positive slaughtered	% of all cows	% of infected
1981-1984	115	38.3	23	20	64
1985	185	61.7	13	7	36
Total	300	100	36	12	100

In January 1989, two Simmental cows aborted in the dairy farm's parturient pen, group B (Table 27-9), and *B. melitensis* was isolated in their aborted fetuses. These cows constituted a secondary source of infection on the farm. From this period on, the main occurrence was among groups of dry and parturient cows. Simmental cows were also infected from the primary source, but at a much lower rate of infection. The highest infection rate in this group was in January. This group was isolated and removed from the dairy herd.

In February and March 1989, 27 Simmental cows parturated. During that period, 21 cows serologically seroconverted from negative to positive within three weeks and were slaughtered. The incidence in this group reached the rate of 40% (Table 27-5). Yet 28 cows were at the pre-calving stage. The prognosis for the Simmental cows was extremely poor, and the potential risk for the dairy cattle was high. It was therefore decided to slaughter all the remaining Simmental cows and calves.

The B.H. dairy cattle herd is still being treated, and the results are as yet unclear. Only after the outbreak has completely passed, will it be possible to properly evaluate all the factors involved and to reach the appropriate conclusions regarding policies for protecting brucellosis-free herds and areas from reinfection.

SUMMARY

In summary, bovine brucellosis has been eradicated in Israel. The history of the disease and the evolution of modes of control are described. The eradication scheme in Israel was based on the "test and slaughter" system together with a vaccination program.

The protection of brucellosis-free areas is the key to a successful control program. Knowledge of the potential sources of infection is indispensable for the selection of the appropriate measures for preventing reinfection. Given the importance of this event, it is described here in detail.

Table 27-8. Agglutination Titers of Infected Cows - B.H.

Month	No. slaughtered	Titers								
		1:2560	1:1280	1:640	1:320	1:160	1:80	1:40		
November 1988	11	5	2	2	-	2	-	-		
December 1988	12	1	1	1	-	-	5	4		
January 1989	20	-	-	-	1	8	3	8		
February 1989	6	-	-	-	-	-	4	2		
March 1989	8	-	-	-	-	-	6	2		
April 1989	14	-	-	-	-	-	12	2		

Table 27-9. Slaughtered cows according to month and location - B. H.

Month	No. culled	Group A	Group B	Group C	Group D	Group E	Group F	Heifers insemin.	Heifers pregnant	Simmental
Nov.	11	-	-	3	-	6	-	-	1	1
Dec.	12	-	-	2	3	3	2	1	1	-
Jan.	20	4	2(Sim)*	2	2	2	1	1	-	8
Feb.	6	-	1*	-	-	-	1	-	1	3
March	8	-	2	1	-	-	-	-	-	4
April	14	-	-	-	-	-	-	-	-	14

* Aborted

References

1. Animal Health Yearbook 1987.
2. Fensterbank. Brucellosis in cattle, sheep and goats. *Technical Series* No. 6, 1987: 9-35.
3. Gur S. Bovine contagious abortion (brucellosis) in Palestine. *Refuah Veterinarith* 1949;6:45.
4. Smith JM. Dept. of Agric. & Fisheries, Vet. Service. *Annual Report* 1927-1930.
5. Dafni I. Problems of bovine brucellosis control in Israel. *Refuah Veterinarith* 1961;18:89-92.
6. Dafni I. Bovine brucellosis. *Refuah Veterinarith,* Special Jubille Issue 1972:18-29.
7. Feinhaken D, Dafni I. Identification of *Brucella* isolates in Israel 1970-1979. *Refuah Veterinarith* 1980;37:117-121.
8. Shimshony A. Activities of the Israeli Veterinary Servies 1973-1982. *Refuah Veterinarith* 1983;40:161-164.
9. Landau M. Brucellosis of sheep and goats in Israel. *Bull Off Int Epiz* 1974;82:61-68.
10. Kellar J, Maria R, Martin W. Brucellosis in Ontario: A case control study. *Can J Comp Med* 1976;40:119-128.
11. Wilesmith JW. The persistence of *Brucella abortus* infection in calves. *Veterinary Record* 1978;103:149-153.
12. Blood DL, Radostits OM, Henderson, JA. Brucellosis caused by *Br. abortus, Veterinary Medicine,* Bailliere Tindall, 1985;605-615.
13. Luchsinger DW, Anderson K. Longitudinal studies of naturally acquired *Br. abortus* in sheep. *Am J Vet Res* 1979; 40:1307-1312.
14. Prior MG. Isolation of *Br. abortus* from two dogs. *Can J Comp Med* 1976;40:117-118.
15. Hemashettan BM. Isolation of *Br. melitensis* from a cow. *Indian Vet J* 1987;64:822-825.
16. Mustafa AA, Corbel, MJ. An epidemiological association between ovine-caprine and bovine brucellosis in Libya. *Bull Anim Prod Afri* 1988;36:93-94.
17. Dukes TW, Nielsen K, Eagleson M, Speckmann G, Corner A. Etiology of *Br. abortus* Singleton reactors, *Can J Comp Med* 1980;44:366-373.
18. Crawford RP, Adams LG, Childers A.B. Value of serologic reactions following Strain 19 vaccination. *Preventive Veterinary Medicine* 1988;5:275-280.
19. National Research Council. Brucellosis research: An evaluation. Washington, D.C. *National Academy of Science* 1977.
20. Afshar A. Bovine abortion. *Veterinary Bulletin* 1965;35:673-677.
21. Crawford RP, Adams G, Richardson B. Correlation of field strain exposure in beef herds vaccinated with Strain 19. *J Am Vet Med Assoc* 1988;192:1550-1552.
22. Blasco JM. Immunization with *Br. melitensis* against *Br. ovis* infection in rams. *Vet Microb* 1987;14:381-392.
23. Dafni I. *Br. melitensis* in dairy herd. *Veterinary Symposium* 1980, The Hebrew University, Rehovot.
24. Garin B, Trap D, Gaumont R. Assessment of the EDTA sero-agglutination test. *Veterinary Record* 1985;117:444-445.

Rapid and Accurate Detection of
Brucellosis in Infected Areas

Hugh E. Metcalf

In 1920, Pennsylvania began a voluntary testing program for brucellosis in cattle.[1] Participation in the program was strictly voluntary but the program became the basis of the current Brucellosis Certified Free Herd program in the United States, which is still voluntary.

By 1934 15 states had voluntary state plans for herd certification: Delaware, Illinois, Indiana, Maryland, Massachusetts, New Hampshire, New York, Ohio, Oklahoma, Rhode Island, Texas, Virginia, West Virginia, Wisconsin, and Wyoming.[2] Wisconsin used demonstration herds in counties to encourage cattlemen to have their herds blood tested and become certified free. Wisconsin's demonstration program started in 1928 with 8 to 10 demonstration herds and by 1934 there had been 70 demonstration herds in the state.[3]

In 1934, the LaFollette amendment to the Jones-Connally bill for the relief of the cattle industry, including the reduction of the cattle population, provided for testing and payment of indemnity for cattle that were reactors to a brucellosis test. Participation in the plan was voluntary but between July 1 and November 1, 1934, blood tests had been completed in over 12,000 herds with 900,000 herds on the waiting list to be tested. Almost 50% of those herds tested were infected.[4]

The 1933-1934 Virginia legislature passed laws requiring compulsory testing of cattle, compulsory slaughter of reactors, and payment of indemnity. Virginia started a county testing program in June 1935 in one county. In 1936 a quarantine was placed on all counties in the state in which the cattle had not been tested.[5] This was the first use of a systematic active surveillance procedure for brucellosis in the United States. In 1935 Oregon also passed a compulsory Bang's Disease Test Law that became effective January 1, 1937.[6]

In 1923, the South Carolina Guernsey Breeders Association would not allow animals to be placed in sale unless they tested negative for brucellosis. This was the first known use of a market testing requirement in the United States for brucellosis. The state of South Carolina adopted regulations in 1924 requiring cattle sold in that state to be tested for brucellosis. If they were positive they would be quarantined to the premises or sold to slaughter.[7] By 1934, 33 states required a negative agglutination test on cattle entering the state.[8]

Surveillance Methods and Procedures

Surveillance for disease may be either *active* or *passive.* Passive surveillance occurs when the investigator does not initiate the investigation. It is based upon some action related to the disease condition which is initiated by the herd owner or someone else besides the primary investigator. Active surveillance occurs when the investigator takes some positive action to find the affected individual or herd. The herd owner of the affected individual may or may not take any action because of the disease until contacted by the investigator.'

Most procedures are not purely active or passive but represent a mixture of each. For instance, a herd owner may report to his veterinarian that he has had an abortion in his herd and thinks he may have brucellosis. As far as the investigator (the state or federal animal health official) is concerned this is strictly a passive action. But if the owner was made aware of the condition of brucellosis because of an active public information campaign on the disease conducted by the investigator then this would have both passive and active actions involved.

Passive Surveillance Methods

Culling a cow because she is old or doesn't have a calf is not sufficient to be considered a specific action by a herd owner. Reporting an abortion to a private veterinarian or state or federal official would be considered a positive action by the owner.

Voluntary participation in a program is generally considered a passive surveillance procedure. The cooperative State-Federal Brucellosis Control Program from 1934 to 1954 was primarily a voluntary program. Owners participated in the program voluntarily with some incentive provided by the state and federal government, such as free cattle testing and indemnity payments to owners for prompt removal of any reactors found. Voluntary participation with incentives is effective in reducing the prevalence of the disease when prevalence is high, as demonstrated by the change in percent of reactors found in the United States from fiscal year 1935 through fiscal year 1940.

Rate for Brucellosis in the United States from
1934 through 1940 Under Voluntary Control Program

Fiscal year	Cattle tested	Number	Reactors percent
1935	3,317,860	381,010	11.5
1936	6,674,709	457,104	6.8

1937	8,021,167	397,864	5.0
1938	7,837,443	324,532	4.1
1939	7,591,398	219,165	2.9
1940	6,937,428	171,953	2.5

Voluntary area participation was used widely in the early area accreditation (certification) plans. It was usually done as the result of a countywide petition or vote of all cattlemen in the county. If the required number or percentage of cattlemen approved the area test then it became mandatory for all the rest of the cattle owners in the county to have their herds tested.

In 1947, the United States Livestock Sanitary Association (USLSA) recommended standard provisions for complete testing of any county when 65% of the owners holding at least 51% of the cattle in the county have voluntarily placed their herds under a voluntary herd plan.[10] This was modified in 1948 to state that when 75% or more of the livestock owners holding 95% or more of the cattle in a given area sign up under any one of a combination of four plans, the livestock sanitary official may require the remaining livestock owners to individually select and participate under one of the four plans.[11] By 1948, 41 states and Puerto Rico had signed memorandums of understanding based on the 1947 USLSA recommendations.[12]

Reports of diagnostic tests because of abortion in a herd by the owner or his private veterinarian has been a traditional means of surveillance since the disease was first recognized as a contagious disease and reporting procedures were established. Making brucellosis a reportable disease requires that any owner or veterinarian who is aware of brucellosis or suspects brucellosis in a herd must report it to the state or federal authorities. General screening of all aborted feti and/or serum samples in diagnostic laboratories for brucellosis is an important adjunct to the present brucellosis surveillance program in the United States.

For passive surveillance programs to work for any disease, the investigator must have an active public education and information program developed to inform individual farmers and private veterinarians about the need to be alert for possible existence of the disease. Some investigators think that actions such as public information programs and incentives make a program an active surveillance program. Even with these adjuncts it is still up to the cattle owner to decide if he or she will participate. Being fully informed about the nature of a disease and its potential losses does not guarantee that the individual will participate in a program. Failure to participate may be due to psychological or sociological factors that have nothing to do with the disease. Public information programs will overcome ignorance but indifference, apathy, and plain obstinance all play a role in individuals not participating in a program.

When disease prevalence and losses from the disease are high, passive surveillance programs can be effective in controlling the disease. If coupled with incentives such as free testing and indemnity for animals destroyed because of disease, passive surveillance programs can effectively reduce the disease prevalence to a relatively low level.

Active Surveillance Methods

To eradicate a disease from a population it is necessary to develop some form of active surveillance with compulsory participation in the program. A number of active surveillance programs have been used in animal disease programs. These generally depend upon doing a complete census of the livestock population in an area or repeated sampling of the population at a very high rate so no infected herd has a chance to escape detection for a long period of time.

The first active surveillance procedure used in the brucellosis eradication program was down-the-road testing of all herds in a county. The concept did not begin with the brucellosis program, however, as area testing of counties had been developed by the Bovine Tuberculosis Eradication Program in the United States. The concept of area testing for bovine tuberculosis (TB) was first used by the Bureau of Animal Industry in 1909 in the District of Columbia; when all cattle in the district were tested and 19% were found to be infected. Several district-wide tests of all cattle were done until 1925 when the infection rate was reduced to zero. The first county in the United States to have a complete county-wide area test for TB was Hillsdale County, Michigan, in 1921. Following this demonstration, county-wide testing became an official part of the TB-accreditation program in 1923.

Area tests for brucellosis were first done in Del Norte County, California, when three county-wide area tests were conducted starting in 1930.[13] Virginia started a county-wide testing program in June 1935 in one county. In 1936 a quarantine was placed on all counties in the state in which the cattle had not been tested.[5]

In 1936 the USLSA established provisions to recognize areas as bangs disease-accredited based on an area-wide test of all cattle herds. To be accredited for one year, less than 0.5% percent of the cattle tested could be infected and all infected herds had to be retested until free of infection. Provision allowed for reaccreditation for three additional years on a test of 10% of the herds in the area including a retest of all previously infected herds.[14]

The first Uniform Methods and Rules for Brucellosis Eradication (UM&R) was approved by the USLSA in 1949. This plan recognized a modified certified area plan for areas based on voluntary participation in one of 4 herd plans.[15] The plan called for a blood test of all cattle herds in the area with less than 1% of the cattle and 5% of the herds being reactors. By 1951, 24 states had laws or regulations that permitted the state authorities to require blood tests of all cattle in an area when a majority of the cattle owners had voluntarily placed their herds under supervision.[16] In 1952, the UM&R was modified to allow modified certified-free brucellosis status in range or semi-range areas based on a test of all dairy and purebred cattle and 20% of the range or semi-range cattle over three years of age in each herd. If infection was found in any of the tested cattle the entire herd had to be tested.[17]

Area testing continued to be the principle means of initially certifying counties and modified certified brucellosis areas until 1973 when the last county in the United States was initially modified certified.[18] Partial area testing with use of the Brucellosis Milk Ring Test (BRT) to monitor dairy herds was used in many states starting in 1952[19] and monitoring with the Market Cattle Identification (MCI) was accepted for initial certification in range or semi-range areas in 1959 with an herd test of all herds not adequately covered by the MCI testing or BRT.[20] This was extended to all states in 1966.[21]

Limited area testing of counties with high infection rates is still recommended as the best method for rapidly locating all the infection in an area. Since 1977, limited area testing has been used extensively in several of the south-eastern states to accelerate the eradication of brucellosis in the United States. In 1977, 18,700 herds were tested in two states (Georgia and Tennessee) and 460 new infected herds were found.[22] The accelerated program was extended to include Alabama and Kentucky in 1978[23] and Arkansas in 1979.[24] There was a dramatic reduction in the number of new infected herds found between the second and third years following area testing in these states. Five years after the start of the accelerated program these states showed an average 45% decrease in numbers of new infected herds found as compared to all other states in the United States which showed a 1% reduction from 1977 through 1981. (See Figure 28-1)

Although county-wide area testing was a very effective method of reducing disease in an area, it was very expensive and required a large number of personnel. A search for more efficient methods of surveillance resulted in development the BRT and the MCI programs which used to provide continuous monitoring of cattle populations in the United States at less cost.

The BRT was first described in Germany in 1937[25] and was used widely for surveillance in Sweden and Denmark in the 1940s.[26,-31] Workers in Sweden and Denmark demonstrated the relative sensitivity and specificity of the ring test to detect infected herds as compared to the whey agglutination tests which had been in use as a surveillance test in Europe.

Preliminary studies on use of the BRT in United States dairies were

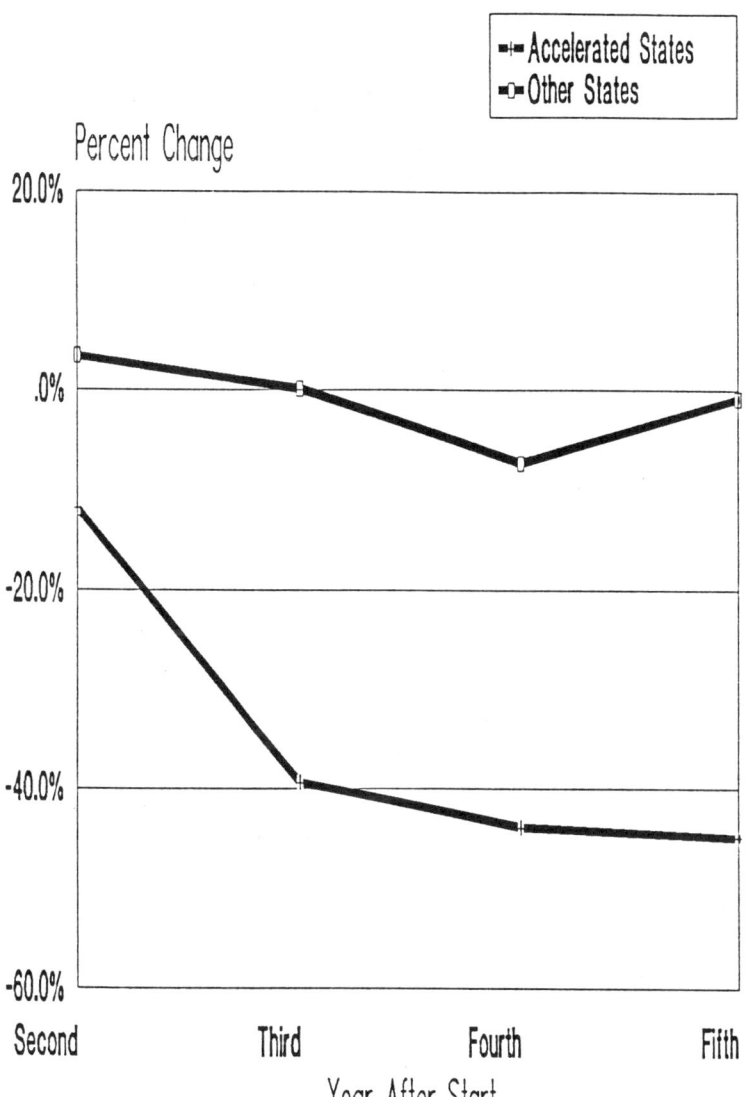

ACCELERATED ERADICATION PROGRAM
Percent Change from Start of Acceleration or 1977

Figure 28-1. Percent New Herds Found During Second through Fifth Years after Beginning of Accelerated Eradication Program in Five States Compared to all other States in United States from 1977 through 1981.

done in Minnesota beginning in 1947[32] and Ohio in 1950.[33] The first studies were done in Minnesota in nine counties on 8,469 herds with 385 (4.5%) reactor herds found in the area-wide herd blood test. There were 121 reactor herds missed by the BRT and 198 herds were BRT-suspicious and negative on the blood test. Of the missed herds, 107 were investigated and, in 69 (64%) of the herds, the reactors found on the blood test were not in production when the BRT sample was collected.[33-35] Additional studies were done in Minnesota in 14 counties and 188 reactor herds were found on an area-wide blood test that had been missed by the BRT done prior to the blood test. Of the BRT missed herds, 165 had single reactors.[36] Studies on the BRT in Wisconsin compared the test with a complete county-wide herd blood test of two counties. Reactor cattle were found in 54 herds in the two counties on the herd tests and 30 of these were ring test suspicious. Of the 24 missed herds three were beef herds or missed on the ring test, the reactors in 10 herds were not lactating at the time of the ring test, and the single reactors in nine of the remaining herds were culture negative for *Brucella abortus*. Only one herd with a *Brucella abortus*-infected animal was missed by the BRT. There were 259 herds in the two counties that were ring test suspicious but did not have animals with significant serological titers for brucellosis.[37]

In 1949, the USLSA recommended that USDA develop a standardized BRT antigen.[15] USDA produced a uniform antigen and made it available only through official channels in 1950.[38]

In 1951, the USLSA Brucellosis committee provided that an area may be declared modified certified brucellosis-free by the semi-annual application of milk tests and blood testing of herds. All non-milk tested herds must be blood tested. To be declared modified certified brucellosis-free an area must have two milk tests not less than six months apart. All herds reacting to the milk test and all non-milk tested herds must be blood tested. The number of reactors (exclusive of officially vaccinated animals under 30 months of age) must not exceed one percent and the herd infection must not exceed five precent. Infected herds were quarantined until they passed at least two consecutive blood tests not less than 60 days apart. This certification was indefinite if semi-annual milk tests were applied and all milk reactor herds were blood tested. Twenty percent of non-milk tested herds were to be blood tested biannually. Continuance of certification depended on the disease incidence not exceeding the maximum required for initial certification.[33]

In 1951, 10 states were using the BRT extensively and three states were using it exclusively for initial survey purposes.[16] By 1953, the BRT was being conducted in 23 states and Puerto Rico with 670,532 herds representing 12 million cattle being tested, and 26.2% of the herds being suspicious.

In the early 1960s it became apparent that the BRT test was missing too many infected herds, particularly the large herds. The test was modified to make it more sensitive.[39] At the present time the low prevalence of brucellosis infection in dairy herds in the United States creates a problem with low specificity of the test for detecting *Brucella* infection in dairy herds. In 1988, 680,223 BRT tests were done representing 37,380,339 head of cattle, and 2,592 (0.38%) of the herds tested were suspicious. Many of the suspicious samples in 1988 would have been repeat samples from herds already under quarantine but more than 90% of the BRT suspicious samples in 1988 were from herds that were not infected (See Figure 28-2).

Market testing of cattle was the other surveillance procedure that was developed to monitor cattle without the costs associated with area testing. Tests for sale of cattle was the first type of market testing done. In 1951, 15 states required a negative blood test for all cattle moved within the state except for immediate slaughter or those otherwise excepted by the regulations.[16] In 1956, federal regulations were adopted which required breeding cattle to be tested for brucellosis within 30 days before interstate movement except for the following: those consigned to immediate slaughter or to public stockyards, animals from certified free herds, animals from modified certified-free areas, official vaccinates under 30 months of age, and official vaccinates under 36 months of age with less than a complete reaction at 1:100 to a blood serum agglutination test.[40]

The community auction market was recognized in 1950 as one of the most potent means of dissemination of animal disease. Legislation to regulate these markets for interstate movement was passed in 1951.[41] Change of ownership testing was considered one of the principle requirements of the accelerated eradication plan in certain high incidence states of the United States in 1977.[22] This included first-point testing of all cattle at stockyards or other points of concentration even if they were going to slaughter. First point testing allows more rapid identification of the herd of origin and also prevents exposed cattle from the same herd of origin from being sold into breeding herds.

The earliest known report of surveillance of brucellosis infection at slaughter was in 1934 in Sardinia, Italy.[42] Blood samples were taken from 127 adult cattle and 46 calves at a slaughter house in Cagliari province, Italy. Ninety-six (75.3%) of the adult cattle and 28 (60.8%) of the calves had serum agglutination titers of 1:100 or greater for *Brucella*.

In 1955, the state of Washington started doing experimental work on a cull and dry cow testing program.[43] In 1956, 10 states reported on preliminary results of tests conducted at auction markets and slaughtering establishments. Effectiveness of tracing in the various states varied from no reactors traced to 91% traced.[44] The USLSA recommended changes in the UM&R to allow range and semi-range areas to qualify as a Modified Certified Brucellosis-free area if, for five years, at least 80% of the retained heifer calves were vaccinated and at least 5% of the breeding cows in the area were subjected to a blood agglutination test for brucellosis collected

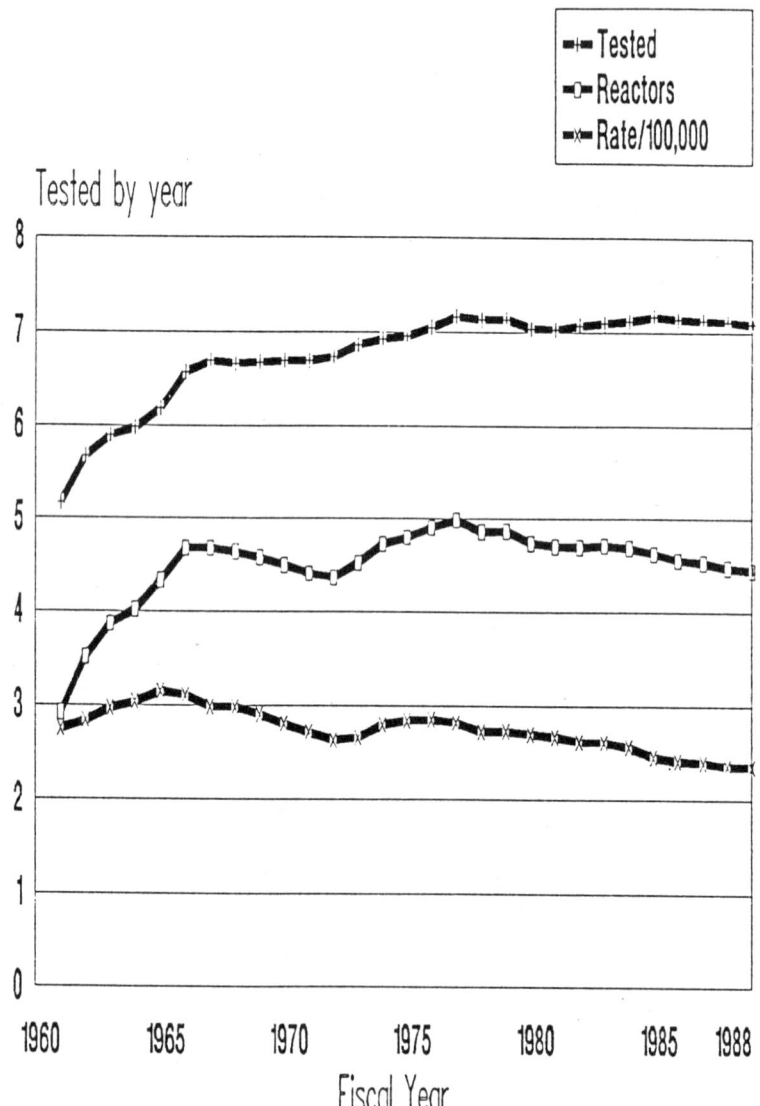

MARKET CATTLE SAMPLES TESTED IN U.S.A.
FISCAL YEAR 1960 THROUGH FISCAL YEAR 1988

Figure 28-2. Log 10 of Number of Brucellosis Milk Ring Tests (BRT) Done, Number BRT Suspicious Herds and Rate of BRT Suspicious Tests per 100,00o Tests Done from Fiscal Year 1952 through Fiscal Year 1988.

from cull and slaughter cows at ranches, sale yards, or slaughtering establishments. Any herds without sufficient numbers of animals tested at the markets, any dairy herds not covered by the BRT, and purebred beef herds were to be subjected to an official blood test within the five-year period.[20] In 1959 the USLSA Brucellosis Committee removed the provisions for initial certification of an area by the cull and dry cow testing from the UM&R but the provision was restored again in 1966.[21]

Recertification of an area during each year beginning in 1956 required that blood samples be taken from cull and slaughter cows at ranches, sale yards, or slaughtering establishments from at least 5% of the breeding cows in the area, or a total of 15% during a three-year period. Any herds of origin of cattle reacting at a titer of complete at 1:100 were subjected to an official blood test.[20] Changes were also made in the addition of certified-free areas allowing them to be recertified based on blood tests of cows and bulls over 30 months of age consigned to market for breeding, feeding, slaughter or other purposes, whether of dairy or beef breeds. At least 5 % of the animals over three years of age in the herd (25 percent over a five-year period or 30 percent over a six-year period) must be tested each year.[21]

With various modifications, the above requirements remained the standards for certifying and recertifying areas until 1982 when the method of classifying states and areas was changed to the current Class Free, Class A, Class B, and Class C. The current requirements for the MCI program require that at least 95% of all cows and bulls over two years of age must be sampled at each slaughter plant. In Class B and Class C areas, 80% of the MCI reactors found must be traced to the herd of origin and 90% must be traced in Class Free and Class A areas.[48]

In 1959, 18 states indicated some degree of participation in the MCT project. There were 29,240 back-tags applied and 39,914 blood samples collected. Of the 120 reactors disclosed, 110 were traced promptly to herds of origin.[44] By 1960 there were 14 states back-tagging cattle for MCT and samples were being collected at slaughter plants in 26 states. By 1962 all states except Alaska were participating in the program (See Figure 28-3).

Classification of cattle as MCT (MCI) reactors was based on a complete reaction at 1:100 on the standard plate or standard tube test without regard to the animal's vaccination status. Studies done on the use of supplemental tests indicated that a card positive test on animals known not to vaccinated and a Rivanol positive test on vaccinated animals was a better criteria for requiring a herd test.[47]

In the early control and eradication program little effort was made to determine the source of infection in herds found to be infected. Many herds had been infected for so many years that it was impossible to trace the source. The herd prevalence rate was also so high there did not appear to be any point in assuming there had been disease transmission from one particular herd to another. With county-wide area testing all the local

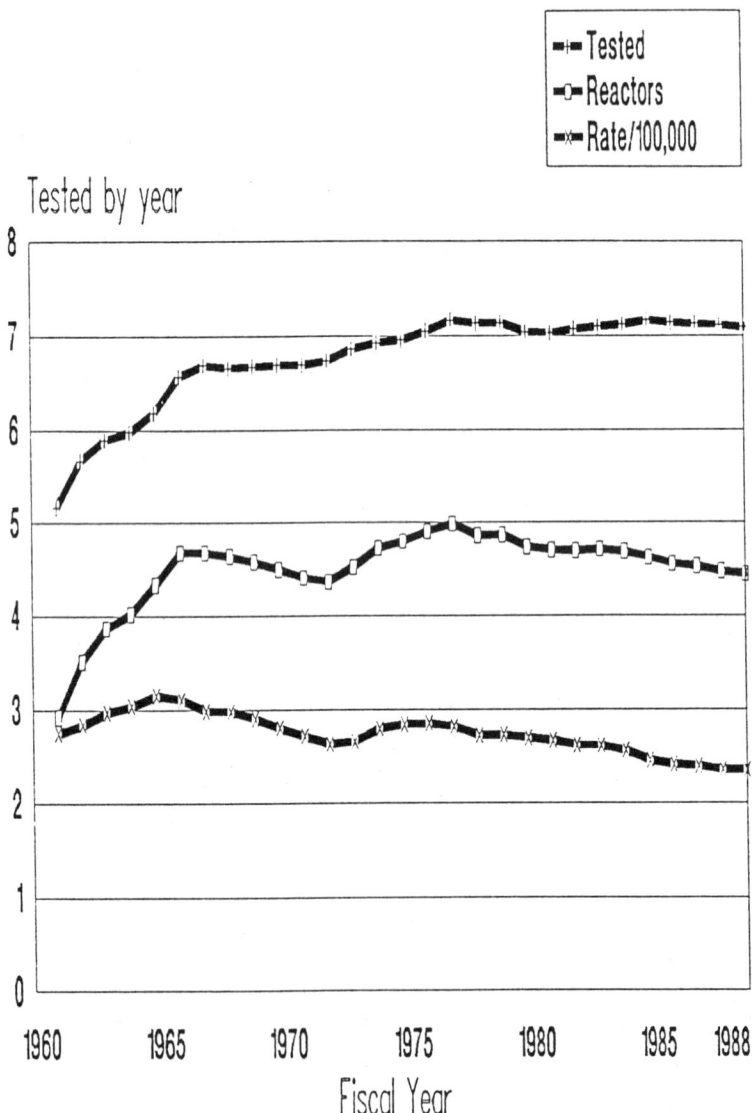

Figure 28-3. Log 10 of Number of Cattle Tested Under the Market Cattle Identification (MCI) Program, Number of Reactors Disclosed, and Reactor Rate per 100,000 Cattle Tested.

herds were being tested for brucellosis anyway so there was little concern about how the disease had been introduced into any infected herd.

As disease prevalence was reduced and particularly in certified-free areas when herds previously known to be free of disease became reinfected then interherd transmission became a concern. Epidemiological tracing of infection into and from infected herds became a standard secondary surveillance procedure in the 1960s. It includes testing of herds adjacent to or in contact with any new infected herd, limited area testing of entire neighborhoods, testing herds from which animals have moved into an infected herd or herds that may have acquired animals from an infected herd.

Adjacent herd testing consists of testing those herds that have an adjoining fence line or are across the road from an infected herd. Contact herds may include adjacent herds but may also include herds with some known contact with the infected herd such as through a shared pasture, grazing association or some other contact. Adjacent and contact herd testing are important means of surveillance and become particularly important in the final stages of eradication. In some cases up to 20% of the adjacent and contact herds tested may be infected although in recent years the rate tends to be less.

Neigborhood testing may be considered an extension of adjacent or contact herd testing or an area test of a limited area. Some states have required that all herds within a certain radius from 1/2 to 5 miles of an infected herd must be tested. The farther the herd is from the infected herd the less successful the herd test is in finding new infection.

Tracing movements into and out of infected herds is an important surveillance tool in low incidence areas and becomes a necessity to be able to qualify an area as free of brucellosis. In some cases it may be necessary to test several herds to find the source herd. In other cases it may be necessary to test several herds to find a possible source. A dealer cannot usually be considered a source but instead a distributor of infection and it may be necessary to trace all his sources. Brucella infection in a herd always has to have a source.

Equally important as tracing source animals into a herd is the identification of animals that may have moved out of the herd into other herds. It is important in any eradication program that these herds be identified and tested.

Discussion

Economic, statistical, diagnostic, and sociological criteria are all important in choosing a surveillance procedure.

To eradicate a disease in the shortest possible time it is necessary to do a census. Although the goal of any census is to sample 100% of the population at a single point in time we rarely ever achieve that goal. To control a disease, a large sample of the population is usually sufficient, particularly if the sample can be biased toward the subset of the population most likely to be affected.

Area testing of all the cattle in a specified area is a form of census taking. To complete the census and test all cattle the following criteria must be met:

1. The area test must be conducted in as short a time frame as possible. The longer it takes for an area test to be done the greater the probability that herds which tested negative early during the area test will come in contact with infected cattle and become infected. The theoretical ideal would be to have every herd in the area tested on one day. In actual practice the ideal time for completing an area test is 30 to 90 days. The eighteen months allowed for completing an area test under the early certification programs was far too long a period of time.

2. All movements from untested herds must be stopped until the area test is completed. After a herd is tested and negative the owner may be allowed to sell cattle to other herds and to buy cattle from other negative tested herds. Exceptions may be allowed for movements to slaughter if the shipped cattle are tested either before or at the time they are slaughtered. Ideally when an area test is started an individual herd quarantine on each herd in the area should be issued at the beginning of the area test. Each individual herd quarantine would be released only when the herd has had a negative complete herd test.

3. Legal authority must be available to require testing of the herd belonging to any uncooperative owner. Law enforcement officials such as the sheriff and district attorney should be alerted when an area test is about to begin so they can be prepared to handle any legal contingencies.

4. Resources must be available and committed to accomplish the above three criteria.

The cost of doing a herd test is one of the principle faults of extensive area testing. The cost of collecting samples on a farm is much greater than the costs of collecting blood samples at markets or slaughter plants or collecting milk samples at a central collection point. Costs that need to be considered are not only the direct costs to the governmental agency collecting the samples but the costs to the livestock producer for confining and handling his animals. Laboratory and record keeping costs do not vary a great deal for each sample tested but will vary per herd if a sample of a herd is tested instead of the complete herd.

Personnel requirements for area testing are high. In the 1930s and 1940s there were frequently more herds signed up waiting to be tested under the voluntary testing program than there were veterinarians available to do the testing. With the beginning of the accelerated program in 1954 one of the frequent problems with area testing in the United States was the lack of sufficient personnel where the herd owners had volunteered or requested an area wide test.[38,48,49]

Market sampling procedures are the best example we have of use of a sampling procedure to try to eradicate a disease. Testing cull cows at slaughter is not a random sampling procedure of all herds as cows that abort or that fail to raise a calf are more likely to be culled than cows that have normal calves. Various factors have been identified that affect the effectiveness of the MCI program, including the following:[50]

1. The number of animals culled and sent to slaughter. The rate of herd turnover varies from herd to herd and also varies with market and feed conditions which are affected by weather, etc.

2. The size of the herd. A large herd with the same turnover rate as a small herd will send more animals to market and thus have a greater chance of having a reactor detected.

3. The amount of infection in the herd. The higher the rate of infection in the herd the greater the probability that a culled animal will be a reactor.

4. The rate of MCI coverage of cull animals. The objective of the MCI program is to cover 100% of all the cull animals sent to slaughter. It isn't sufficient to collect samples from all these animals, however, if they are not identified and not traceable to a herd of origin. The current UM&R requires collection of samples from at least 95% of the eligible cattle slaughtered.

5. The marketing patterns or chance that cull animals from individual herds being identified and going to slaughter plants where blood samples are collected. The current UM&R requires that all slaughter plants in an area collect at least 95% of the eligible cattle slaughtered.

Testing cattle for change of ownership either at markets or for direct farm to farm sales has a lower probability of finding infection in the herd of origin since barren cows or cows that are otherwise diseased would usually not be marketed as breeding animals.

Brucellosis milk ring testing is a form of census of the milk-producing cattle population. Repeat sampling several times during the year will ensure that all milk-producing herds are included. Individual herds may be missed because they are out of production or because of other factors.

Diagnostic test criteria are important for any surveillance program. Laboratory diagnostic procedures used on collected samples must be sufficiently sensitive so that infected herds are not missed and at the same time be sufficiently specific so that heterologous or vaccination antibody does not initiate an investigation and test of a herd which is not infected. The tests must also be reproducible and relatively inexpensive to conduct on a large volume of samples.

Increasing the sensitivity of the diagnostic test used in a surveillance program will result in fewer infected animals being missed but will also result in more non-specific heterologous reactions and more interference from vaccination. The result is an increase in effectiveness of the surveillance program but with some loss of efficiency.

Increasing the specificity of the diagnostic test will result in less interference from vaccination and non-specific reactions while risking missing more infected animals. The result is an increase in efficiency but with some loss of effectiveness.

Reproducibility of tests is a factor that is often overlooked when a test is evaluated for use in a surveillance program. A test that is not reproducible is a poor test for use in any part of a surveillance program. Loss of public confidence in a program is probably more affected by tests that are not consistent than by any other procedure employed.

The time it takes to test a sample and get a result is less important for slaughter samples than it is for samples collected at a market or occasionally on the farm.

Cost is probably the most significant criteria in determining which surveillance method will be used. Area testing is probably the most rapid method we have of achieving rapid eradication in an area but it is also the most expensive. First-point testing of marketed cattle has several advantages over slaughter testing since the origin of the animal can be immediately identified and any associated exposed animals can be immediately prevented from being sold and moved into clean herds. Cost determines that we rely heavily on slaughter surveillance because it is still the most cost-effective despite its other inefficiencies.

The support of the livestock industry for any type of surveillance procedure does play a role in acceptance of the procedure. Herd owners will usually not accept repeated on-farm bleeding of their herds especially if the test results are usually negative. Industry acceptance of the BRT and MCI has been a major factor in their success. One of the problems with these relatively unobtrusive procedures when the the disease incidence becomes very low is that the majority of unaffected herd owners do not even know they exist. Industry support for the entire program will tend to wane at this point.

Reliability of the surveillance procedure is critically important to its success. Heterospecific serological reactions and vaccination antibody tend to reduce the reliability of many the surveillance procedures as the disease incidence is reduced to a very low level. Slaughter surveillance has many points at which it can fail and thus become unreliable. Identification of animals, proper identification and collection of samples at the slaughter plant and maintaining the identification at the laboratory are critical to the success of the program. These are areas that cannot be left to attend to themselves but must be constantly monitored and necessary corrections made if they are to continue to succeed.

There is a need for continued surveillance after an area is free of known brucellosis. As long as animals can be moved into a free area from an infected area either legally or illegally there will always be the possibility of reinfection. Even after an area has been free from all known infection there may be some residual infection in a few herds within the free area. In areas where brucellosis in wild animals is not controlled and these wild animals can come in contact with domestic animals, surveillance must be continued indefinitely to prevent re-establishment of infection in the domestic livestock population. How long do we need to continue surveillance without finding infection before we can declare a disease eradicated? When a disease has been determined to be eradicated then further surveillance and preventive measures within the local eradication area should end. In theory there should be a complete population changeover to a completely unvaccinated susceptible population without any evidence of the disease before a disease could be declared eradicated. In actual practice the time interval before eradication is declared is usually much shorter and is influenced more by political, sociological and economic factors than theory.

In summary, a number of surveillance procedures have been used in the United States since 1920 when the first voluntary testing program for brucellosis control started. The early systems were largely passive with minimal involvement of the state and federal goverments. As the prevalence of the disease was reduced the state and federal governments have become more active in seeking out and eliminating the last vestiges of the disease. The background and development of the various passive and active surveillance procedures is discussed.

References

1. Barnes MF, Church HR. Progress of Bang Bacillus Disease Control in Pennsylvania. *Proc* U S Livestock Sanit Assn 1927;901-918.
2. Robinson TE. Symposium on Bang's Disease. *Proc* U S Livestock Sanit Assn 1934; 312-341.
3. Larsen VS. Bang's Disease Control Project. *Proc* U S Livestock Sanit Assn 1934;303-310.
4. Wight AE: Symposium on Bang's Disease. *Proc* U S Livestock Sanit Assn 1934; 312-313.
5. Givins HC, Brookbank RE. Area Work in Bang's Disease Control. *Proc* U S Livestock Sanit Assn 1936;273-287.
6. Foster SB. Bang's Disease Control in Oregon. *Proc* U S Livestock Sanit Assn1935;253-257.
7   Lewis WK. Experiences and Results of State Quarantine Against Abortion Disease. *Proc* U S Livestock Sanit Assn 1931;333-336.
8. Fitch CP, chairman. Report of Committee on Bang's Disease. *Proc* U S Livestock Sanit Assn 1934;311-312.
9. Anderson RK. Surveillance: Criteria for Evaluation and Design of Epidemiologiic Surveillance Systems for Animal Health and Productivity. *Proc* U S Livestock Sanit Assn 1982;321-340.
10. Smith RW, chairman. Report of the Committee on Brucellosis. *Proc* U S Livestock

Sanit Assn 1947;166-169.

11. West R, chairman. Report of the Committee on Brucellosis. *Proc* U S Livestock Sanit Assn 1948;193-197.

12. Kuttler AK. Report on Brucellosis Eradication Project. *Proc* U S Livestock Sanit Assn 1948;188-192.

13. McKay K. Experiences in the Control of Bang's Disease in California. *Proc* U S Livestock Sanit Assn 1936;292-301.

14. Fitch CP, chairman. Report of Committee on Bang's Disease. *Proc* U S Livestock Sanit Assn 1936;301-305.

15. Clark CF, chairman. Report of Committee on Brucellosis. *Proc* U S Livestock Sanit Assn 1949;63-73.

16. Kuttler AK. Report on Brucellosis Eradication Project. *Proc* U S Livestock Sanit Assn 1951;245-248.

17. Driver FC, chairman. Report of Committee on Brucellosis. Proc U S Livestock Sanit Assn 1952;135-137.

18. Fichtner GJ. Progress of the State-Federal Brucellosis Eradication Program. U S Livestock Sanit Assn 1973;100-108.

19. Geyer HG, chairman. Report of Committee on Brucellosis. *Proc* U S Livestock Sanit Assn 1951;249-254.

20. Smith RW, chairman. Report of the Committee on Brucellosis. *Proc* U S Livestock Sanit Assn 1956;119-130.

21 Smith RW, chairman. Report of the Committee on Brucellosis. *Proc* U S Livestock Sanit Assn 1959;104-119.

22. Johnson B.G. Progress of the Cooperative State-Federal Brucellosis Eradication Program. U S Livestock Sanit Assn 1977;97-113.

23. Johnson BG. Status of the Cooperative State-Federal Brucellosis Eradication Program. U S Livestock Sanit Assn 1978;157-172.

24. Johnson B.G. Status of the Cooperative State-Federal Brucellosis Eradication Program. U S Livestock Sanit Assn 1979;105-117.

25. Fleishauer G. Die Abortus-Bang-Ringprobe (ABR) sur Feststellung von bangverdachtigen Vollmilchproben. Berl. tierarztl. Wschr.: 53:527, 1937

26. Bruhn PA. The Abortus-Bang Ring Test Compared to Whey and Serum Agglutination Titer. *Medlemsbl danske DyrLegeforen* 1944;27:477-502.

27. Bruhn PA. The Brucella Abortus Ring Test. *Am J Vet Res* 1948;9:360-369.

28. Christiansen MJ. Om Abortus-Bang-Ringpro/ven og den Anvendense i den praktiske Kastingsbekaempelse.[On the use of the Ring Test in Combating Bovine Brucellosis. Maanedsskr Dyrl 1948;59:193-230.

29. Norell NO, Olson A. On the value of Serological Investigations of Milk According to "ABR" (Abortus-Bang-Ringprobe). *Skand Vettidsskrl* 1943; 33:321-341.

30 Seit B, Jorgensen K. Abortus-Bang-Ringpro/vens Vaerdi som diagnostisk Hjaelpemiddel. *Maanedsskr Dyrl* 1944;56:277.

31. Winther O, Hansen AC. Investigations of the Abortus-Bang Ring Test.*Maanedsskr Dyrl* 1946;33:401-416.

32. Roepke MH, Clausen LB, Walsh AL. The Milk and Cream Ring Test for Brucellosis. *Proc* U S Livestock Sanit Assn 1948;147-159.

33. Geyer HG, Edgington BH, Bond HG. Application of the (A.B.R.) Ring Test in Area Brucellosis Control. *Proc* U S Livestock Sanit Assn 1950;84-86.

34. Driver FC, Roepke MH. Field Studies on the Diagnosis of Animal Brucellosis with Special Emphasis on the Ring Test. Third Int-amer Congr on Brucellosis 1950;133-143.

35. Roepke MH, Paterson KG, Driver FC, Clausen LB, Olson L, Wentworth JE. The *Brucella abortus* Ring Test. *Am J Vet Res* 1950;11:199-205.

36. Roepke MH, Stiles FC, Driver FC. The Efficacy of the Brucellosis Ring Test in Certifying Areas. *J Am Vet Med Assn* 1958;133:93-96.

37. Janney GC, Berman DT, Erdmann AA. The Relative Efficiency of the Milk Ring Test and Area Blood Tests for Bovine Brucellosis. *J Am Vet Med Assn* 1958;133:586-589.

38. Winter A. Report on Brucellosis Eradication Project. *Proc* U S Livestock Sanit Assn 1952;131-134.

39. Kimberling CV. Increased sensitivity of the Brucellosis Ring Test. *Proc* 4th Ann Conf Bruc Epidem-1964. 1966:108-112.

40. West R, chairman. Report of the Committee on Brucellosis. *Proc* U S Livestock Sanit Assn 1953;144-153.

41 Winter A. Report on Brucellosis Eradication Project. *Proc* U S Livestock Sanit Assn1950;78-80.

42. Castelli A. La frequence de la Brucellose chez les animaux d'abattoir dans la province de Caglari. [Frequency of Brucellosis in Slaughterhouse animals of Cagliari Province]. *Boll Soc Internsz. Microbiol* 1934;6:456- 458.

43 Mulhern FJ. Outline Review of the Market Cattle Testing Program. USDA ARS ADE Division Notice (Mimeo.) 1962.

44. Mingle CK. Report of the Cooperative Brucellosis Control and Eradication Program. *Proc* U S Livestock Sanit Assn 1956;82-88.

45 United States Department of Agriculture, Animal and Plant Health Inspection Services, Veterinary Services. *The Uniform Methods and Rules for Brucellosis Eradication* APHIS 91-1, Hyattsville, MD. 1986.

46. Mingle CK. Report of the Cooperative Brucellosis Control and Eradication Program. *Proc* U S Livestock Sanit Assn 1959;76-82.

47. Metcalf HE. *An Evaluation and Study of the Market Cattle Testing Program for Brucellosis Eradication.* MPH Thesis, Univ. of Minn. 1966.

48 Kuttler AK. Status of Federal-State Brucellosis Eradication. *Proc* U S Livestock Sanit Assn 1955;116-124.

49. Mingle CK. Report of the Cooperative Brucellosis Control and Eradication Program. *Proc* U S Livestock Sanit Assn 1953;110-116.

50. Beal VC Jr. *Regulatory Statistics* Volume 1. 6th Ed. USDA APHIS VS, Hyattsville, MD, 1983.

Chapter Twenty-nine

Initiation of a National
Brucellosis Control Program
in Egypt

Mohamed K. Refai,
Samira El-Gibaly and
Ahmed T. Adawi

Brucellosis in animals has been recorded in Egypt since 1939.[1] The prevalence of serological reactors on limited surveys has varied however from one author to the other. In cows it was reported to be 16.5%,[2] 18.8%,[3] 20%,[4] 22.2%,[5] and 23.3%.[6] The prevalence among buffaloes varied from 7 to 10%.[1,6,7] Isolations of *Brucella abortus* from cattle were made by various workers as early as 1943.[8-10] Since 1970, *Brucella melitensis* has also been isolated.[11-14]

During the 1960s, with the importation of Friesian cows for the establishment of governmental farms with large numbers of animals, the incidence of brucellosis in cattle reached 37% on some farms. This increase took on an alarming nature during the early 1980s with the increased creation of farms with large number of animals on relatively small areas of land.

The aim of the present work was to gain experience with the use of the reduced dose S19 vaccine in calves.

Materials and Methods

During the years 1985 to 1987, 15,815 adult cattle on 16 farms in 6 governorates were tested periodically by the tube agglutination test and positive cases were confirmed by rivanol or complement fixation test (CFT). In 1988, a total of 29,823 cows, 809 buffalo, 3,355 calves, and 192 sheep in large farms were tested. In addition, 2,528 blood samples obtained from animals from small farms, markets, and abattoirs, and tested.

During the years 1987 and 1988, 8,709 calves, 3 to 7 months old, were vaccinated with the reduced dose S19 vaccine obtained from the United States. Before application of the vaccine, each batch was subjected to viability counts to be sure that the used dose (2 ml) was between 3 and 10 billion organisms.

Results

Serosurvey During the Years 1985 to 1987

As shown in Table 29-1, the prevalence of cattle with positive and suspicious titers animals reached up to 34% in some farms; however, this percentage dropped drastically following the slaughter of reactors. This is clearly demonstrated in Table 29-2 concerning Farm no. 7 in Damietta. This farm contained 980 imported Friesian cows. The percentage of reactors was very high (34.5%) when the animals were tested in March 1986. The gradual slaughtering of reactors almost cleaned up the farm so that the incidence at the end of the year was 9.2%. However, it increased again and reached up to 11.4%.

In Qena Farm no. 1 there were 590 imported Friesian cows. During December 1985, the rate of infection was 32.9%. Following the slaughter of reactors, the rate of infection dropped to 3.5%. Four of 50 persons working on the farm contracted the disease.

In one of the private farms in Sharkia, Friesian cows were vaccinated annually with H38 vaccine so that some animals received up to five doses. The serological testing of 446 animals revealed 317 positives and 64 suspicious animals. Titers of 1/40-1/320 (tube agglutination), 1/50-1/400 (Rivanol) and 1/40-1/160 (CFT) were obtained. Another private farm in the Giza governorate had a similar pattern.

Calfhood Vaccination

Only calves proved to be serologically negative when vaccinated. The serological follow-up of the vaccinated calves revealed a variable pattern. In general, about 55% of the calves had agglutinins one month after vaccination. A titer of 1/10 was detected in 7%, 1/20 in 13.7%, 1/40 in 16.9% and 1/80 in 18%. Three months after vaccination, the calves showing titers between 1/10 - 1/40 increased to 62%; however, all animals tested negative seven to eight months after vaccination.

Serosurvey in the Year 1988

As shown in Table 29-3, 1.6% of cows had positive reactions and 0.9% were suspicious. On the other hand, all 809 buffalo tested were negative. In calves, 2.6% were positive and 3.3% were suspicious. Sheep had high percentages (31.7% and 10.4%) of positive and suspicious samples. Table 29-4 demonstrates the absence of reactors in animals in abattoirs of three governorates (Damietta, Sharkia and Kalubia) and markets in Sharkia and Kalubia. Only one positive and three suspicious cases were detected among 1,731 animals owned by small farmers.

Table 29-1. Incidence of *Brucella* Reactors in 16 Farms of Adult Cattle

Farm	No. of Animals	First Report of Brucellosis	Percent of Reactors	Dates of Testing
Quena 1	596	17.12.1985	32.9%	1985
			3.5%	1986
Quena 2	652	16.07.1985	0.4%	1985
Quena 3	195		0.0%	1987
G. Sami Assad	1,271	23.05.1982	0.5%	1986
			0.8%	1987
Damietta 1	1,067	10.03.1986	0.1-0.6%	1986
			0.2-0.3%	1987
Damietta 2	1,181	10.03.1986	0.8-0.0%	1986
			0.3-2.8%	1987
Damietta 7	980	10.03.1986	34.5-0.2%	1986
			0.22-0.0%	1987
Shalakan	137	8.12.1985	2.8%	1985
			3.4-14.0%	1986
			1.7-0.7%	1987
W. Shalaby	295	16.12.1986	21.3%	1987
El-Asakra	760	—	0.0%	1987
Abo-Gabre	4,687	17.07.1986	1.8-7.6%	1986
			5.1%	1987
El-Tounsy	2,806	21.10.1985	34.2%	Jan.-April, 1987
				Jan.-Nov., 1987
Labana	146	13.01.1987	23.4%	1987
El-Samanoudy	73	24.11.1985	16.4%	1985
El-Katta prison	120	4.03.1985	15.5-9.0%	1986
Touch Tanbesha	848	1969	83%	1984
			22.8%	1985
			6.8-6.2%	1986
			6.3-29.%	1987

Discussion

Reviewing the literature concerning brucellosis in Egypt indicates that the disease was found at levels of 16 to 23% in cattle and 7 to 10% in buffaloes. However, during the sixties, with importation of Friesian cows, the prevalence on some farms became very high. In Touch Tanbesha, for example (Table 29-1), it reached up to 38% in 1984. Such a high incidence was observed only in farms with a large number of animals concentrated on relatively small amount of land.

Parallel with the open door policy in the late seventies and early eighties, there was a marked increase in the number of intensive breeding farms, both governmental and private. This was based on importation of

Table 29-2. Periodical Testing of Animals on Farm 7

No. of Animals	Date	Result Positive	Suspicious	Percent
713	3/86	232	14	34.5
829	4/86	146	15	19.4
703	3/86	78	15	13.2
157	6/86	37	5	26.7
380	8/86	38	6	11.8
497	9/86	32	5	7.4
326	11/86	1	—	0.3
628	12/86	—	1	0.2
235	1/87	9	7	6.8
531	2/87	8	10	3.4
710	3/87	1	—	0.1
730	4/87	11	22	4.5
686	6/87	3	75	11.4
21	7/87	—	—	
77	8/87	—	—	

large numbers of Friesian cows from different countries. As an example, 8,136 breeding animals were imported in the year 1983. The appearance of brucellosis among these newly established farms in most governorates was alarming. It was in fact a dilemma for the owners as well as the veterinary authorities. The load on the diagnostic laboratory in Dokki was great. The quarantine measures were applied on farms having positive reactors. The owners sought advice from all possible sources with the result that several types of vaccines were used, sometimes in the same animal. This led to the surprising finding on the aforementioned private farm in Sharkia where 71.0% of the animals had positive titers in addition to 14.0% suspicious cases. In such cases, the policy of test and slaughter was a burden on the government. Therefore, it was decided to compensate only farms with infection less than 10%.

The initiation of a control program based on calfhood vaccination with the reduced dose of S19 vaccine was made possible through the American-Egyptian Project (EG-APHIS-217). However, when we started practicing this type of vaccination several problems emerged:

a. Differences in opinion of veterinary officials regarding the policy of brucellosis control, such as vaccine to be used, age of vaccination, type of tests to be used.

b. Lack of exact information about the incidence of brucellosis and the prevailing *Brucella* spp. and biotypes among animals in Egypt.

Table 29-3. Serosurvey of Animals in Large Farms in 10 Governorates

Animals	No. tested	Positive	%	Suspicious	%
Cows	29,823	573	1.6	289	0.9
Buffalo	809	-	-	-	-
Calves	3,355	85	2.6	112	3.3
Sheep	192	61	31.7	20	10.4

Table 29-4. Serosurvey of Farmers' Animals, Animals in Markets and in Abbatoirs

	Cows	Result +	±	Buffaloes	Result +	±
Farmer's animals	878	1	3	853	—	—
Markets	152	—	—			
Abbatoirs	158	—	—	487	—	—

    c. Confusion among field veterinarians and herd owners about brucel losis control.

    d. Shortage of vaccines and diagnostic reagents.

    Accordingly, a National Brucella Committee was established representing the General Organization of Veterinary Services, Animal Health Research Institute, Animal Reproduction Research Institute, Serum and Vaccine Research Institute, and universities. Through this committee the following decisions were made.

    1. It was decided to use U.S. reduced-dose S19 vaccine (3-10 billion organism per dose) in serologically negative calves, 3 to 7 months old. The adult vaccination (0.5 billion) was not approved, instead the adults were are allowed to be vaccinated with the killed 45/20 vaccine. The application of S19 was planned initially to be used in selected farms in five governorates. Use of the vaccination was expanded in the first year to 28 farms and in the second year to 37 farms. All other vaccines are officially not allowed at present.

2. It was decided to use the buffered acidified plate antigen (BAPA) as a presumptive test. Positive samples were then tested with the tube agglutination and Rose Bengal (card) tests; Rivanol and, if possible, CFT were used as confirmatory tests.

3. For evaluation of the vaccine a titer follow up was suggested. Challenge experiments were not accepted. Calves should be negative before breeding age.

4. In dairy farms, the milk ring test (MRT) was to be applied to bulk milk tank samples every 3 to 4 months and positive herds were to be subjected to blood testing of individual animals.

5. Because of the increased volume of laboratory work in the central laboratory at Dokki, selected provincial laboratories were strengthened as far as possible with facilities and trained personnel so that they can carry out the screening tests.

6. To eliminate any confusion concerning brucellosis epidemiology and control, training courses for field veterinarians were conducted and a guide covering the most essential facets of brucellosis in cattle was printed and distributed.

7. All imported animals were to be kept in quarantines for at least 30 days. Pregnant imported animals should be negative when tested 14 days after calving. Herds containing even one positive animal were put under quarantine and all animals were to be subjected to periodical testing every 21 days. Quarantine measures were released if the animals pass three consecutive negative tests at 21-day intervals.

In our opinion, all these measures (namely, the periodical testing, slaughtering of positives, calfhood vaccination with the reduced dose S19, adult vaccination with 45/20, strict quarantine measures and testing of imported animals and infected herds) have led to the drastic drop in incidence of brucellosis in cattle and buffalo at some farms. In order to get better results, this system needs to be expanded to cover all governorates in Egypt.

The problem of a high incidence of *B. melitensis* infection in sheep and goats remains to be considered. This is alarming as *B. melitensis* has been recorded[3,11-14] to be predominant in the cattle and buffalo samples cultured in the last three years.

In our opinion, this situation requires, that more attention be given to sheep and goats with regard to testing, slaughtering, and vaccination to control the disease among them and to eliminate the potential spread of the infection from sheep and goats to cattle and buffalo.

More studies are needed to determine the role of S19 vaccine in protecting cattle from *B. melitensis* infection and to decide if *B. melitensis* vaccine such as Rev. 1 should be used.

Summary

Before starting the application of the reduced dose S19 calfhood vaccination 15,815 adult cattle in 16 selected farms were serologically tested. The incidence of positive reactors reached 34% at some farms. The policy of test and slaughter and calfhood vaccination of calves in these and adjacent farms (8,709 calves in 29 farms) resulted in a drastic drop in the rate of positive reactors. Sheep and goats, which are not yet considered in the program, had a high incidence of reactors (31%). Isolation attempts with positive cattle and buffalo revealed the frequent recovery of B. *melitensis*. This finding suggests to us that sheep and goats, and possibly other animals should be included in the control program.

References

1. Ahmed MR. The incidence of brucellosis in different domesticated animals in Egypt. *Tech Bull* 1939;2310:210-231.
2. Goniem NH, Mowafy LE, Marzouk MA, Abdel Karim, AM. Sero-epidemiological study on B. *abortus* infection in some dairy farms. *Vet Med J* 1985; 11-15.
3. Hamada S, Sherief I, El-Sawaf H, Youssef M. A survey done on brucellosis. *J Arab Vet Ass*, 1963; 23:175-179.
4. Gohar MA, El-Kohly S, Elyan A. Incidence of brucellosis in human beings in Egypt. *J Bact* 1940: 54:101-109.
5. Shalaby MN. A survey on brucellosis as a cause of reproductive disorders in farm animals in Egypt. Ph.D. Thesis, Faculty of Vet. Med. Cairo Univ. 1986.
6. Kamel HM and Abd El-Fattah,AH. Incidence of brucellosis. *J Arab Vet Ass* 1971; 31:409-415.
7. Yehia SI. Trials for application of rapid tests in the detection of brucellosis. Second Ann. Vet. Congress, Cairo, Egypt, 1961.
8. Zaki R. B. *abortus* infection in buffaloes, ewes and camels. Isolation of the organism from milk. M.V.Sc. thesis, Faculty of Vet. Med., Cairo Univ. 1943.
9. Roushdy A. Incidence of pathogenic bacteria in market milk in Cairo. M.V.Sc. thesis, Faculty of Vet. Med., Cairo Univ. 1944.
10. Kamel HM. Incidence of brucellosis. *J Arab Vet Ass* 1971; 21:510-519.
11. El-Gibaly, SM. Studies on brucellosis in dairy animals in UAR. Ph.D. thesis, Faculty of Vet. Med., Cairo Univ. 1969.
12. El-Gibaly, SM. Preliminary studies on epidemiology of brucellosis as a zoonotic disease in an infected area in Egypt. First Arab Biologist Congress, Alexandria, Egypt, 1977.
13. Sayour EM, El-Gibaly, SM and El-Naasan A. Investigation on the common *Brucella* strains in UAR. *J Egypt Vet Med Ass* 1970; 30:109-120.
14. Refai M, El-Gibaly, SM and Salem, ThF. Studies on brucellosis in cows and buffaloes in Egypt. International Buffalo Congress, New Delhi, 1988.

Chapter Thirty

Construction of National Epidemiological Data Bases: Data Acquisition, Storage, Retreival, Analysis and Accessibility   *Steve Weber*

Use of computers to assist in the management of a national disease control program began with the Brucellosis Information System in 1981. Since then data from other national disease programs, including Tuberculosis and Pseudorabies, have been automated. Many of the ideas presented in this paper though, will be based on the initial concepts learned during implementation of the Brucellosis Information System.

Attention will be given to all aspects of integration of automation with an existing animal disease program-including the need for automation, the initial design of an applicable data base, accurate data collection and entry onto the data base, retrieval and analysis of the collected data, and finally a redesign of the entire process.

Need for Automation

For 50 years information on Brucellosis was collected through clinical studies at universities, field trials, and through the U.S. Department of Agriculture (USDA) and industry sponsored research. These data proved invaluable in defining the disease and determining methods of controlling its transmission.

Unfortunately, at the same time, some of the most epidemiologically relevant data derived from Brucellosis testing, surveillance and eradication procedures lay unreferenceable in a multitude of filing cabinets in state and federal offices throughout the United States.

Perhaps these data are in part, what Dr. Winthrop Ray was referring to in 1977 at the International Symposium on Bovine Brucellosis when he said, "Much of the basic epidemiology (of brucellosis) was described by 1930 and remains to be discovered by each succeeding generation."[1]

That fact was also recognized by the National Academy of Sciences Subcommittee on Brucellosis and the Brucellosis Technical Commission in 1977. Both groups determined that greater use could be made of the information that had been generated from the brucellosis program. The

Technical Commission went further and suggested that the Animal and Plant Health Inspection Service (APHIS) investigate automation of the data.

The Administrator of APHIS endorsed the concept of automation and in 1980 the Brucellosis Information System (BIS) project was initiated.

Design of an Automated System

The initial concept of the application of automation did not incorporate a need to change the existing methods of operation within the Brucellosis eradication program. Rather, the data base was designed primarily to serve as a reservoir for all data which was requested on brucellosis test charts. Since then, experience has shown that the application of automation to a national disease control program can be a catalyst for analyzing and optimizing operational methods that may have been considered standard.

The data base design team, including epidemiologists, veterinarians, systems analysts and computer programmers, interviewed potential users and beneficiaries of the system to provide the background necessary to understand the Brucellosis program. They traveled with veterinarians to view the various brucellosis testing procedures and went to laboratories and State offices to follow the processing of the data collected. They also analyzed existing national and local reports to determine potential uses for the data collected.

Because reasons were not provided to modify the type of information collected, the data elements for the designed data base included all information currently collected during brucellosis testing in the field and at market and slaughter plants. These data elements encompassed both epidemiological and administrative aspects of the brucellosis program.

The design process basically defined the relationship between each of the data elements to most efficiently process, store and retrieve them. Computer hardware and software were also assessed to determine the technological architecture that would best accommodate the program procedures and data base as defined. The necessary constraints for this determination included the potential volume of national brucellosis data and the type of computer technology available for purchase by government agencies.

The tremendous volume of expected data dictated the processing capability of a mainframe computer. Due to this volume, a centralized data processing environment was designed. A Sperry/Univac mainframe computer was purchased and installed within an existing USDA computer facility in Ft. Collins, Colorado, to serve as the central computer.

The design included entry of brucellosis testing data onto Harris minicomputers located in state or federal offices and laboratories. The data would then be transmitted to the mainframe computer. The USDA contracted with Telenet communications to facilitate the data transmission. The telecommunications network also provided a means for retrieving information from the central site by the state and federal offices and field locations.

Unfortunately, computer hardware and software choices were made without adequate consideration of future needs and the user's desire for additional unique data elements. This proved to be a limiting factor in progressive utilization of BIS due to a lack of alternative uses for the system as designed. Nevertheless, programming for the system was initiated and, in 1981, New Mexico became the first state to enter and transmit brucellosis data to the Brucellosis Information System.

Throughout the next 4 years, other aspects of the brucellosis program were automated. The complete automated program included 10 data entry modules: herd, market and slaughter testing, vaccination, brucellosis milk ring test (BRT), indemnity, transportation, importation, herd status and epidemiology. These data were stored in six separate data bases for each state using the specific modules. Data from all states were not integrated because of initial concerns about privacy of information.

Automation for all aspects of the brucellosis program was completed in 1985 and at the height of its use there were 200 various modules being used by 47 different states.

Data Acquisition

As stated previously, data for BIS was acquired mainly from brucellosis test charts completed by accredited practitioners and regulatory personnel. These test charts included testing performed in the field and at market and slaughter. All data present on the test chart could be entered. Some data elements were mandatory because they were key fields of the data base and therefore needed to be present for all records.

Other data fields were edited at the time of entry to increase the integrity of the data. These fields included those data elements that were of a prescribed format, such as eartags, or those elements limited to specific values, such as sex or breed.

Obtaining test chart data that was complete, accurate and legible was one of the greatest difficulties to be overcome in order to ensure reliability. This problem was addressed in different manners and to different degrees by the various managers in each state. In many states, training classes were held specifically for completion of brucellosis test forms for veterinarians.

It was easy to achieve cooperation by regulatory personnel in most cases but letters and withholding of payments for testing to fee-basis veterinarians were sometimes required.

The aspect of data integrity remains vital to any automation. Effective decision making can only be done if the data on which the decisions are based is as accurate as possible. Additional efforts made within BIS to increase accuracy of data have included bar coding of information and the investigation of data entry devices to be used in the field thus avoiding data transcription errors.

Although brucellosis test charts were the primary source of information, data were also generated from health certificates, restricted movement permits, vaccination charts, indemnity claims, and epidemiology forms.

Most states entered data generated only after they came onto the system. Others though, took the time to enter all data previously collected on infected herds.

The herd status portion of the program was the most subjective portion of the program. It could be used as a dynamic list of classifications of herds, i.e., infected or quarantined. It was also used as a scheduling calendar for procedures that needed to take place such as investigation or retesting. Many times there were no documents for data entry that listed this particular information.

Because of this, the herd status module was one of the more difficult BIS modules. But once understood and utilized, it was a significant benefit to brucellosis program managers because it provided a means of tracking activities that previously were unmonitored.

Data entry was new for those who had not yet used an automated system. Changes had to be made in personnel responsibility assignments to allow for data entry. Processing time guidelines were established and documents to be entered were prioritized to ensure reasonably prompt entry of necessary data.

Data Storage

The data entered by the states were scheduled to be transmitted on a routine basis from the state's minicomputers to the Fort Collins Computer Center through the USDA telecommunications network. Once at the Center, additional data integrity checking was performed as the data were loaded nightly onto each state's data base. The following morning, a report was sent to each transmitting site listing the number of records processed and any errors that had been detected.

Although all BIS data bases were located on a Sperry/Univac 1180 mainframe, the modules of herd, market, slaughter, herd status, and import were integrated on a single DMS 1100 data base. The remaining modules each had a separate DMS 1100 hierarchial data base, with the exception of the vaccination module which was programmed for a DB4 relational data base. The lack of integration of all data bases for a state caused additional difficulty when information was retrieved.

The volume of data accumulated within the first 5 years of operation was enormous. So much so, that to conserve the costs of data storage, archiving techniques were proposed by a user group and initiated in 1985. The archived data were still accessible through microfiched reports and through the reloading of taped information but the utility of the system was subsequently decreased.

The volume of information on the system at the time of archiving was approximately 15 million records and annual costs for access and storage of information at the Fort Collins Computer Center were about $2,000,000.

To date, approximately 50 million brucellosis test records have been entered onto the system. However, the costs and amount of on line data have increased only slightly due to data archiving, alternative initiatives by state agricultural departments, and the distributed processing efforts by Veterinary Services.

Retrieval, Analysis, and Accessibility

The major learning problem to overcome in initiating an automated system was not data acquisition or entry. It was retrieval and use of the data once they were on the system. Early in the process of automation, the states were almost mandated to use the system. Later use was primarily due to necessity rather than decree.

Although data retrieval classes were held, the initial target audience was not at the correct level. To increase use of the systems, the managers and epidemiologists needed to understand the available information.

A similar lack of understanding in relation to surveillance systems in general is identified by Schwabe in his book, *Veterinary Medicine and Human Health* "Recognition of the need is there on the part of many veterinarians and so is the desire, but knowledge of what the tools are is still too frequently lacking."[2]

Unfortunately, because veterinarians were not the targeted audience, they grew to depend on data entry clerks and program records supervisors for retrieval of information. Their initial lack of understanding of the system and the information it could provide potentiated a fear of sharing data between states and a continued reliance on hard copy documents rather than the data base for answers.

Numerous reports were written and specialized retrieval statements were formatted to assist in data retrieval. These reports could be transmitted to the office or to anywhere a portable terminal was taken that had access to a phone line. For the most part, data was accessible 24 hours a day, except during the period when a data base was being updated.

Inaccuracies in data often became more visible as that data was aggregated and retrieved in an automated report type format. Those not in favor of an automated system were quick to point out those inaccuracies without realizing that many of those same inaccuracies existed on the hard copy documents from which the data were entered.

Correct user identification numbers and passwords were required for data retrieval from a state's database. The state's password could be shared among users but initially was not. As Veterinary Services regional epidemiologists began using the system, they generally were provided with passwords for all states within their region.

The single most valuable function within BIS that caused epidemiologists and program managers to increasingly use the system was the capability of tracing eartags or other forms of animal identification within and between states. This capability more than anything else has created a dependence on automation in some states and the willingness to share data in many.

Unfortunately, there is still not a major emphasis on the brucellosis data in an epidemiologic sense. Few, if any, theories have been proposed or substantiated on the basis of the data that has been automated. Few requests for data have been received from industry or university entities. In-depth analysis of data for specific trends or other epidemiologic elements has not occurred.

Overall, though, the creation of a national data base has been invaluable for the Brucellosis Eradication Program. The widespread use of BIS represented for the first time in many years a consistency in the way data were reported. The automated scheduling of retests, follow up on investigations, and identification of milk patrons needing to be resampled have been made routine in some States. Also, as previously mentioned, many program directors have grown dependent on the system for the tracing of animals.

Perhaps the most significant indicator of the benefit that a potential change could provide to a program is the willingness to redesign the operational procedures of the program to optimize the incorporation of that change. The recognized benefit of automation of brucellosis data is now evidenced by the redesign of the operational aspects of the brucellosis program that has occurred at some state levels and the reconsideration of data necessary for disease control which is now occurring at the national level.

Summary

As national epidemiologic data bases are constructed for other animal disease control programs, several concepts may be applied from the experiences gained during construction of the data base for brucellosis.

First of all, the use of an effective national automated program cannot be mandated but must be generated on the basis of the benefits it can provide. The automation has to provide a recognizable benefit for a previously determined resource cost which the users are willing to pay. This includes both short-term and long-term benefits and should be presented as such. The benefits can be incorporated into the program based upon users' needs and with their input.

User input is desireable from all levels of potential use but is essential from those who are directing and managing the animal disease program. It is their understanding and acceptance of the system that will result in a recognition of the system is potential and therefore increase its use and effectiveness.

Secondly, the system has to be developed with a specific data set in mind. It is too expensive in development time and data acquisition costs, in data entry resources, and in data base storage costs, to try to automate all available data.

A consistent data set among all states needs to be specified by program managers on the basis of epidemiological and statistical principals to accurately represent the status of the disease control program and emerging trends. The data requested should be considered on the basis of their relationship to the program, their obtainability, and the cost of acquisition. As data trends develop, the existing data set may then be modified to further clarify specific aspects. The length of time that on-line access will be required for these data elements must be determined initially, as well as the need for potential automated integration of data. Computer hardware and software should be chosen on the basis of these potential volumes of data, processing and output specifications, and the requirements for data access.

Thirdly, it is important that national systems be developed with a balance of data integrity and consistency and with a flexibility that will accommodate minor variations in an overall operational program. User's needs differ throughout the country. Additional incentive for use of the program can be provided by allowing such flexibility. However, it is extremely important to have consistency and integrity in the central core of data so that statistics can be relied on and trends accurately interpreted. Codes that are initiated for data elements need to be easily interpreted to avoid additional integrity problems.

Fourthly, training and support of an automated system are vital for its initial and continued use. A system must be designed for ease of use and understanding, but thorough training and prompt attention to problems are also necessary. Feedback from users is vital, and appropriate action on the feedback is required. The appropriate audience must be trained initially by those who understand both the disease program and the automated application. Others should be trained as back-up personnel and additional support. Easy-to-follow documentation is necessary to supplement the training and additional implements such as tutorials are helpful.

It is critical that the automated data base systems which are developed and implemented become part of a routine procedure in disease management. Not only do the data need to be acquired and reported by a method that ensures integrity, but they must be entered onto the system in a timely fashion with attention to accuracy. Routine management of the data bases is also necessary to ensure data integrity and timely access to the data.

Finally, and probably of most importance in the construction of national data bases, the automated data have to be routinely used by program managers and epidemiologists. It is the use of data that gives credence to the arduous and costly task of collecting and entering that data. And it is the interpretation of the data that is necessary to assess the status of the disease program and to specify modifications that need to be made to the automated or operational programs. These modifications, once determined, allow the adaptation of a static automated and operational program to a dynamic disease environment to provide continued efficiency and effectiveness.

References

1. *Bovine Brucellosis An International Symposium.* College Station, Texas: Texas A&M University Press, 1977.
2. Schwabe CW. *Veterinary Medicine and Human Health.* Third edition. Baltimore: Williams & Wilkins, 1984.

Abstracts

Epidemiology and Control of Brucellosis in North China

Jian-Lin Zhang
Department of Brucellosis
Institute of Epidemiology and Microbiology
Chinese Academy of Preventive Medicine
Beijing, China

Around 1960, there was a high incidence of human and animal brucellosis in China, particularly in the 11 provinces and regions of northern China. The main sources of infection for human brucellosis were infected sheep and goats. The relative frequency and routes of shedding *Brucella* by infected female sheep and goats were found as follows: aborted litter 100%, milk 38.4%, placenta 27%, vaginal discharge 20.5%, urine 3.4%; it was not found in blood or feces. The *Brucella* excreted from milk lasted over 90 days while the *Brucella* in vaginal discharge and urine persisted no longer than 90 days after abortion. It could be isolated from 65% of vaginal discharges within 30 days after abortion. From 1950 to 1960, the so-called "comprehensive measure" could not be successfully applied in China. Later, a new measure for control of animal brucellosis was used in China. The major procedure was to vaccinate all livestock (without testing whether they were positive or negative) by inoculation once a year and 4 to 5 years later and to slaughter all the old sheep and goats including the positives. An experimental field study was carried out in a county of Inner Mongolia for seven years. The positive rate of *Brucella* isolated from aborted litters before vaccination was 59%. After vaccination, positive levels were 12.2% in the first year; 0.3% the second year, and 0% last year. Almost the same results were obtained as those after taking a set of so called "comprehensive measure." After that, the above-mentioned measure was applied to all areas where brucellosis-infected sheep and goats were found in China. The morbidity of brucellosis in humans and animals so far has been found to decline sharply.

A Comparative Study of Different Species of *Brucella* on the Immunosuppression Effect of Plaque Forming Cells in Inbred Mice

Jian-Lin Zhang, Lian-Fan Yang, Bao-Lan Guo,
and Chun-Huai Chui
Department of Brucellosis
Institute of Epidemiology and Microbiology
Chinese Academy of Preventive Medicine,
Beijing, China

The pathogenesis of brucellosis is not yet completely clear. In general, the clinical pictures of the patients infected with *B. melitensis* are more serious than those infected with *B. abortus*. The mechanism of the phenomenon is rather complicated. An experimental study on the plaque-forming cell (PFC) responses in inbred mice was carried out. The mice were infected with one million viable cells of *B. melitensis* and *B. abortus*, Five days later the sheep red blood cells (SRBC) were injected intraperitoneally into five mice per group of BALB/c mice. Four days later the mice were killed and the spleen cells were used in the PFC assay by using the Yamada method.

It was found that there was a significant immunosuppression of PFC with *B. melitensis*. In contrast, there was no effect on PFC in the case of *B. abortus*. The average number of plaques per drop was 21.4-5.8 in *B. melitensis;* 41.6-7.3 in *B. abortus;* and 49.4-5.8 in the positive control. The p value of *B. melitensis* was less than 0.01 when compared with the control, while the p value of *B. abortus* was more than 0.05 when compared with the positive control. When the effects on the supernatants of the culture medium of these two strains were studied, a similar significant difference was revealed between them. On the contrary, 100 to 500 µg dose of the endotoxin was found to stimulate PFC response in BALB/c mice.

A kinetics study on the suppressive effects of the above *Brucella* on PFC responses in C57/BL mice was also undertaken. The initial time and degree suppression were different. *B. melitensis* had a significant suppression at the earlier stage of infection while the suppressive effect of *B. abortus* started only at the middle stage of infection.

The data provided a lead for studying the question of why there are different clinical pictures of *B. melitensis* and *B. abortus* infections in human brucellosis.

DNA Polymorphism in Strains of the Genus *Brucella* as Shown by Restriction Fragment Analysis and Partial Physical Map

A.A. Servent, M.J.N. Carles, S. Michaux, G. Bourg, and M. Ramuz
Institut National de la Santé et de la Recherche Médicale
Nîmes, France

The purpose of this study was to determine the genomic support of the differences between species in the genus *Brucella* and to establish a partial physical map of five *Brucella* strain chromosomes. Preparations of DNA from 23 *Brucella* strains including 19 reference strains were compared by restriction endonuclease analysis. Pulsed-field gel electrophoresis resulted in optimal resolution of fragments generated by digestion with low-cleavage-frequency restriction enzymes such as XbaI. By this technique, five electrophoretypes were distinguished in five reference strains of the different species, i.e. *B. abortus, B. melitensis, B. suis, B. canis* and *B. ovis*. Minor profile differences allowed us to discriminate between most biovars within a species. However, the differences in the DNA patterns of different field strains of biovar 2 of *B. melitensis* were not sufficient to serve as markers for epidemiological studies. From the XbaI fragments, we were able to estimate the size of the genomes of *B. abortus* 544[T], *B. melitensis* 16M[r] and *B. suis* 1330[T]. This method revealed a relationship between DNA fingerprints, species, and pathovars that could shed light on problems concerning the classification and evolution of members of the genus *Brucella*.

Furthermore, six recombinant clones have been isolated from a *Brucella* DNA library in the λgt11 bacteriophage with four monoclonal antibodies and a polyclonal serum. Recombinant-derived probes were hybridized with Southern blots of the XbaI digests of the five species *B. melitensis, B. abortus, B. suis, B. canis,* and *B. ovis*. Restriction fragments from the five strains were labeled with different probes, which made it possible to map several fragments corresponding to almost one-fourth (564 to 618 kb according to the strain) of the 2600-kb-long *Brucella* chromosome. This study demonstrated some differences in the distribution of the XbaI restriction sites between these five species.

Brucella Antibodies in Veterinarians Exposed to Strain 19

E.J. Young

Veterans Administration
Medical Center and Baylor College of Medicine
Houston, Texas

Veterinarians and others whose occupations place them in close contact with animals are at increased risk of contracting brucellosis. The risk of disease from exposure to Strain 19 vaccine remains less well defined. We studied the prevalence of antibodies to *Brucella* in the sera of veterinarians engaged in bovine brucellosis eradication with attention to exposure to Strain 19. Sera from this group was compared with sera from patients with pathogens other than *Brucella* and with normal volunteers. Antibodies were determined using the serum agglutination test (SAT) and 2-mercaptoethanol (2ME) in order to distinguish between IgM and IgG agglutinins.

We studied 42 individuals (37 veterinarians, five technicians) ranging in age from 27-66 years (mean age 45 years). The 36 men and six women had from one to 40 years of brucellosis experience (mean 14.8 years). Six reported previous brucellosis (five diagnosed serologically, one proven bacteriologically). Fifteen of 42 (37.7%) reported known accidental exposure to Strain 19 (nine needle stick, three eye splashes, three unspecified); 32 (76%) were negative by SAT and 41 (97.6%) were negative by 2ME-agglutination. Of the 10 SAT positive sera, six had low ($\leq$1:40) titers of IgM antibodies. Of interest, four had titers $\geq$1:80, which is in the range generally considered "suspicious" for brucellosis; however, these antibodies were also of the IgM class. Only one sample contained IgG (2ME-resistant) antibodies, and this was in low titer (1:20), not suggestive of active infection. There was no correlation between a history of prior brucellosis, previous positive serology, or exposure to Strain 19 and the presence of antibodies at the time of the study. No patients with other infections, and no normal volunteers had antibodies to *Brucella*.

Conclusions: 1) More than one-third of veterinarians sampled reported accidents using Strain 19 vaccine; 2) despite such exposure, only 10 of 42 individuals at risk had antibodies to *Brucella* when tested; 3) there was no correlation between a history of vaccine accidents and the presence of antibodies at the time of survey; 4) antibodies detected were predominantly IgM agglutinins, suggesting residual titers from past exposure. In view of the millions of doses of vaccine administered, the product appears safe and poses limited risk to vaccinators.

Bovine Brucellosis: A Sero-Epidemiological Survey in Morocco

A. Benkirane,* A. Tber,* B Faïk,*** R. Azilaf,**
A. Fikri,**and D.W. Johnson*
*Department of Microbiology, Immunology and Infectious Disease
Institut Agronomique et Veterinaire Hassan II, Rabat;
**Division of Animal Health- Ministry of Agriculture, Rabat; and
***National Veterinary Laboratory, Casablanca, Morocco

The purpose of the survey was to evaluate the prevalence of bovine brucellosis in Morocco in 1987-1988. Based on the epidemiological situation of bovine brucellosis in Morocco (presented at this symposium), a national eradication program was set up. Due to the infection rate and for economic reasons, the principle of "test and slaughter" at the initial phase of the program has been ruled out. A discrimination has been made between regions according to their infection rate at the herd level:

In the first group of 21 highly infected provinces (more than 2% herds infected) it has been decided to:

1. vaccinate female calves aged 4 to 7 months with B19 Vaccine

2. indelibly mark male reactors with the letter "B" and prohibit their use in reproduction.

3. systematically record bovine abortions; test the aborting cows for brucellosis (bacteriology and Rivanol test). Mark the positive animals with the letter "B" and slaughter them within two months.

The second group includes eight provinces which have an infection rate of less than 2%. In this group, each herd is to be individually checked for brucellosis, first with the Ring test (RT) (bulk tank 8 to 30 individuals) then with Rose Bengal Test (RBT) and Complement Fixation Test (CFT) for positive reactors on R.T:

1. Negative herds will be submitted to the same test yearly.

2. Positive herds will be handled like those of the first group.

The third group (11 provinces) is supposed to be brucellosis free. To maintain this status, the movements of animals must be controlled and a sero-epidemiological study conducted every two years.

Furthermore, during the fifth year of the program, a new sero-epidemiological study at the national level will be performed and the eradication program reconsidered and economically evaluated. We expect that by that time the infection rate will have been brought to a level low enough to stop vaccination and to continue improved sanitation.

A Diagnostic Test for Brucellosis Using Polymerase Chain Reaction

A. Fekete,* M.R. Sanborn,**S.M. Halling,**** and J.A. Bantle*

Departments of Zoology* and Microbiology**
Oklahoma State University, Stillwater, Oklahoma
United States Department of Agriculture/
Agricultural Research Service,*** Ames, Iowa

We are exploring the possibility that the recently developed technique of polymerase chain reaction can be used as a diagnostic test for brucellosis. Polymerase chain reaction offers the advantage of amplifying only a portion of the genome of *Brucella* so that it can be readily detected using agarose gel electrophoresis. Because the amplification factor is greater than 100,000, a signal can be observed even though the *Brucella* DNA is only a small portion of the DNA extracted from the infected host. In our present study we cloned an outer membrane protein gene of *Brucella abortus* Strain 19 into a pUC19 vector. The ends of an EcoR I fragment 635 bp in length were sequenced and 25 bp primers on opposite strands were synthesized making sure that there were no internal complementary regions present. The plasmid served as a template DNA for the first set of reactions. The resulting signal was great enough to immediately attempt an amplification of *Brucella* Strain 19 DNA (1μg) as a template even though we had not yet optimized the reaction. This amplification was successful and a similar amount of *Escherichia coli* K12 DNA tested negative except for some small fragments with sizes less than 635 bp. In another experiment we successfully amplified an 810 bp region of the lac Z gene out of this sample of *E. coli* DNA showing that the Taq polymerase could work on this sample. Despite these limited experiments, the amplification was fast and easy to perform.

Our next series of experiments dealt with adjusting the components of the assay. We found the optimum Mg^{++} ion concentration to be 3mM Mg^{++}/ 0.8 3 mM dNTP (a ratio of 3.75 to 1). The optimal Taq polymerase concentration is 2.5 U Taq polymerase (AmpliTaq-Perkin Elmer Cetus) per 100 ml of reaction mixture. The optimum primer concentration was 1 mM primer. The thermocycler settings are denaturation 90.5°C- 1.5 minutes, primer annealing 60°C- 1 minute, and primer extension 72°C- 1 minute (inside tube measurements). We can amplify the template up to 50 cycles on the thermocycler.

We have only tested *Escherichia coli* K12 and HB101 DNA as a heterologous template. No significant cross-reaction was observed. Before continuing the testing with heterologous DNAs we wanted to confirm the presence of the 635 bp sequence in all species and some of the strains of

Brucella first. By successfully detecting the gene in all species, we would prove that the test would not produce false negatives. The samples for this test included *B. melitensis, B. abortus* 544, *B. abortus* S19, *B. abortus* 2308, *B. canis, B. abortus* f.s. 8-0840, *B. abortus* f.s. 8-1070, *B. ovis, B. suis, B. neotomae.* We successfully amplified the 635 bp region in each sample. We have learned from preliminary testing of the *B. abortus* S19 DNA that the DNA needs to be very pure in order for the reaction to work. We used a special CTAB purification to remove lipopolysaccharide from the preparation.

We have detected as little as 5 pg of purified S19 *Brucella* DNA but we should be able to detect the gene fragment in even smaller quantities of *Brucella* DNA. In summary, the outlook for a polymerase chain reaction test for brucellosis appears promising.

Epidemiological Study of Abortions in Cattle Infected with *Brucella melitensis*

M.Banai,* I. Mayer,* R. Versano,* E. Katz,* A. Cohen,*
M. Davidson,** and H. Adler**
*Dept. of Bacteriology, Kimron Veterinary Institute and
**Veterinary Field Services, Ministry of Agriculture, Beit Dagan, Israel

In November 1988, *Brucella melitensis* infection of a cattle herd in Kibbutz Bat-Haemek, in Israel was identified. Unpasteurized ovine whey used to water the animals was the suspected source of infection. At the time, the herd included 300 *B. abortus* S19 vaccinated Israeli Holstein milking cows and 132 vaccinated heifers, and 75 imported nonvaccinated Simmental heifers. At first, nine animals from the Israeli breed and one Simmental were identified positive and slaughtered. Subsequently, a test and slaughter program was implemented using bacteriological and conventional serological tests to diagnose infected animals. *B. melitensis* biotype 3 was isolated in all cases of bacteriological confirmation of the disease. In spite of eliminating the infected animals at first notice of infection, new positive reactors have continuously been identified. Since 1988, 15 (20%) Simmental and 42 (9.7%) Israeli cows were found positive reactors, and have been slaughtered.

The rate of abortions in the Israeli breed, assuming 371 pregnant cows during 1988, was 4.5%, resembling normal values of abortions in other healthy cattle herds in the area. Compared with *B. abortus* infection, this annual value indicates a trend of a lower abortion percentage. However, in view of the fact that the disease was confirmed in the herd only by the last term of the year and because positive pregnant cows were eliminated before due term, this value may not represent accurately the real contribution of *B. melitensis* infection to abortions in cattle. Therefore, we attempted direct isolation of *Brucella* from serologically positive reactors amongst pregnant cows and heifers and aborted fetuses. One of three cows that had aborted prior to the outbreak period and were later found to be positive reactors had excreted *Brucella* in its milk. Also *Brucella* was isolated from aborted fetuses belonging to two Simmental cows and one 6-year-old Israeli cow. In other cases, animals slaughtered at pregnancy were confirmed bacteriologically positive and *Brucella* was not isolated from their fetuses.

We concluded: a) The manifestation of *B. melitensis* infection in cattle is not synchronous with the contamination event, and is enhanced in pregnancy, b) *B. melitensis* can cause abortions in cattle especially in nonvaccinated animals or when vaccination immunity is decreased, c) Abortions contribute to the spread and perpetuation of infection in the herd, d) In the very last days, when this abstract was already concluded, 16 more previously negative Simmental cows have been identified serologically positive after normal calving. Therefore, all the animals belonging to this breed were slaughtered.

Smooth Lipopolysaccharide Heterogeneity Among *Brucella* Biovars Related to A and M Specificities: Sodium Dodecyl Sulfate-Polyacrylamide Gel Electrophoresis and Immunoblotting Analysis with Murine Monoclonal Antibodies and Rabbit, Bovine, or Caprine Polyclonal Mono- and Poly-specific Sera

B. Garin-Bastuji,* R. Bowden,**G. Dubray,** J. Limet,***
*Centre National d'Etudes Vétérinaires et Alimentaires, Laboratoire
Central de Recherches Vétérinaires, Maisons-Alfort, France,
**Institut National de la Recherches Agronomique
Station de Pathologie de la Reproduction Nouzilly, France,
***Unit of Experimental Medicine, International Institute of Cellular
and Molecular Pathology, Brussels, Belgium

The purpose of this study was to determine the relationship between A and M specificities and sodium dodecyl sulfate-polyacrylamide gel electrophoresis (SDS-PAGE) profiles of various smooth lipopolysaccharide

(S-LPS) fractions of *Brucella*. S-LPS-enriched fractions from reference and field strains of various biovars of *Brucella abortus, B. melitensis,* or *B. suis* were prepared 1) by the hot phenol-water method (LPS-F5); or 2) by hot SDS extraction and proteinase K digestion (LPS-PK); or 3) dimethyl sulfoxide extraction (LPS-DMSO). The fractions were then analyzed by SDS-PAGE coupled with periodic oxidation and silver staining or immunoblotting, either with LPS -A or -M specific monoclonal antibodies or polyclonal mono- or poly-specific sera from rabbit, cattle, or goats.

Molecular weights of the most represented subunits of S-LPS were estimated between 30-60kD and two electrophoretypes were distinguished according to A or M immunodominance regardless of the fraction tested: a close succession of regularly spaced narrow bands for A>M strains and regularly spaced triplets of bands including either 1) a first thin band followed by two thick bands for *B. abortus* M>A strains or 2) one thick band between two thin bands for *B. melitensis* and *B. suis* M>A strains.

This assesses the reproducibility of distinct S-LPS molecular, patterns for A and M specificities in relation to Wilson and Miles description and confirmed here by sandwich enzyme immunoassay and latex agglutination inhibition with monoclonal antibodies and polyclonal sera.

Cloning of *Brucella abortus* Genes Coding for Proteins Immunologically Active Cows

O.L. Rossetti, S.G. Rossi, P.A. Oszlak, S.L. Cravero
Instituto de Biologia Molecular, CICV-INTA
Buenos Aires, Argentina

Little is known about the immune response elicited by constituent proteins of *Brucella abortus* due to the difficulty in obtaining LPS-free proteins. Recombinant DNA technology offers the possibility of having high-purity proteins without contaminants from *Brucella*.

The purpose of this study was to isolate of genes from a λgt11 library coding for proteins which could induce a measurable immune response.

A *B. abortus* S19 DNA library was obtained by cutting the DNA with AluI and RsaI and cloning the 200 to 7000 bp pieces in the λgt11 vector system. Rabbit antisera against a whole lysate of Brucella's cells was prepared, which together with *E. coli* Y1090 was used to screen the library. More than 100 positive clones were isolated and lysogenized in *E. coli* Y1089.

All the clone lysates from isopropyl-thio-galactopyranoside (IPTG)-induced recombinant lysogens show prominent protein bands in the molecular weight range of 116 to 170 KD, as seen by SDS-PAGE. When the lysates were analyzed by Western blotting, fusion and non-fusion proteins were detected; some of the proteins were negative.

Clone 31 gave a strong reaction when tested against the rabbit antisera. The same result was obtained when assayed against a cow antisera prepared by immunizing an animal with 5×10^{10} cells of the vaccinial strain *B. abortus* S19. Specific antibodies against the protein expressed by clone 31 were purified from the polyclonal rabbit antisera by their affinity to the protein bound to nitrocellulose. SDS-PAGE of whole, membrane, and soluble fractions of *B. abortus* prepared by differential centrifugation, were run and a western blot was performed using the antibodies purified by affinity. One band of 60 KD was seen in the whole and soluble fractions, but no band appeared in the membrane fraction. The 60 KD was coincident with a band present in a western blot of whole bacterial proteins developed with bovine sera. When the 31 insert was subcloned in pP06 and induced with IPTG, a 50-KD positive band was seen when tested with polyclonal or affinity purified rabbit sera.

These results show that a 50-KD protein expressed by a clone derived from a *B. abortus* DNA library is recognized by antibodies elicited by a 60-KD protein present in the soluble fraction of *B. abortus* S19.

The gene coding for this protein is being mutagenized to be later inserted by conjugation and recombination into the *B. abortus* genome to obtain a new vaccinial strain able to induce an immune response different from that elicited by the field strains.

Cloning and Expression of *Brucella abortus* 60 and 66 Kilodalton Immunogenic Proteins in *Escherichia coli*

R.M. Roop II, * S.M. Boyle,* ** N. Sriranganathan,* **
and G.G. Schurig, **

*Department of Microbiology and Immunology
University of Arkansas for Medical Sciences, Little Rock, Arkansas,
**Department of Pathobiology, Virginia-Maryland Regional College of
Veterinary Medicine, Blacksburg, Virginia

The purposes of this study were 1) to express *Brucella abortus* antigens in recombinant *Escherichia coli* clones, and 2) to determine the potential immunologic significance of these recombinant antigens. Because they do not share the problems associated with contamination by immunodominant LPS that are often observed in native *B. abortus* fractions, recombinant *B. abortus* antigens should be provide useful tools for evaluating the role of individual antigens in the protective immune response to brucellosis. *Sau*3A fragments of *B. abortus* 2308 DNA were ligated into the *Bam*HI site of the plasmid vector pUC9 and the recombinant plasmid bank used to transform *E. coli* DH5-α. Approximately 4000 transformants were screened for the production of *B. abortus* antigens using a colony blot enzyme linked immunosorbent assay (ELISA). We obtained 14 independent clones that reacted with *B. abortus*-specific hyperimmune goat serum. To assess the potential immunologic importance of the *B. abortus* antigens expressed by these clones, the clones were tested in both colony blot ELISA and immunoblots with sera from mice experimentally infected with *B. abortus* 2308 and dogs naturally and experimentally infected with *B. canis*. Two clones producing recombinant *B. abortus* antigens reactive with sera from infected animals were further characterized. Clones designated II-16 and III-2 produced *B. abortus* antigens with apparent molecular weights of 60,000 and 66,000 daltons, respectively. Restriction enzyme analysis of the recombinant plasmids isolated from these clones indicated the presence of a 16-kilobase insert in II-16 and a 12-kilobase insert in III-2. The recombinant antigens expressed by both clones reacted strongly in immunoblots with sera from both *B. abortus*-infected mice and *B. canis*-infected dogs. These latter observations suggest that the recombinant *B. abortus* antigens expressed by clones II-16 and III-2 are potentially important in the immune response to brucellosis.

Cloning the Gene for Glucokinase from *Brucella abortus* Strain 19

R.C. Essenberg
Department of Biochemistry, Oklahoma State University,
Oklahoma Agricultural Experiment Station, Stillwater, Oklahoma

The means by which *Brucella abortus* cells obtain nutrients from their environment, especially that in the macrophage, have not been determined. In order to learn something of the cells, an attempt was made to isolate the genes for uptake and metabolism of glucose by complementing an *Escherichia coli* strain unable to transport and phosphorylate glucose. A library was constructed in the vector pUC9, using *Brucella* DNA partially cleaved with restriction endonuclease EcoRI. From this library were found plasmids that complemented the defect in the *E. coli* strain, either allowing growth on glucose, or leading to color production on indicator plates. Restriction maps and Southern blot analysis showed at least two different plasmids isolated in this way. One gives a much more positive phenotype. The part of it giving rise to the positive growth phenotype has been isolated to 2000 bp by subcloning and exonucleaseIII-produced deletions from both ends. A smaller fragment, 1500 bp, still gives an indicator medium positive phenotype. The insert works in either orientation in the vector and does not require isopropyl-thio-galactopyranoside (IPTG) for induction, so may be operating from a *Brucella* promoter. Glucokinase activity has been restored in the *E. coli* mutant by this plasmid.

Cloning and Expression in *Escherichia coli* of Seven *Brucella* Outer Membrane Proteins

Ph. de Wergifosse, * *J. Van Broeck,* * *F. de Sauvage,* *
J.M. Verger, * * *A. Cloeckaert,* * *G. Dubray,* * * *J.N. Octave,*
and J.N. Limet *
*Catholic University of Louvain, Belgium, ''Institut National de la Recherche Agronomique, Nouzilly, France

Antibodies to *Brucella* induced by vaccination or infection are nearly indistinguishable by classical tests. A vaccine and a diagnostic test, using different recombinant antigens, will solve this problem and speed up brucellosis eradication.

Identification of protective or potential diagnostic antigens is made difficult by the inadequacy of classical purification techniques to produce native outer membrane proteins (OMP) devoid of lipopolysaccharide (LPS) contamination. The 25-27 and 36-38 kDa OMPS are the major constituents of the vaccinal sodium dodecyl sulfate (SDS)-insoluble fraction of the cell walls and could be implicated in cellular immunity. Cloning of the corresponding gene was therefore undertaken.

Fragments (0.5-6 Kb) of *B. abortus* DNA were first cloned in the λgt11 expression vector. The genomic library was screened with monoclonal antibodies (MAbs), (described in the accompanying poster, Cloeckaert et al.) directed against 4 OMPs of apparent molecular weight 25-27, 31, 36-38, and 89 kDa. As the proteins were expressed as β-galactosidase fusion proteins, a partial digest (Sau3A) of *B. abortus* DNA (9-32 Kb fragment) was ligated to λEMBL3 arms. Positive plaques were also detected in this genomic library by the MAbs raised against the 10, 16.5, 19, 25-27, 36-38 and 89 kDa OMPs. For the 25-27 and 36-38 kDa major OMPs, one of the λgt11 inserts hybridized with all the λgt11 and λEMBL3 phages DNA coding for corresponding OMP. A 1.2 Kb λgt11 DNA fragment coding for part of the 36-38 kDa porin was sequenced and among these 1.2 Kb, 152 nucleotides of the insert correspond to the partial sequence published by Ficht et al. (1988). When full genes became available, they will be subcloned in a suitable expression vector, purified and used for a protection assay after active and passive immunization.

As for the gene of the 31 kDa protein cloned by Mayfield et al. (1988), the expression of all these OMPs genes is apparently under the control of a *Brucella* DNA sequence which functions as a promoter in *E. coli*.

A Competition Enzyme Immunoassay for Brucellosis Diagnosis

A.P. MacMillan, I. Greiser-Wilke,** V. Moennig,** and L.A. Mathias**
*Food Agricultural Organization/World Health Organization Collaborating Centre for Brucellosis Reference and Research, Central Veterinary Laboratory, Weybridge, United Kingdom. **Institut für Virologie, Tierarztliche Hochschule Hannover, Federal Republic of Germany

The purpose of the study was to evaluate a competition enzyme immunoassay (cEIA) for the diagnosis of brucellosis in a variety of domestic animals.

Lipopolysaccharide (LPS) extracted from *Brucella abortus* Strain 99 by the hot phenol-hot water method was used to coat the wells of polystyrene micro titer plates. Test sera and controls were titrated in doubling dilutions from 1/2 to at least 1/128, and immediately either of two peroxidase conjugated murine monoclonal antibodies, BM38 or BM40, was added to each well. Both BM38 and BM40 had been raised following inoculation of mice with *B. melitensis* and had been shown previously to bind to *Brucella* LPS. Following incubation for 2 hours at 37°C, OPD was added and the optical density (OD) read after 10 minutes.

The complement fixation test, serum agglutination test and indirect EIA were carried out in parallel and in some cases *Brucella* was cultured.

Samples were tested from over 1,000 cattle, 1,000 pigs, 200 sheep, and 50 goats, including infected, vaccinated, and known *Brucella*-free animals. The cEIA showed a significantly superior sensitivity and specificity and was more simple to carry out than the other tests studied. The technique appears to offer great promise, particularly for use in developing countries.

Expression of *Brucella abortus* Cell-envelope Proteins in the Outer Membrane of *Escherichia coli*

H. Marquis,* S.W. Bearden,* B.A. Sowa,** T.A. Ficht*
Departments of Veterinary Microbiology and Parasitology,
**Veterinary Pathology, Texas A&M University,
College Station, Texas

Ficht et al. (*Infect. Immun.* 56: 2036-2046, 1989, submitted) cloned and sequenced a *B. abortus* gene locus (*omp* 2) coding for 33-kDa (*omp* 2a) and a 36-kDa (*omp* 2b, the *B. abortus* porin) proteins having 96% sequence homology over their shared length. The genes are situated on opposite strands and separated by 900-bp. Under laboratory conditions and in the original gene organization, only *omp* 2b is expressed in *B. abortus* or in *E. coli* transformed cells (ECB611/pAGF201). When the 900 bp DNA fragment separating both genes is inverted, *omp* 2a is expressed in ECB611/pAGF211.

The purpose of the present investigation is to determine the exact location of *omp* 2 gene products in the cell envelope of transformed *E. coli*. Cell envelopes of ECB611/pAGF201 and 211 are fractionated according to the technique described by Osborn et al. (*J. Biol. Chem.* 247: 3962-3972, 1972). Cells are harvested at mid-log growth phase, plasmolysed in sucrose, and treated with lysozyme and EDTA-forming spheroplasts which are lysed by an osmotic shock. Cell envelopes are fractionated on a sucrose gradient, and collected fractions are tested for NADH oxidase activity and protein concentration. Selected fractions are pooled according to their ratio of enzyme activity to protein concentration, the smaller value being attributed to the outer membrane fraction and the larger value to the inner membrane fraction. To evaluate the efficiency of separation, the ketodeoxy octenoate (KDO) content and the NADH oxidase activity of purified fractions are measured. Each fraction is resolved by SDS-PAGE and the proteins are electroblotted on nitrocellulose. Rabbit hyperimmune serum raised against *omp* 2b is absorbed with *E. coli* λgt11 lysate, and used to probe *B. abortus* proteins expressed in ECB611/ pAGF201 and 211. Both proteins have been detected in the outer membrane fraction of ECB611/ pAGF211 and 201 respectively. *Omp* 2a appears to be expressed at a much lower level than *omp* 2b. This result is not an artifact due to a lower affinity of the rabbit hyperimmune serum for *omp* 2a, since it has been previously demonstrated in *E. coli* maxicells that this protein is in fact expressed at a lower level than *omp* 2b in ECB611 transformed cells (Ficht et al. *Infect. Immun.*, submitted). Traces of both proteins have been detected in the respective IM fractions because of some cross-contamination with the OM fractions.

From these results, we can conclude that *omp* 2a and 2b code for outer membrane proteins of *B. abortus*. We hypothesize that *omp* 2a expression may be subject to coordinate regulation responding to a specific environmental signal, as has been reported for other virulent bacteria (Miller et al. *Science* 243: 916-922, 1989). In subsequent experiments, we will investigate the potential expression of *omp* 2a in *B. abortus* under various growth conditions.

Analysis of *Brucella* Genomic DNA for Polymorphism and Plasmids

S.M. Halling and E.S. Zehr
United States Department of Agriculture
Agricultural Research Center,
National Animal Disease Center, Ames, Iowa

DNA-DNA hybridization studies of Brucellae species show that the *Brucella* spp. are closely related. It has been reported that the expression level of two Brucellae cell surface proteins (BCSP), BCSP20 and BCSP31, which are conserved among the various Brucellae species, is variable. We wanted to study the relatedness of Brucellae strains by probing the BCS20 and BCS31 loci with characterized DNA probes.

Genomic DNA was isolated from each of the species of *Brucella* and from several *B. abortus* biovars, vaccine strains, and field strains. The DNA was treated with Eco RI or Hind III restriction endonuclease, electrophoresed through agarose, blotted onto nytran, and probed with biotin or radioactive labeled BCSP20 and BCSP31 gene sequences. A single instance of DNA polymorphism was found among the strains. No differences were found between the strains when the sizes of each of the labeled bands were analyzed when BCSP20 was used as a probe. However, when BCSP31 was used as a probe, *B. ovis* genomic DNA had two Hind III fragments that hybridized. One band was 1,250 base pairs (bp), and the other was 1,400 bp. The larger fragment was cloned and analyzed by restriction endonuclease mapping, and the polymorphism was found to map downstream of the coding region for BCSP31. Why one of the bands of *B. ovis* is the same size as the bands in the other strains of *Brucella* analyzed is being investigated.

The polymorphism noted at the BCS31 loci in genomic *B. ovis* DNA was analyzed further. This time, an Eco RI *B. ovis* genomic blot, rather than a Hind III blot, was probed. While the control, *B. abortus* Strain 19 (S19), had a single band, *B. ovis* had two bands. One of the bands was the same size as that labeled in the *B. abortus* S19 control. The other band was approximately 1,000 bp larger. When the *B. ovis* and *B. abortus* blots were stripped and probed with the 2.2 kilo-bp downstream sequences, the labeled fragment pattern did not change. The polymorphism may be the result of the insertion of approximately 1,000 bp.

When genomic DNA from 25 strains of Brucellae was analyzed by agarose gel electrophoresis, a large molecular weight DNA species was noted in the genomic DNA from all 25 strains. The data are consistent with all the species of Brucellae containing a large singe copy number plasmid. Mapping and cloning studies are in progress.

Brucellae strains are genetically closely related, even when DNA hybridization was used to study specific loci. A single polymorphism was noted. We believe Brucellae strains carry a large low-copy-number plasmid.

A Comparison of Proteins and Genomic DNA of Species and Biovars of *Brucella*

E.S. Zehr and S.M. Halling
United States Department of Agriculture
Agricultural Research Center,
National Animal Disease Center, Ames, Iowa

The genus *Brucella* is divided into six species, each having a different natural host. DNA-DNA hybridization studies have revealed that all the species are closely related. As differences noted in protein banding and in DNA fingerprinting may be linked to host virulence, we analyzed whole-cell lysates and genomic DNA of 25 *Brucella* strains for differences. All *Brucella* species and biovars, as well as several *B. abortus* vaccine and field strains, were included in the study.

For protein analysis, cultures were grown in the presence of carbon dioxide on tryptose agar plates supplemented with 0.5% agar and 5% bovine serum. Cells were killed with methanol and boiled in sample buffer in the absence of reducing agent. Whole-cell lysates were analyzed on 10 to 20% gradient sodium dodecyl sulfate-polyacrylamide gels. Gradient gel results showed differences between all strains; however, fewer differences were noted when members within the same species were compared with each other.

Genomic DNA was isolated from methanol-killed cells. Cells were suspended in sucrose Tris EDTA (STE) buffer, washed in acetone, freeze-thawed three times, and treated with lysozyme, proteinase K, 10% sarkosyl, and EDTA. The lysate was treated with RNase A, extensively extracted with phenol/chloroform/isoamyl alcohol, extracted with chloroform/

isoamyl alcohol, and dialyzed against Tris EDTA (TE) buffer.

Genomic DNA from all 25 strains of *Brucella* was fingerprinted with Hind III. While others have reported no differences between Hind III fingerprints of various strains of *Brucella*, we found differences, most notably between 6,000 and 9,000 base pairs.

Restriction endonuclease cleavage of genomic DNA of *B. abortus* Strain 19 (S19) was studied using 24 enzymes. This DNA was highly fragmented with many of these restriction enzymes. Methylation of adenosine was not detected by digestion with *Sau*3AI and MboI.

The *Brucella* species are closely related, but protein profiles and DNA fingerprints of *Brucella* species and biovars show differences between strains. When strains of a *Brucella* species are compared with each other, only minor differences are seen. However, when strains of different species are analyzed, more differences are found.

Comparison of *Brucella* Species and *Brucella abortus* Field Strains by Gradient Sodium Dodecyl Sulfate-Polyacrylamide Gel Electrophoresis

C.A. Belzer,* D.R. Ewalt,** and L.B. Tabatabai*
*United States Department of Agriculture
Agricultural Research Center, National Animal Disease Center,
**United States Department of Agriculture/Animal and Plant Health
Inspection Service/Veterinary Service,
National Veterinary Services Laboratories, Ames, IA

Conventional methods for differentiating species and biotypes of *Brucella* species are time consuming. The DNA band restriction endonuclease analysis (BRENDA) patterns of *Brucella* species and biotypes requires the isolation and purification of DNA and enzymatic hydrolysis with enzymes each under specific buffer requirements. The BRENDA patterns with the currently available restriction enzymes are not always feasible. We describe here the results obtained using gradient sodium dodecyl sulfate-polyacrylamide gel electrophoresis (SDS-PAGE) of *Brucella* whole-cell lysates representative of all species and commonly found biotypes, and various field strain isolates. The results suggest that silver-stained gradient SDS-PAGE gels can be used to distinguish between *Brucella* species and between *B. abortus* biovars 1, 2, and 4. We also show that differences exist between the vaccine strain (Strain 19) of *B. abortus* and the virulent Strain 2308, and other field strains. Most of the major differences between the protein profiles of the *Brucella* species and bio-vars occur in the molecular weight range of 20 to 34 kilodaltons (kDa). Protein profiles obtained from *B. abortus, B. melitensis, B. suis,* and *B. canis* grown on iron-depleted medium differed from the protein profiles of *Brucella* species grown in tryptose-serum agar. The major differences occurred in the molecular weight range between 10 and 30 kDa and, in one case, at >66 kDa. *Brucella ovis* and *B. neotomae* did not grow on the iron-depleted medium. These results imply that it is feasible to develop a definitive *in vitro* test within 48 hours after obtaining a culture.

Titration of *Brucella* Cell Surface Protein and Lipopolysaccharide Response in Mice

G.W. Pugh, Jr., L.B. Tabatabai, T.J. McDonald,
and M. Phillips
United States Department of Agriculture
Agricultural Research Service, National Animal Disease Center,
Ames, Iowa

A study was conducted to determine the immune and protective responses induced in BALB/c mice by a: (i) single vaccinal inoculation using varying concentrations of *Brucella* cell surface protein (BCSP) or lipopolysaccharide (LPS); (ii) primary inoculation using a standard concentration of BCSP; and (iii) primary inoculation using a standard concentration of BCSP or LPS followed by a secondary inoculation using varying concentrations of BCSP or LPS. Four weeks after the primary inoculation, mice were challenge-exposed with approximately 1×10^4 colony forming units (CFU) of *Brucella abortus* Strain 2308 and all mice were sacrificed at six weeks. Reduced splenic weights and reduced CFU in vaccinated mice, when compared with non-vaccinated mice, were the criteria of protectiveness; an increase in serum immunoglobulin IgM and IgG was the criterion of immunity.

Both BCSP and LPS induced protection and immune responses that were proportional to the dose given up to an optimal limit. However, once the optimal was reached, additional amounts of the respective antigen perturbed both the protective and immune responses. This was true for mice given either one or two vaccinal inoculations. Enhanced secondary protective responses were seen only when suboptimal doses were used in the primary inoculation. Excessive or optimal doses in the secondary inoculation obscured the protectiveness and immunity by primary inoculations. When suboptimal doses were used in the primary and secondary inoculations, the protective effects appeared to be additive. When subimmunogenic doses were used, there was a relative reduction in the antibody concentration after challenge exposure when compared with non-vaccinated mice.

The overall results indicated that the protective responses induced by BCSP were due to a functional LPS component. The results also indicated that there was a linear increase in protectiveness and immunity corresponding to increasing doses up to an optimum dose, and this stoichiometric optimum may be achieved by the use of one or more vaccinal inoculations. However, once this optimum was obtained, additional amounts of LPS cause perturbation of both the protective and serologic responses.

A 20-Kilodalton Protein from *Brucella abortus* is a Cu-ZN Superoxide Dismutase

B.L. Beck,* L.B. Tabatabai,* and J.E. Mayfield**
*United States Department of Agriculture
Agricultural Research Center National Animal Disease Center
**Zoology Department,
Iowa State University, Ames, Iowa

Soluble salt-extractable *Brucella* proteins, which can be used by Western blotting to distinguish vaccinated from infected cattle, are promising components for a non-viable subunit vaccine and a complimentary diagnostic test for bovine brucellosis. A salt-extractable protein preparation from *B. abortus* Strain 19 has previously been shown to be antigenic and immunogenic in cattle (Tabatabai and Deyoe, *Dev. Biol. Stand.*, 56:199-211, 1984). The gene for a 20-kilodalton (kDa) protein from the antigenic *Brucella* protein preparation has been cloned and expressed in *Escherichia coli* [Bricker et al., 1989 (submitted)]. The present study reports the amino acid sequence of the recombinant 20 kDa protein from *B. abortus*. Through homology searches and enzyme activity studies, we have determined that the *Brucella* 20-kDa protein is a Cu-Zn superoxide dismutase. *Brucella* Cu-Zn superoxide dismutase is 53.6% homologous to *Photobacterium leiognathi* and 27.4% homologous to bovine and human Cu-Zn superoxide dismutase. To date, Cu-Zn superoxide dismutase has only been found in five species of bacteria. The function of superoxide dismutase is to protect aerobic bacteria by scavenging harmful superoxide radicals generated during aerobic metabolism. We propose that *Brucella* Cu-Zn superoxide dismutase may provide one of the mechanisms by which the organism can survive as an intracellular parasite within host macrophages and neutrophils. One of the ways that macrophages and neutrophils destroy invasive organisms is by generation of superoxide radicals. The presence of a novel Cu-Zn superoxide dismutase in *Brucella* may be a critical virulence associated factor allowing for the organism's survival in the host.

Monoclonal Antibodies Directed to *Brucella* O-Antigens: Protection in a Mouse Model

M. Phillips and B.L. Deyoe
United States Department of Agriculture
Agricultural Research Center, National Animal Disease Center
Ames, Iowa

Lipopolysaccharides (LPS) are the immunodominant surface structures on *Brucella abortus* cells. The effectiveness of LPS as a protective immunogen has been demonstrated in mouse models where protection against *B. abortus* was defined as clearance of organisms from the spleen and livers, as well as reduced splenomegaly. The formation of antibodies (Ab) directed to the O-antigen moiety of LPS indicated that humoral responses had an important role in protection, in addition to the cellular mechanisms, for the protection of the mice.

Monoclonal antibodies recognizing the O-polysaccharide portion of *B. abortus* Strain 2308 provided passive protection against challenge by the homologous strain in BALB/c mice. Spleen colony forming organisms were reduced by both the immunoglobulin (Ig) M and IgG monoclonals. Active immunization of mice by *B. abortus* Strain 2308 LPS provided production of IgM antibody at 14 days. Clearance of organisms in the actively immunized mice after challenge at 14 days was nearly identical to that of passively immunized mice. Mice either passively immunized or actively immunized were effectively protected from 0 to 28 days. Spleen colonization was observed to increase in both groups of mice at 56 days, and indicated that humoral responses were effective in eliminating the organism in the early stages of infection, but other immune mechanisms are necessary for protection of mice in the later stage of infection against the virulent strains of *B. abortus*.

Lysis of *Brucella abortus* Pulsed Monocytes by a Subpopulation of Bovine Peripheral Blood Mononuclear Cells

A.M. Likos-Burkhart and J.H. Wyckoff III
Department of Veterinary Parasitology, Microbiology, and Public Health, Oklahoma State University, Stillwater, Oklahoma

Both helper and cytolytic T cells may contribute to acquired resistance against intracellular bacterial pathogens. The purpose of this study was to investigate the presence and nature of effector cells in the peripheral blood from bovines that recognize and lyse target cells displaying *Brucella abortus* antigens. Monocytes were cultured with and without gamma-irradiated *B. abortus* for 24 hours prior to use as assay targets. Nylon wool-passaged peripheral blood mononuclear cells were used as effector cells in a 4-hour cytolytic assay. Target lysis was detected by kinetic assay of released lactate dehydrogenase and percent antigen-specific lysis was determined. Antigen-specific lysis was observed only if effector cell donors had been previously immunized with *B. abortus* Strain 19. Effectors from unimmunized cattle were unable to produce detectable antigen-specific lysis. Furthermore, reduction in the antigen-specific lysis when nonautologous effector and target combinations were used indicated genetic restriction of the lysis observed. Results demonstrate an effector cell population of nylon wool-nonadherent, peripheral blood mononuclear cells in the bovine capable of exerting lytic activity against *B. abortus*-pulsed monocytes in an antigen-specific and genetically restricted manner.

Polymorphism of Periplasmic Proteins in the Genus *Brucella*

R. Cortey and R. Caravano
Unite INSERM 65, Montpellier, France

The genus *Brucella* is generally recognized as a very homogeneous taxon. DNA hybridization studies have confirmed this notion to such an extent that proposals have been made that only one species be recognized within the genus (Verger et al., *Int. J. Syst. Bacteriol.* 1985, 35:292). However, since clearcut subdivison of field strains are needed, especially for epidemiologic studies, we have for some time attempted to document significant differences between various fractions from *Brucella* strains. The pooled proteins extracted from whole bacteria by low-molarity buffers, or plain water, after plasmolysis by sucrose, or by chloroform, are most interesting in this respect. Ultrastructural examination of bacteria treated that way confirmed the involvement of the periplasmic space, and gave some information on the relationship of the cytoplasmic membrane with the wall-outer membrane complex. Bacteria in the rough phase were more prone to plasmolysis and periplasmic protein (PP) extraction than those in the smooth phase.

Periplasmic protein of the various nomenspecies within the genus *Brucella* (*melitensis, abortus, suis,* and *ovis*) were studied by the current electrochemical methods. Sodium dodecylsulphate-polyacrylamide gel electrophoresis (SDS-PAGE) revealed several discriminating peptidic bands and isoelectric focusing (IEF) gave even more selective patterns. All the strains belonging to a nomenspecies currently recognized gave identical patterns, irrespective of their biovar, and differences between nomenspecies were clear enough to be visibly identified. The vaccinal Strain Rev. 1 gave a pattern identical to that of *B. melitensis,* but *B. ovis* is quite different, interestingly, to that of *B. melitensis.* The smooth and rough variant of a same strain gave identical patterns. This suggests that the method could identify strains isolated directly in the rough phase, a goal that the classical identification methods used cannot reach.

More detailed studies are needed to confirm if these differences are due to isoforms of periplasmic enzymes, as suggested by the bidimensional titration curves.

These results confirm that a polymorphism may be demonstrated in the pool of periplasmic proteins of four nomenspecies belonging to the genus *Brucella.* With this group of bacteria, careful phenotypic classification keeps all its interest, at least with regard to the tracking of the strains for epidemiological analysis.

Functional Properties of Murine Anti-*Brucella* Monoclonal Antibodies

P. Vendrell, A. Delobbe, M.F. Huguet, S. Cabane, F. Peraldi, A. Serre, A. Cannat, and R. Caravano
Unite INSERM 65, Montpellier, France

Although cellular immunity is known to be central to immune protection against facultative intracellular bacteria, humoral immunity participates in the immune resistance to *Brucella* infections, and immune sera or polyclonal anti-*Brucella* antibodies transfer good protection to non-immunized mice. This led us to test a panel of monoclonal anti-*Brucella* antibodies (MAbs) for their protective properties. The nine MAbs chosen for this study belong to different immunoglobulin isotypes and subclasses: three IgG2a, three IgG3, two IgM, and one IgA. Six of the MAbs reacted with the same band on electrotransfers of sodium dodecylsulphate-polyacrylamide gel electrophoresis (SDS-PAGE) of the vaccinating fraction SF and shared the same specificity for an antigen designated "Ag 311." Protection was assessed by estimating of the acceleration of the blood clearance of intravenously inoculated *Brucella* and the reduction of splenic infection on day 7 after infection. Four "strongly protective," three "weakly protective" and two "non-protective" MAbs were identified. As a first step towards the study of the mechanism of this humoral protection, these MAbs were further compared for structural and functional properties such as immunoglobulin isotype, anti-*Brucella* specificity, anti-*Brucella in vitro* direct or macrophage-dependent bacteriostasis, *Brucella* agglutination and complement fixation when complexed with tyndallized *Brucella*. No correlation was found between protection and either agglutination or direct bacteriostasis. On the other hand, the results observed suggest that isotypes (and especially the IgG2a isotype) could play an important role in *in vivo* immune protection and that both "antibody and macrophage-dependent" and "antibody-and complement-dependent" mechanisms could be involved. However, the fact that one of the protective MAbs belongs to the IgA isotype, does not cross-react with the others in anti-*Brucella* epitopic specificity, and does not fix complement underlines the probable diversity of the mechanisms involved.

Immunological Reactions Elicited by *Brucella abortus* Rough Strain RB51 and Its Antigen and Biochemical Characteristics

G. Schurig, R.M. Roop,** D. Buhrman,*
N. Sriranganathan,* and F. Enright****
*Dept. of Pathobiology, Virginia-Maryland Regional College of Veterinary Medicine, Blacksburg, Virginia, **Dept. of Microbiology and Immunology, University of Arkansas for Medical Science, Little Rock, Arkansas; ***Dept. of Veterinary Sciences, LSU, Baton Rouge, Louisiana

The purpose of this study was to determine if the rifampin-resistant mutant of *Brucella abortus* Strain 2308, denominated Strain RB51, is devoid of the O-side chain and if its characteristics change after passage in animals.

B. abortus lipopolysaccharide (LPS) was analyzed by SDS PAGE electrophoresis and Western blotting. Antisera to Strain RB51 was prepared by injecting animals with 1×10^8 (mice) or 1×10^{10} to 1×10^9 (cattle) viable plategrown, colony forming units (CFU) of RB51 intraperitoneally (mice) or subcutaneously (cattle). Additional sera were obtained by injecting goats, cattle, and rabbits with killed *B. abortus* cells or cell fractions. Sera were collected before and after treatment and analyzed by Western blotting using *B. abortus* and *Yersinia enterocolitica* (serotypes 0:0 and non-09) LPS and whole cells. Conventional *Brucella* serology was also performed. Isolates from infected animals were obtained from spleen (mice) and lymph nodes (cattle). *B. abortus* strains were tested for urease activity, nitrate reduction, and utilization of erythritol and glucose using conventional methods. Sensitivity to 21 antibiotics was also tested. All strains were tested in colony blot ELISA.

RB51 resembled parentral Strain 2308 in its cell and colony size and in its ability to utilize erythritol. However, the other biochemical characteristics of RB51 more closely resembled these of Strains 45/20 and 19. RB51 was originally selected. Colonies of RB51 were stained with crystal violet and also autoagglutinated in acriflavin and physiological saline indicative of their rough nature. Silver staining of SDS-PAGE gels indicated that LPS extracted from RB51 appears to be devoid of the O-chain component. Western blot analysis with a monoclonal antibody (BRU38=specific for the perosamine homopolymer O-chain of smooth *Brucella* LPS) as well as with selected rabbit and bovine sera with strong anti-O-chain reactivity did not demonstrate the presence of the O-chain antigen. Colony blot ELISAs with BRU38 were negative. Isolates obtained from both infected mice and cattle retained the characteristics of Strain RB51 even after several passages through mice. Sera obtained from RB51-infected mice and cattle did not show anti-O-chain activity as demonstrated by negative tube agglutination tests and Western blot analysis using LPS from *Brucella* and *Y. enterocolitica* serotype O:9. Nevertheless, sera obtained from cattle immunized twice with cell walls from fermentor grown RB51 induced a transient response to the O-chain.

These observations suggest that fermentor-grown RB51 organisms may express a small amount of O-chain antigen which can induce an anti-O-chain antibody response in cattle. In contrast, injection of viable, plate grown, RB51 organisms does not lead to the production of detectable O-chain antibodies.

Identification of Four Distinct Epitopes on *Brucella* Lipopolysaccharides by Monoclonal Antibodies

J.T. Douglas and D.A. Palmer

Department of Microbiology, University of Hawaii, Honolulu, Hawaii

The major serological response occurring with infections resulting from smooth *Brucella* is due to the lipopolysaccharide (LPS) complex. The type and quantity of epitopes involved are determined by the class of LPS exposed on the surface of the infecting organisms, vaccine or strain representing a specific biotype. Among smooth *Brucella* we have found three classes of LPS represented by different biotypes: "M-LPS", *B. melitensis* biotype I; "A-LPS", *B. abortus* biotype I; and "A&M LPS", represented by *B. suis* biotype IV. With our monoclonal antibodies (MAbs designated 12AE6 ("A" type) and 33.1 ("M" type), we have demonstrated that the old concept of rations of A:M antigens on different strains of *Brucella* is no longer appropriate. The exception is the "A&M" type found with *B. suis* biotype IV. The use of dot blot and indirect ELISA with "A" type and "M" type MAbs demonstrate the absence of M determinants of *B. abortus* biotype I and the absence of A determinant on *B. melitensis* biotype I.

In spite of these findings, the original work of Wilson, Miles, and Pirie is not in doubt. The cross absorption techniques used in the past to produce monospecific "A" and "M" sera has prevented analysis of common or shared epitopes. In support of this hypothesis, we found that two additional determinants are common to *B. abortus*, *B. suis*, and *B. melitensis*. These epitopes are classified by MAbs as "C" for common within the *Brucella* species and "C/Y" for common within the *Brucella* species and shared with *Y. entercolytica* type 0:9. These MAbs are designated 9.1.2 ("C" type) and 6.9D ("C/Y" type). Application of Western blot procedures indicate that these epitopes may reside on different molecules within a highly purified LPS complex. This is further confirmed by Limilus assay determinations which show differential activity with precipitates produced by complexes of highly purified LPS and the four different MAb types. In another application with whole organisms, variations in MAb binding patterns to *Brucella* species treated with acetone or chloroform indicated that these MAbs may be of use in determining ratios of LPS epitopes on organisms prepared for serological reagent or on vaccines.

This work is a summary of our laboratory's efforts in investigating the epitopes of *Brucella* LPS. We have established a set of four monoclonals antibodies which can characterize the distribution of LPS epitopes on *Brucella* species. In addition, these monoclonal antibodies have provided a means to classify *Brucella* LPS types based on "M," "A," and common epitopes.

Reproducibility of *Brucella abortus* Strain 19 Vaccine Counts and Stability of *Brucella abortus* Vaccine

L.A. Elsken and G.G. Christianson
United States Department of Agriculture,
Animal and Plant Health Inspection Service, Science and Technology/
National Veterinary Services Laboratory, Ames, Iowa

This study evaluated the reproducibility of *Brucella abortus* Strain 19 live culture vaccine bacterial counts and the stability of desiccated *B. abortus* vaccine. Viability counts were conducted according to the CFR9, Part 113.65 on serials of *B. abortus* vaccine. The count procedure was conducted by rehydrating two final container vials with accompanying diluent, serially diluting aliquots from each vial to 10^{-7} with 1% peptone broth, and inoculating 0.1 ml onto each of four tryptose agar plates per vial. Plates were incubated 96 hours at 35 to 37° C, and colonies per plate were enumerated and averaged. This average was then used to calculate the number of colony forming units (CFU) per dose.

The reproducibility of viability counts was compared in 30 replicate assays. Correlation (r^2) between the average count and individual counts averaged 0.933, with a range of 0.770 to 0.999. Correlation between laboratories was 0.997 for replicate assays. When all serials (n=117) for 1986 through 1988 were analyzed, correlation between laboratories was found to be 0.807.

Vaccine stability was evaluated with a total of 79 serials. Sixty-four serials had initial counts between 3 and 10 billion CFU per dose, and were retested once approximately 12 months later. Fifteen serials had initial counts above 10 billion, and were retested until counts fell below 10 billion per dose (3 to 6 times). Linear regressions, expressed as log decrease in counts per week, were calculated for each serial. The mean slope for all serials was found to be -0.00382 log per week. The difference in slope between the serials with initial counts above 10 billion CFU per dose (slope = -0.00434) and serials with initial counts between 3 and 10 billion (slope = -.0.00348) was not significant. The formula used was:

$$x = y - (0.00382 * w),$$

where $x = \log^{10}$ current count, $y = \log^{10}$ initial count, and w = weeks since initial count.

This could be used to estimate current counts from a known initial count, or to estimate the time required to reach the maximum allowable count (10 billion CFU per does) for a serial with an initial count above 10 billion.

Brucella Outer Membrane Protein Epitopes Involved in Vaccination and Diagnostic Tests

P. Uerkhofs,*R.A. Bowden,**H. Bosseray,**
Pr. de Wergifosse,* M. Plommet,** G. Dubray,**
and J.N. Limet*
*Catholic University of Louvain, Belgium,
**Institut National de la Recherche Agronomique, Nouzilly, France.

Brucellosis eradication would be made easier if vaccinal antigens did not induce immunological responses to antigens involved in diagnostic tests.

Because the lipopolysaccharide (LPS) which confers protection to mice is also the main antigen involved usually in diagnostic tests, we looked for other antigens potentially protective and/or of diagnostic significance. Twenty-eight monoclonal antibodies (MAbs) against seven outer membrane proteins (OMP) were obtained from mice immunized with living or killed rough Brucella abortus 45/20 and B. melitensis 115, cells or cell-wall fractions. MAbs recognized the two major OMPs of 25-27 kDa (glycoprotein) and 36-38 kDa (porin) and minor OMPs of 10, 16.5, 19, 31-34, and 89 kDa. All MAbs, except the 89 kDa, bind to whole rough Brucella cells, indicating that OMP are exposed to the cell surface. In contrast on smooth Brucellae, only the two major OMPs (on Strains 2308 or H38) were accessible to MAbs. The 31-34 kDa OMP only binds to the cell surface of B. melitensis.

Protection was tested by transfer of MAbs to mice that were challenged with virulent Strain B. abortus 544. Spleen counts performed one week later indicated that one 25-27 MAb and one 36-38 MAb conferred a significant protection, lower however than that conferred by anti-LPS MAbs.

Most MAbs do not react with cross reacting bacteria E. coli 0157 and Yersinia enterocolitica 09 cell-walls and may thus be of value to develop new specific diagnostic tests. Antibodies from infected cows and goats bind to epitopes 10, 19 and 89 kDa and some to 16.5, 25-27 and 36-38 kDa. Thus, to detect all infected animals an appropriate OMP mixture should be used, since immune response to infection is not uniformly directed against one protein.

Study of Lymphohematopoietic Changes in Mice in Response to *Brucella* Antigens: Virulent versus Avirulent Strains

A.V. Sanin and V.E. Malikov

The Gamaleya Institute of Epidemiology and Microbiology
Moscow 123098, USSR.

We conducted a comparative study of the effects produced by different lipopolysaccharide (LPS) preparations obtained from *Brucella melitensis* virulent Strain 565, and *B. abortus* vaccine Strain 19-BA on hematopoiesis, and suppressor T cell generation in mice. The LPS preparations were obtained 1) by Boivin's technique, 2) by Westphal's method, and 3) by mild alkaline hydrolysis of Boivin's active complex, the latter technique having originally been developed at the Brucellosis Laboratory of the Gamaleya Institute.

The total numbers and concentration of hematopoietic stem cells (CFUs) in spleen, bone marrow, and peripheral blood were assessed, as well as the proportion of endogenous and cycling CFUs.

By all criteria tested, LPS from *B. melitensis* virulent Strain 565 had a more pronounced, disturbing effect on hematopoiesis than LPS from *B. abortus* vaccine Strain 19-BA. After a single injection of *B. melitensis* 565 LPS, a massive, early dose-dependent wave of CFU proliferation was observed, accompanied by a dramatic increase in blood CFU concentration. Bone marrow and thymus cellularity was depressed. In thymus, predominance of suppressor T cells was shown. Treatment with polymyxin B, but not with Cetavlone, was shown to abolish the acute effects of *B. melitensis* 565 LPS upon hematopoiesis. Among the LPS preparations obtained by different methods, the one obtained with the use of the technique developed at the Gamaleya Institute (3), proved to have the mildest effects on hematopoiesis, probably due to the partial saponification of the lipid component of LPS.

Polysaccharide moiety of *Brucella* LPS stimulated hematopoiesis in mice when taken at a larger dose than lipid A.

A correlation between the virulence of *Brucella* strains and their effects on lymphohematopoiesis in mice is noted.

Elaboration of Gene Transfer Techniques in *Brucella*: Plasmid Transformation and Chromosome Marker Transduction

V.N. Gorelov, D.F. Selyutina, U.D. Kulakov,
and Z.G. Skavronskaya
The Gamaleya Institute for Epidemiology and Microbiology, AMS
Moscow, USSR

To elaborate the genetic analysis techniques for *Brucella*, genetically marked strains of *Brucella* have been collected. The strains include auxotrophic mutants induced by EMS (1%) and selected by the penicillin or carbenicillin selection techniques. Auxotrophs for histidine and agrinine have been registered with high frequency. The auxotrophs for methionine, tryptophane, and adenine were also obtained.

The known methods of genetic transformation were applied to *Brucella* in order to construct a means of genetic transfer for this microorganism. The high efficiency of modified cryotransformation has been registered in *Brucella*. The transformation frequency was DNA-isolation source, species, and plasmid dependent. ColE1 plasmid derivatives are not inherited by *Brucella* cells, while RP4, RSF1010 plasmids and their hybrids transform *Brucella* with the frequencies 1.10^1 -$2.10^4/\mu g$.

Using *Brucella* bacteriophages of various origins and *Brucella* auxotrophs, we attempted to elaborate the transduction technique. The genetic intergeneric and intrageneric transduction was registered for bacteriophages S708 and JP32A/3 used with m.o.i. 0.1-10.0. The highest efficiency of transduction was obtained for Trp+ and Str^R markers (4.10^{-8} and $2.4.10^{-9}$).

Some Indices of Physico-Chemical Characteristics and Immunobiological Activity of *Brucella* S-LPS and its Components

V.E. Malikov
Gamaleya Institute of Epidemiology and Microbiology,
AMS, USSR, Moscow

Among antigenic *Brucella* complexes that interact with the immune system of macroorganisms, one should regard lipopolysaccharide (LPS) which is characterized by a number of biological properties and specific composition and therefore is greatly distinguished from the LPS of other gram negative bacteria. For this study, LPSs were obtained from *Brucella* strains (*B. melitensis* 16-M, *B. abortus* 19 BA and *B. suis* 1330) by the hot phenol-water extraction. Bacterial cells were extracted by 45% phenol at 70°C for 30 minutes. To purify the LPS, gel chromatography was employed on column of sepharose CL-4B, reprecipitated with ethanol, treated with RNase, DNase, and proteinase K. The *Brucella* LPS preparations differed not only in the structure of O-specific polysaccharide (O-PS), but in the contents of lipid A fatty acids as well. The lipid components of the LPS differed greatly both in quantity and quality. In particular, lipid A of *B. abortus* 19 BA had no heptadecanoic (17:0) acid in its composition, while this acid was found in LPS of *B. melitensis* 16-M and *B. suis* 1330. Physical and chemical methods of investigation revealed that *Brucella LPS* may exist there in an aggregated state, the ability to form large micella being more displayed in the LPS of *B. abortus* 19 BA. In an immunodiffusion test, according to Ouchterlony, the LPS of *B. melitensis* 16-M and *B. suis* 1330 showed clearly expressed precipitation lines after 18 to 24 hours, whereas the LPS of *B. abortus* 19 BA remained at the starting point. Use of sodium thiocyanate as a chaotropic agent allowed for demicellated preparations of the LPS which were easily soluble, and preserved serological activity and the basic biological characteristics. Thus, in hemagglutination inhibition tests the LPS of *B. melitensis* 16-M responded to polyvalent serum in concentrations of 1 µg/ml. The evaluated toxicity for mice of the LPS studied was 1-10 µg in a test with actinomycin D. In experiments with guinea pigs, the protective properties of *Brucella* LPS were studied. The purified LPS preparations were demonstrated to display no immunogenicity, whereas alkali-treated LPS (0,5 NaOH, 10 min, 56°C) was found to be able to protect from virulent *Brucella* culture. One of the possible explanations of the obtained data may be the well known ability of *Brucella* LPS to induce T-suppressors. Such LPS activity may be due to its lipid component since *Brucella* LPS treated with NaOH acquired not only immunogenic properties but a more manifest ability for antibody formation 2 to 4 weeks after introduction of the preparation. We have also studied protective properties of O-PS. The O-PS introduced to guinea pigs, at a dose of 100 µg in a complete Freund adjuvant was shown to induce specific immunity in 62.5% of experimental animals. Thus, the physical and chemical properties and manifestations of immunobiological activity of *Brucella* LPS should be taken into account in considering questions of development of protective preparations.

Protective *Brucella* Antigen and Development of Chemical Vaccine

E.A. Dranovskaya
Gamaleya Research Institute for Epidemiology and Microbiology,
AMS, USSR, Moscow

The purpose of this work was to obtain *Brucella* protective antigen (BPA), and study its structure, and immunobiological functions in order to construct a *Brucella* chemical vaccine (BCV). BPA was obtained with the help of acetic acid hydrolysis from the cell wall of S-*Brucella* and is represented by protein-polysaccharide complex. By electron microscopy study, BPA was found to be localized in the surface layers of microbial cells. There were no manifest toxic and pyrogenic properties, or sensitizing effect after multiple BPA injections. Introduction of optimal immunogenic dose (600 µg) to animals was followed by induction of specific immunity of the same intensity as in case with live vaccine *B. abortus* 19 BA for 3 or 4 months. By this time, the levels of specific antibodies and serum-preventive activity were found to decrease. The results of experiments and consequent tests in volunteers were studies of BPA as a chemical vaccine in a limited epidemiologic experiment. The optimal immunizing dose of vaccine was determined for a single intramuscular injection (1 µg BPA) and much less expressed sensitizing effect as compared with *B. abortus* 19 BA live vaccine was registered provided that the antigenic activity of the vaccines compared was identical during 4 months after vaccination. The optimal interval for revaccinating was estimated at 10 to 12 months and the optimal revaccinating dose was estimated at 1 µg.

The New Tool for *Brucella* Identification: Genus-Specific DNA Probe

V.N. Gorelov, U.K. Kulakov, and A.G. Skavronskaya
The Gamaleya Institute for Epidemiology and Microbiology,
AMS, Moscow USSR

DNA of the recombinant plasmid coding for synthesis of 38 Kd protein in *E. coli* cells was used to construct the *Brucella* genus-specific DNA probe. Since the protein is analogous to a major outer membrane protein of *B. melitensis* 565 (biovar 1) donating the DNA for cloning in the recombinant plasmid, the latter was used as the source of the probe.

The molecular probe is a 1,1 kb DNA fragment labelled by ^{32}P dCTP and hybridization with DNA of all biovars from different species of *Brucella*, i.e. *B. melitensis, B. abortus, B. suis* as well as with DNA of *B. neotomae* and *B. canis.* Negative response was registered in the probe hybridization with the DNA from *Brucella ovis, Franciscella tularensis, Yersinia enterocolitica* 0:9, *E. coli* 0:157, and other bacteria. Thus, the constructed molecular probe is specifically hybridizable with typical representatives of *Brucella* genus and may be recommended for their identification.

Fate of *Brucella* in Macrophages and their Effect Upon the Ultrastructure of Cells in Phagocytosis

N.A. Grekova, E.A. Gubina, V.L. Popov, and V.V. Gosteva
Gamaleya Research Institute for Epidemiology and Microbiology,
AMS, USSR, Moscow

Up to now the effect of both virulent and L-forms of *Brucella* on the ultrastructure of macrophages in phagocytosis has not been sufficiently studied even though this information seems important from the view point of understanding the conditions that are necessary for the chronic-course of brucellosis infection.

All the processes taking place in the cell are known to have a morphological equivalent, and morphological changes of organellas may serve an evidence of dysfunction in phagocytes. The effect of virulent *Brucella abortus* on macrophage ultrastructure in phagocytosis was studied in experiments on peritoneal macrophages of guinea pigs with the help of electron microscopy. Macrophages were found to phagocytize small amounts of *Brucella*, as a rule. In *Brucella* phagocytosis, interfusion of phagosomes containing bacterial cells frequently results in formation of large phagosomes, in which *Brucella* may multiply (in such instances phagosomes were not observed to fuse with lysosomes).

Brucella absorption by macrophage was followed by a number of cytopathic changes in macrophage ultrastructure. By the first day after infection, macrophages were observed to have accumulations of some parasitophoric phagosomes, ribosomes, and polyribosomes near the outer surface of the membrane (a phenomenon that is quite unusual for facultative intracellular parasites), and mitochondria of the host not infrequently contacted with phagosome membrane. Changes were also observed in the structure of endoplasmic reticulum which is responsible for formation of lysosomal enzymes.

L-transformation of *Brucella* was followed by the loss of cell wall lipopolysaccharide, considerable changes in chemical composition and antigenic properties of the microbe, as well as by the surface charge reduction. Therefore one may suggest that the effect of L-forms of *Brucella* on macrophage ultrastructure will be less manifest than that of *Brucella* of the original virulent culture.

ELISA - A Universal Method for Brucellosis Diagnosis

M.M. Zheludkov
Gamaleya Research Institute for Epidemiology and Microbiology,
AMS, USSR, Moscow

The available methods for laboratory diagnosis of brucellosis need further improvement. The search for unique universal method for detecting of specific antibodies and antigen which could become a substitute for the available routine tests is underway.

We have determined levels of specific antibodies belonging to different classes in blood sera from 42 patients with acute, 25 with subacute, 39 with primary-chronic, and 217 patients with secondary-chronic brucellosis. For sensitization of microtiter plates, we used LPS from *B. abortus* 99. In this work alkaline phosphatase-labelled anti-IgG, A, M-conjugates were used. The investigations indicated that acute and subacute forms of brucellosis are characterized by the high titers-specific antibodies of all three classes in all the patients. In the case of the primary-chronic form we noticed some decrease of IgG and IgA antibodies (94.9 and 92.3% respectively) and a significant decrease of IgM antibodies (69.2%). The level of titers of IgG antibodies was 1:2560, IgA-1:640, IgM-1:160. The secondary chronic form is characterized by much more significant lowering of IgM antibodies-54.4%, while IgG and IgA antibodies were detectable in a higher percentage of cases (89.4 and 88.5% respectively). In this form of brucellosis, the antibody titer was low with anti-IgM (1:256), higher with anti-IgA (1:640), and rather high with anti-IgG (1:4000) conjugates.

Antigen freely circulating and bound in circulating immune complexes (CIC) was determined in blood sera of 147 patients with chronic form of brucellosis. For CIC detection, used plates sensitized with anti-C_{1q} fragment of human complement; and for detection of free antigen, IgG fraction of rabbit anti-brucellosis serum. The amount of the present free and CIC-bound brucellosis antigen was calculated in ng/ml according to LPS-associated calibrating curve. Specific antigen was detected by ELISA technique in 35.4% and CIC in 26.5% of the cases at a dose of 2.85 ±0.63 and 1.51 ±0.59 ng/ml respectively. Both freely circulating antigen and CIC were detected in 25 (17%) patients, CIC alone in 9.5%, and free antigen-in 18.37% of the cases. Comparative reviews of the values of CIC and specific antibody titers did not reveal any correlation.

The performed investigation indicated a high effectiveness of ELISA for detection of various classes of specific antibodies antigen and circulating immune complexes.

Cloning in *Escherichia coli* and Immunochemical Characterization of *Brucella melitensis* and *Brucella abortus* Proteins

V.N. Gorelov, V.A. Chibisova, D.F. Selyutina, L.E. Tokareva,
and E.A. Dranovskaya
The Gamaleya Institute for Epidemiology & Microbiology,
AMS, USSR, Moscow, USSR

The genes from *B. melitensis* 565 and *B. abortus* 99 were cloned in *E. coli* cells. The clones producing the specific *Brucella* antigens were isolated. The obtained antigens were characterized using sonicated cells of the clones in the reaction of two dimensional immunodiffusion in PAAG, immunoblotting with the specific antiserums.

The cloned antigens are the 38-Kd and-15Kd proteins. They are thermostable, possess stable immunochemical properties when affected by HCL, sodium periodate, disrupted by NaOH, papain, and proteinase K. The electrophoretical mobility of 38-Kd protein is changed by trypsin digestion: it migrates from anode to catode zone in immunoelectrophoresis. The protein is possibly analogous to a major outer membrane protein of *Brucella*. The immunochemical properties of the 15-Kd protein are trypsin-proof.

Isolation and purification of antigens was fulfilled by affinity chromatography using versions of immunosorbents on columns or in the "sandwich" technique. Optimal conditions were found for the isolation of antigens having kept their immunochemical activity. The possibility of use the purified 38-and 15-Kd proteins as immunoprotectors and components of diagnostics test systems is being studied.

Index